Arthritis: Pathophysiology and Therapeutics

Arthritis: Pathophysiology and Therapeutics

Editor: Mary Kellar

FOSTER ACADEMICS

www.fosteracademics.com

www.fosteracademics.com

FOSTER ACADEMICS

Cataloging-in-Publication Data

Arthritis : pathophysiology and therapeutics / edited by Mary Kellar.
p. cm.
Includes bibliographical references and index.
ISBN 978-1-63242-486-0
1. Arthritis. 2. Rheumatoid arthritis. 3. Arthritis--Pathophysiology. 4. Arthritis--Treatment. I. Kellar, Mary.
RC933 .A78 2017
616.722--dc23

Foster Academics,
118-35 Queens Blvd., Suite 400,
Forest Hills, NY 11375, USA

ISBN 978-1-63242-486-0 (Hardback)

Printed and bound in the United States of America.

Contents

Preface

This book has been a concerted effort by a group of academicians, researchers and scientists, who have contributed their research works for the realization of the book. This book has materialized in the wake of emerging advancements and innovations in this field. Therefore, the need of the hour was to compile all the required researches and disseminate the knowledge to a broad spectrum of people comprising of students, researchers and specialists of the field.

Arthritis is musculoskeletal disorder that affects the joints. This book on arthritis discusses the physiology and treatment methods of this disease. Technological advancement has enabled better diagnosis of this disease. The aim of this book is to present researches that have transformed this discipline and aided its advancement. Different approaches, evaluations, methodologies and advanced studies on arthritis have been included in this book. Students, researchers, experts and all associated with this will benefit alike from this book.

At the end of the preface, I would like to thank the authors for their brilliant chapters and the publisher for guiding us all-through the making of the book till its final stage. Also, I would like to thank my family for providing the support and encouragement throughout my academic career and research projects.

Editor

SKLB023 Blocks Joint Inflammation and Cartilage Destruction in Arthritis Models via Suppression of Nuclear Factor-Kappa B Activation in Macrophage

Caifeng Xie[9], **Liang Ma**[9], **Juan Liu, Xiuxia Li, Heying Pei, Mingli Xiang*, Lijuan Chen***

State Key Laboratory of Biotherapy, West China Medical School, Sichuan University, Chengdu, China

Abstract

Rheumatoid arthritis (RA) is the most common arthritis and is mainly characterized by symmetric polyarticular joint disorders. Our previous study demonstrated a novel small molecule compound (Z)-N-(3-Chlorophenyl)-2-(4-((2,4-dioxothiazolidin-5-ylidene) methyl) phenoxy) acet-amide (SKLB023) showed potently anti-arthritic effects in a rat arthritis model, however, the underlying mechanisms for this are largely unknown. Both NF-κB and macrophages were reported to play important roles in the pathologic processes of RA. The purposes of this study were to indicate whether NF-κB and macrophages contributed to anti-arthritic effects of SKLB023 in two experimental arthritis models. Our results showed that SKLB023 could significantly improve joint inflammation and cartilage destruction both in adjuvant induced arthritis (AIA) and collagen-induced arthritis (CIA) models. We further found that the binding activation of NF-κB to DNA in joint tissues and RAW264.7 macrophages were suppressed by SKLB023. SKLB023 also inhibited the NF-κB activity in peritoneal macrophages by luciferase assay. Furthermore, the number of macrophages in synovial tissues was decreased after the treatment of different doses of SKLB023. The levels of TNF-α, IL-1β, and IL-6 in plasma, and the levels of TNF-α, NO, and IL-1β in peritoneal macrophages were down-regulated by SKLB023. Finally, SKLB023 attenuated the expression of iNOS and COX-2 in vivo and suppressed the phosphorylations of components of the mitogen-activated protein kinases (MAPKs). These observations identify a novel function for SKLB023 as an inhibitor of NF-κB in macrophages of RA, highlighting that SKLB023 was a potential therapeutic strategy for RA.

Editor: Dominique Heymann, Faculté de médecine de Nantes, France

Funding: This work is supported by the National Key Programs of China during the 12th Five-Year Plan period (grant 2012ZX09103101-017). The funders had no role in study design, data collection and analysis, decision to publish, or preparation of the manuscript.

Competing Interests: The authors have declared that no competing interests exist.

* E-mail: tmkxiang@gmail.com (MX); lijuan17@hotmail.com (LC)

[9] These authors contributed equally to this work.

Introduction

Rheumatoid arthritis (RA), which afflicts about 1% of the world's population, is a systemic, chronic, autoimmune inflammatory disease that preferentially attacks the synovial lining cells of the joints, destroys local articular structures, and further affects related tissues and organ systems [1,2]. Therefore, therapy to joint inflammation and cartilage destruction is a logical strategy for preventing the progression of RA [3,4].

In RA, the joint synovial tissue is abnormally infiltrated by a variety of specific cells such as macrophage, T cell, B cell, granulocyte, and monocyte [5]. Among these inflammatory cells, macrophages are abundantly present in the inflamed synovial membrane and at the cartilage-pannus junction, contributing to joint inflammation and cartilage destruction in the acute and chronic progression of RA [6–8]. The infiltration/activation of macrophages stimulates the over-expression of several proinflammatory cytokines including TNF-α, IL-1β, and IL-6 which are, at least in part, dependent on the activation of NF-κB [9]. Additionally, large numbers of synovial lining macrophages in RA represent a source of nitric oxide (NO) that promote the highly expression of TNF-α production and further induce the incidence of synovitis [10], and the transcription of proinflammatory cytokine genes in lipopolysaccharide (LPS)-stimulated macrophages is usually regulated by the activation of NF-κB signaling pathway [11].

The activation of members of NF-κB transcription family is proven to be a crucial factor for contributing to chronic inflammatory responses in the pathogenesis of RA [12–14]. NF-κB is highly activated in synovial tissue of patient with RA [15,16] and NF-κB binds to DNA sequence and further induces the transcription and production of cytokines, chemokines, and inducible nitric oxide [17,18]. Besides, activation of NF-κB usually has great effect on other signal transduction proteins, many of which are relevant to RA, including iNOS, COX-2 and components of the mitogen-activated protein kinase (MAPK) [19,20]. Thus, the modulation of NF-κB pathways may be effective approaches for the treatment of RA and other chronic inflammatory disorders.

In the present study, we demonstrate that systemic administration of SKLB023 effectively ameliorates the chronicity and progression of RA both in AIA and CIA experimental models. The potential mechanisms of SKLB023 in RA may be inhibiting the activation of NF-κB signaling pathways in macrophages.

Materials and Methods

Ethics and Statement

Animal experiments were carried out in strict accordance with the recommendations in the Guide for the Care and Use of Laboratory Animals of the National Institutes of Health. The protocol was approved by our Institutional Animal Care and Use Committee of the Sichuan University in China (IACUC number: 20100318). All surgery was performed under chloral hydrate anesthesia, and all efforts were made to minimize suffering.

Reagents, Cell Line and Cell Culture

SKLB023 was prepared as previously described [21]. Indomethacin, LPS (*Escherichia coli*, O111: B4), and other analytical grade chemicals were purchased from Sigma. RAW264.7 cell line was obtained from the American Type Culture Collection (TIB 71, Rockville, MD, USA). Dulbecco's modified Eagle medium (DMEM), penicillin, streptomycin, and fetal bovine serum were purchased from Gibco Life Technologies (Rockville, MD, USA). RAW264.7 cells were grown in DMEM with 10% fetal bovine serum, 100 U/ml penicillin, and 100 μg/ml streptomycin at 37°C in a humidified atmosphere of 5% CO2 in air.

AIA Model in Lewis Female Rats

Seven-week-old female Lewis rats were purchased from Tengxin Laboratory Animal Co. Ltd. (Chongqing, China). Freund's complete adjuvant (CFA, Chondrex) was prepared at 10 mg/ml by suspending heat-killed *Mycobacterium tuberculosis (Mt) H37Ra* (Difco, Detroit, USA) in incomplete Freund's adjuvant (IFA, Chondrex). Lewis female rats were injected subcutaneously at the tail base with a 100 μl of CFA emulsion, and randomly divided into five groups with each containing 8 animals. Treatment was initiated on day 14 after the immunization. Different dosages of SKLB023 suspended in 1.0% methylcellulose/PBS (10, 20, 50 mg/kg) were daily administrated by oral gavage (o.g.). The clinical score for the progression of AIA was examined every three day and the scoring for each limb ranged from 0 to 4 (0 = no arthritis; 1 = redness or swelling of one toe/finger joint; 2 = redness and swelling of more than one toe/finger joints; 3 = involvement of the ankle and tarsal-metatarsal joints; 4 = redness or swelling of the entire paw). The arthritis score was calculated by summing the scores from all paws [22]. Animals were sacrificed on day 28, and the plasma samples were collected and the concentration of TNF-α, IL-1β, and IL-6 was determined using commercial ELISA kits (R&D Systems).

CIA Model in DBA/1J Male Mice

DBA/1J male mice (6–7 weeks old) were obtained from Shanghai SLAC Laboratory Animal Co. Ltd (Shanghai, China). CIA was induced by subcutaneous injection with a 100 μL emulsion which contained 100 μg of bovine CII (Chondrex) and 100 μg of CFA (2 mg/ml) at the base of the tail. On day 21, 50 μl of booster emulsion containing 50 μg of bovine CII and IFA was injected subcutaneously at the tail, but at a different location from

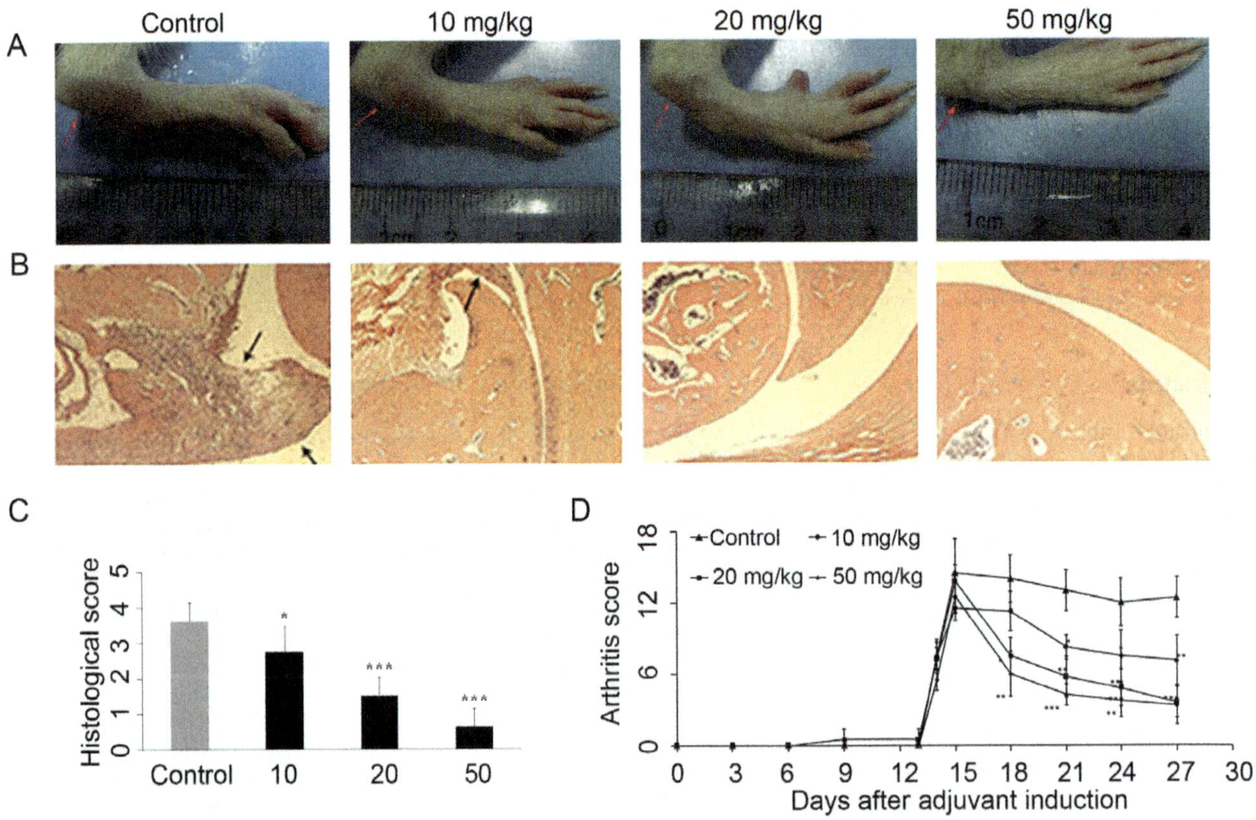

Figure 1. SKLB023 improved histological changes and arthritis scores in Lewis rats. (A) Representative photographs of tarsotibial joint swelling of the hind paws in rats treated with or without SKLB023 in AIA (n = 8). (B) Representative histopathologies of the ankle joints stained with hematoxylin and eosin (H&E) in AIA. (C) Histological examinations of a total of 8 rats for each pair were scored from 0 to 4 as described in Materials and Methods. (D) Arthritis scores during the progression of AIA. Error bars represented SEM, *P<0.05, **P<0.01, and ***P<0.001 indicated significant differences from the control group.

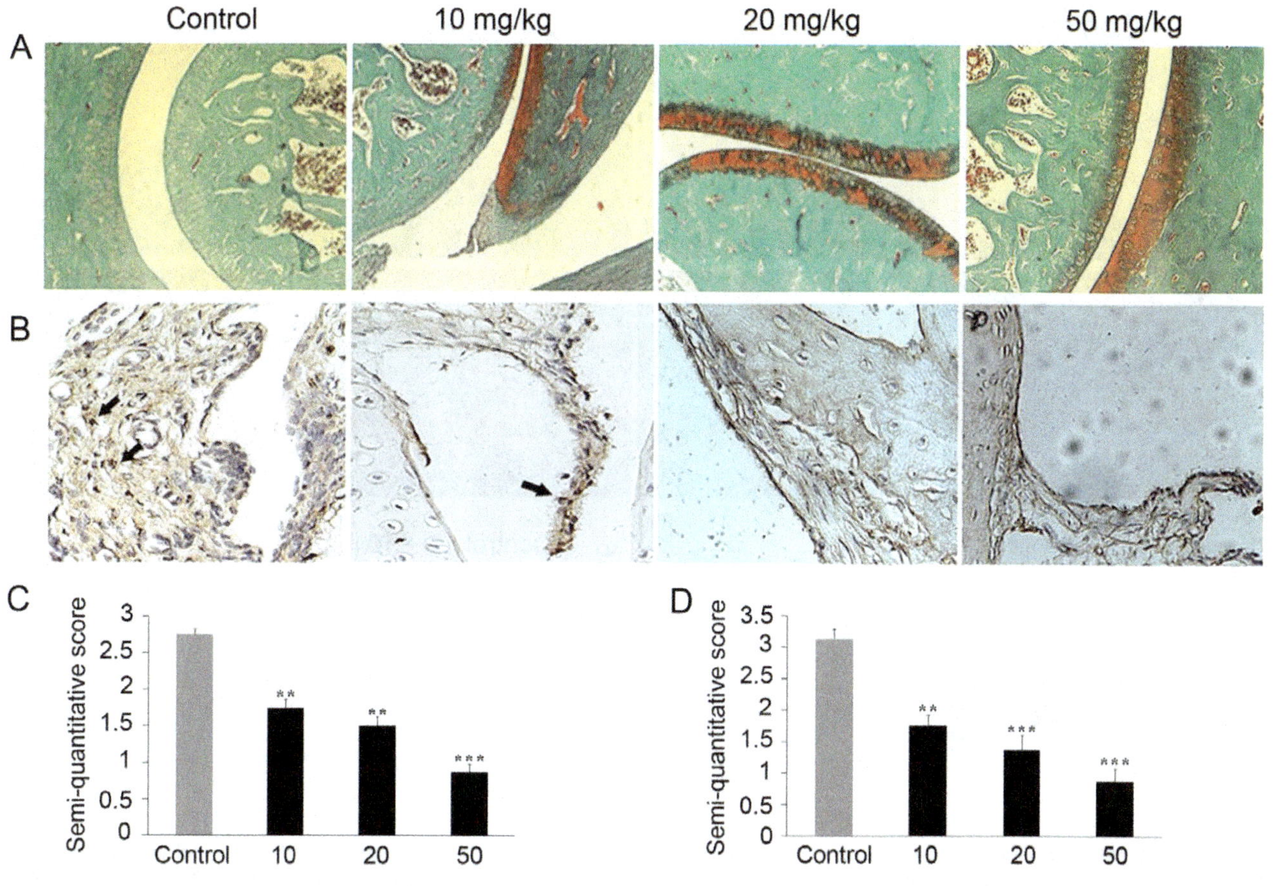

Figure 2. SKLB023 improved cartilage destruction and macrophages infiltration in AIA model. (A) Representative histopathologies of the ankle joints stained with Safranin-O in AIA. (B) SKLB023 inhibiting the infiltration of CD68 positive cells in synovial tissue of AIA model. Synovial tissue sections were analyzed for the expression of CD68 using immunohistochemical method as described in Materials and Methods. (C) Histologic analysis of cartilage in AIA rats after SKLB023 therapy. Sections were scored in a blinded manner on a 4-point scale as described in Materials and Methods. Significantly less loss of safranin O staining was observed in the animals treated with SKLB023 than in controls, indicating inhibition of cartilage destruction. (D) CD68 expression was measured by immunohistochemistry in rats with AIA. It was scored in a blinded manner on a scale of 0 to 4 as described in Materials and Methods. A statistically significant reduction of CD68 expression was observed in the rats treated with different doses of SKLB023. Error bars represented SEM, $^{**}P<0.01$, and $^{***}P<0.001$ indicated significant differences from the control group.

the site of first injection. Mice were randomly divided into four groups with each containing 8 animals and then treated with 2.5 mg/kg Indomethacin (Indo), 10 mg/kg, and 20 mg/kg SKLB023, respectively. The treatment continued for 27 days, during which the arthritis index was measured every three days. To determine the arthritis index, each paw was graded on a scale of 0–4 (0 = no visible signs; 1 = edema and erythema of a single joint or digit; 2 = 2 joints; 3 = more than 2 joints; and 4 = severe arthritis of the entire paw). The arthritis score was calculated by summing the scores from all paws [23]. Animals were all sacrificed on day 67, and the plasma samples were collected. The serum concentration of TNF α, IL 1β, and IL-6 was analyzed using ELISA kits (R&D System).

Histologic Examination and Immunohistochemical Analysis

Both legs and hind paws of Lewis rats and DBA/1J mice were removed, fixed with 4% paraformaldehyde in PBS, decalcified for 15 days with EDTA, and then embedded in paraffin. The paraffin sections were stained with H&E and Safranin O-fast green. For the immunohistochemical analysis, the ankle joints were cut into 5 μm sections and fixed in cold acetone for 20 min. Endogenous peroxidase was quenched with 3% H_2O_2 for 5 min. Sections were pretreated with 3% goat serum for 1 h at 37°C before the application of primary antibody. Indirect immunoperoxidase staining was performed at 37°C for 1 h. Specimen was treated with anti-CD68 monoclonal antibodies (Cell Signaling Technology, Beverly, MA) to identify the synovial macrophages.

All sections were evaluated histologically by two independent observers. For H&E, the gradation of arthritis was scored from 0 to 4 according to the intensity of lining layer hyperplasia, mononuclear cell infiltration, and pannus formation, as described previously [24]: 0, normal ankle joint; 1, normal synovium with occasional mononuclear cells; 2, definite arthritis, a few layers of flat to rounded synovial lining cells and scattered mononuclear cells; 3, clear hyperplasia of the synovium with three or more layers of loosely arranged lining cells and dense infiltration with mononuclear cells; 4, severe synovitis with pannus and erosions of articular cartilage and subchondral bone. Safranin O staining was scored with a semiquantitative scoring system (0–3), where 0 represents no loss of proteoglycans and 3 indicates complete loss of staining for proteoglycans [25]. For immunohistochemical staining, expression of the CD68 in the synovial tissue of all ankle joints present was scored semiquantitatively on a 5-point scale

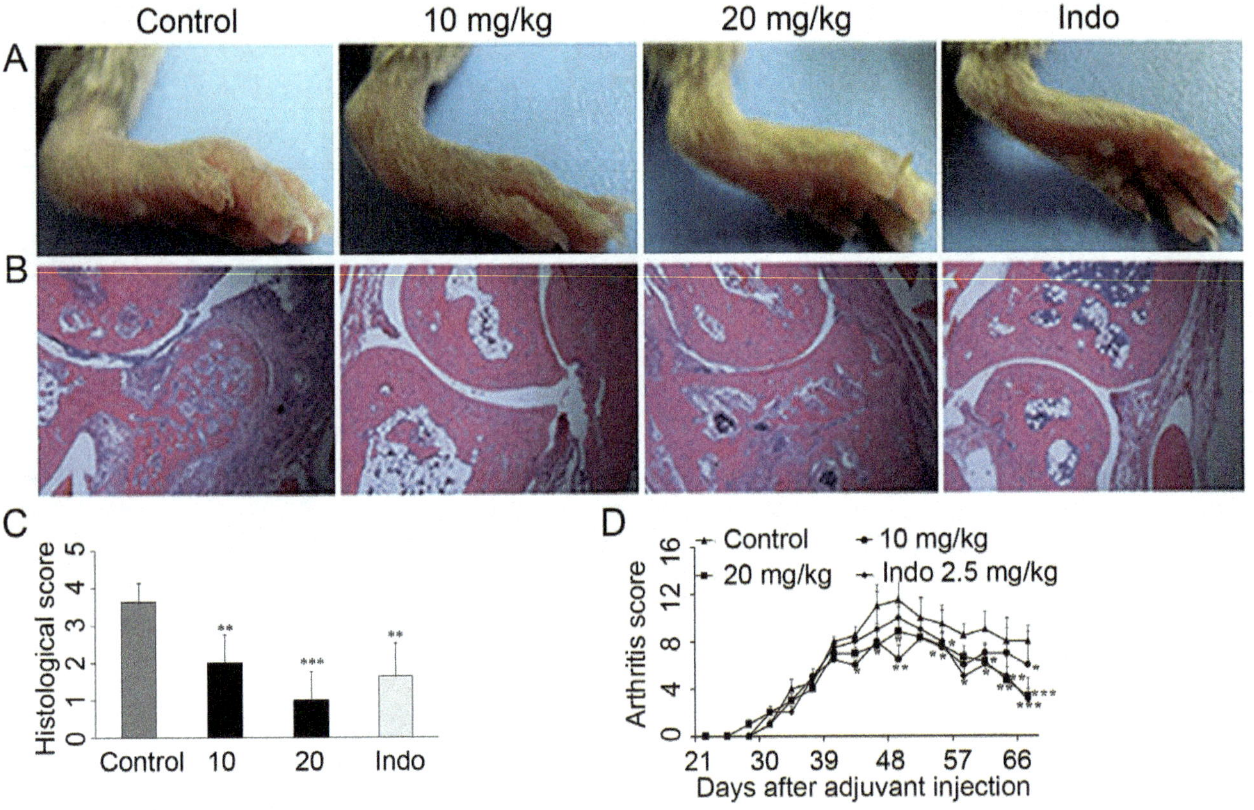

Figure 3. SKLB023 improved histological changes and arthritis scores in DBA/1J mice. (A) Representative photographs of tarsotibial joint swelling of the hind paws in mice treated with or without SKLB023 (n = 8). (B) Representative histopathologies of the ankle joints stained with hematoxylin and eosin (H&E) in CIA. (C) Histological examinations of a total of 8 mice for each pair were scored from 0 to 4 as described in the Methods. (D) Arthritis scores during the progression of CIA. Error bars represented SEM, *P<0.05, **P<0.01, and ***P<0.001 indicated significant differences from the control group.

[26]. A score of 0 represented minimal expression, while a score of 4 represented abundant expression of a marker.

Electrophoretic Mobility Shift Assay

Nuclear proteins were extracted from AIA joint tissues and RAW264.7 cells incubated with LPS (1 μg/ml) and 20 μM of SKLB023 for 10, 30, and 60 min as previously described [27]. The following oligonucleotides were used: NF-κB sense, 5-AGCTTCAGAGGGGACTTTCCGAGAGG-3, and NF-κB, antisense 5-TCGACCTCTCGGAAAGTCCCCTCTGA-3. Gel mobility-shift assay and super shift assay were performed as described [28].

NF-κB luciferase Reporter Assay

NF-κB-luc transgenic mice on a Balb/c background (Xenogen Corp., Alameda, CA) were injected with 2–3 ml of 3% thioglycollate and peritoneal exudated cells were harvested after 3 days. Peritoneal macrophages were adhered onto six-well plates (2×10^6 cells) for 3 h. Non-adherent cells were removed, and then the attached cells were cultured with LPS (1 μg/ml) alone or with 20 μM of SKLB023 for 10, 30, and 60 min [29]. Activated macrophages were harvested and lysed in lysis buffer, and then lysate was used in accordance with luciferase assay kit (E1500, Promega, Madison, WI).

Isolation of Peritoneal Macrophages and Cytokine Analyses in vitro

BALB/c mice were injected with 2–3 ml of 3% thioglycollate and peritoneal exudated cells were harvested after 3 days. Peritoneal macrophages were adhered onto six-well plates (2×10^6 cells) for 3 h. Non-adherent cells were removed, and then the attached cells were cultured with DMEM medium alone or activated with LPS (1 μg/ml) and 20 μM of SKLB023 for18 h. Culture supernatants were analyzed for NO using the Greiss reagent, and for TNF-α, IL-1β, and IL-6 using ELISA kits (R&D Systems, Minneapolis, MN) as recommended by the manufacturer.

Western Blot Analysis

RAW264.7 macrophages (ATCC), were cultured in 6-well plates (1×10^6 cells/well) overnight, and then incubated with LPS (1 μg/ml) and 20 μM of SKLB023 for 10, 30, and 60 min. Cells were washed with PBS, and lysed in lysis buffer containing 0.1% Triton X-100, 20 mM Tris (pH 8.0), 100 mM KCl, 1 mM dithiothreitol, 1 mM phenylmethylsulfonyl fluoride, and protease inhibitor cocktail. Total cell lysates were electrophoresed, and transferred to PVDF membrane. The membrane was incubated with antibodies overnight at 4°C, and 1 h at room temperature with anti-rabbit or anti-mouse secondary antibodies linked to horseradish peroxidase. Proteins were visualized using the chemiluminescence system (Bio-Rad) and autoradiography. Proteins extracted from the ankles of AIA and CIA was subjected to

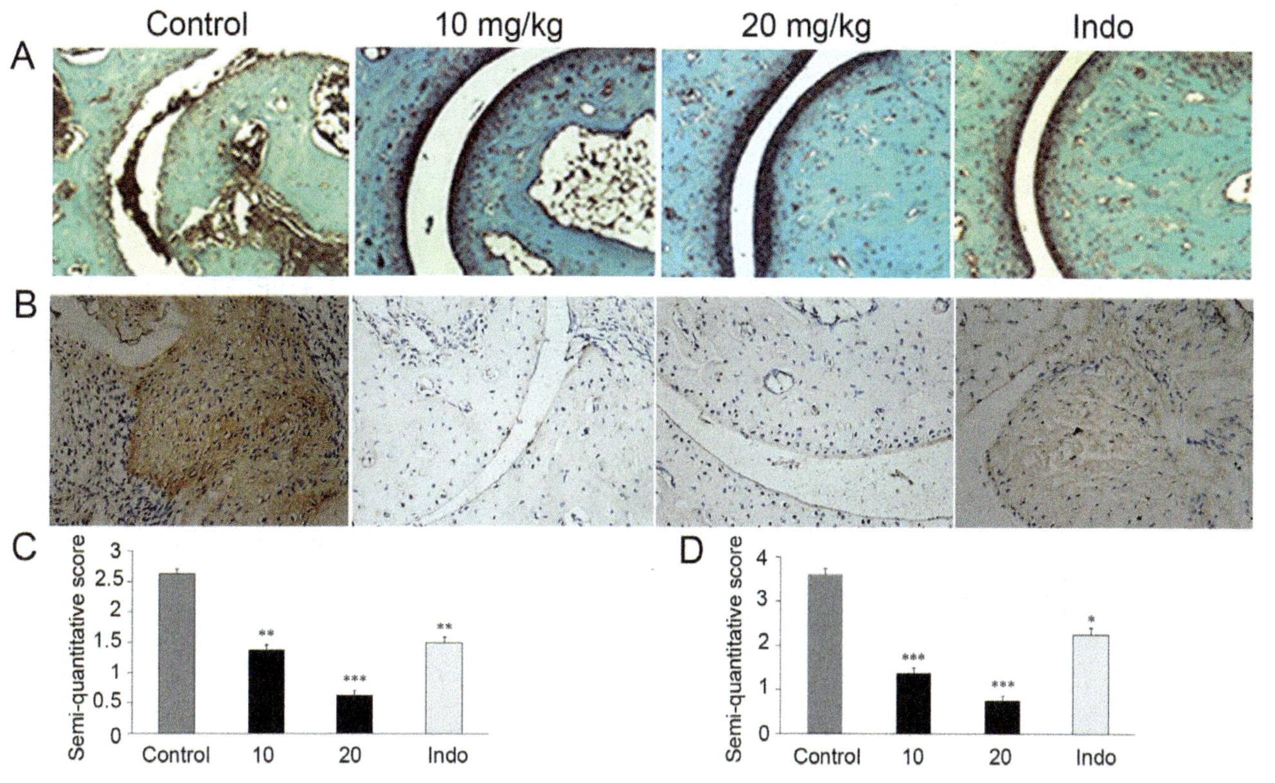

Figure 4. SKLB023 improved cartilage destruction and macrophages infiltration in CIA model. (A) Representative histopathologies of the ankle joints stained with Safranin-O in CIA. (B) SKLB023 inhibiting the expression of CD68 in synovial tissue of CIA model. Synovial tissue sections were analyzed for the expression of CD68 using immunohistochemical method as described in Materials and Methods. (C) Histologic analysis of cartilage in CIA mice after SKLB023 therapy. Sections were scored in a blinded manner on a 4-point scale as described in Materials and methods. Significantly less loss of safranin O staining was observed in the animals treated with SKLB023 than in controls, indicating inhibition of cartilage destruction. (D) CD68 expression was measured by immunohistochemistry in rats with CIA. Expression of CD68 was scored in a blinded manner on a scale of 0 to 4 as described in Materials and Methods. A statistically significant reduction of CD68 expression was observed in the rats treated with different doses of SKLB023.Error bars represented SEM, *P<0.05, **P<0.01, and ***P<0.001 indicated significant differences from the control group.

8% SDS-PAGE and then incubated with anti-iNOS (1:1000), anti-COX-2 (1:1000), and anti-β-actin (1:1000) antibodies (Cell Signaling Technology, Beverly, MA) for 60 min.

Statistical Analysis

Data are presented as means ± s.d. for each group. The Mann–Whitney U test was used for comparison of medians from

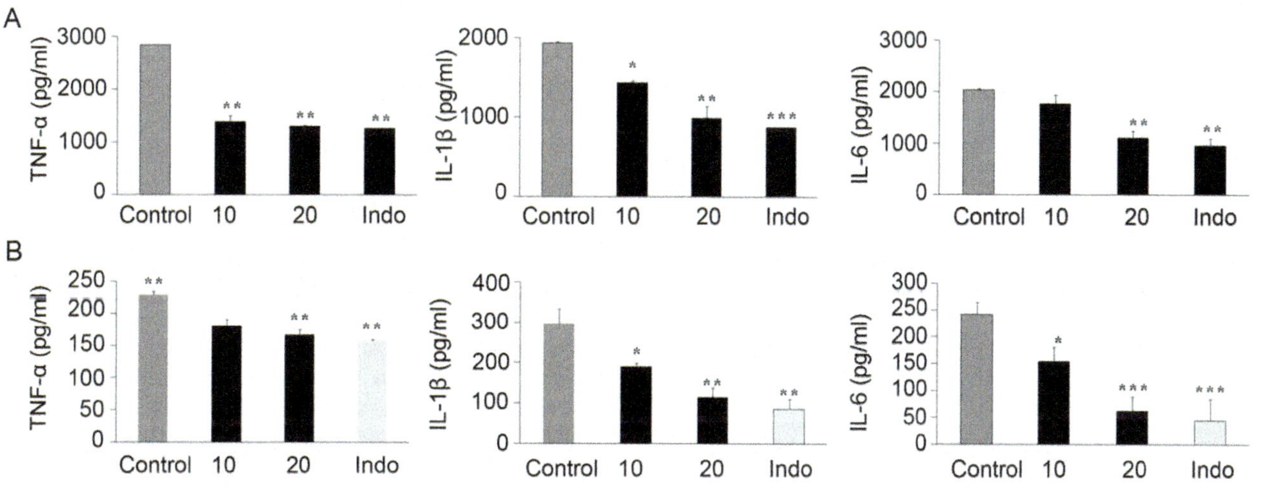

Figure 5. SKLB023 decreased the level of proinflammatory cytokines in two animal models of arthritis. (A) Serum levels of TNF-α, IL-6, and IL-1β in AIA. (B) Serum levels of TNF-α, IL-6 and IL-1β in CIA. Error bars represented SEM, *P<0.05, **P<0.01, and ***P<0.001 indicated significant differences from the control group.

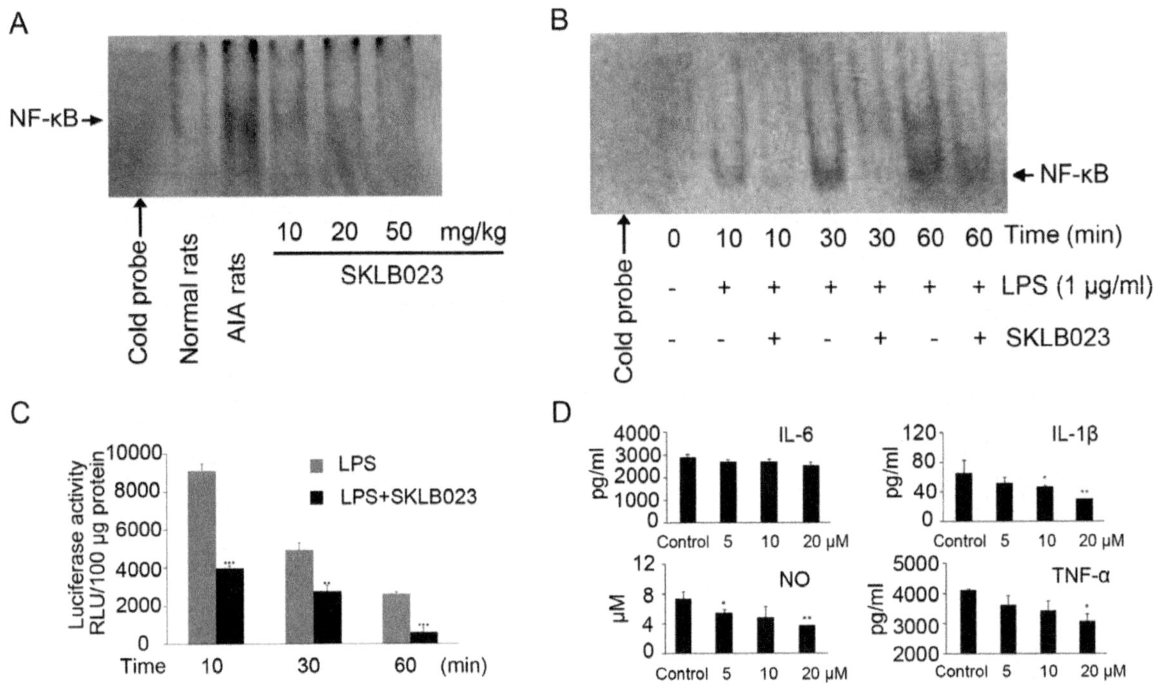

Figure 6. SKLB023 suppressed the activity of NF-κB both in vivo and in vitro. (A) EMSA assay using an NF-κB probe on nuclear extracts of each group rats, different doses of SKLB023 blocked the binding of DNA and NF-κB in vivo. (B) EMSA assay using an NF-κB probe on nuclear extracts of RAW264.7 cells stimulated with LPS (1 μg/ml) and incubated with SKLB023 (20 μM) for the indicated time. (C) Luciferase activity in extracts of peritoneal macrophages from NF-κB luciferase transgenic mice incubated with LPS(1 μg/ml)and then treated with SKLB023(20 μM) for 10,30 and 60 min. (D) Peritoneal macrophages from BALB/c mice were not activated or activated with LPS/IFN-γ, and then cocultured with SKLB023. Culture supernatants were assayed for TNF-α, IL-6, and IL-1β by ELISA kits, and NO production by Greiss assay. Error bars represented SEM, *P<0.05, **P<0.01, and ***P<0.001 indicated significant differences from the control group.

independent samples, in all cases, *P* values less than 0.05 were considered significant.

Results

SKLB023 Ameliorates AIA

To assess different doses of SKLB023 in the development of arthritis, the AIA model in Lewis female rats was initially performed. After the oral administration of SKLB023 at a dosage of 50 mg/kg for two weeks, the arthritic signs characterized by erythematous oedema appearing in limbs and joint swelling were markedly improved (**Figure 1A**). The treatment with SKLB023 contributed to a gradual suppression of these histopathological changes, and inhibited the mononuclear cell infiltration and pannus formation in synovial tissues. There was a statistically significant difference in scores for H&E staining between the SKLB023-treated group and control group (**Figure 1B, 1C**). Importantly, these treated rats access SKLB023 displayed delayed onset, lower incidence and decreased severity of AIA compared to untreated rats (**Figure 1D**). The articular scores, especially at a dose of 20 and 50 mg/kg, were both ≤ 4 at the end point of treatment (both P<0.01).

The degradation and destruction of articular cartilage tissues was assessed by Safranin O-fast green staining, a method to detect the matrix proteoglycan depletion. Proteoglycan loss in the ankle joints of groups treated with SKLB023 was significantly decreased than that of control groups (**Figure 2A, 2C**), stating that the cartilage profiles in RA have been significantly improved after the daily administration of SKLB023 as illustrated by the increased deep red Safranin O staining in cartilage tissues (**Figure 2A**).

CD68 is the major phenotype of macrophage-like synovial cells which played a critical role in the progression of RA. Representative analysis of the infiltration of CD68 positive cells in synovial tissue of AIA rats were displayed using immunohistochemical methods (**Figure 2B**). Large numbers of CD68 positive cells in the control groups were detected in the lining layers of synovium. In contrast, the number of CD68 positive cells in SKLB023-treated groups was markedly decreased to 52.0% (P<0.01), 43.4% (P<0.001), and 24.9% (P<0.001) at a dose of 10, 20, and 50 mg/kg, respectively (**Figure 2D**).

SKLB023 Ameliorates CIA

Previously, 20 mg/kg of SKLB023 exhibited similar activity to 50 mg/kg of that in AIA model. And then, the CIA model in DBA/1J male mice was further evaluated for the effects of SKLB023 on preventing autoimmune arthritis at the dosages of 10, and 20 mg/kg. Representative photographs of the tarsotibial joint swelling of the hind paws from DBA/1J mice were shown in **figure 3A.** 20 mg/kg/day of SKLB023 inhibited the erythematous oedema in CIA mice, which was comparable to indomethacin at a dose of 2.5 mg/kg/day. H&E staining of the ankle joints indicated that administration of SKLB023 at a dose of 20 mg/kg resulted in a significant suppression of these histopathological changes compared to control group (**Figure 3B, 3C**). These SKLB023-treated mice (20 mg/kg) exerted similar therapeutic results to the ones treated with indomethacin (2.5 mg/kg). However, a 10 mg/kg/day dose of SKLB023 reduced the arthritic severity, but did not block the arthritic onset (**Figure 3D**). Additionally, the SKLB023-treated CIA mice at a dose of 20 mg/

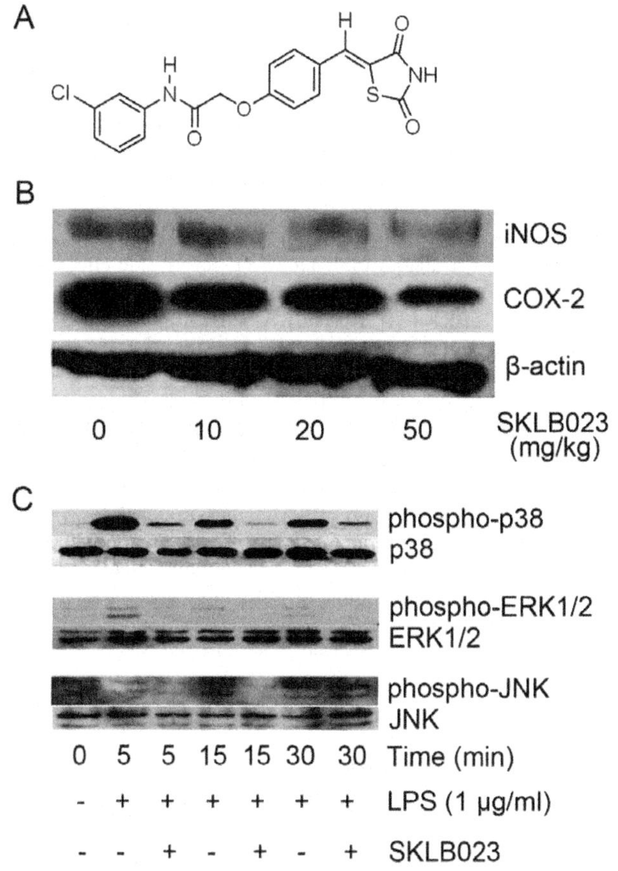

Figure 7. SKLB023 inhibited the phosphorylation of MAPKs. (A) Chemical structure of SKLB023. (B) iNOS and COX-2 expression in the ankle joints of AIA rats untreated or treated with various doses of SKLB023. (C) RAW264.7 cells were stimulated with LPS (1 μg/ml) and incubated with SKLB023 (20 μM) for the indicated time. Cell lysates were prepared and blotted with total or phosphospecific antibodies to ERK1/2 (Thr202/Tyr204), p38 MAPK (Thr180/Tyr182), and JNK (Thr183/Tyr185).

kg approximately recovered to the normal levels by the analysis of Safranin O-fast green staining (**Figure 4A, 4C**).

Representative analysis of the infiltration of CD68 positive cells in synovial tissue of CIA mice were presented in **figure 4A**. Mice treated with 10, and 20 mg/kg SKLB023 decreased the infiltration of CD68 positive cells to respective 51, and 19% compared to untreated mice, while mice treated with indomethacin only decreased to 62%.

SKLB023 Inhibited Proinflammatory Cytokines Production in vivo

As shown in **figure 5A**, the serum levels of TNF-α, IL-1β, and IL-6 in AIA rats were significantly increased compared to the control ones while the levels (especially IL-1β) were decreased in a dose-dependent manner after the treatment with SKLB023 (10, 20, and 50 mg/kg). In addition, the plasma concentrations of these proinflammatory cytokines were also effectively down-regulated by SKLB023 and close to the ones of indomethacin in CIA model (**Figure 5B**).

SKLB023 Suppressed the Activation of NF-κB Both in vivo and in vitro

To confirm that SKLB023 blocked NF-κB activity in vivo, we carried out electrophoretic mobility shift assay (EMSA) using tissue samples prepared from the ankle joints of the AIA mice. NF-κB DNA-binding activity was decreased in the joints of rats treated with different dosages of SKLB023, in contrast to untreated rats (**Figure 6A**).

To determine the effects of NF-κB inhibition by SKLB023 on RA in vitro, we obtained the nuclear extracts from LPS-stimulated RAW264.7 cells in the presence or absence of SKLB023. The EMSA results showed that LPS could significantly increase the NF-κB-DNA binding affinity at 10, 30, and 60 min, whereas the binding activity was suppressed by the pretreatment of SKLB023 at the concentration of 20 μM (**Figure 6B**). The densitometry data for both in vivo and in vitro NF-κB-DNA binding affinity were showed in **Figure S1**. Furthermore, SKLB023 dose-dependently inhibited LPS-induced NF-κB transcriptional activity in peritoneal macrophage derived from NF-κB-luciferase transgenic mice (**Figure 6C**).

SKLB023 Decreased Proinflammatory Cytokines Production in vitro

Our previous studies indicated that SKLB023 inhibited the production of NO in RAW264.7 cells. In present investigation, we evaluated the in vitro anti-inflammatory effects of SKLB023 on the activation of peritoneal macrophage by ELISA analysis (**Figure 6D**). We demonstrated that the inducible production of several important proinflammatory cytokines such as TNF-α, IL-1β, and NO were reduced by SKLB023 in a dose-dependent manner, whereas IL-6 seemed to be not sensitive to SKLB023 in vitro.

SKLB023 Attenuated the Expression of iNOS and COX-2 and the Phosphorylations of MAPKs

As the activation of NF-κB plays a crucial role in LPS-induced transcriptional regulation of iNOS and COX-2 gene expressions in macrophages, we determined whether SKLB023 inhibited the expressions of iNOS and COX-2 proteins in AIA rats. In normal Lewis rats, iNOS and COX-2 proteins were rare and even undetectable. Importantly, SKLB023 (**Figure 7A**) dose-dependently blocked the iNOS and COX-2 protein expressions (**Figure 7B**), stating that the down-regulation of iNOS and COX-2 proteins by SKLB023 were favorable for the treatment of RA in rats.

Activation of MAPKs pathway is widely involved in aberrant inflammatory responses. Thus, the total expression of MAPKs proteins (ERK1/2, p38 MAPK, and JNK) and their corresponding phosphoproteins (p-ERK1/2, p-p38 MAPK, and p-JNK) were subsequently analyzed by Western blot. Previous report demonstrated that the maximal levels of MAPKs phosphoproteins expressed during 30 min after the stimulation of LPS in human and murine monocytes/macrophages [30]. In our study, RAW264.7 cells were pretreated with SKLB023 at a concentration of 20 μM for 30 min, stimulated by LPS (1 μg/ml, for 0, 5, 10, and 30 min), and then performed for the analysis of MAPKs activation. As depicted in **figure 7C**, the phosphorylated effects of ERK1/2, p38 MAPK, and JNK were gradually up-regulated by the induction of LPS. However, SKLB023 attenuated the phosphorylations of ERK1/2, p38 MAPK at 5, 10, and 30 min, and of JNK at 10 min, suggesting that SKLB023 attenuated the expression of the phosphorylations of MAPKs.

Discussion

In this study, we have shown that SKLB023 improved the severity of RA in a dose-dependent manner in two animal models of arthritis. We found that SKLB023 decreased the number of macrophages in the synovial tissues and suppressed the activity of NF-κB in AIA rats. We also demonstrated that SKLB023 blocks joint inflammation and cartilage destruction in arthritis models via suppression of nuclear factor-kappa B activation in macrophage.

Activation of macrophages plays a pivotal role in the development and progression of joint inflammation and cartilage destruction in RA. And further these activated cells secreted high levels of proinflammatory cytokines (NO, IL-1β, TNF-α, and IL-6) in the joint synovial tissues of RA [31]. Our studies have shown that SKLB023 suppressed the infiltration of CD68 (macrophage marker) positive cells in ankle joints of AIA rats and CIA mice. Besides, all the serum levels of IL-1β, TNF-α and IL-6 were decreased by the treatment with different doses of SKLB023 compared to those of the control groups in vivo. Thus, SKLB023 could protect joints from inflammation through its influence on macrophages. However, SKLB023 significantly inhibited the expression of IL-1β, TNF-α, NO but not IL-6 in peritoneal macrophages in vitro. This may indicate that SKLB023 inhibited the IL-6 production in a different pathway responsible for the in vivo effects.

NF-κB could regulate cell proliferation, apoptosis, cytokine expression, and metalloproteinase production. In addition, they modulate various genes through both transcriptional and post-transcriptional mechanisms in RA and play key roles in adaptive immune inflammatory responses [32,33]. The functions of NF-κB suggest that the inhibition of NF-κB activity would reduce the production of proinflammatory cytokines and further modulate the related inflammatory reactions [34,35]. Therefore, an alternative targeting to the signal pathways of NF-κB was proposed [36]. In the present study, we found that SKLB023 suppressed the DNA-binding activity to NF-κB in ankle joints of AIA rats. In addition, we demonstrated that the activity of NF-κB also be inhibited by SKLB023 in peritoneal macrophages and macrophage cell line, RAW264.7. Furthermore, Additional activation of p38 and extracellular-signal–regulated kinase mitogen-activated protein kinases (MAPKs) was necessary to trigger destructive inflammation on top of the already active NF-κB [37]. It is interesting that we observed SKLB023 attenuated the phosphorylations of ERK1/2, p38 MAPK, and JNK in RAW264.7. NF-κB is activated in the synovium of patients with RA and regulates genes that contribute to inflammation, including iNOS and COX-2. In our previous study, SKLB023 inhibited the expression of iNOS and COX-2 in vitro. Accordingly, in our present study, we further demonstrated that SKLB023 decreased the expression of iNOS and COX-2 in vivo. These results indicated that SKLB023 not only affected the binding activity of NF-κB to DNA, also the expression of proteins related with NF-κB signaling pathways in RA, which warrant the amelioration of SKLB023 on the RA and other inflammatory diseases.

During the past 15 years, the improved understanding of the pathophysiology of RA has led to a series of dramatic changes in the therapeutic strategies [38]. However, severe side effects have been observed in the long-term administration of many drugs for the treatment of RA [39]. Recently, a better understanding of the signal transduction systems and gene regulation by transcription factors involved in cytokine production has opened the way for the discovery of novel therapeutic compounds useful in treating patients with RA [40,41]. Our experiments shown that inhibition of transcription factor NF-κB in the specific cell type macrophage improved the condition of RA decreased the production of cytokines and the expression of RA related proteins.

In conclusion, inhibition of NF-κB in macrophages by SKLB023 ameliorated the joint inflammation and cartilage destruction in the progression of RA, and it serves as a novel therapeutic strategy for rheumatoid arthritis. Future works are required to identify how SKLB023 inhibits the NF-κB signaling cascade, and how SKLB023 decrease the production of IL-6 in vivo.

Supporting Information

Figure S1 The densitometry data for NF-κB-DNA binding affinity. (A) The densitometry data for NF-κB-DNA binding affinity in AIA rats. Error bars represented SEM, $^{**}P<0.01$, and $^{***}P<0.001$ indicated significant differences from the AIA rats group. (B) The densitometry data for NF-κB-DNA binding affinity in RAW264.7 cells. Error bars represented SEM, $^{*}P<0.05$, and $^{***}P<0.001$ indicated significant differences from the group treated with LPS alone.

Acknowledgments

We thank Zheng Hao, Ma Yinghua, and Wen Ti for technical assistance.

Author Contributions

Conceived and designed the experiments: LJC MLX. Performed the experiments: CFX LM. Analyzed the data: CFX JL. Contributed reagents/materials/analysis tools: XXL HYP. Wrote the paper: CFX LM.

References

1. Firestein GS (2003) Evolving concepts of rheumatoid arthritis. Nature 423: 356–61.
2. Weissmann G (2006) The pathogenesis of rheumatoid arthritis. Bull NYU Hosp Jt Dis 64: 12–5.
3. Van Vollenhoven RF (2009) Treatment of rheumatoid arthritis: state of the art 2009. Nat Rev Rheumatol 5: 531–41.
4. Emery P (2006) Treatment of rheumatoid arthritis. BMJ 332: 152–5.
5. Choy EH, Panayi GS (2001) Cytokine pathways and joint inflammation in rheumatoid arthritis. N Engl J Med 344: 907–16.
6. Kinne RW, Brauer R, Stuhlmuller B, Palombo-Kinne E, Burmester GR (2000) Macrophages in rheumatoid arthritis. Arthritis Res 2: 189–202.
7. Bondeson J (2011) Are we moving in the right direction with osteoarthritis drug discovery? Expert Opin Ther Targets 15: 1355–68.
8. Thurlings RM, Wijbrandts CA, Bennink RJ, Dohmen SE, Voermans C, et al. (2009) Monocyte Scintigraphy in Rheumatoid Arthritis: The Dynamics of Monocyte Migration in Immune-Mediated Inflammatory Disease. PLoS ONE 4(11): e7865.
9. Feldmann M, Maini SR (2008) Role of cytokines in rheumatoid arthritis: an education in pathophysiology and therapeutics. Immunol Rev 223: 7–19.
10. Kinne RW, Stuhlmuller B, Burmester GR (2007) Cells of the synovium in rheumatoid arthritis. Macrophages. Arthritis Res Ther 9: 224.
11. Firestein GS, Manning AM (1999) Signal transduction and transcription factors in rheumatic disease. Arthritis Rheum 42: 609–21.
12. Hammaker D, Sweeney S, Firestein GS (2003) Signal transduction networks in rheumatoid arthritis. Ann Rheum Dis 62 Suppl 2: ii86–9.
13. Tak PP, Firestein GS (2001) NF-kappaB: a key role in inflammatory diseases. J Clin Invest 107: 7–11.
14. Marok R, Winyard PG, Coumbe A, Kus ML, Gaffney K, et al. (1996) Activation of the transcription factor nuclear factor-kappaB in human inflamed synovial tissue. Arthritis Rheum 39: 583–91.
15. Tak PP, Gerlag DM, Aupperle KR, van de Geest DA, Overbeek M, et al. (2001) Inhibitor of nuclear factor kappaB kinase beta is a key regulator of synovial inflammation. Arthritis Rheum 44: 1897–907.
16. Baldwin AS, Jr (1996) The NF-kappa B and I kappa B proteins: new discoveries and insights. Annu Rev Immunol 14: 649–83.
17. Miagkov AV, Kovalenko DV, Brown CE, Didsbury JR, Cogswell JP, et al. (1998) NF-kappaB activation provides the potential link between inflammation and hyperplasia in the arthritic joint. Proc Natl Acad Sci USA 95: 13859–64.

18. Bondeson J, Foxwell B, Brennan F, Feldmann M (1999) Defining therapeutic targets by using adenovirus: blocking NF-kappaB inhibits both inflammatory and destructive mechanisms in rheumatoid synovium but spares anti-inflammatory mediators. Proc Natl Acad Sci USA 96: 5668–73.
19. Amin AR, Attur M, Abramson SB (1999) Nitric oxide synthase and cyclooxygenases: distribution, regulation, and intervention in arthritis. Curr Opin Rheumatol 11: 202–9.
20. Thalhamer T, McGrath MA, Harnett MM (2008) MAPKs and their relevance to arthritis and inflammation. Rheumatology (Oxford) 47: 409–14.
21. Ma L, Xie C, Ma Y, Liu J, Xiang M, et al. (2011) Synthesis and biological evaluation of novel 5-benzylidenethiazolidine-2,4-dione derivatives for the treatment of inflammatory diseases. J Med Chem 54: 2060–8.
22. Bendele A (2001) Animal models of rheumatoid arthritis. J Musculoskelet Neuronal Interact 1: 377–85.
23. Hegen M, Keith JC Jr, Collins M, Nickerson-Nutter CL (2008) Utility of animal models for identification of potential therapeutics for rheumatoid arthritis. Ann Rheum Dis 67: 1505–15.
24. Brackertz D, Mitchell GF, Mackay IR (1977) Antigen-induced arthritis in mice. Arthritis Rheum 20: 841–850.
25. Dudler J, Renggli-Zulliger N, Busso N, Lotz M, So A (2000) Effect of interleukin 17 on proteoglycan degradation in murine knee joints. Ann Rheum Dis 59: 529–532.
26. Tak PP, Smeets TJ, Daha MR, Kluin PM, Meijers KA, et al. (1997) Analysis of the synovial cell infiltrate in early rheumatoid synovial tissue in relation to local disease activity. Arthritis Rheum 40: 217–225.
27. Schreiber E, Matthias P, Müller MM, Schaffner W (1989) Rapid detection of octamer binding proteins with 'mini-extracts', prepared from a small number of cells. Nucleic Acids Res 17: 6419.
28. Fritsche G, Dlaska M, Barton H, Theurl I, Garimorth K, et al (2003) Nramp1 functionality increases inducible nitric oxide synthase transcription via stimulation of IFN regulatory factor 1 expression. J Immunol 171: 1994–8.
29. Sinha P, Clements VK, Bunt SK, Albelda SM, Ostrand-Rosenberg S (2007) Cross-talk between myeloid-derived suppressor cells and macrophages subverts tumor immunity toward a type 2 response. J Immunol 179: 977–83.
30. Bian ZM, Elner SG, Yoshida A, Elner VM (2003) Human RPE-monocyte co-culture induces chemokine gene expression through activation of MAPK and NIK cascade. Exp Eye Res 76: 573–83.
31. Kinne RW, Bräuer R, Stuhlmüller B, Palombo-Kinne E, Burmester GR (2000) Macrophages in rheumatoid arthritis. Arthritis Res 2: 189–202.
32. Simmonds RE, Foxwell BM (2008) Signalling, inflammation and arthritis: NF-kappaB and its relevance to arthritis and inflammation. Rheumatology (Oxford) 47: 584–90.
33. Brown KD, Claudio E, Siebenlist U (2008) The roles of the classical and alternative nuclear factor-kappaB pathways: potential implications for autoimmunity and rheumatoid arthritis. Arthritis Res Ther 10: 212.
34. Amin AR, Attur M, Abramson SB (1999) Nitric oxide synthase and cyclooxygenases: distribution, regulation, and intervention in arthritis. Curr Opin Rheumatol 11: 202–9.
35. Bingham CO, 3rd (2002) The pathogenesis of rheumatoid arthritis: pivotal cytokines involved in bone degradation and inflammation. J Rheumatol Suppl 65: 3–9.
36. Gilmore TD, Garbati MR (2011) Inhibition of NF-kappaB signaling as a strategy in disease therapy. Curr Top Microbiol Immunol 349: 245–63.
37. Guma M, Stepniak D, Shaked H, Spehlmann ME, Shenouda S, et al. (2011) Constitutive intestinal NF-κB does not trigger destructive inflammation unless accompanied by MAPK activation. J Exp Med 208: 1889–900.
38. Olsen NJ, Stein CM (2004) New drugs for rheumatoid arthritis. N Engl J Med 350: 2167–79.
39. Emery P (2006) Treatment of rheumatoid arthritis. BMJ 332: 152–155.
40. Drosos AA (2002) Newer immunosuppressive drugs: their potential role in rheumatoid arthritis therapy. Drugs 62: 891–907.
41. Barnes PJ, Karin M (1997) Nuclear factor-kappaB: a pivotal transcription factor in chronic inflammatory diseases. N Engl J Med 336: 1066–71.

2

An Antibody-Based Leukocyte-Capture Microarray for the Diagnosis of Systemic Lupus Erythematosus

Ming-Wei Lin[1,2¤], Joshua W. K. Ho[3], Leonard C. Harrison[4], Cristobal G. dos Remedios[5], Stephen Adelstein[1,2*]

1 Department of Clinical Immunology, Royal Prince Alfred Hospital, Sydney, New South Wales, Australia, **2** Discipline of Medicine, Sydney Medical School, The University of Sydney, Sydney, New South Wales, Australia, **3** Division of Genetics, Department of Medicine, Brigham and Women's Hospital, Harvard Medical School, Boston, Massachusetts, United States of America, **4** The Walter and Eliza Hall Institute of Medical Research, Department of Clinical Immunology and Burnet Clinical Research Unit, The Royal Melbourne Hospital, Parkville, Victoria, Australia, **5** Discipline of Anatomy, Bosch Institute, The University of Sydney, Sydney, New South Wales, Australia

Abstract

The diagnosis of Systemic Lupus Erythematosus (SLE) is challenging due to its heterogeneous clinical presentation and the lack of robust biomarkers to distinguish it from other autoimmune diseases. Further, currently used laboratory tests do not readily distinguish active and inactive disease. Several groups have attempted to apply emerging high throughput profiling technologies to diagnose and monitor SLE. Despite showing promise, many are expensive and technically challenging for routine clinical use. The goal of this work is to develop a better diagnostic and monitoring tool for SLE. We report a highly customisable antibody microarray that consists of a duplicate arrangement of 82 antibodies directed against surface antigens on peripheral blood mononuclear cells (PMBCs). This high-throughput array was used to profile SLE patients (n = 60) with varying disease activity, compared to healthy controls (n = 24), patients with rheumatoid arthritis (n = 25), and other autoimmune diseases (n = 28). We used a computational algorithm to calculate a score from the entire microarray profile and correlated it with SLE disease activity. Our results demonstrate that leukocyte-capture microarray profiles can readily distinguish active SLE patients from healthy controls (AUROC = 0.84). When combined with the standard laboratory tests (serum anti-dsDNA, complements C3 and C4), the microarrays provide significantly increased discrimination. The antibody microarrays can be enhanced by the addition of other markers for potential application to the diagnosis and stratification of SLE, paving the way for the customised and accurate diagnosis and monitoring of SLE.

Editor: Frederic Rieux-Laucat, Pavillon Kirmisson, France

Funding: Studies were supported by the NWG Macintosh Memorial Fund of the Department of Anatomy & Histology, University of Sydney and the Special Purposes Trust Fund and generous donors to the Department of Clinical Immunology, Royal Prince Alfred Hospital. The funders had no role in study design, data collection and analysis, decision to publish, or preparation of the manuscript.

Competing Interests: The authors have declared that no competing interests exist.

* E-mail: stephen.adelstein@sydney.edu.au

These authors contributed equally to this work.

¤ Current address: Department of Clinical Immunology, Westmead Hospital, New South Wales, Australia

Introduction

Systemic Lupus Erythematosus (SLE) is an immune-mediated, multisystem, inflammatory disease characterised by autoantibody production. Its diagnosis relies on identification of combinations of clinical features and laboratory tests to distinguish it from other autoimmune disorders [1]. This is often problematic in clinical practice as some of the features required to fulfill the diagnostic criteria may take years to develop and some individuals with pathognomonic features do not meet all the established criteria. The clinical course of the disease is typified by unpredictable flares manifest by the onset of new organ involvement, worsening of existing disease, and periods of remission. Although several laboratory measurements, such as serum complement C3 and C4 levels, anti-dsDNA antibody titers and erythrocyte sedimentation rate (ESR) are routinely used in the clinic to help with disease management, individually they are not diagnostic of SLE and do not on their own give an accurate indication of disease activity. Consequently, assessment of disease activity and response to therapy remains largely clinical. The development of reliable biomarkers would enable us to distinguish between SLE and other autoimmune or infective conditions with similar clinical presentations, and would assist in the diagnosis and management of the condition. Such markers would ideally stratify the condition, predict flares, determine disease severity and activity, and response to therapy, and thereby limit unnecessary investigation and exposure to the side effects of immunosuppressive agents.

By using gene transcripts grouped into modules, Chaussabel *et al.* [2] developed a bioinformatics system to monitor disease activity in SLE. Their results raise the possibility of more precise characterisation of disease activity based on the pathogenesis of the condition and its molecular expression. However, the high cost, need for batch analysis and the delays in acquisition of results of molecular analyses using current technology limits the clinical utility of this approach for individual patients.

Autoantibodies are the hallmark of many autoimmune diseases. To circumvent the limitations of the DNA gene array, many groups [3–6] have employed miniaturised formats of parallel detection of autoantibodies using antigen microarrays. Of particular interest, Robinson *et al.* [4] fabricated 1152-feature arrays containing 196 distinct biomolecules representing major autoantigens targeted by autoantibodies from patients with autoimmune rheumatic diseases and found them to be of comparable sensitivity and specificity to conventional assays. Fattal *et al.* [7] used an array to measure antibodies to 930 different antigens including viral proteins in 40 SLE patients and successfully identified particular combinations of markers specific for the disease at various levels of activity. They quoted a sensitivity of >93% and specificity of >88% in distinguishing SLE from normal controls.

Belov *et al.* demonstrated the utility of leukocyte-capture antibody microarrays in the diagnosis, monitoring and stratification of patients with lymphoproliferative diseases [8,9]. The concept was co-invented by one of the authors (CGdR) and has been successfully employed to identify different clonally expanded leukocytes populations that are characteristic of human leukaemias [8,9]. However, it soon became clear that these cell capture microarrays could also be used to detect more subtle changes in leukocyte populations, for example cell activation or inflammatory changes in patients with heart disease and other inflammatory diseases [10–15]. We postulated that inflammatory diseases such as SLE would also cause changes to the expression of leukocyte surface molecules that could be detected by the cell array. To demonstrate the potential utility of this microarray in the diagnosis and stratification of SLE, we conducted a study of patients with SLE and demonstrated that the leukocyte capture array profile of these patients is readily distinguishable from that of healthy controls. By generating an immunophenotypic fingerprint for each patient, the cell capture microarray can identify common patterns that permit identification of subgroups based on disease activity. Notably, we show that our microarray can on its own distinguish SLE from healthy controls and can complement standard laboratory tests to improve stratification of SLE patients based on disease activity. Further customisation with other antibodies, based on knowledge of leukocytes surface antigen expression related to pathogenesis of SEL, is likely to improve the sensitivity and specificity of the array.

Methods

Microarray construction

Antibody microarrays (DotScan^{TM}) were purchased from Medsaic Pty. Ltd., Sydney. The construction of the antibody microarray has been described previously [8]. It consists of a duplicate set of 82 mouse monoclonal antibodies directed against human cluster of differentiation (CD) antigens that are robotically placed on the surface of a nitrocellulose-coated glass slide (Schleicher and Schuell, FAST slides). The slides and the antibodies, including the appropriate isotype control antibodies, are listed in Figure S1. Unoccupied binding sites on the remaining surface of the slide are then blocked using powdered skim milk to minimise non-specific binding. A set of mouse isotype control antibodies is included, and the perimeter of the CD antibody array is marked by anti-CD44, a pan-leukocyte CD antibody, used to show that leukocytes are evenly distributed across the antibody area. Only 10 nL of each antibody is required for each spot, which, once deposited on the nitrocellulose surface, spreads to a diameter of 450–500 μm. This is large enough to accommodate up to 1500 leukocytes, providing an acceptable statistical sampling of the population of cells applied to the array surface. After 30 minutes any leukocytes that are not immobilized at the antibody dots are removed by gentle washing, the slide is scanned, and the attached cells are quantified by light scattering [8]. We previously reported a good correlation between the dot intensities on antibody microarrays and flow cytometry with the same antibodies [8], but both the production of the microarrays and the nitrocellulose slides have changed since this was published. Accordingly, we have included new data from the batch of antibody microarrays to those used in the experiments report in this paper. PBMCs from a healthy blood donor were stimulated by overnight exposure to anti-CD3 monoclonal antibody and then applied to microarrays and quantified by densitometry as described above and also monitored by flow cytometry. The microarray spot densities for four randomly selected expressed antigens (CD25, CD69, CD71 and HLA-DR) are well matched by the cell numbers determined by flow cytometry from the same sample (Figure S2).

Patients

Written informed consent was obtained from 117 subjects attending clinics of the Royal Prince Alfred Hospital. 137 assessments were performed: 60 on patients with SLE, 53 with other autoimmune diseases including rheumatoid arthritis (RA) (N = 25), vasculitis (N = 9), polymyositis (N = 1), seronegative arthritis (N = 8), scleroderma (N = 3), Sjogren's syndrome (N = 1), undifferentiated connective tissue diseases (N = 6), and 24 healthy controls. All SLE patients fulfilled at least four of the American College of Rheumatologists (ACR) criteria for the disease [1] and their disease activity was determined according to the SLE Disease Activity Index (SLEDAI) score [16]. We assigned patients into three disease activity groups according to their SLEDAI score with ≥8 defined as clinically active, 5–7 as intermediate (semi-active) activity and, ≤4 as inactive. The details of their immunosuppressive medications were recorded at the time of each clinic visit. Thirty three (55%) patients had inactive disease, 16 (27%) had intermediate disease activity, usually following treatment of a disease flare, and 11 (18%) were clinically active. There were no differences between the demographics of the patients in any of the clinical categories, their use of immunosuppressants at the time of study or the number of ACR criteria fulfilled during the course of their illness (Table 1). The results of anti-dsDNA antibodies (Farr assay, Trinity Biotech, Ireland) and serum complements C3 and C4 levels (Immage® 800, Beckman Coulter) were recorded at each visit. The project was approved by the Royal Prince Alfred Hospital Ethics Committee (Approval number X06-0089).

Blood processing and microarray profiling

Anticoagulated whole blood was collected in EDTA tubes from each participant and maintained at room temperature until use within 24 hours. Leukocytes from peripheral blood mainly consisting of peripheral blood mononuclear cells (PBMCs) were isolated using Histopaque (Sigma-Aldrich), washed in PBS, resuspended in PBS containing 1 mM EDTA to a density of 10^7 cells/ml, and incubated on the cell array for 30 min at room temperature; unbound cells were then gently washed off with PBS. Arrays were then fixed for at least one hour in PBS containing 1% (v/v) formaldehyde (Sigma-Aldrich) washed in PBS, scanned, and the light scattering by the attached cells recorded in an image file. The microarray data is accessible at National Center for Biotechnology Information (NCBI)'s Gene Expression Omnibus (Accession number: GSE27293).

Preprocessing of microarray expression data

The raw intensity light scatter values at each spot on the slide were scale-normalised such that the expression value for each CD antigen is between 0 and 10. This normalisation method has been

Table 1. Demographic and clinical characteristics of the patients.

	SLE active	SLE intermediate	SLE inactive
Number	11	16	33
Demographics			
Age, mean (range), years	43 (36–59)	36 (28–48)	47 (24–80)
Female (%)	10/11 (91%)	14/16 (88%)	29/33 (88%)
Caucasian	8 (73%)	11 (69%)	26 (79%)
Asian	3 (27%)	5 (31%)	7 (21%)
No of ACR criteria fulfilled	6	6	7
Laboratory criteria			
Anti dsDNA positive*	10(91%)	9 (56%)	8 (24%)
C4*	7 (64%)	7 (44%)	7 (21%)
C3*	7 (64%)	10 (63%)	8 (24%)
Medications			
No immunosuppressants	3(27%)	2 (13%)	10(30%)
Prednisone alone	1(9%)	3 (19%)	7 (21%)
Immunosuppressants alone	2(18%)	1 (6%)	3 (9%)
Prednisone+immunosuppressants	5(45%)	10 (63%)	13(39%)

*at time of assessment

shown to generate antigen expression levels that correlate linearly with corresponding cell counts by flow cytometry [11]. Further, we applied two filtering criteria to the data: Firstly, antigens that had low expression across all samples were excluded. An antigen was deemed to have low expression if its median expression value among the 20% most highly expressed samples was less than 1, since this is approximately the lower limit of the technology to reliably detect antigen binding [11]. Secondly, CD antigens that had a low signal-to-noise ratio (SNR) were rejected. The SNR of an antigen was defined as the ratio of the standard deviation of its mean expression value across all samples against the mean absolute difference between the two intra-slide replicate measurements across all samples. CD antigens with a SNR less than 1.2 were filtered out since this ratio appeared to be a conservative threshold that filtered out most of the negative control spots on the array.

Individual CD antigen biomarkers for SLE

To identify CD antigens that individually showed strong evidence of association with the class label (*e.g.*, SLE or control), we performed a linear model analysis using the R package, *limma* [17], which is a program specifically designed for microarray analysis. A p value was calculated using the moderated t statistics for each CD antigen to determine whether it was statistically significant. We also calculated the Area Under the Receiver Operating Characteristic (AUROC) curve for each CD antigen. This analysis was performed using the R package *ROCR* [18].

We tested whether the expression levels of each individual CD antigen were significantly associated with SLE activity using a moderated t test and AUROC. Six sets of comparisons were performed to assess whether each individual marker was good for diagnosis or stratification of SLE. A CD antigen qualified as a singleton biomarker if it had $p<0.05$ and AUROC>0.7 in any comparison.

Measurement of SLE activity based on the multiple biomarkers

We used an advanced classification algorithm, Support Vector Machine (SVM) [19,20] to create an SLE activity score from the entire antigen expression profile. We used the SVM implementation in the R package *e1071* with default parameters (kernel = - radial basis kernel, cost = 1). Briefly, a SVM uses labelled training examples to construct a non-linear decision rule (*i.e.*, a decision boundary) that can best distinguish the expression profiles of SLE patients from those of healthy controls. We assumed there is a linear trend in SLE disease activity; therefore we trained the SVM model using profiles from healthy controls and active SLE patients only. Once the SVM model was trained we calculated an SLE activity measure, which we refer to as an S-score, for every expression profile, x, based on the profile's distance, $f(x)$, from the decision boundary as determined by the SVM classifier. The S-score is calculated by the following formula:

$$Sscore = \exp(-f(x))$$

Cross-validation

We used a three-fold repeated sub-sampling cross-validation strategy to assess the performance of the SLE activity score. Briefly, we iteratively performed the following steps 100 times: randomly partitioned the samples into three equal portions and used two of these portions as the training set to build a SVM model. The remaining portion was a testing set to assess the model's sensitivity and specificity for each of the three SLE activity states. An ROC curve and an AUROC value were generated at each iteration and the mean and standard deviation of AUROC of the 100 iterations were recorded.

Table 2. A list of the CD antigens that exhibit statistically significant SLE-activity dependent expression patterns.

CD antigens	Category	Inactive vs. healthy		Semi-active vs. healthy		Active vs. healthy		Active vs. inactive		Semi-active vs. inactive		Active vs. semi-active	
		p	*AUROC*	*p*	*AUROC*	*p*	*AUROC*	*p*	*AUROC*	*p*	*AUROC*	*p*	*AUROC*
Down regulated in SLE													
TCR a/b	T cells	0.24	0.60	0.01	0.73	0.19	0.62	0.63	0.54	0.09	0.65	0.37	0.59
CD2	T cells	0.00	0.74	0.00	0.86	0.00	0.82	0.22	0.58	0.12	0.64	0.92	0.52
CD3	T cells	0.09	0.64	0.00	0.79	0.01	0.75	0.16	0.62	0.07	0.66	0.86	0.53
CD4	T cells	0.04	0.65	0.01	0.76	0.02	0.73	0.38	0.58	0.24	0.60	0.89	0.51
CD5	T cells	0.01	0.68	0.00	0.86	0.00	0.82	0.11	0.63	0.02	0.69	0.64	0.54
CD7	T cells	0.01	0.71	0.00	0.89	0.00	0.80	0.13	0.62	0.03	0.69	0.73	0.53
CD8	T cells	0.28	0.62	0.02	0.79	0.03	0.77	0.16	0.68	0.11	0.66	1.00	0.59
CD28	T cells	0.03	0.63	0.01	0.71	0.15	0.61	0.85	0.51	0.32	0.59	0.34	0.60
CD45RA	Naïve T and B cells	0.17	0.62	0.01	0.78	0.02	0.72	0.15	0.63	0.09	0.68	0.95	0.52
CD56	NK cells	0.00	0.67	0.00	0.78	0.01	0.75	0.57	0.58	0.26	0.59	0.71	0.50
CD57	NK cells	0.72	0.59	0.03	0.75	0.05	0.75	0.07	0.65	0.04	0.66	0.98	0.52
CD52	Membrane glycopeptide	0.01	0.70	0.00	0.82	0.06	0.67	0.99	0.51	0.35	0.58	0.48	0.59
kappa 1/4 IM	B cells	0.16	0.64	0.02	0.74	0.28	0.66	0.96	0.55	0.22	0.56	0.36	0.51
lambda 1/4 IM	B cells	0.22	0.63	0.05	0.68	0.15	0.70	0.58	0.56	0.30	0.57	0.76	0.50
Up regulated in SLE													
CD66c	Platelets	0.11	0.69	0.07	0.73	0.03	0.73	0.33	0.58	0.60	0.61	0.64	0.51
CD95	Granulocytes	0.30	0.59	0.76	0.52	0.04	0.70	0.16	0.64	0.22	0.61	0.03	0.74
Conventional laboratory tests													
dsDNA	dsDNA							0.01	0.80	0.12	0.70	0.22	0.62
C3	Complement C3							0.01	0.79	0.01	0.74	0.69	0.66
C4	Complement C4							0.54	0.65	0.11	0.69	0.49	0.57

Significant SLE-activity dependent expression patterns are determined based on moderated *t*-test and AUROC ($p<0.05$ and AUROC >0.7 in at least one comparison). All p-value less than 0.05 and AUROC value greater than 0.7 are highlighted in bold.

Results

Analysis of singleton biomarkers for SLE

After the normalisation and filtering steps, 57 antibody spots passed our quality filters and were used in subsequent analyses. The results demonstrate (Table 2) that many T and NK-cell surface markers are down-regulated in SLE. Another important observation was that, although many of these CD antigens have statistically significant associations with the disease, none are good biomarkers of SLE activity because the AUROC values are not sufficiently high (<0.85), and do not positively correlate with disease activity. This indicates that no CD antigen alone, as measured by our antibody microarray, can be used as a reliable biomarker for monitoring the activity of SLE. We performed the same moderated *t* test and ROC analysis for each of the conventional laboratory markers (anti-dsDNA, complement C3 and C4), and found that they can generally differentiate patients with inactive SLE from those with active forms of SLE, but cannot reliably distinguish semi-active patients and active ones (Table 2). In particular, anti-dsDNA and C3 show reasonable discriminatory ability that no single marker in the current version of the microarray can match.

The heat map in Figure 1A shows the expression pattern of singleton CD antigen biomarkers. Hierarchical clustering reveals two large clusters of profiles, one dominated by SLE patients (left hand side of Figure 1A), and one dominated by healthy subjects (right side of Figure 1A). Although the clustering analysis cannot perfectly separate the SLE patients from healthy controls, the results suggest that the antigen profiles contain useful discriminatory information for building a diagnostic test.

To investigate whether the set of CD biomarkers contained redundancy (by having multiple biomarkers with highly correlated expression patterns), we performed a Pearson's correlation coefficient among the expression profile of all singleton CD antigen biomarkers listed in Table 2. Figure 1B shows that there are several strongly co-expressed clusters of CD antigens among T cell (CD7, CD5, CD3, and CD2), NK cell (CD56, CD57) and B cell markers (kappa, lambda). Some of the CD antibodies that produced highly correlated antigen expression profiles can therefore be selectively removed from the microarray without decreasing its predictive value. It is well known in the machine learning literature that the best feature sets for classification are those that individually are strongly associated with the class label, but are unrelated to each other. The conventional serum biomarkers such as C3, C4 and anti-dsDNA measured in the patient cohort have little correlation with other CD biomarkers in the study, suggesting that they can provide complementary information in the assessment of SLE.

Leukocyte capture arrays can discriminate SLE from healthy subjects

Next we explored whether building a SLE classification rule based on the expression of multiple antigens can result in a more accurate and robust diagnostic assay. We built a multivariate classifier for our microarray profile using SVM, and validated the classification performance using rigorous cross-validation. We used this SVM classification approach to construct a SLE diagnostic score, called the S-score, using expression of all the 57 CD antigens measured, and assessed the quality of the S-score using cross-validation. The ROC plots in Figure 2A demonstrate that inactive SLE cannot be reliably separated from healthy controls, but semi-active and active SLE patients can (AUROC = 0.83 and 0.84 respectively). In addition, we also investigated whether the S-score is positively correlated with SLE disease activity. The average S-score of the samples belonging to the four classes (healthy, SLE inactive, SLE semi-active and SLE active) from the 100 rounds of cross-validation are summarised in Figure 2B, and demonstrate a positive correlation between the S-score and disease activity. This is a particularly encouraging finding since the SVM model was trained using samples from healthy subjects and active SLE patients only, but it correctly identified the relative disease activity of semi-active and inactive patients, which supports the robustness of this approach.

We also investigated whether the antibody array can distinguish SLE patients from patients with other autoimmune diseases. In this analysis, we independently built a two-class SVM classifier for each comparison (RA vs. healthy, RA vs. SLE inactive, RA vs. SLE semi-active and so on) as shown in Figure 2C. These analyses show that active and semi-active SLE can be reliably distinguished from healthy controls with an AUROC greater than 0.8 (black

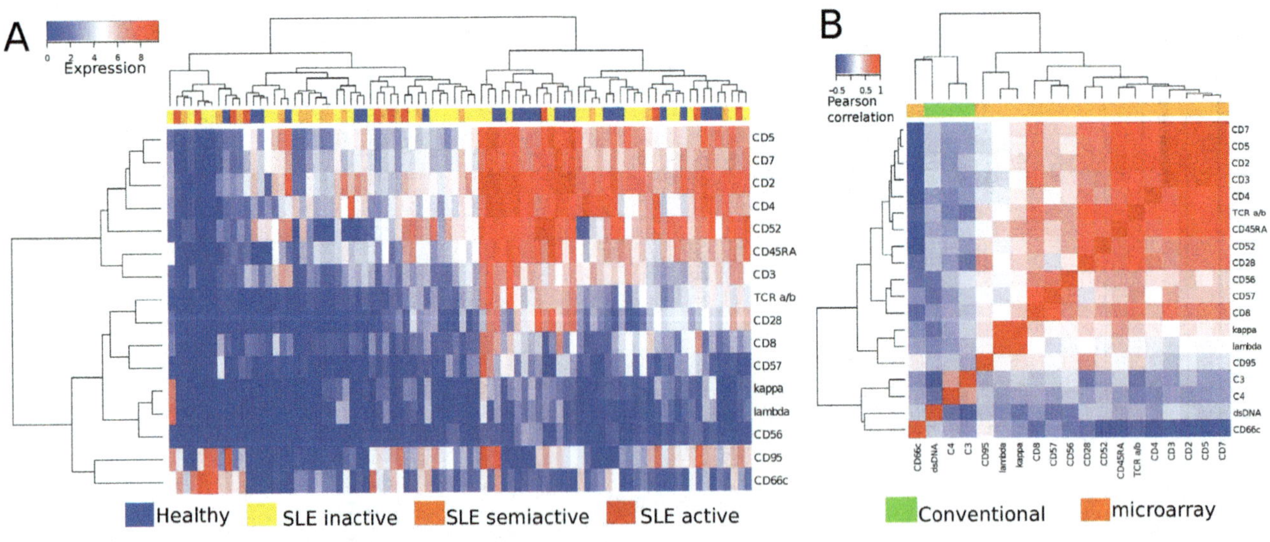

Figure 1. SLE singleton biomarker analysis. (A) Heat map of singleton CD biomarkers from SLE patients and healthy controls. (B) Heat map of Pearson's correlation coefficient between each pair of CD biomarkers and conventional laboratory biomarkers.

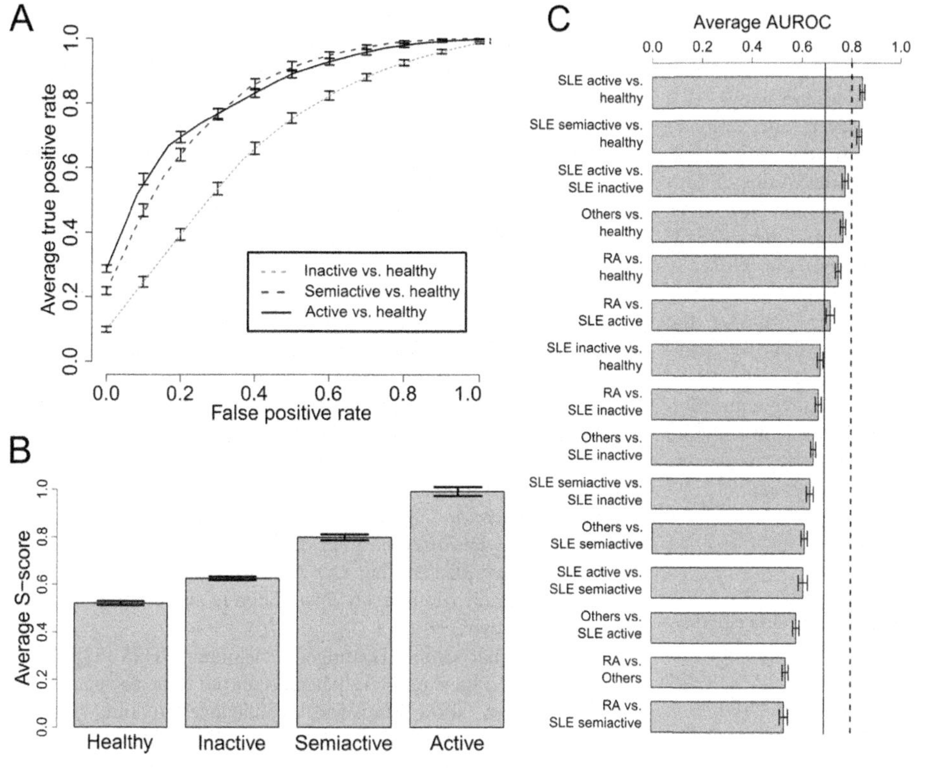

Figure 2. Cross-validation analysis of a SVM based classifier for diagnosis and stratification of SLE. (A) ROC analysis of the SLE classification measure. **(B)** The average S-score of test samples from 100 rounds of cross-validation (error bar represents S.E.M). **(C)** Average AUROC of comparisons between SLE, healthy controls, rheumatoid arthritis (RA) and other autoimmune diseases (others). The black dotted line at AUROC = 0.8 indicates a classifier that can readily separate the two classes, and a black solid line at AUROC = 0.7 indicates a classifier that is moderately effective for separating two classes (error bar represents S.E.M).

dotted line). Active SLE compared to inactive disease, other autoimmune diseases and RA compared to healthy subjects and RA compared to active SLE, have AUROC values between 0.7 and 0.8 (between the black solid and dotted lines) that indicate discrimination with less certainty, while the remainder of the diseases with AUROC values <0.7 (to the left of the solid black line (*e.g.*, RA and other autoimmune diseases vs. SLE inactive etc) cannot be reliably distinguished.

Leukocyte capture arrays improve the discriminative ability of conventional laboratory tests in SLE

Currently the assessment of SLE activity is based on a combination of clinical symptoms, signs, and laboratory tests. Since discriminating inactive SLE from more active forms of SLE (*i.e.*, semi-active or active) may be important in management, we evaluated the discriminatory ability of combination of tests including antibody arrays and the serological and immunochemical tests performed. For each of the datasets, we trained a classifier using the SVM approach, and its discriminatory ability was

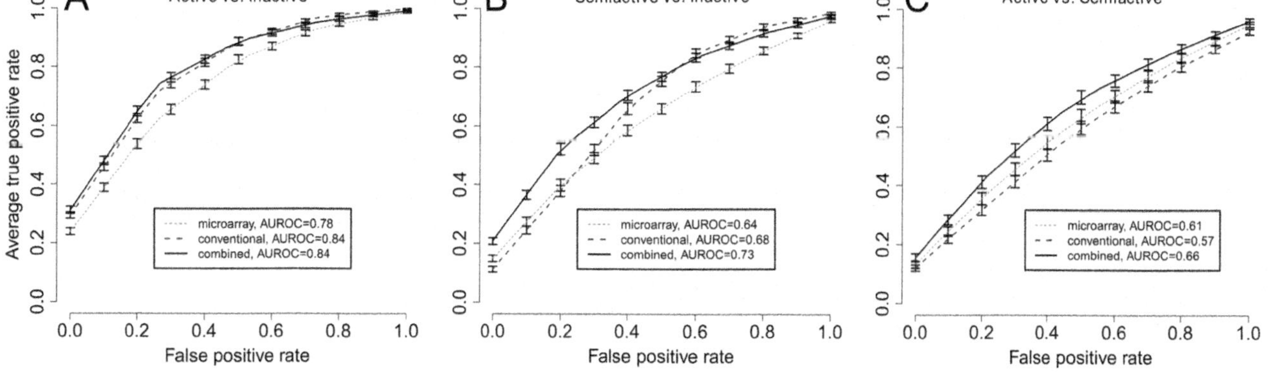

Figure 3. Comparison of discriminatory ability of CD antibody microarray and conventional laboratory tests.

evaluated with 100 rounds of three-fold cross validation (Figure 3). The serum tests, anti-dsDNA antibodies, C3, and C4 levels, are more discriminating than our antibody microarray ($p<0.001$, one-sided paired t test) in distinguishing semi-active and active SLE from inactive SLE (Figure 3A and B). However, our antibody microarray can better distinguish active from semi-active SLE ($p<0.001$). When we trained a SVM based on the results of both microarray and the serum tests, we achieved a significantly better separation of semi-active SLE from inactive and active SLE ($p<0.001$ for both classification tasks). Given the clinically heterogeneous presentation of SLE patients, it is particularly encouraging to note that the microarray can improve the discriminative ability of conventional laboratory tests for semi-active vs. inactive SLE. Taken together with the observation that nearly all singleton CD biomarkers have very low expression correlation with the measurements from the three conventional laboratory tests (Figure 1B), we believe that the leukocyte microarray does indeed provide additional information.

Discussion

This antibody microarray yields comparable diagnostic sensitivity and specificity to the DNA microarray system described by Chaussabel *et al.* [2]. The antibody microarray we described is, however, a potentially more practical platform for use in the diagnostic laboratory, since the analytical equipment required is less technically challenging and much less expensive (cost per microarray is ~US$90) than gene expression microarrays or flow cytometry for the same number of antibodies, and it can be performed rapidly on an *ad hoc* basis. Traditionally, cellular markers and populations (and more importantly the changes in these populations) are detected by flow cytometry. This is generally a technically challenging, slow and expensive method that, when performed in a sophisticated laboratory with large sample volumes of sera and reagents and skilled technicians, can analyze no more than 17 CD antigens in a single analysis. The cell capture microarrays, in contrast to flow cytometry, can be performed on the bench in any laboratory and can simultaneously determine the presence of more than 100 antigens expressed on the surface of leukocytes. Furthermore, the microarray provides a semi-quantitative method of monitoring the numbers of cells in a sample since the light scattering from the cells is proportional to the number of cells immobilized on the arrays [8,11]. In our experience, the method requires minimal training and uses only small volumes of antibodies and peripheral blood. In addition to the discriminatory ability demonstrated in this study, the technical simplicity of this profiling technology makes it attractive for clinical use.

The high-throughput nature of this microarray is also particularly attractive because it allows rapid identification of an immunophenotype for each patient based on the expression of multiple cell surface molecules that have been perturbed due to current or previous activation events in SLE. In principle, combinations of expressed surface membrane proteins (CD antigens and other membrane proteins) characterise functional subsets of leukocytes. One key idea of this study is that such leukocyte surface markers carry useful information about SLE activity. Our data represent a proof of concept only and will need to be validated using a much larger sample size before the microarray is applied in a clinical setting.

It is possible to turn our antibody microarray approach on its head, namely to immobilize the antigen and capture the antibodies as undertaken by Fattal *et al.* [7] and Robinson *et al.* [4]. Although these methods can distinguish SLE from healthy controls, their clinical performance in distinguishing SLE from other autoimmune and rheumatic has not been demonstrated and performance characteristics in the clinic are not yet reported. Our pilot study demonstrates that leukocyte surface markers contain information that may be used alone or in combination to other markers (such as anti-dsDNA) to distinguish SLE from normal controls, stratify disease activity, and may even distinguish SLE from other autoimmune and rheumatic conditions, although the later requires further study.

We show that a disease activity score can be constructed based on the entire antigen expression profile through a state-of-the-art machine learning technique. Similar supervised machine learning approaches for clinical diagnostic support using microarray technology have been reported extensively in the last decade, particularly in the field of cancer classification [21,22]. Unlike a traditional singleton biomarker, the calculation of our S-score depends on the size and quality of the training examples. Different SVM decision functions are generated by using different training samples. Therefore, we performed a cross-validation analysis to estimate the sensitivity and specificity of this classifier for SLE. This analysis indicates that our approach for generating the S-score is generally robust even when different subsets of the training samples are used.

We note that some CD antigens, including CD95 [23], CD86 [24,25], which have previously been reported to be associated with SLE, do not show statistical significance in our singleton biomarker analysis. This is surprising given their role in co-stimulation and cell activation. We suspect this may reflect the lack of specificity of the clone of antibodies used in this version of the microarray. From our experience, different clones of antibodies have different antigen-binding characteristics, and further experiments using different antibody clones will determine if alternative antibodies will contribute to the discriminatory ability of the array.

Although the discriminatory ability of the current version of the microarray on its own is no better than conventional tests, the fact that the microarray provides additional information for clinical assessment of SLE is an important finding. The expression values from about 40% of the antibody spots in the current version of the microarray were filtered out because of low expression or high variability in performance. This is not surprising as this version of microarray was originally designed for the diagnosis of lymphoproliferative diseases [8]. It is likely that a customised antibody microarray containing rationally selected antibodies that target CD antigens known to reflect the pathogenesis and activity of SLE will improve the sensitivity and specificity of the antibody microarray [26]. In particular, we propose that a customised SLE antibody microarray can be developed by retaining only those informative biomarkers in the current generation of the array, and augmenting the array with other antibodies directed to cell surface markers whose expression has been reported to be perturbed in patients with SLE. These could include antibodies related to innate immunity (CD1a, CD14, CD83), adaptive immunity (CD161), adhesion molecules (CD166 and CD6), other markers (CD279 and other chemokines *e.g.*, CCR6). These and other molecules have been shown to be potentially involved in the pathogenesis of SLE and may therefore also be useful markers of the disease and level of activity [26,27].

Conclusion

Our observations using a first-generation antibody microarray demonstrate that SLE patients can be distinguished from healthy controls based on the differential expression of CD markers on PBMCs. Our analysis indicates that the current version of PBMC

CD antibody microarray can be combined with current laboratories tests to provide superior discriminatory ability to stratify SLE patients according to disease activity. We postulate that the addition of rationally selected antibodies based on reports of their altered expression in SLE will result in an even higher discriminatory ability than currently used tests, with potential benefits both for diagnosis and monitoring of disease and tailoring of therapy.

Supporting Information

Figure S1 An image of the scanned microarray from a healthy control and SLE patients with different disease activity.

Figure S2 Validation of expressed microarray CD antigen markers using flow cytometry. (A) Unnormalized microarray spot intensity of four randomly selected expressed CD antigens in CD3 stimulated leukocytes. **(B)** Flow cytometry analysis of the same four antibodies in the same cell population, and also controls. All four measured expressed CD antigens detected by the microarray are also detected as being expressed by flow cytometry.

Acknowledgments

We thank members of the Department of Rheumatology at the Royal Prince Alfred Hospital for recruiting patients with rheumatoid arthritis for the study.

Author Contributions

Conceived and designed the experiments: SA CGdR. Performed the experiments: MWL LCH. Analyzed the data: JWKH. Wrote the paper: MWL JWKH CGdR SA.

References

1. Tan EM, Cohen AS, Fries JF, Masi AT, McShane DJ, et al. (1982) The 1982 revised criteria for the classification of systemic lupus erythematosus. Arthritis Rheum 25: 1271–1277.
2. Chaussabel D, Quinn C, Shen J, Patel P, Glaser C, et al. (2008) A modular analysis framework for blood genomics studies: application to systemic lupus erythematosus. Immunity 29: 150–164. doi:10.1016/j.immuni.2008.05.012.
3. Joos TO, Schrenk M, Höpfl P, Kröger K, Chowdhury U, et al. (2000) A microarray enzyme-linked immunosorbent assay for autoimmune diagnostics. Electrophoresis 21: 2641–2650. doi:10.1002/1522-2683(20000701)21:13<2641::AID-ELPS2641>3.0.CO;2-5.
4. Robinson WH, DiGennaro C, Hueber W, Haab BB, Kamachi M, et al. (2002) Autoantigen microarrays for multiplex characterization of autoantibody responses. Nat Med 8: 295–301. doi:10.1038/nm0302-295.
5. Huang RP, Huang R, Fan Y, Lin Y (2001) Simultaneous detection of multiple cytokines from conditioned media and patient's sera by an antibody-based protein array system. Anal Biochem 294: 55–62. doi:10.1006/abio.2001.5156.
6. Hueber W, Kidd BA, Tomooka BH, Lee BJ, Bruce B, et al. (2005) Antigen microarray profiling of autoantibodies in rheumatoid arthritis. Arthritis Rheum 52: 2645–2655. doi:10.1002/art.21269.
7. Fattal I, Shental N, Mevorach D, Anaya J-M, Livneh A, et al. (2010) An antibody profile of systemic lupus erythematosus detected by antigen microarray. Immunology 130: 337–343. doi:10.1111/j.1365-2567.2010.03245.x.
8. Belov L, Vega O de la, Remedios CG dos, Mulligan SP, Christopherson RI (2001) Immunophenotyping of Leukemias Using a Cluster of Differentiation Antibody Microarray. Cancer Res 61: 4483–4489.
9. Belov L, Mulligan SP, Barber N, Woolfson A, Scott M, et al. (2006) Analysis of human leukaemias and lymphomas using extensive immunophenotypes from an antibody microarray. Br J Haematol 135: 184–197. doi:10.1111/j.1365-2141.2006.06266.x.
10. Lal S, Lui R, Nguyen L, Macdonald P, Denyer G, et al. (2004) Increases in leukocyte cluster of differentiation antigen expression during cardiopulmonary bypass in patients undergoing heart transplantation. Proteomics 4: 1918–1926. doi:10.1002/pmic.200300756.
11. Brown A, Lattimore J-D, McGrady M, Sullivan D, Dyer W, et al. (2008) Stable and unstable angina: Identifying novel markers on circulating leukocytes. Proteomics Clin Appl 2: 90–98.
12. Lui R, Brown A, Wu B, Lin M-W, Thompson J, et al. (2008) Use of Antibody Microarrays in the Analysis of Inflammation, Autoimmunity, Viral Infection, and Cancer Metastases. In: Eyk JEV, Dunn MJ, editors. Clinical Proteomics. Wiley-VCH Verlag GmbH & Co. KGaA. pp. 571–592. Available:http://onlinelibrary.wiley.com/doi/10.1002/9783527622153.ch31/summary.Accessed 30 June 2012.
13. Lal S, Brown A, Nguyen L, Braet F, Dyer W, et al. (2009) Using antibody arrays to detect microparticles from acute coronary syndrome patients based on cluster of differentiation (CD) antigen expression. Mol Cell Proteomics 8: 799–804. doi:10.1074/mcp.M800335-MCP200.
14. Mohamed A, Lal S, Brown A, Lui R, Ho J, et al. (2010) How to Interrogate the cellular immune system in patients with ischemic heart disease. Myocardial Ischemia: Causes, Symptoms and Treatment. Nova Biomedical Press. pp. 195–216.
15. Ho JWK, Koundinya R, Caetano T, Remedios CG dos, Charleston MA (2008) Inferring differential leukocyte activity from antibody microarrays using a latent variable model. Genome Informatics 21: 126–137.
16. Bombardier C, Gladman DD, Urowitz MB, Caron D, Chang CH (1992) Derivation of the SLEDAI. A disease activity index for lupus patients. The Committee on Prognosis Studies in SLE. Arthritis Rheum 35: 630–640.
17. Smyth GK (2004) Linear models and empirical bayes methods for assessing differential expression in microarray experiments. Stat Appl Genet Mol Biol 3: Article3. doi:10.2202/1544-6115.1027.
18. Sing T, Sander O, Beerenwinkel N, Lengauer T (2005) ROCR: visualizing classifier performance in R. Bioinformatics 21: 3940–3941. doi:10.1093/bioinformatics/bti623.
19. Cortes C, Vapnik V (1995) Support-Vector Networks. Mach Learn 20: 273–297.
20. Cristianani N, Shawe-Taylor J (2000) An Introduction to Support Vector Machines: and other kernel-based learning methods. Cambridge University Press, UK.
21. Ramaswamy S, Tamayo P, Rifkin R, Sayan Mukherjee, Yeang C-H, et al. (2001) Multiclass cancer diagnosis using tumor gene expression signatures. Proc Natl Acad Sci USA 98: 15149–15154.
22. Golub TR, Slonim DK, Tamayo P, Huard C, Gaasenbeek M, et al. (1999) Molecular classification of cancer: Class discovery and class prediction by gene expression monitoring. Science 286: 531–537.
23. Bijl M, Horst G, Limburg PC, Kallenberg CG (2001) Fas expression on peripheral blood lymphocytes in systemic lupus erythematosus (SLE): relation to lymphocyte activation and disease activity. Lupus 10: 866–872.
24. Bijl M, Horst G, Limburg PC, Kallenberg CG (2001) Expression of costimulatory molecules on peripheral blood lymphocytes of patients with systemic lupus erythematosus. Ann Rheum Dis 60: 523–526.
25. Morris DL, Graham RR, Erwig L-P, Gaffney PM, Moser KL, et al. (2009) Variation in the upstream region of P-Selectin (SELP) is a risk factor for SLE. Genes Immun 10: 404–413. doi:10.1038/gene.2009.17.
26. Ho JWK, Lin M-W, Braet F, Su YY, Adelstein S, et al. (2010) Customising an antibody leukocyte capture microarray for systemic lupus erythematosus: beyond biomarker discovery. Proteomics Clin Appl 4: 179–189. doi:10.1002/prca.200900165.
27. Tsokos GC (2011) Systemic lupus erythematosus. N Engl J Med 365: 2110–2121. doi:10.1056/NEJMra1100359.

3

Functional Annotation of Rheumatoid Arthritis and Osteoarthritis Associated Genes by Integrative Genome-Wide Gene Expression Profiling Analysis

Zhan-Chun Li[1], Jie Xiao[2], Jin-Liang Peng[3], Jian-Wei Chen[1], Tao Ma[1], Guang-Qi Cheng[1], Yu-Qi Dong[1], Wei-li Wang[1], Zu-De Liu[1]*

1 Department of Orthopaedic Surgery, Ren Ji Hospital, School of Medicine, Shanghai Jiao Tong University, Shanghai, P. R. China, **2** Department of Anesthesiology, Ren Ji Hospital, School of Medicine, Shanghai Jiao Tong University, Shanghai, P. R. China, **3** School of Biomedical Engineering/MED-X Research Institute, Shanghai Jiao Tong University, Shanghai, P. R. China

Abstract

Background: Rheumatoid arthritis (RA) and osteoarthritis (OA) are two major types of joint diseases that share multiple common symptoms. However, their pathological mechanism remains largely unknown. The aim of our study is to identify RA and OA related-genes and gain an insight into the underlying genetic basis of these diseases.

Methods: We collected 11 whole genome-wide expression profiling datasets from RA and OA cohorts and performed a meta-analysis to comprehensively investigate their expression signatures. This method can avoid some pitfalls of single dataset analyses.

Results and Conclusion: We found that several biological pathways (*i.e.*, the immunity, inflammation and apoptosis related pathways) are commonly involved in the development of both RA and OA. Whereas several other pathways (*i.e.*, vasopressin-related pathway, regulation of autophagy, endocytosis, calcium transport and endoplasmic reticulum stress related pathways) present significant difference between RA and OA. This study provides novel insights into the molecular mechanisms underlying this disease, thereby aiding the diagnosis and treatment of the disease.

Editor: Ted S. Acott, Casey Eye Institute, United States of America

Funding: This study was supported by Shanghai Natural Science Foundation, China (No. 13ZR1424900) and Medical-Engineering Joint Fund of Shanghai Jiao Tong University (No. YG2011MS41). The funders had no role in study design, data collection and analysis, decision to publish, or preparation of the manuscript.

Competing Interests: The authors have declared that no competing interests exist.

* E-mail: zudeliu001@163.com

Introduction

Rheumatoid arthritis (RA) is a common chronic systemic autoimmune disease that mainly affects the flexible joints. It is characterized by the inflammation of articular synovial. The lasting recurrent inflammation of synovial can lead to the deformation and destruction of cartilage and bones, which could result in disability of the patients [1,2]. RA mainly occurs in the 30~70 years old people and is more frequent in females than males. More than 1% of the world's population may be affected by RA [3,4]. This disease brings great physiological and psychological burden to patients. However, the biological causes for RA remain largely unknown. Although infectious agents including viruses, bacteria and fungi have long been suspected, none has been comprehensively proved [5,6]. Previous researches have also investigated the potential associations between RA and environmental factors, such as smoking, vitamin D deficiency, etc [7,8]. It is now generally believed that the pathogenesis of RA is closely related to genetic factors. Certain genes such as the human leukocyte antigen (HLA). HLA-DR4 and DW4 antigen, were identified in more than 90% of the patients. These pathological factors are referred to as the RA-shared epitope [3,9].

Osteoarthritis (OA) is another main type of chronic disease that affects the joints. The major pathological feature of OA is the degradation of articular cartilage and subchondral bone, and this may lead to the rigidity deformity and dysfunction of the joints [10]. The incidence of this disease in more than 50 years old people is as high as 80%. Etiological factors of OA include the mechanical injury, overweight, impairment of peripheral nerves, etc [11]. Osteoarthritis is different from rheumatoid arthritis in that there are extra-articular manifestations for rheumatoid arthritis. In addition, these diseases have different pathological manifestations for the synovial. RA is characterized by synovial cell hypertrophy and hyperplasia, infiltration of lymphocytes and inflammatory cells, whereas OA has fewer leukocytic infiltrates [12,13].

Recently, large efforts have been made to screen the genetic factors involved in RA and OA by high-throughput methods [14,15]. Several key genes and diagnostic markers have been identified for these diseases. However, the integrative analysis of multiple factors that contribute to the development of RA and OA appears to be a challenging task, and the underlying pathogenesis of RA and OA remain far from being understood. In this study, we compiled several whole-genome gene expression profiling datasets from RA and OA. Then we used a meta-analysis method to identify the aberrantly expressed genes. The subsequent functional annotation of these genes was performed based on gene ontology (GO) and Kyoto Encyclopedia of Genes and Genomes (KEGG) analysis [16,17]. We demonstrated that several biological pathways are highly enriched in both RA and OA associated genes, such as chemokine signaling pathway, regulation of autophagy, focal adhesion, etc. Whereas other pathways, including regulation of autophagy, endocytosis, calcium transport and endoplasmic reticulum stress related pathways, are differentially influenced in the RA and OA respectively. This analysis provides a novel insight into the pathophysiological processes involved in these diseases. In addition, it would help to prioritize putative targets for further experimental studies and develop novel therapeutic strategies in preventing the RA and OA.

Materials and Methods

Sample Collection

We first queried the PubMed and related literatures to collect the expression profiling datasets from RA, OA and the corresponding normal control (NT) tissues. The following key words and their combinations were used: "rheumatoid arthritis, osteoarthritis, gene expression, microarray". We only retained the original experimental works that analyzed the gene expression profiling between RA, OA and NT samples, respectively. Non-human studies, review articles and integrated analysis of expression profiles were excluded (**Figure 1**). At last, a total of 15 expression profiling datasets from 11 studies were collected (**Table 1**).

Data Preprocessing

In this study, a global normalization method to minimize the data inconsistency and heterogeneity was used. We used the *Z-score* transformation approach to calculate the expression intensities for each probe of the gene expression profiles [18]. *Z-scores* were calculated according to the following formula:

$$Z-score=\frac{x_i-\bar{x}}{\delta}.$$

where x_i represents raw intensity data for each gene; $\bar{x}$ represents average gene intensity within a single experiment and δ represents standard deviation (SD) of all of the measured intensities.

Statistical Analysis

To give an overview of the global shifts of gene expression between pathological and normal tissues, we first calculated the pairwise Euclidean distances for samples from RA, OA and NTs according to the following the formula:

$$D=\sqrt{\sum_{i=1}^{n}(x_{i1}-x_{i2})^2}.$$

The significance analysis of microarray (SAM) algorithm was then used to identify the differentially expressed genes between pathological and control samples. The SAM procedure first calculate the "relative difference" score for each gene based on a modified *t-test* method, then a subsequent permutation analysis was

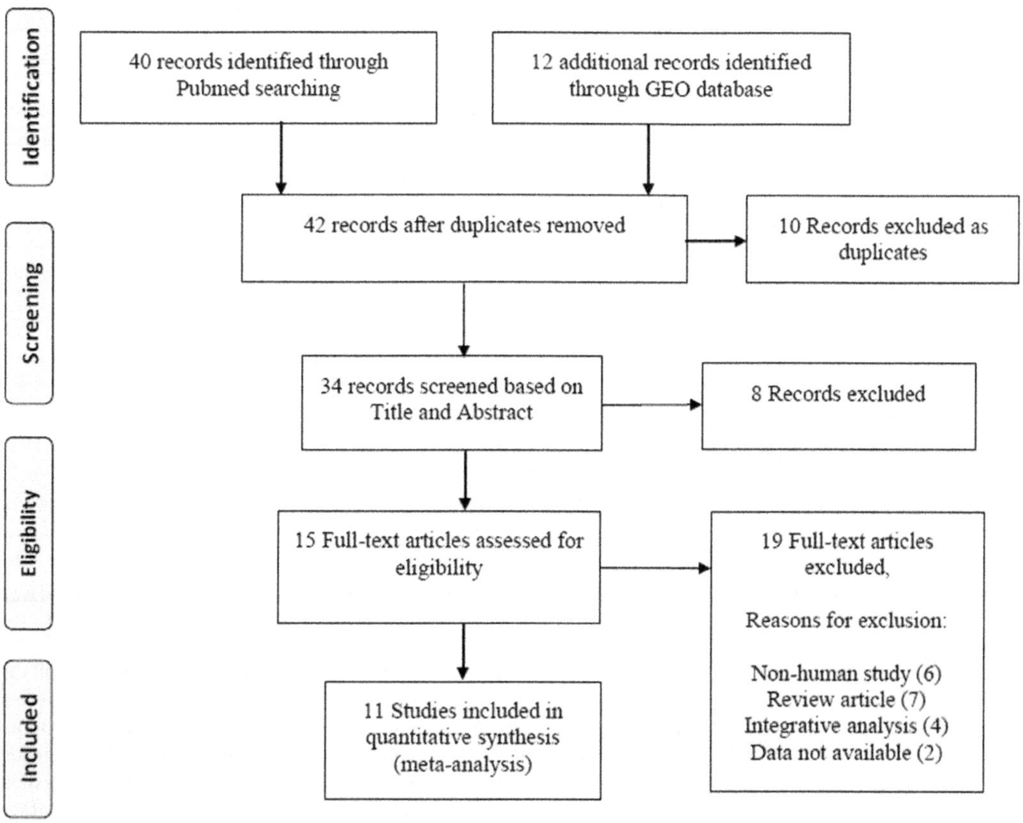

Figure 1. Flowchart of the selected process of microarray datasets for the meta-analysis.

Table 1. Characteristics of analyzed datasets.

GEO Acc	PMID	Publish date	tissue type	Platforms	Number of samples
GSE1919	20858714	4-Nov-04	synovial	Affymetrix HGU95A	5 OA
					5 NC
					5 RA
GSE2053	20858714	10-Dec-04	synovial	HUMAN UNIGENE SetI Part 1	4 NC
					4 RA
GSE3698	16508983	6-Jun-06	synovial	Human Unigene3.1 cDNA Array 37.5K v1.0	18 RA
					19 OA
GSE7669	21474483	30-Aug-07	synovial	Affymetrix HGU95 2.0	6 RA
					6 OA
GSE9027	17665400	13-Sep-07	synovial		28 RA
GSE12021	18721452	2-Sep-08	synovial	Affymetrix HGU133A HGU133B Array	20 OA
					22 RA
					13 NC
GSE17755	21496236	21-Aug-10	peripheral blood	Hitachisoft AceGene Human Oligo Chip 30K 1 Chip Version	112 RA
					8 NC
					45 NC
GSE27390	21679443	31-May-11	bone marrow	Affymetrix HGU133 Plus 2.0	9 RA
					11 OA
GSE29746	22021863	25-Oct-11	synovial	Whole Human Genome Microarray 4x44K G4112F	9 RA
					11 OA
GSE36700	17469140	27-Mar-12	synovial	Affymetrix HGU133 Plus 2.0	6 OA
					7 RA
GSE39340		22-Oct-12	synovial	Illumina HumanHT-12 V4.0 expression beadchip	10 RA
					7 OA

A total of 11 expression profiles comparing RA, OA and NTs samples were collected in this study. Their GEO accession number, PubMed ID, publish date, tissue type, expression platform and number of samples were listed.

used to compute false discovery rate (*FDR*) [19]. To get the best balance between the number of significant calls and the lowest *FDR* for the dataset tested, we used *FDR* <0.05 and $|\log$ fold change$| >1$ as the criteria for significant difference.

Functional Annotation

In order to examine the biological significance of the differentially expressed genes, we performed GO and KEGG enrichment analysis to investigate their functional and pathway implications. The online based software GeneCoDis3 was used to perform this analysis [20]. The differentially expressed genes and all the expressed genes were submitted as the gene list and background list, respectively. The 5% cut-off of the FDR was used.

Results

Short Overview of the Studies Included

In recent years, many studies have used microarray technology to analyzed the whole genome expression proofing in samples of RA and OA. In this study, a total of 11 expression profiling datasets were collected, which include 383 samples. The characteristics of all these datasets included in this analysis were listed as **Table 1**. Among the 11 datasets, nine studies focused on synovial tissues and two studies focused on peripheral blood and bone marrow-derived mononuclear cells, respectively. More than half (six) of these studies focused on the differentially expressed genes between RA and OA samples, whereas four studies focused on the expression profiling of RA or OA and the corresponding NT samples, and one study only provided the expression profiling from RA samples.

Global Changes in Gene Expression in RA and OA Samples

Normalization is an important issue for comparison of microarray datasets. The heterogeneity of different datasets may lead to difficulties for comparing the results directly. The improperly normalized data used in microarray comparisons may run a high risk of skewing comparison results and reduces the credibility of individual gene change measurements. Towards this end, a global transformation of *z-score* was used to normalize all the expression profiling data retrieved for RA and OA. After filtering the normalized data, a total of 14,047 genes were detected in more than 60% of the samples. By using the assembled expression compendium, we investigated the global shifts of gene expression between RA, OA and NTs samples respectively. The average Euclidean distance was calculated to measure expression divergence between individual samples. As indicated in **Figure 2**, the expression divergence between OA and corresponding NT samples is significantly larger than that between RA and NT samples (Mann-Whitney U test, *P-value* <1e-6). We found that expression divergence between pathological samples and NTs is significantly larger than the distance between pathological samples of RA and OA samples (Mann-Whitney U test, *P-value*: 2.37e-57 and 1.12e-83 respectively,). This indicates that the similarities of expression signatures between RA and OA and several pathogenesis in common may contribute to the development of these diseases.

Identification of Differentially Expressed Genes from RA *vs.* NT Samples

To obtain the genetic markers involved in the development and progression of RA and OA, the SAM method was used to identify the differentially expressed genes between pathological and control samples. At last, a total of 201 genes were found to be differentially expressed between RA and NT samples with the threshold of *FDR* <0.05 and minimal two-fold changes of expression. Among those differentially expressed genes, 35 genes were up-regulated and 166 genes were down-regulated in RA samples compared with the NT samples, respectively. The full list of these genes was provided in **Table S1**. The top 10 up-regulated and down-regulated genes for RA *vs.* NT were listed in **Table 2**, which include the *DCTN1, GABRR3, SOX18, ALPK2, UCP2, GGTL3, GNGT2, ABHD11, ETV3, NPCDR1,* etc. The gene with the most significant expression difference between RA and OA is Dynactin subunit 1 (*DCTN1*), which presents a ~1437.67 fold higher expression in RA samples. *DCTN1,* encoding the largest subunit of dynactin, is involved in a diverse array of cellular functions, including the centripetal movement of lysosomes and endosomes, spindle formation, chromosome movement, nuclear positioning, and axonogenesis. Conversely, the gene with the most significant expression divergence and higher expression in RA samples (151.59 fold) is *NPCDR1*. Some of the deregulated genes have been previously reported to be closely related to the development of RA.

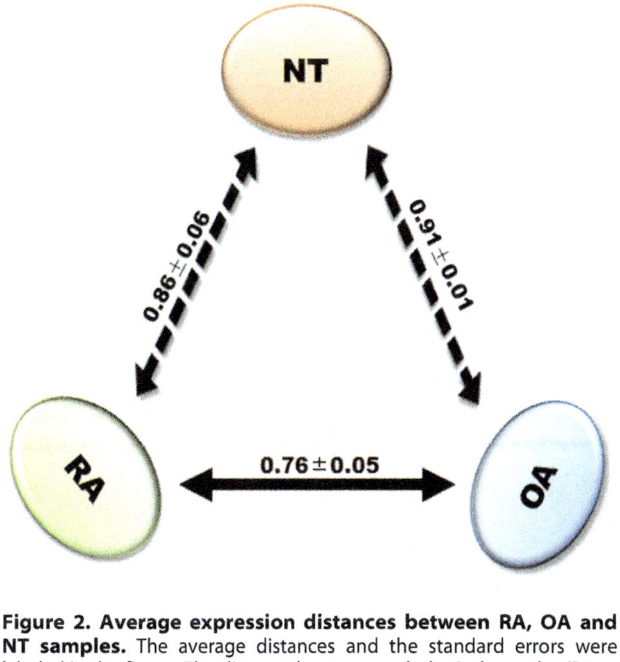

Figure 2. Average expression distances between RA, OA and NT samples. The average distances and the standard errors were labeled in the figure. The distance between pathological samples (RA or OA) and NTs is significantly larger than the distance between RA and OA samples.

For example, the single nucleotide polymorphism within the *UCP2* gene was identified to associate with many chronic inflammatory diseases including RA and systemic lupus erythematosus (SLE) [21]. Activated *PIAS1* gene was identified to repress the transcription of inflammatory genes [22], repression of *PIAS1* related pathways have some effects for the treatment of inflammatory disorders such as RA and atherosclerosis [23].

Identification of Differentially Expressed Genes from OA *vs.* NT Samples

With the same analytic procedure described above, we identified 244 genes to be differentially expressed in OA samples comparing with NT samples, which include 45 up-regulated and 199 down-regulated genes. The full gene list and the top deregulated gene list for OA *vs.* NT samples were listed in **Table S2** and **Table 3**, respectively. Specifically, the top deregulated genes for OA *vs.* NT samples include the *DPM2, MUS81, VAMP2, ZBTB33, NUP62, RHBDD1, PDZD7, PLEKHG4, ABCG1, TCEA3,* etc. Several of these genes have been identified to be involved in the development RA or OA samples, including *COL2* [24], *Gal-9* [25,26], *MUS81* [27] and *ABCG1* [28].

Functional Annotation of Differentially Expressed Genes

To gain insights into the biological roles of these differentially expressed genes from RA and OA *vs.* NT samples, we performed a GO categories enrichment analysis. GO category provides a descriptive framework of functional annotation and classification for gene sets analysis. GO categories are organized into three groups: biological process, molecular function and cellular component. In our work, only biological process and molecular function categories were considered. The functional enrichment work was performed by a web-based software, GeneCoDis3. With the *FDR* <0.05, we found GO terms for molecular functions significantly enriched in protein binding (GO:0005515), metal ion binding and DNA binding (GO:0003677), while for biological processes, the enriched GO terms were regulation of transcription (GO:0006355), embryonic limb morphogenesis (GO:0030326) and otic vesicle development (GO:0071599) (**Figure 3**).

To further evaluate the biological significance for the differentially expressed genes, we also performed the KEGG pathway enrichment analysis. The top enriched biological pathways associated with RA and OA include chemokine signaling pathway, glycosaminoglycan biosynthesis-chondroitin sulfate, SNARE interactions in vesicular transport, endocytosis, autophagy, etc. (**Table 4**). The chemokine pathway, for example, has long been suspected to involve in the development of RA. The chemokines are a family of small cytokines or signaling proteins secreted by cells, which function is to control cells of the immune system during processes of immune surveillance. Many chemokines could participates in the inflammatory response and attracts immune cells to the site of inflammation [29]. The genes involved in chemokines signaling pathway was identified to be altered in both RA *vs.* NT and OA *vs.* NT. The *CXCL2*, for example, also known as *GRO2*, is implicated in the recruitment of neutrophils from the circulation system to the sites of inflammation [30], it is constitutively expressed in resting OA cells, which supports the idea that some circumstances OA can be considered inflammatory disease [31].

As for apoptosis, genes involved in the regulation of cell survival and anti-apoptosis and autophagy related pathways are significantly affected, such as the mitogen-activated protein kinases (MAPK) pathways. MAPK comprises a family of serine/threonine protein kinases that implicated in the regulation of key cellular processes including cell survival, proliferation, differentiation and

Table 2. Summary of differentially expressed genes between RA *vs.* NT samples.

Gene Symbol	Description	Score (D)	Fold Change	Status
DCTN1	dynactin 1	3.46	1437.67	down-regulated
GABRR3	gamma-aminobutyric acid (GABA) A receptor, rho 3	3.23	130.1	down-regulated
SOX18	SRY (sex determining region Y)-box 18	4.32	70.33	down-regulated
ALPK2	alpha-kinase 2	3.96	64.95	down-regulated
UCP2	uncoupling protein 2	3.85	52.75	down-regulated
MITD1	microtubule interacting and transport, domain containing 1	3.15	46.12	down-regulated
SMEK1	SMEK homolog 1, suppressor of mek1	3.64	35.59	down-regulated
BANF1	barrier to autointegration factor 1	3.46	33.62	down-regulated
PIAS1	protein inhibitor of activated STAT, 1	3.25	33.18	down-regulated
GFOD2	glucose-fructose oxidoreductase domain containing 2	3.38	30.77	down-regulated
TSPAN1	tetraspanin 1	−3.13	−48.9	up-regulated
HSPB2	heat shock 27kDa protein 2	−4.52	−50.67	up-regulated
NEK6	NIMA-related kinase 6	−10.5	−56.03	up-regulated
COL2	collagen, type II, alpha 1	−3.62	−62.02	up-regulated
LGALS9	lectin, galactoside-binding, soluble, 9	−4.85	−64.47	up-regulated
GGTL3	gamma-glutamyltransferase 7	−3.23	−79.05	up-regulated
GNGT2	guanine nucleotide binding protein (G protein), gamma transducing activity polypeptide 2	−9.81	−89.35	up-regulated
ABHD11	abhydrolase domain containing 11	−4.03	−95.86	up-regulated
ETV3	ets variant 3	−3.66	−106.96	up-regulated
NPCDR1	nasopharyngeal carcinoma, down-regulated 1	−4.79	−151.59	up-regulated

The symbol name, description, D score and the expression fold change were provided.

Table 3. Summary of differentially expressed genes between OA *vs.* NT samples.

Gene Symbol	Description	Score (D)	Fold Change	Status
DPM2	dolichyl-phosphate mannosyltransferase polypeptide 2	4.18	697.61	down-regulated
MUS81	MUS81 structure-specific endonuclease	4.3	236.6	down-regulated
VAMP2	vesicle-associated membrane protein 2	6.38	220.45	down-regulated
ZBTB33	zinc finger and BTB domain containing 33	3.67	25366	down-regulated
NUP62	nucleoporin 62kDa	3.24	157.76	down-regulated
LOXL3	lysyl oxidase-like 3	4.84	111.57	down-regulated
LIMK2	LIM domain kinase 2	3.88	76.61	down-regulated
ZNF593	zinc finger protein 593	3.73	65.5	down-regulated
MRPS5	mitochondrial ribosomal protein S5	4.24	54.33	down-regulated
SMYD2	SET and MYND domain containing 2	3.62	31.41	down-regulated
MAN2	alpha Mannosidase II	−4.51	−87.45	up-regulated
SDCCAG1	NEMF nuclear export mediator factor	−6.12	−97.84	up-regulated
IGSF8	immunoglobulin superfamily, member 8	−6.9	−100.79	up-regulated
PBX1	pre-B-cell leukemia homeobox 1	−5.22	−133.75	up-regulated
KIAA1128	CCSER2 coiled-coil serine-rich protein 2	−6.9	−195.25	up-regulated
RHBDD1	rhomboid domain containing 1	−6.18	−231.9	up-regulated
PDZD7	PDZ domain containing 7	−4.48	−286	up-regulated
PLEKHG4	pleckstrin homology domain containing, family G (with RhoGef domain) member 4	−8.78	−337.12	up-regulated
ABCG1	ATP-binding cassette, sub-family G (WHITE), member 1	−3.87	−441.27	up-regulated
TCEA3	transcription elongation factor A (SII), 3	−8.37	−1241.14	up-regulated

The symbol name, description, D score and the expression fold change were provided.

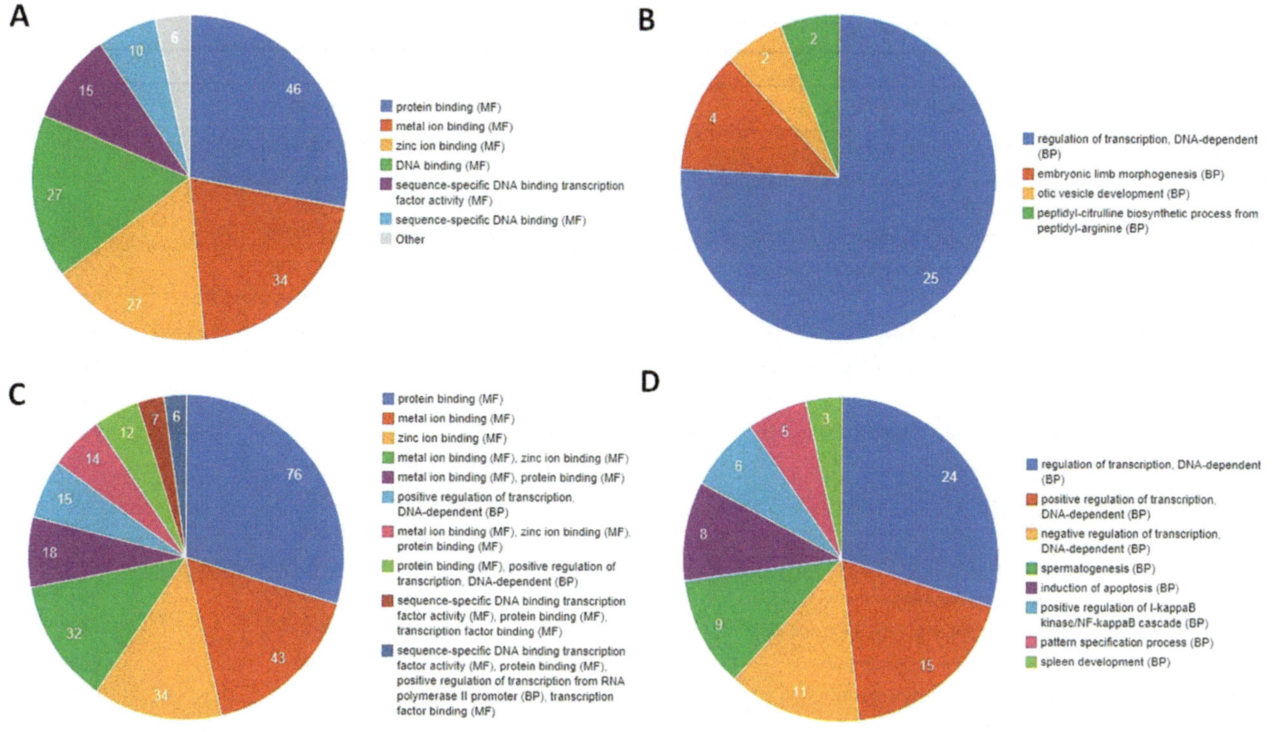

Figure 3. Enriched GO terms of differentially expressed genes between RA and OA *vs.* NT samples. (A) molecular functions for differentially expressed genes of RA *vs.* NT samples; (B) biological process for differentially expressed genes of RA *vs.* NT samples; (C) molecular functions for differentially expressed genes of OA *vs.* NT samples; (D) biological process for differentially expressed genes of OA *vs.* NT samples.

apoptosis as well as cellular stress and inflammatory responses. The respective genes in MAPK pathway showed altered expression levels in RA and OA patients of this study. Involvement of MAPK in the regulation of the synthesis of inflammation mediators and the development of RA have been widely identified [32]. Inhibitors targeting MAPK related pathways have been developed and the preclinical data indicated that they exhibit anti-inflammatory activities. This makes them the potential targets of anti-inflammatory therapy for these diseases [33].

Focal adhesion kinase (FAK) is another pathway that known to play a key role in cell proliferation and migration. Members of this family, which include FAK and PYK2 and their associated signaling intermediates, have been implicated in cell adhesion, migration and osteoclast differentiation [34]. GRB2 is one of the interaction factors of FAK that facilitate intracellular signaling [35]. This gene was found to be up-regulated in both of the diseases, and this may be responsible for the activation of the FAK family signaling and results in the adhesion and migration of the pathological cells.

Discussion

Rheumatoid arthritis and osteoarthritis are the most commonly observed types of arthritis. However, the underlying causes of RA and OA remain largely unknown. Understanding the pathogenesis could have important implications for drug development and treatment for these diseases. Genetic researches on RA and OA have pursued throughout the last years. For example, the whole genome expression profiling studies by using microarrays. Gene expression profiling studies are capable of identifying differences in transcription of thousands of genes on a genome-wide scale. This technique may investigate the pathophysiology of complex genetic tracts and the altered molecular pathways. The first genome wide comparisons of gene expression of RA and OA was performed by Ungethuem *et al.* in 2006. To date, a total of 11 microarray mRNA profiling studies comparing RA and OA with control tissue have been published. Combination and comparison of these studies may have the potential to substantiate and filter the results of each single study and may provide further insights into the pathogenesis of these diseases. However, the heterogeneity of the datasets may run a risk of skewing comparison results and reduces the credibility of gene expression change measurements. To this end, we collected those published expression profiling datasets and used a global normalization method to calculate the expression level for each gene. This algorithm used in this study could reduce heterogeneity of different datasets and make them comparable. Then we performed a systemic meta-analysis based on re-analysis of primary data sets to retrieve RA and OA associated genes. Followed functional implication analysis was performed to investigate their physiological impact in development of these diseases. To our knowledge, no other systematic meta-analysis of gene profiling has been performed to investigate the differences and similarities between RA and OA. The present study suggests several promising genes and may provide a clue to the role of these genes played in the development of these diseases.

Based on our results, it is evident that inflammation as well as apoptotic processes are key elements in the development and progression of RA since several inflammation- and apoptosis-associated genes were identified. For example, the *Gal-9*. *Gal-9* is a kind of immunity associated gene that plays a role in inflammatory responses. This gene has previously been proved to be a ligand of T cell Ig and mucin domain (*Tim-3*). It was reported that *Tim-3* expression is higher in patients with inflammatory disorders such as RA compared to controls [36]. In this case, up-regulation of

Table 4. KEGG pathway enrichment of genes differentially expressed RA and OA *vs.* NT samples.

Sample type	KEGG pathway	Number of genes	Entrez gene ID	*P-value*
OA vs. NT	Chemokine signaling pathway	5	2920 2869 409 9844 2309	0.0168
OA vs. NT	Endocrine and other factor-regulated calcium reabsorption	5	56302 6546 490 793 8766	0.0179
OA vs. NT	Glycosaminoglycan biosynthesis - chondroitin sulfate	3	55501 64132 10090	0.0286
OA vs. NT	SNARE interactions in vesicular transport	3	6844 53407 113189	0.0462
OA vs. NT	NF-KAPPA B signaling	5	27040 29760 8915 10015 2637	0.0439
OA vs. NT	PPAR signaling pathway	3	1376 364 10999	0.0726
OA vs. NT	Protein processing in endoplasmic reticulum	4	50613 9695 3300 4217	0.0726
OA vs. NT	Phagosome	3	53407 23673 30835	0.0726
OA vs. NT	Pathogenic Escherichia coli infection	3	9181 999 10092	0.0726
OA vs. NT	MAPK signaling pathway	3	999 9844 6197	0.0726
OA vs. NT	Focal adhesion	3	6844 3783 3912	0.0974
OA vs. NT	Oxidative phosphorylation	4	9997 4519 28487 4512	0.0981
OA vs. NT	Endocytosis	3	2869 23096 409	0.0996
RA vs. NT	Vasopressin-regulated water reabsorption	3	6844 51164 1639	0.0175
RA vs. NT	Glyoxylate and dicarboxylate metabolism	3	4190 48 847	0.0275
RA vs. NT	Chemokine signaling pathway	3	2885 2793 2829	0.0493
RA vs. NT	Regulation of autophagy	3	25989 5562 9474	0.0339
RA vs. NT	NF-KAPPA B signaling	4	29760 8915 8091 9020	0.0339
RA vs. NT	SNARE interactions in vesicular transport	3	6844 9527 9482	0.0339
RA vs. NT	Oxidative phosphorylation	5	4508 9997 4519 28487 4512	0.0421
RA vs. NT	Citrate cycle (TCA cycle)	3	4190 48 945406	0.0421
RA vs. NT	mTOR signaling pathway	3	25989 5562 1978	0.0421
RA vs. NT	Adherens junction	3	81 6615 7414	0.0781
RA vs. NT	Wnt signaling pathway	4	56998 6093 9475 51176	0.0781
RA vs. NT	MAPK signaling pathway	4	9448 4773 7151 4217	0.0793
RA vs. NT	Pathogenic Escherichia coli infection	3	9181 999 4690	0.0793
RA vs. NT	Focal adhesion	3	81 2885 3912	0.0841
RA vs. NT	Bacterial invasion of epithelial cells	3	10163 999 9844	0.0841

The number of differentially expressed genes in a specific pathway, enriched gene ID and adjusted *P-values* calculated by fisher's exact test were included.

Gal-9 may enhance the *Tim-3-Tim-3L* interactions in synovial and improve the symptoms of inflammation.

In addition, we found that the NF-κB signaling pathway may play significant role in these diseases. NF-κB is a key transcription factor that regulates a variety of genes involved in immune response, cell differentiation and proliferation. Incorrect activation of NF-κB was suggested to associate with cancer, inflammatory and autoimmune diseases, septic shock and viral infection [37]. It has previously indicated that Interleukin-1 beta (*IL-1β*) gene was induced in the RA patient-derived synovial fibroblast cell line MH7A by cigarette smoke condensate [38]. NF-κB binding sites were found in the promoter region of *IL-1β* gene. Therefore, this indicated that aberrant expression of the genes relevant of NF-κB signaling pathway may play a pathological role in the development of RA and OA.

Abnormalities in the mitochondria have been a topic of interests into the study of arthritis. It has been reported that mutation frequency of mtDNA is significantly higher in the inflamed synovial compared with normal synovial. This high mutation frequency is caused by the inflammatory mediators of TNFα and interferon γ (IFNγ) and eventually results in the changes of microenvironment and function of mitochondria [39]. Here, we reported that expressions of certain genes related to the function of mitochondria were altered in RA patients. Notably, the relevant genes, which include the *ATP6, SCO2, CYTB, DN1, COX1, ANT1*, are mainly function in oxidative phosphorylation, whereas dysfunction in oxidative phosphorylation related genes is closely related to the systemic juvenile idiopathic arthritis and endemic osteoarthritis [40,41]. This largely indicates that both RA and OA can be classified as mitochondrial disorder.

Although RA and OA samples share many similarities of their respective gene expression profiles and a number of pathways show comparable variance in both of these diseases, thus reflecting basic common pathomechanism of these joint diseases. However, RA and OA samples can be clearly differentiated regarding gene expression variances in other pathways. In OA, the pathways affected by expression variances include calcium ion transport, PPAR signaling pathway, protein processing in endoplasmic reticulum (ER), phagosome and endocytosis related pathways, etc. Calcium is the essential structural component of the skeletal system. Adequate calcium intake is the basis of osteoblast growth. Observation of the dysregulated expression of calcium related gene may partially explain why calcium pyrophosphate dihydrates accumulate in synovial of OA patients [42,43]. Endocytosis and autophagy are the major pathways for materials to be transported into the lysosomes in cells. The former is responsible for uptake of extracellular constituents and the latter for degradation of cytoplasmic constituents. Several common factors and pathways that regulate the endocytosis and autophagy has been identified [44]. Since there is a high correlation between autophagy activation and the severity of experimental osteoarthritis [45], we may speculate the causal relationship between the deregulation of endocytosis related genes and the development of OA.

ER stress refers to as the enhanced expression of normal or folding-defective proteins and the accumulation of unfolded protein in ER by stimuli. This process has been shown to participate in many disease, including diabetes, inflammation, and neurodegenerative disorders [46]. It was also indicated that ER stress may contribute to chondrocyte apoptosis along with OA progression, which was closely associated with an enhanced apoptotic response and a reduced protective response by cells [47]. Therefore, molecules that regulate the ER stress response would be candidate targets for treatment of this disease.

In contrast to OA, RA-specific pathways are involved in vasopressin-regulated water reabsorption, adherens junction, etc. As a proinflammatory hormone, vasopressin can stimulate the cell proliferation in chondrocytes that derived from patients with RA [48]. Adherens junctions are protein complexes that occur at cell-cell junctions in epithelial tissues to create ephemeral connections with counterparts from adjacent cells. The inflamed synovial tissue undergoes remodeling during the course of RA, the synovial lining becomes hyperplastic and forms a condensed tissue [49]. Genes related to the adherens junctions pathway is speculated to involve in this process and their abnormal expression may enhance the development of RA. Identification of interferon signaling and bacterial invasion related pathways suggests that some of the cases are indeed caused by microbial infection. In addition, other canonical pathways that involved in the RA development, such as the Wnt signaling and mTOR signaling pathways, were also identified in this analysis [50,51]. These affected pathways and the respective genes reported here may provide the basis for further analyses of the pathogenesis and the differences between RA and OA on a cellular and molecular level.

In conclusion, by collecting the whole genome expression data sets from different platforms, multiple biological markers were identified for RA and OA. This work is important to characterize the specific roles of those genes involved in the pathogenesis of RA and OA. Functional analysis of these genes may provide additional insights into the complex process of these diseases. In addition, this analysis may help to improve the diagnosis and treatment of these diseases.

Supporting Information

Table S1 Full lists of the differentially expressed genes between RA *vs.* NT samples. The symbol name, D score and the expression fold change were provided.

Table S2 Full lists of the differentially expressed genes between OA *vs.* NT samples. The symbol name, D score and the expression fold change were provided.

Acknowledgments

We thank the two anonymous reviewers for their valuable suggestions.

Author Contributions

Conceived and designed the experiments: ZCL ZDL. Performed the experiments: ZCL JX JP JC TM GC YD WW. Analyzed the data: ZCL JX. Contributed reagents/materials/analysis tools: JX JP. Wrote the paper: ZDL.

References

1. Huber LC, Distler O, Tarner I, Gay RE, Gay S, et al. (2006) Synovial fibroblasts: key players in rheumatoid arthritis. Rheumatology (Oxford) 45: 669–675.
2. Bartok B, Firestein GS (2010) Fibroblast-like synoviocytes: key effector cells in rheumatoid arthritis. Immunol Rev 233: 233–255.
3. Scott DL, Wolfe F, Huizinga TW (2010) Rheumatoid arthritis. Lancet 376: 1094–1108.
4. Firestein GS (2003) Evolving concepts of rheumatoid arthritis. Nature 423: 356–361.
5. Alvarez-Lafuente R, Fernandez-Gutierrez B, de Miguel S, Jover JA, Rollin R, et al. (2005) Potential relationship between herpes viruses and rheumatoid arthritis: analysis with quantitative real time polymerase chain reaction. Ann Rheum Dis 64: 1357–1359.
6. Balandraud N, Roudier J, Roudier C (2004) Epstein-Barr virus and rheumatoid arthritis. Autoimmun Rev 3: 362–367.
7. Albano SA, Santana-Sahagun E, Weisman MH (2001) Cigarette smoking and rheumatoid arthritis. Semin Arthritis Rheum 31: 146–159.
8. Wen H, Baker JF (2011) Vitamin D, immunoregulation, and rheumatoid arthritis. J Clin Rheumatol 17: 102–107.
9. Plenge RM, Seielstad M, Padyukov L, Lee AT, Remmers EF, et al. (2007) TRAF1-C5 as a risk locus for rheumatoid arthritis–a genomewide study. N Engl J Med 357: 1199–1209.
10. Kingsbury SR, Conaghan PG (2012) Current osteoarthritis treatment, prescribing influences and barriers to implementation in primary care. Prim Health Care Res Dev 13: 373–381.
11. Brandt KD, Dieppe P, Radin E (2009) Etiopathogenesis of osteoarthritis. Med Clin North Am 93: 1–24, xv.
12. Baecklund E, Iliadou A, Askling J, Ekbom A, Backlin C, et al. (2006) Association of chronic inflammation, not its treatment, with increased lymphoma risk in rheumatoid arthritis. Arthritis Rheum 54: 692–701.
13. Franklin J, Lunt M, Bunn D, Symmons D, Silman A (2006) Incidence of lymphoma in a large primary care derived cohort of cases of inflammatory polyarthritis. Ann Rheum Dis 65: 617–622.
14. Heruth DP, Gibson M, Grigoryev DN, Zhang LQ, Ye SQ (2012) RNA-seq analysis of synovial fibroblasts brings new insights into rheumatoid arthritis. Cell Biosci 2: 43.
15. Zhang R, Fang H, Chen Y, Shen J, Lu H, et al. (2012) Gene expression analyses of subchondral bone in early experimental osteoarthritis by microarray. PLoS One 7: e32356.
16. Ashburner M, Ball CA, Blake JA, Botstein D, Butler H, et al. (2000) Gene ontology: tool for the unification of biology. The Gene Ontology Consortium. Nature Genetics 25: 25–29.
17. Kanehisa M, Araki M, Goto S, Hattori M, Hirakawa M, et al. (2008) KEGG for linking genomes to life and the environment. Nucleic Acids Res 36: D480–484.
18. Cheadle C, Vawter MP, Freed WJ, Becker KG (2003) Analysis of microarray data using Z score transformation. J Mol Diagn 5: 73–81.
19. Tusher VG, Tibshirani R, Chu G (2001) Significance analysis of microarrays applied to the ionizing radiation response. Proc Natl Acad Sci U S A 98: 5116–5121.
20. Tabas-Madrid D, Nogales-Cadenas R, Pascual-Montano A (2012) GeneCodis3: a non-redundant and modular enrichment analysis tool for functional genomics. Nucleic Acids Res 40: W478–483.
21. Yu X, Wieczorek S, Franke A, Yin H, Pierer M, et al. (2009) Association of UCP2-866 G/A polymorphism with chronic inflammatory diseases. Genes Immun 10: 601–605.
22. Liu B, Shuai K (2008) Targeting the PIAS1 SUMO ligase pathway to control inflammation. Trends Pharmacol Sci 29: 505–509.
23. Sikora KA, Fall N, Thornton S, Grom AA (2012) The limited role of interferon-gamma in systemic juvenile idiopathic arthritis cannot be explained by cellular hyporesponsiveness. Arthritis Rheum 64: 3799–3808.
24. Fraser A, Fearon U, Billinghurst RC, Ionescu M, Reece R, et al. (2003) Turnover of type II collagen and aggrecan in cartilage matrix at the onset of inflammatory arthritis in humans: relationship to mediators of systemic and local inflammation. Arthritis Rheum 48: 3085–3095.
25. Seki M, Sakata KM, Oomizu S, Arikawa T, Sakata A, et al. (2007) Beneficial effect of galectin 9 on rheumatoid arthritis by induction of apoptosis of synovial fibroblasts. Arthritis Rheum 56: 3968–3976.
26. Lee J, Park EJ, Noh JW, Hwang JW, Bae EK, et al. (2012) Underexpression of TIM-3 and blunted galectin-9-induced apoptosis of CD4+ T cells in rheumatoid arthritis. Inflammation 35: 633–637.

27. Daouti S, Latario B, Nagulapalli S, Buxton F, Uziel-Fusi S, et al. (2005) Development of comprehensive functional genomic screens to identify novel mediators of osteoarthritis. Osteoarthritis Cartilage 13: 508–518.
28. Collins-Racie LA, Yang Z, Arai M, Li N, Majumdar MK, et al. (2009) Global analysis of nuclear receptor expression and dysregulation in human osteoarthritic articular cartilage: reduced LXR signaling contributes to catabolic metabolism typical of osteoarthritis. Osteoarthritis Cartilage 17: 832–842.
29. Reedquist KA, Tak PP (2012) Signal transduction pathways in chronic inflammatory autoimmune disease: small GTPases. Open Rheumatol J 6: 259–272.
30. De Filippo K, Dudeck A, Hasenberg M, Nye E, van Rooijen N, et al. (2013) Mast cell and macrophage chemokines CXCL1/CXCL2 control the early stage of neutrophil recruitment during tissue inflammation. Blood.
31. Scaife S, Brown R, Kellie S, Filer A, Martin S, et al. (2004) Detection of differentially expressed genes in synovial fibroblasts by restriction fragment differential display. Rheumatology (Oxford) 43: 1346–1352.
32. Thalhamer T, McGrath MA, Harnett MM (2008) MAPKs and their relevance to arthritis and inflammation. Rheumatology (Oxford) 47: 409–414.
33. Kaminska B (2005) MAPK signalling pathways as molecular targets for anti-inflammatory therapy–from molecular mechanisms to therapeutic benefits. Biochim Biophys Acta 1754: 253–262.
34. Shahrara S, Castro-Rueda HP, Haines GK, Koch AE (2007) Differential expression of the FAK family kinases in rheumatoid arthritis and osteoarthritis synovial tissues. Arthritis Res Ther 9: R112.
35. Schlaepfer DD, Broome MA, Hunter T (1997) Fibronectin-stimulated signaling from a focal adhesion kinase-c-Src complex: involvement of the Grb2, p130cas, and Nck adaptor proteins. Mol Cell Biol 17: 1702–1713.
36. Lee J, Oh JM, Hwang JW, Ahn JK, Bae EK, et al. (2011) Expression of human TIM-3 and its correlation with disease activity in rheumatoid arthritis. Scand J Rheumatol 40: 334–340.
37. Gilmore TD (1999) The Rel/NF-kappaB signal transduction pathway: introduction. Oncogene 18: 6842–6844.
38. Adachi M, Okamoto S, Chujyo S, Arakawa T, Yokoyama M, et al. (2013) Cigarette Smoke Condensate Extracts Induce IL-1-Beta Production from Rheumatoid Arthritis Patient-Derived Synoviocytes, but Not Osteoarthritis Patient-Derived Synoviocytes, Through Aryl Hydrocarbon Receptor-Dependent NF-Kappa-B Activation and Novel NF-Kappa-B Sites. J Interferon Cytokine Res 33: 297–307.
39. Harty LC, Biniecka M, O'Sullivan J, Fox E, Mulhall K, et al. (2012) Mitochondrial mutagenesis correlates with the local inflammatory environment in arthritis. Ann Rheum Dis 71: 582–588.
40. Ishikawa S, Mima T, Aoki C, Yoshio-Hoshino N, Adachi Y, et al. (2009) Abnormal expression of the genes involved in cytokine networks and mitochondrial function in systemic juvenile idiopathic arthritis identified by DNA microarray analysis. Ann Rheum Dis 68: 264–272.
41. Li C, Wang W, Guo X, Zhang F, Ma W, et al. (2012) Pathways related to mitochondrial dysfunction in cartilage of endemic osteoarthritis patients in China. Sci China Life Sci 55: 1057–1063.
42. Kumarasinghe DD, Sullivan T, Kuliwaba JS, Fazzalari NL, Atkins GJ (2012) Evidence for the dysregulated expression of TWIST1, TGFbeta1 and SMAD3 in differentiating osteoblasts from primary hip osteoarthritis patients. Osteoarthritis Cartilage 20: 1357–1366.
43. Robier C, Neubauer M, Fritz K, Lippitz P, Stettin M, et al. (2013) The detection of calcium pyrophosphate crystals in sequential synovial fluid examinations of patients with osteoarthritis: once positive, always positive. Clin Rheumatol 32: 671–672.
44. Lamb CA, Dooley HC, Tooze SA (2013) Endocytosis and autophagy: Shared machinery for degradation. Bioessays 35: 34–45.
45. Carames B, Hasegawa A, Taniguchi N, Miyaki S, Blanco FJ, et al. (2012) Autophagy activation by rapamycin reduces severity of experimental osteoarthritis. Ann Rheum Dis 71: 575–581.
46. Yoshida H (2007) ER stress and diseases. FEBS J 274: 630–658.
47. Takada K, Hirose J, Senba K, Yamabe S, Oike Y, et al. (2011) Enhanced apoptotic and reduced protective response in chondrocytes following endoplasmic reticulum stress in osteoarthritic cartilage. Int J Exp Pathol 92: 232–242.
48. Petersson M, Bucht E, Granberg B, Stark A (2006) Effects of arginine-vasopressin and parathyroid hormone-related protein (1–34) on cell proliferation and production of YKL-40 in cultured chondrocytes from patients with rheumatoid arthritis and osteoarthritis. Osteoarthritis Cartilage 14: 652–659.
49. Kiener HP, Lee DM, Agarwal SK, Brenner MB (2006) Cadherin-11 induces rheumatoid arthritis fibroblast-like synoviocytes to form lining layers in vitro. Am J Pathol 168: 1486–1499.
50. Kudryavtseva E, Forde TS, Pucker AD, Adarichev VA (2012) Wnt signaling genes of murine chromosome 15 are involved in sex-affected pathways of inflammatory arthritis. Arthritis Rheum 64: 1057–1068.
51. Laragione T, Gulko PS (2010) mTOR regulates the invasive properties of synovial fibroblasts in rheumatoid arthritis. Mol Med 16: 352–358.

4

Anti-TNF Therapy Reduces Serum Levels of Chemerin in Rheumatoid Arthritis: A New Mechanism by Which Anti-TNF Might Reduce Inflammation

Marieke M. J. Herenius[1]*, Ana S. F. Oliveira[1,2], Carla A. Wijbrandts[1], Daniëlle M. Gerlag[1], Paul P. Tak[1¤], Maria C. Lebre[1,2]

1 Department of Clinical Immunology and Rheumatology, Academic Medical Center, University of Amsterdam, Amsterdam, The Netherlands, **2** Department of Experimental Immunology, Academic Medical Center, University of Amsterdam, Amsterdam, The Netherlands

Abstract

Background: Chemerin is a specific chemoattractant for macrophages and dendritic cells (DC). In addition, it can rapidly stimulate macrophage adhesion to extracellular matrix proteins and adhesion molecules and is able to activate fibroblast-like synoviocytes (FLS), suggesting a role in the pathogenesis of rheumatoid arthritis (RA). Chemerin is also an adipocytokine that has been related to the inflammatory state of endothelial cells and as such could be involved in the changes in endothelial cells in RA and perhaps increased cardiovascular morbidity. We investigated whether anti-Tumor Necrosis Factor (TNF) treatment affects chemerin levels.

Materials and Methods: 49 patients with active RA (disease activity score evaluated in 28 joints (DAS28) ≥3.2) were started on adalimumab therapy. Blood was drawn from patients while fasting at baseline and 16 weeks after initiation of treatment. Chemerin serum levels were measured by ELISA and related to disease activity, mediators of inflammation and known risk factors for cardiovascular disease.

Results: Adalimumab therapy reduced chemerin serum levels, which was correlated with the reduction in DAS28 ($r = 0.37$, $p = 0.009$). In addition, the decrease in chemerin serum levels after anti-TNF treatment was associated with the decrease in serum levels of IL-6 ($r = 0.39$, $p = 0.033$) and macrophage migration inhibitory factor (MIF) ($r = 0.31$, $p = 0.049$). Baseline chemerin serum levels were not related to traditional risk factors for atherosclerosis, except perhaps for smoking ($p = 0.07$).

Conclusions: This exploratory study shows that adalimumab therapy lowers chemerin levels, which is associated with the reduction in disease activity parameters, and inflammatory mediators IL-6 and MIF. This suggests a possible involvement of chemerin in the migration/retention of macrophages in the synovium.

Trial Registration Nederlands Trial Register: NTR 857

Editor: Oliver Frey, University Hospital Jena, Germany

Funding: The clinical part of this study was funded by Abbott Laboratories. The funders had no role in study design, data collection and analysis, decision to publish, or preparation of the manuscript.

Competing Interests: The study was financed by Abbott Laboratories. There are no patents, products in development or marketed products to declare.

* E-mail: m.m.herenius@amc.uva.nl

¤ Current address: Academic Medical Center/University of Amsterdam, Amsterdam, The Netherlands and GlaxoSmithKline, Stevenage, United Kingdom

Introduction

The synovium in rheumatoid arthritis (RA) is characterized by a dense infiltrate, consisting of T and B cells, plasma cells, macrophages, dendritic cells (DC), and other cells. [1] Inflammatory chemokines present in the synovium contribute to the migration and/or retention of these immune cells.[2–4] Chemerin is a recently discovered chemokine that specifically modulates chemotaxis and activation of macrophages and DC (in particular plasmacytoid DC (pDC) and monocyte-derived DC). [5] Furthermore, it can contribute to inflammation by stimulating macrophage adhesion to extracellular matrix proteins and adhesion molecules. [6] The expression of chemerin receptor chemokine-like receptor 1 (CMKLR1) or ChemR23 on antigen-presenting cells (macrophages and DC) suggests that chemerin constitutes an important link between innate and adaptive immunity. Both the innate and adaptive immune responses are implicated in the pathogenesis of RA and might even occur in a parallel fashion. Related to this it was recently reported [7] in RA that endothelial cells and synovial lining and sublining cells express chemerin while its receptor ChemR23 was expressed on macrophages, immature DCs and fibroblast-like synoviocytes (FLS). Interestingly, chemerin induced the release of IL-6, chemokine (C-C-motif) ligand 2 (CCL2) and matrix metalloproteinase-3 (MMP-3) by RA FLS. [7] These data suggest that blockade of chemerin represents an attractive candidate for future drug development as it could disrupt disease perpetuation. Interestingly, chemerin has also been implicated in the pathogenesis of another immune-mediated inflammatory disease, psoriasis. Chemerin expression in psoriatic skin lesions preceded and paralleled accumulation of pDC and clinical expression of psoriasis. [8].

Chemerin also belongs to the novel adipocytokine family together with omentin, visfatin, nesfatin and vaspin. [9] As such, it has been associated with the metabolic syndrome, which is defined by dyslipidemia, abdominal obesity, elevated blood pressure, elevated plasma glucose levels and a pro-inflammatory state promoting atherosclerotic cardiovascular disease. [10] In RA the prevalence of the metabolic syndrome is increased. [11] In addition, ChemR23 is expressed by vascular endothelial cells and it is regulated by pro-inflammatory cytokines, including TNF. [12] These observations may suggest the involvement of chemerin in the changes in the endothelial cells of RA patients and as such in increased vascular morbidity in RA patients.

In this exploratory study, we aimed to provide insight into the mechanism of action of anti-TNF therapy on synovial inflammation and vascular disease in RA, Therefore, we investigated the effects of adalimumab treatment on chemerin levels. Primary questions were the relationship between chemerin serum levels, DAS28, markers of inflammation (IL-6 and MIF) and traditional factors of atherosclerosis.

Materials and Methods

Patients and Clinical Assessments

The details of this cohort were previously described. [13] The study was performed according to the Declaration of Helsinki and approved by the medical ethics committee. All participants gave written informed consent. Patients (n = 49) were selected for the current study based on the availability of serum at baseline combined with standardized follow up data on the response to adalimumab treatment 16 weeks after the initiation of adalimumab. The protocol for this trial and information on patient enrollment are available as supporting information; see Checklist S1, Protocol S1 and Enrollment log S1. Briefly, all patients had an indication for the use of anti-TNF therapy according to the guidelines of the Dutch Society for Rheumatology, which is active disease status (DAS28≥3.2) despite previous treatment with at least 2 conventional disease-modifying anti-rheumatic drugs (DMARDs). All patients started adalimumab (40 mg subcutaneously every other week). Clinical response at week 16 was determined according to the European League Against Rheumatism (EULAR) criteria. [14] Patients with EULAR good and EULAR moderate response were considered responders. Primary study endpoints were the relationship between the change in chemerin serum levels and the change in DAS28, ESR and CRP, and the change parameters of inflammation (MIF and IL-6 serum levels). Secondary endpoints were the relation between chemerin serum levels at baseline and DAS28, ESR and CRP and traditional risk factors for atherosclerosis as assessed by recording medical history including cardiovascular events, body mass index (kg/m^2), smoking (current smoking and ever smoking), current medication, hypertension, lipid profile ((TC, HDL, LDL, TG, Apo A-I, Apo B, Lp(a)) and diabetes. In addition, we assessed the relationship between the change in chemerin serum levels and the change in lipid profile.

Lipid Profiles and Assessment of Radiological Damage

Blood was drawn from patients while fasting at baseline and 16 weeks after initiation of adalimumab treatment. Lipid levels were measured as described previously. [13] Radiographs of the hands and feet were obtained at baseline and were scored using the Sharp/van der Heijde score. [15].

Serum Enzyme-linked Immunosorbent Assay (ELISA)

Chemerin serum levels were determined using a commercially available DuoSet ELISA Development kit (DY2324; R&D systems Inc, Minneapolis, MN). The serum levels of IL-6 and MIF were assessed as described previously. [13] As stated above, fasting serum samples were stored at −80°C until use.

Statistical Analysis

When indicated, a paired t-test or the Wilcoxon signed ranks test was used to determine significant changes from baseline. Probability values <0.05 were considered statistically significant. The Mann Whitney U test was used to detect differences between groups (sex, prior cardiovascular events, anti-citrullinated peptide antibody (ACPA) and IgM-rheumatoid factor (RF)-status or users vs. non-users of non-steroidal anti-inflammatory drugs (NSAIDs), statins or anti-hypertensive drugs). Correlations were assessed with the Pearson product-moment or Spearman rank-order correlation coefficients, whichever was appropriate. The calculations were performed with SPSS 18.0 for Windows (SPSS, Chicago, IL). To avoid multiple testing comparisons for the primary objective were tested formally, (i.e. change in chemerin and its' association with the change in DA28, ESR, CRP, IL-6 and MIF) while secondary comparisons were described.

Results

Patients and Clinical Response

The baseline patient characteristics are described in Table 1.The DAS28 score decreased significantly 16 weeks after initiation of adalimumab treatment from 5.4 (±1.1, mean±SD) to 3.6 (±1.2, mean±SD). According to EULAR response criteria 33%, 45%, and 22% of patients, respectively, achieved good, moderate or no response. There was no association between baseline chemerin serum levels and baseline Sharp van der Heijde score.

Anti-TNF Treatment Decreases Chemerin Serum Levels, which is Associated with the Decrease in Disease Activity, Serum Levels of IL-6 and Macrophage Migration Inhibitory Factor

At baseline chemerin serum levels varied from a minimum of 99 ng/ml to a maximum of 217 ng/ml. There was no relationship between chemerin serum levels at baseline and the use of low doses of corticosteroids, NSAIDs or the use of methotrexate (MTX). In addition, chemerin serum levels at baseline were not related to IgM-RF- or ACPA-status. Sixteen weeks after the initiation of adalimumab treatment chemerin levels showed a reduction from 154 ng/ml±28 ng/ml (mean±SD) to 141 ng/ml±29 ng/ml (mean±SD) (Figure 1A; p = 0.025). The decrease of chemerin serum levels 16 weeks after initiation of adalimumab treatment was seen only in EULAR responders (relative change −11.2±43.4 (mean±SD) and −11.3 [−30.3–3.9] (median, IQR)) and not in EULAR non-responders (relative change 2.0±33.8 (mean±SD) and 1.9%, [−23.3–33.7] (median, IQR) (Figure 1B). The decrease in chemerin serum levels was associated with decrease in parameters of disease activity DAS28 (r = 0.37, p = 0.009), ESR (r = 0.55 p<0.001) and CRP (r = 0.40, p = 0.005) (Fig. 2A–C, respectively). In addition, we found an association between the reduction in chemerin levels and the decrease in serum levels of IL-6 (r = 0.39, p = 0.033) and MIF 16 weeks

Table 1. Baseline characteristics.

Demographics	
Age (years)	50±14
Female (%)	39 (81)
Baseline characteristics	
Disease duration (months)	61 (32 - 142)
Sharp/van der Heijde score	6.6 (0 - 25.5)
Rheumatoid factor positive (%)	34 (71)
Anti-CCP positive (%)	33 (67)
DAS28	5.4±1.1
Use of corticsteroids (%)	13 (26)
Use of NSAIDs (%)	36 (71)
ESR (mm/hour)	20 (11 - 35)
C-reactive protein (mg/L)	7.7 (4.8 - 18.5)
Cardiovascular characteristics	
BMI kg/m2	26.7±6.0
Smokers, current (%)	11(22)
Diabetes mellitus type 2 (%)	4 (8)
Prior cardiovascular event (%)	6 (12)
Systolic blood pressure	132±16
Diastolic blood pressure	80±9
Plasma triglycerides level	1.0±0.5
Total cholesterol level	4.8±1.1
HDL cholesterol level	1.5±0.4
LDL cholesterol level	2.9±1.0
Statin use (%)	7 (14)

Mean values ± standard deviation (SD), median and interquartile range or percentages are shown. BMI = body mass index, ESR = erythrocyte sedimentation rate.

after initiation of anti-TNF antibody treatment ($r = 0.31$, $p = 0.049$) (Figure 2 D and E, respectively).

Chemerin Serum Levels at Baseline are not Related to Traditional Risk Factors of Atherosclerosis

Chemerin serum levels at baseline were not related to sex, age, BMI, lipid profile (TC, HDL, LDL, TG, Apo A-I, Apo B, Lp(a)), systolic or diastolic blood pressure, cardiovascular events in the medical history, diabetes or the use of statins and anti-hypertensive drugs, or was the change in chemerin levels 16 weeks after initiation of adalimumab treatment related to the change in lipid profile. Of interest, we found a trend towards higher levels of serum chemerin in current smokers (n = 11, 162 ng/ml, IQR154–183 ng/ml) than in non-smokers (n = 38, 143 ng/ml, IQR 129–175) ($p = 0.07$) (Figure 3). In this cohort smoking was not associated with increased disease activity or a diminished response to therapy.

Discussion

In this exploratory study chemerin serum levels decreased significantly after initiation of adalimumab treatment and this decrease was modestly associated with the decrease in disease activity parameters DAS28, ESR and CRP and with the inflammatory mediators IL-6 and MIF. Of importance, chemerin serum levels only showed a statistically significant decrease in EULAR responders. In accordance with our findings, previous studies reported positive associations of chemerin serum levels and markers of inflammation [16,17] and correlations between the decrease in chemerin serum levels and the decrease in CRP levels. [18] Furthermore, the reduction in chemerin levels was modestly associated with the reduction in IL-6 serum levels and MIF serum levels. Of importance, in RA macrophages are a source of IL-6 and MIF and the decrease in the number of synovial macrophages is consistently associated with clinical improvement after initiation of anti-TNF therapy. [19] As chemerin is a potent chemoattractant for macrophages, TNF antagonists might partly exert their effect by reducing chemerin levels, thereby reducing the number of synovial macrophages. In addition to its chemotactic function it was recently shown that chemerin can induce the release of IL-6 by RA FLS. [7] Thus, the decreased IL-6 serum levels observed after TNF blockade might be partly explained by decreased chemerin levels resulting in decreased FLS-derived IL-6. On the

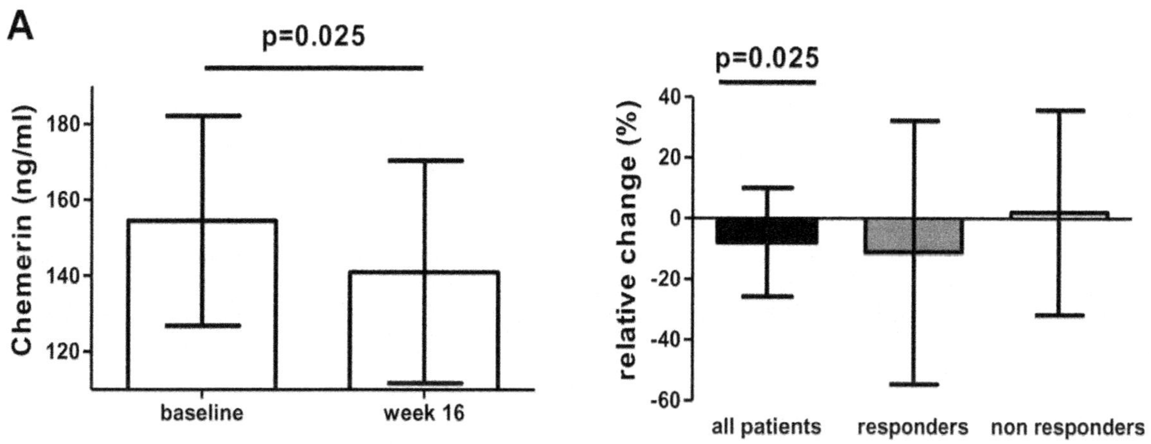

Figure 1. Changes in chemerin serum levels 16 weeks after initiation of treatment with adalimumab. (A) Absolute change in all patients (n = 49). Data are represented as mean values with standard deviation. (B) Relative change for all patients (n = 49), EULAR responders (n = 38) and EULAR non- responders (n = 11). Data are presented as mean values with standard deviation.

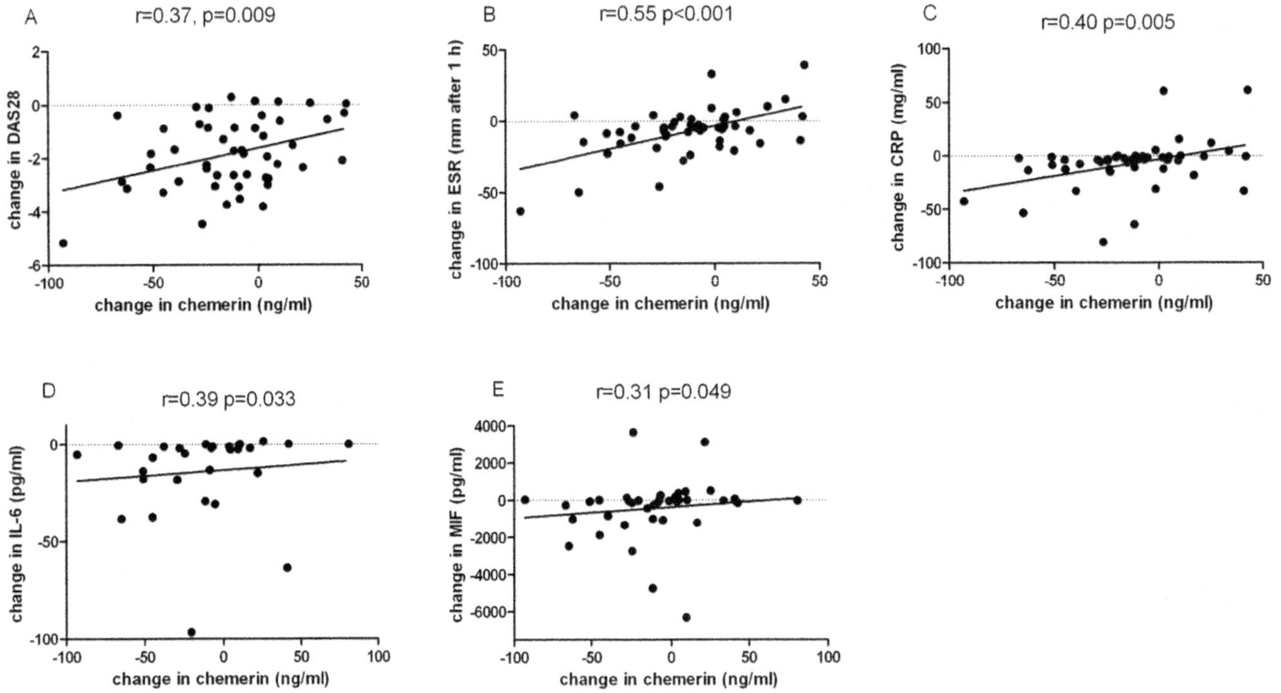

Figure 2. Changes in chemerin serum levels 16 weeks after initiation of treatment correlate with changes in disease activity parameters DAS28 (A, n = 49), ESR (B, n = 49) and CRP (C, n = 49) and changes in IL-6 (D, n = 29) and MIF (E, n = 41) serum levels, respectively.

other hand, as TNF upregulates chemerin production by RA FLS [7], by blocking TNF, this cytokine will not be able to induce chemerin production by FLS, resulting in decreased chemerin serum levels.

In contrast to some previous studies [16,17], we did not find a clear cut relationship between traditional risk factors for athero-

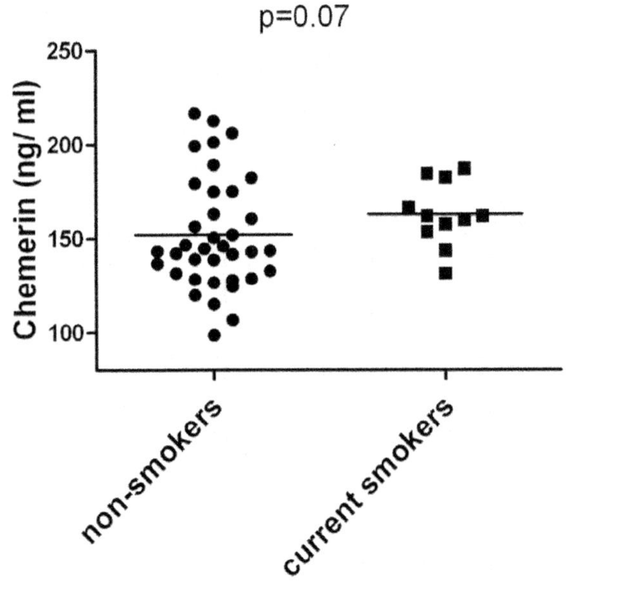

Figure 3. Chemerin levels at baseline tend to be higher in current smokers (n = 11) than in non-smokers (n = 38). Data are presented as median values.

sclerosis and chemerin serum levels, suggesting that chemerin might represent an independent risk factor. Interestingly, the prevalence of traditional risk factors does not account for the increased risk of cardiovascular morbidity and mortality in RA patients and chronic inflammation, characterizing RA, is considered to play a key role in accelerating atherosclerosis. [20].

We also found a modest association between the decrease in chemerin serum levels and the decrease in MIF serum levels 16 weeks after initiation of TNF blockade. Interestingly, MIF has recently emerged as an important cytokine possibly linking RA and atherogenesis [13,21]. It is tempting to speculate that the decrease of chemerin levels after TNF blockade will result in the decreased of MIF by inhibiting the recruitment of MIF-producing cells (i.e. macrophages and DC), contributing to reduced vascular inflammation.

Consistent with data obtained in a murine model for cigarette smoking [22], our data suggest that smoking might elevate chemerin serum levels. Furthermore, in ChemR23 knockout mice, exposure to cigarette smoke resulted in diminished recruitment of inflammatory cells (neutrophils, inflammatory monocytes, DC and T cells) and decreased levels of chemokines (CCL2, CXCL1 and CCL20) in bronchoalveolar lavage fluid and lung tissues compared to those from wild-type mice, suggesting involvement of the chemerin/ChemR23 axis in inflammation secondary to to smoking. In RA cigarette smoking is a well-recognized risk factor for the development of the disease and it has also been associated with more severe disease. [23] Thus, elevated expression of chemerin might represent one of the underlying mechanisms by which smoking increases disease activity in RA patients.

An obvious limitation to this study is the relatively small number of patients, allowing only univariate analysis. However, it is important to mention that treatment and response evaluation were conducted according to a stringent treatment protocol.

In conclusion, we have shown that adalimumab treatment reduced chemerin serum levels which are associated with the reduction in disease activity parameters (DAS28, ESR and CRP), and the inflammatory mediators IL-6 and MIF. As these mediators are produced by macrophages, their reduction might be a consequence of decreased chemerin-dependent accumulation of synovial macrophages. This suggests a distinct role for chemerin in the migration and/or retention of macrophages in the synovium and as such in the pathophysiology of RA. Altogether, the present study suggests that the sustained downregulation of chemerin is associated with mechanisms by which anti-TNF therapy might reduce (vascular) inflammation in RA patients.

Supporting Information

Checklist S1 CONSORT 2010 Checklist.

Enrollment log S1 Trial enrollment log including reason of drop out/harms.

Protocol S1 Trial protocol: "Prospective study on the effects of adalimumab treatment in patients with rheumatoid arthritis who are naïve for TNF-α blocking therapy and patients who do not respond (anymore) to prior treatment with other anti-TNF-α medication."

Acknowledgments

We thank the clinical research team of the division of Clinical Immunology and Rheumatology and especially Mariane Anson for performing the clinical assessments and D. Pots, M. de Boer and I. Fluri for sample handling.

ETHICAL APPROVAL

This study was conducted with the approval of the Medical Ethical Committee of the Academic Medical Center/University of Amsterdam.

Author Contributions

Conceived and designed the experiments: MH AO CW DG PT ML. Performed the experiments: MH AO CW ML. Analyzed the data: MH ML. Contributed reagents/materials/analysis tools: MH AO CA DG PT ML. Wrote the paper: MH ML PT. Obtained ICF: MH CW DG.

References

1. Tak PP, Bresnihan B (2000) The pathogenesis and prevention of joint damage in rheumatoid arthritis: advances from synovial biopsy and tissue analysis. Arthritis Rheum 43: 2619–2633. 10.1002/1529-0131(200012)43:12<2619:AID-ANR1>3.0.CO;2-V [doi].
2. Buckley CD (2003) Why does chronic inflammatory joint disease persist? Clin Med 3: 361–366.
3. Szekanecz Z, Vegvari A, Szabo Z, Koch AE (2010) Chemokines and chemokine receptors in arthritis. Front Biosci (Schol Ed) 2: 153–167. 53 [pii].
4. Tak PP (2006) Chemokine inhibition in inflammatory arthritis. Best Pract Res Clin Rheumatol 20: 929–939. S1521-6942(06)00073-8 [pii];10.1016/j.berh.2006.06.001 [doi].
5. Wittamer V, Gregoire F, Robberecht P, Vassart G, Communi D et al. (2004) The C-terminal nonapeptide of mature chemerin activates the chemerin receptor with low nanomolar potency. J Biol Chem 279: 9956–9962. 10.1074/jbc.M313016200 [doi];M313016200 [pii].
6. Hart R, Greaves DR (2010) Chemerin contributes to inflammation by promoting macrophage adhesion to VCAM-1 and fibronectin through clustering of VLA-4 and VLA-5. J Immunol 185: 3728–3739. jimmunol.0902154 [pii];10.4049/jimmunol.0902154 [doi].
7. Kaneko K, Miyabe Y, Takayasu A, Fukuda S, Miyabe C et al. (2011) Chemerin activates fibroblast-like synoviocytes in patients with rheumatoid arthritis. Arthritis Res Ther 13: R158. ar3475 [pii];10.1186/ar3475 [doi].
8. Albanesi C, Scarponi C, Pallotta S, Daniele R, Bosisio D, et al. (2009) Chemerin expression marks early psoriatic skin lesions and correlates with plasmacytoid dendritic cell recruitment. J Exp Med 206: 249–258. jem.20080129 [pii];10.1084/jem.20080129 [doi].
9. Yamawaki H (2011) Vascular effects of novel adipocytokines: focus on vascular contractility and inflammatory responses. Biol Pharm Bull 34: 307–310. JST.JSTAGE/bpb/34.307 [pii].
10. Grundy SM, Cleeman JI, Daniels SR, Donato KA, Eckel RH, et al. (2005) Diagnosis and management of the metabolic syndrome: an American Heart Association/National Heart, Lung, and Blood Institute Scientific Statement. Circulation 112: 2735–2752. CIRCULATIONAHA.105.169404 [pii];10.1161/CIRCULATIONAHA.105.169404 [doi].
11. Pereira RM, de Carvalho JF, Bonfa E (2009) Metabolic syndrome in rheumatological diseases. Autoimmun Rev 8: 415–419. S1568-9972(09)00004-4 [pii];10.1016/j.autrev.2009.01.001 [doi].
12. Kaur J, Adya R, Tan BK, Chen J, Randeva HS (2010) Identification of chemerin receptor (ChemR23) in human endothelial cells: chemerin-induced endothelial angiogenesis. Biochem Biophys Res Commun 391: 1762–1768. S0006-291X(09)02537-6 [pii];10.1016/j.bbrc.2009.12.150 [doi].
13. Wijbrandts CA, van Leuven SI, Boom HD, Gerlag DM, Stroes EG, et al. (2009) Sustained changes in lipid profile and macrophage migration inhibitory factor levels after anti-tumour necrosis factor therapy in rheumatoid arthritis. Ann Rheum Dis 68: 1316–1321. ard.2007.086728 [pii];10.1136/ard.2007.086728 [doi].
14. van Gestel AM, Anderson JJ, van Riel PL, Boers M, Haagsma CJ, et al. (1999) ACR and EULAR improvement criteria have comparable validity in rheumatoid arthritis trials. American College of Rheumatology European League of Associations for Rheumatology. J Rheumatol 26: 705–711.
15. van der Heijde D (2000) How to read radiographs according to the Sharp/van der Heijde method. J Rheumatol 27: 261–263.
16. Bozaoglu K, Bolton K, McMillan J, Zimmet P, Jowett J, et al. (2007) Chemerin is a novel adipokine associated with obesity and metabolic syndrome. Endocrinology 148: 4687–4694. en.2007-0175 [pii];10.1210/en.2007-0175 [doi].
17. Lehrke M, Becker A, Greif M, Stark R, Laubender RP, et al. (2009) Chemerin is associated with markers of inflammation and components of the metabolic syndrome but does not predict coronary atherosclerosis. Eur J Endocrinol 161: 339–344. EJE-09-0380 [pii];10.1530/EJE-09-0380 [doi].
18. Sell H, Divoux A, Poitou C, Basdevant A, Bouillot JL, et al. (2010) Chemerin correlates with markers for fatty liver in morbidly obese patients and strongly decreases after weight loss induced by bariatric surgery. J Clin Endocrinol Metab 95: 2892–2896. jc.2009-2374 [pii];10.1210/jc.2009-2374 [doi].
19. Haringman JJ, Gerlag DM, Zwinderman AH, Smeets TJ, Kraan MC, et al. (2005) Synovial tissue macrophages: a sensitive biomarker for response to treatment in patients with rheumatoid arthritis. Ann Rheum Dis 64: 834–838. ard.2004.029751 [pii];10.1136/ard.2004.029751 [doi].
20. Bisoendial RJ, Stroes ES, Tak PP (2011) Critical determinants of cardiovascular risk in rheumatoid arthritis. Curr Pharm Des 17: 21–26. BSP/CPD/E-Pub/000305 [pii].
21. Morand EF, Leech M, Bernhagen J (2006) MIF: a new cytokine link between rheumatoid arthritis and atherosclerosis. Nat Rev Drug Discov 5: 399–410. nrd2029 [pii];10.1038/nrd2029 [doi].
22. Demoor T, Bracke KR, Dupont LL, Plantinga M, Bondue B, et al. (2011) The role of ChemR23 in the induction and resolution of cigarette smoke-induced inflammation. J Immunol 186: 5457–5467. jimmunol.1003862 [pii];10.4049/jimmunol.1003862 [doi].
23. Manfredsdottir VF, Vikingsdottir T, Jonsson T, Geirsson AJ, Kjartansson O, et al. (2006) The effects of tobacco smoking and rheumatoid factor seropositivity on disease activity and joint damage in early rheumatoid arthritis. Rheumatology (Oxford) 45: 734–740. kei240 [pii];10.1093/rheumatology/kei240 [doi].

5

Symptoms, the Nature of Fibromyalgia, and *Diagnostic and Statistical Manual 5 (DSM-5)* Defined Mental Illness in Patients with Rheumatoid Arthritis and Fibromyalgia

Frederick Wolfe[1]*, Brian T. Walitt[2], Robert S. Katz[3], Winfried Häuser[4,5]

1 National Data Bank for Rheumatic Diseases and University of Kansas School of Medicine, Wichita, Kansas, United States of America, **2** Washington Hospital Center, Washington, D.C., United States of America, **3** Rush University Medical Center, Chicago, Illinois, United States of America, **4** Department of Psychosomatic Medicine and Psychotherapy Technische Universität München, Munich, Germany, **5** Department Internal Medicine I, Klinikum Saarbrücken, Saarbrücken, Germany

Abstract

Purpose: To describe and evaluate somatic symptoms in patients with rheumatoid arthritis (RA) and fibromyalgia, determine the relation between somatization syndromes and fibromyalgia, and evaluate symptom data in light of the Diagnostic and Statistical Manual-5 (DSM-5) criteria for somatic symptom disorder.

Methods: We administered the Patient Health Questionnaire-15 (PHQ-15), a measure of somatic symptom severity to 6,233 persons with fibromyalgia, RA, and osteoarthritis. PHQ-15 scores of 5, 10, and 15 represent low, medium, and high somatic symptom severity cut-points. A likely somatization syndrome was diagnosed when PHQ-15 score was ≥10. The intensity of fibromyalgia diagnostic symptoms was measured by the polysymptomatic distress (PSD) scale.

Results: 26.4% of RA patients and 88.9% with fibromyalgia had PHQ-15 scores ≥10 compared with 9.3% in the general population. With each step-wise increase in PHQ-15 category, more abnormal mental and physical health status scores were observed. RA patients satisfying fibromyalgia criteria increased from 1.2% in the PHQ-15 low category to 88.9% in the high category. The sensitivity and specificity of PHQ-15≥10 for fibromyalgia diagnosis was 80.9% and 80.0% (correctly classified = 80.3%) compared with 84.3% and 93.7% (correctly classified = 91.7%) for the PSD scale. 51.4% of fibromyalgia patients and 14.8% with RA had fatigue, sleep or cognitive problems that were severe, continuous, and life-disturbing; and almost all fibromyalgia patients had severe impairments of function and quality of life.

Conclusions: All patients with fibromyalgia will satisfy the DSM-5 "A" criterion for distressing somatic symptoms, and most would seem to satisfy DSM-5 "B" criterion because symptom impact is life-disturbing or associated with substantial impairment of function and quality of life. But the "B" designation requires special knowledge that symptoms are "disproportionate" or "excessive," something that is uncertain and controversial. The reliability and validity of DSM-5 criteria in this population is likely to be low.

Editor: Shervin Assassi, University of Texas Health Science Center at Houston, United States of America

Funding: The authors have no support or funding to report.

Competing Interests: Winfried Häuser has received one consulting honorarium by Daiichi-Sankyo and honoraria for educational lectures by Abbott Germany, Eli-Lilly, Janssen-Cilag and Pfizer in the last 5 years. He is the head of the steering committee of the German guideline on FMS. The other authors have declared that no competing interests exist.

* E-mail: fwolfe@arthritis-research.org

Introduction

Fibromyalgia is defined by criteria that depend upon the range and severity of symptoms. Because the defining symptom of fibromyalgia is widely distributed pain, fibromyalgia is usually considered a pain disorder, at least in the rheumatology and pain communities. In the American College of Rheumatology (ACR) 1990 fibromyalgia criteria [1], musculoskeletal pain is the only symptom evaluated, while in the updated 2010 criteria [2,3], only 1 of the 5 criteria items directly concerns musculoskeletal pain. In other disciplines–particularly psychiatry, psychology, psychosomatic medicine and, perhaps, general medicine, fibromyalgia is more often considered to be a symptom or psychosomatic disorder [4,5].

Symptom disorders–simply the presence of many symptoms–are related to the concept of somatization that organizes and attributes meaning to them. Lipowski's often cited summary, defined somatization as "… a tendency to experience and communicate somatic distress and symptoms unaccounted for by pathological findings, to attribute them to physical illness, and to seek medical help for them," adding that "it is usually assumed that this tendency becomes manifest in response to psychosocial stress brought about by life events and situations that are personally stressful to the individual" [4]. In his comprehensive review he warned, however, that "… symptoms are extremely common and do not necessarily indicate that the person experiencing them is under stress or interprets them as suggestive of physical illness and seeks medical help." Moreover, somatization "… is neither a disorder nor a diagnostic category and does not imply that an individual displaying it must suffer from a psychiatric disorder" [4]. But in practical terms, psychological issues are not to be ignored: "the real divide in defining somatization, wrote Kurt Kroenke, centers on the role of psychologic factors" [5]. *Somatization*–the disease not just the concept was officially enshrined as a psychiatric diagnosis in the American Psychiatry Association's Disease and Statistical Manual of Mental disorders versions 3 through 4 as one of the somatoform disorders, (DSM-III. DSM-IV, DSM-IVTR), [6,7,8] but was abandoned in 2013 in DSM-5 [9] and replaced by "Somatic Symptom Disorder" (DSM SSD) (See Table S1).

Somatization as a disorder faltered when it was recognized that the idea of "unexplained" physical symptoms was not intellectually tenable and it became clear that "medically unexplained symptoms" and "symptoms unaccounted for by pathological findings" implied inauthenticity ("It's all in your head)" [10]. In addition, 'somatization' criteria couldn't adequately handle symptoms that were not unexplained but which were potentially "exaggerated." DSM-IV criteria for somatization were so arcane and difficult to satisfy that the diagnosis was almost never made, while DSM-IV "*Undifferentiated Somatoform Disorder*" criteria were too easy to satisfy [10]. The prevalence of undifferentiated somatoform disorder in the general population was 20% [11], 25% in neurology outpatients [12], and 27% in primary care [13]. Still, despite the clear occurrence of patients with somatization and undifferentiated somatoform disorders in the clinic, these DSM-IV illnesses did not gain diagnostic acceptance and were rarely coded [10]. Among researchers there were attempts to rename somatic symptom disorders to somatic symptoms disorder [14], physical symptom disorder [15], functional symptom disorder [16], bodily distress syndrome [17], among others. The idea of somatization–with all that it implied historically–became anathema, and one author went so far as to write: "We recommend that researchers who use self-report instruments do not use the term "somatisation" (even if the instrument is labeled as a "somatisation" scale), but use the term "multiple physical symptoms" instead. The current operational use may unduly lead to a "psychologisation" of physical complaints" [18].

DSM-5 altered the definitional landscape with the release of the American Psychiatry Association's highly influential Disease and Statistical Manual-5 (DSM-5) which defined a "mental disease" called *Somatic Symptom Disorder (SSD)* and eliminated somatoform disorders. Briefly, patients had a DSM somatic symptom disorder if they had at least 1 severe somatic symptom (for example, leg or joint pain, headache, etc.) and it was judged that they had at least one of the following: (1) Disproportionate and persistent thoughts about the seriousness of one's symptoms; (2) Persistently high level of anxiety about health or symptoms; or (3) Excessive time and energy devoted to these symptoms or health concerns. These criteria together with other changes in the DSM unleashed a firestorm of criticism, including the specific concern that the somatic symptom disorder definition would impose a mental illness diagnosis on a large proportion of otherwise normal individuals with physical illnesses [19,20,21]. But the key feature of the somatic symptom disorder is not the symptoms–as almost everyone with any severe symptom will qualify; it is that the symptoms are "disproportionate" or "excessive."

In rheumatic diseases, all patients have symptoms. Patients under the burden of rheumatic illnesses can be overwhelmed and report disproportionate or excessive symptoms. Or they could report severe symptoms that are not disproportionate, or partially disproportionate. Should one believe patients with a "10" score on the 0–10 visual analog pain scale (VAS) when they do not exhibit the behaviors associated with excruciating pain? Does the rheumatoid arthritis patient who doesn't respond to biologics as she would like have symptom concerns that are excessive? When does the patient's concern that rheumatoid arthritis is a disabling disorder with increased mortality and disability become excessive? After all, some patients are worried and some are not. Concerns that symptoms are disproportionate or excessive are of particularly of concern for those with fibromyalgia, where there is considerable data and debate among physicians as to whether the symptoms are at least somewhat exaggerated [22,23,24,25]. For patients, a common and important concern is that others think "it is all in my head" [26,27].

The language of somatization and somatic disorders is confusing. The term *somatization syndrome* disorders has been suggested to identify persons with high levels of somatic symptoms including non-DSM somatoform disorders [28], while DSM-5 somatic symptom disorder implies mental disease and excessive or disproportionate concerns. In this study we describe and evaluate the content and severity of somatic symptoms in patients with rheumatoid arthritis and fibromyalgia. We use the well-regarded Patient Health Questionnaire-15 (PHQ-15) [29] to quantify somatic symptoms and various definitions of somatization syndrome disorders. We explore the DSM-5 criteria and provide some estimates of the proportion of patients who might be considered to have DSM-5 mental illness. Finally we explore the relation of somatic symptoms to fibromyalgia symptoms and diagnosis.

Methods

Ethics

All participants were informed about the study procedures and signed an informed consent form. The study was approved by the Via Christi Institutional Review Board of Wichita, Kansas.

Patients and Diagnosis

In 2012, we administered the PHQ-15 questionnaire to 6, 233 participants with fibromyalgia, rheumatoid arthritis (RA) and osteoarthritis (OA) who were participants in the National Data Bank for Rheumatic Diseases (NDB) longitudinal study of rheumatic diseases outcomes [30]. Participants were volunteers, recruited primarily from the practices of US rheumatologists, who complete mailed or Internet questionnaires at 6-month intervals. They were not compensated for their participation. Diagnoses were made by the patient's rheumatologist or confirmed by the patient's physician in cases that were self-referred [30]. However, to be classified as having fibromyalgia patients were required to satisfy research criteria for fibromyalgia by their responses in the most recent survey questionnaire.

Patients were designated as having criteria positive fibromyalgia if they satisfied research criteria for fibromyalgia. [3] The research fibromyalgia criteria (2011) were a modification of the 2010 American College of Rheumatology preliminary diagnostic criteria for fibromyalgia [2] to allow the use of self-report questionnaires for research. When we use the term ACR criteria or (ACR) research criteria for fibromyalgia, we are referring to the modified criteria. For patients to be diagnosed with fibromyalgia they had to have either a Widespread Pain Index(WPI) ≥ 7 and Symptom Severity Score (SS) ≥ 5, or a Widespread Pain Index between 3–6 and Symptom Severity Score ≥ 9. [2,3] The widespread pain index is a 0–19 count of painful body regions. The Symptom Severity Score is the sum of the *severity* (0–3) of the 3 symptoms (fatigue, waking unrefreshed, cognitive symptoms) plus the sum of the *number* of the following symptoms occurring during the previous 6 months: headaches, abdominal pain, and depression. The final score is between 0 and 12. For fatigue, waking unrefreshed, and cognitive problems, scoring was 0 No problem; 1 Slight or mild problems, generally mild or intermittent; 2 Moderate, considerable problems, often present and/or at a moderate level; 3 Severe: continuous, life-disturbing problems.

Soon after the publication of the 2010 ACR criteria, it was suggested that the 2 components of the 2010 criteria, the 0–19 widespread pain index and the 0–12 symptom severity score, could be combined by addition into a 0–31 index. Originally called the "fibromyalgianess scale" [31], a term that was a little awkward and limiting, it has subsequently been termed the "polysymptomatic distress" scale (PSD). The PSD scale is an excellent measure of the intensity of fibromyalgia symptoms and correlates with all general measures of distress [32]. Because of the scoring rules of the fibromyalgia criteria, criteria positive individuals will always have a PSD score of at least 12. The PSD scale, therefore, provides a way to examine fibromyalgia and fibromyalgia content on a continuous scale.

Diagnostic Groups

Patients groups with RA (N = 4718) and OA (N = 952) were composed of patients with these diagnoses; they were unselected as to the presence of absence of concomitant fibromyalgia. Patients in the fibromyalgia group (N = 440) were fibromyalgia criteria positive, but did not include patients with RA who satisfied fibromyalgia criteria. Some patients with an initial physician diagnosis of fibromyalgia on entry into the NDB (N = 123) no longer satisfied fibromyalgia criteria at the time of this study, a change that occurred primarily because of symptom improvement [33]. To mimic possible "primary" fibromyalgia as it is seen in the clinic, a noninflammatory group (N = 1515) was composed of patients initially diagnosed with fibromyalgia–whether or not they satisfied criteria for fibromyalgia at any time, as well as patients in the OA group, some of whom might also satisfy fibromyalgia criteria. "OA" was composed of patients with various forms of osteoarthritis and back pain syndromes. OA data are reported in Table 1, primarily to provide perspective for the primary analyses of RA and fibromyalgia that follow.

Terminology

We use the recently proposed [28] term "somatization syndromes" to indicate somatization/somatoform disorders when defined by PHQ-15 questionnaire or the PSD scale. DSM-SSD refers to the disorder described by DSM-5. Somatoform disorder is often used in the literature to refer to any somatic symptoms disorder. In this report, somatoform disorder, somatization syndromes, somatic symptom disorders, physical symptoms disorder, bodily distress disorder and functional disorders are terms that have generally similar meanings. When using these terms with the PHQ-15≥10 criterion we do so without implying the presence or absence of psychological reasons for somatic symptoms or a mental disorder, or speculating on whether the symptoms are medically unexplained.

Confusion exists regarding the term "somatic" or "physical" when it is used in the context of somatization syndromes. Each of the syndromes permits consideration of fatigue and sleep problems within its scope of measurement, even if there is uncertainty about whether fatigue and sleep problems are actually "somatic" symptoms. The authors of DSM-5 have also have assessed the DSM-5 somatic symptom disorder diagnosis with the *Somatic Symptom Short Form* that includes fatigue and trouble sleeping [10]. Barsky and Borus indicate that symptoms common to these (functional) somatic syndromes include … problems with memory, attention, and concentration …" [16], thereby including cognitive problems, which are also part of the fibromyalgia criteria [2,3]. Therefore, in this report we use the term somatic symptoms in the broad sense that includes fatigue, sleep and memory/cognitive problems.

Study Assessments

PHQ-15. We used the Patient Health Questionnaire 15 (PHQ-15) to determine somatic symptom severity and to provide a cut-off for a somatization disorder. The PHQ-15 contains 15 somatic symptoms. Each symptom is scored from 0 (not bothered at all) to 2 (bothered a lot). PHQ-15 scores of 5, 10, and 15 represent cutoff points for low, medium, and high somatic symptom severity, respectively. The usefulness of the PHQ-15 in screening for somatization syndromes and in monitoring somatic symptom severity in clinical practice and research has been demonstrated in numerous studies [29].

A level of PHQ-15≥10 was found to be the optimum level to predict the diagnosis of a "somatoform disorder" in primary care, with a sensitivity of 80.2% and specificity of 58.5% [34]. The PHQ-15 at ≥10 was also used in a large population based study of somatization syndromes where 9.3% were found to satisfy the criterion [28]. In the current report we used this PHQ-15 level to estimate the probable presence of a somatic syndrome disorder. In a similar primary care study of 2,147 eligible patients that utilized the PHQ-15, a cutoff level of 3 or more severe somatic symptoms during the past 4 weeks defined a somatoform disorder with a sensitivity of 78% and specificity of 71% [35]. We also used this cut-off to examine somatic syndrome disorders in our patients.

DSM-5 criteria. With respect to the DSM-5 criteria [9], we considered any of the PHQ-15 items that was scored as "bothered a lot" (or "2") to satisfy the DSM-5 "A" criterion: " One or more somatic symptoms that are distressing …" As noted above, we also investigated "3 or more severe somatic symptoms" in the PHQ-15 as a more rigorous measure of somatic symptom severity. To investigate the DSM-5 "B" criteria items of "1) Disproportionate and persistent thoughts about the seriousness of one's symptoms; 2) Persistently high level of anxiety about health or symptoms; and 3) Excessive time and energy devoted to these symptoms or health concerns–we used as a surrogate the reporting of 1, 2 or 3 ACR criteria symptoms that were "3 Severe: continuous, life-disturbing problems." As there are no precise instructions about how to evaluate the DSM-5 "B" criterion, we also examined mean levels of clinical severity variables described below.

Other assessments. Study participants completed the Short-form 36 (SF-36) version 1 from which the physical component summary (PCS) and the mental component summary (MCS) scores were calculated [36,37]. The primary time period of the SF-36 questionnaire was 4 weeks. The MCS and PCS population mean is 50 with a standard deviation of 10. In addition, using a cutoff score of 42, the MCS had a sensitivity of 74% and a specificity of 81% in detecting patients diagnosed with depressive disorder [38]. For the separate SF-36 5-item mental health scale, the mean score in the lowest tertile in the US population was 61, and was associated in a general increase in health services and mental health specialist care [39]. Patients also self-reported current and lifetime "mental illness" (not defined further in the questionnaire), and the presence now and ever of "depression" and "drug or alcohol abuse." We classified a patient as having a "psychiatric illness" (current or past) if any "mental illness," "depression" or "drug or alcohol abuse" was endorsed. These categories were meant to describe self-report patient information about mental health problems, but do not have physician validation.

Table 1. Prevalence of PHQ-15 symptoms in RA, SLE and Fibromyalgia.

PHQ Item	*RA (4718)*	*OA (952)*	*FM (440)*	*RA (4718)*	*OA (952)*	*FM* (440)*
	Bothered a little (%)			**Bothered a lot (%)**		
Feeling tired or having low energy	75.9	75.2	98.2	29.9	27.6	80.5
Pain in arms, legs or joints	82.3	89.8	98.9	33.1	41.6	73.6
Back pain	66.1	75.5	95.2	24.1	32.3	67.3
Trouble sleeping	61.9	63.6	91.6	21.0	19.5	54.6
Constipation, loose bowels, or diarrhea	44.6	45.2	75.5	9.8	10.9	33.9
Nausea, gas, or indigestion	42.5	43.0	73.2	6.8	7.7	24.1
Headaches	38.4	37.4	73.2	5.5	4.4	22.7
Shortness of breath	29.6	31.3	57.1	4.4	5.1	11.4
Stomach pain	27.7	27.5	60.5	4.3	5.2	16.1
Dizziness	23.8	26.8	57.7	2.6	2.8	7.5
Feeling your heart pound or race	17.5	18.1	41.1	1.6	2.0	6.6
Pain or problems during sexual intercourse	11.8	10.2	22.7	3.9	3.1	10.5
Chest pain	9.5	9.3	28.4	1.1	1.0	3.4
Menstrual cramps or other problems with your periods [Women only]	5.5	4.3	8.6	1.4	1.4	3.0
Fainting spells	1.9	2.5	6.8	0.3	0.6	1.1
Summary Scores						
Total PHQ-15 score Mean (SD)	6.9 (4.5)	7.3 (4.3)	14.0 (4.1)			
PHQ-15 score ≥10 (%)	26.4	28.5	88.9			
≥3 "bothered a lot" symptoms (%)	24.2	26.8	77.5			

PHQ-15- Patient Health Questionnaire-15.
*Criteria positive patients.

To measure functional status, we used the Health Assessment Questionnaire disability index (HAQ) [40] and the SF-36 PCS. HAQ scores ≥1 represent substantial functional impairment. Pain over the last week was assessed by a 0–10 visual analog scale. We also used the 5-level Euroqol (EQ-5D) to estimate a preference-based single measure of health status [41]. Lower scores represent worse outcome for the PCS, MCS, and EQ-5D.

Work disability and employment was determined by self-report. We use self-report for disability rather than receipt of a disability pension, as all patients are not eligible for a pension because of age or previous work history limitations. Hospitalization refers to hospitalization for any cause in the previous 6 months and is validated by medical records.

Statistical Methods

To measure the relation and significance between PHQ-15 groups and predictor variables, we used ordered logistic regression. To measure agreement we used the kappa statistic. According to Landis and Koch [42], kappa may be interpreted as: <0 no agreement, 0.0–0.20 very low agreement, 0.21–0.40 low agreement, 0.41–0.60 moderate agreement, 0.61–0.80 full agreement, and 0.81–1.00 almost perfect agreement.

Results

Using PHQ-15 scores as the criterion for non-DSM somatic syndrome disorders, 26.4% and 28.5% of RA and OA patients had PHQ-15 scores ≥10 (Table 1). Generally similar values were obtained by using an allied proposed criterion: the percentage of patients who had at least 3 "bothered a lot" endorsements out of 15 PHQ-15 items: 24.2% and 26.8%. When applied to patients with noninflammatory rheumatic disorders, the kappa for agreement between PHQ-15≥10 and "at least 3 bothered a lot" symptoms was 0.762, 95% CI = 0.728–0.795 (complete agreement). The four highest ranked symptoms by occurrence were *feeling tired or having low energy* (fatigue); *pain in arms legs or joints*; *back pain*; and *trouble sleeping*. When "bothered a lot" symptoms in table 1 were studied, PHQ-15 item percentages were approximately three times greater in fibromyalgia than in other diagnoses, providing an estimate of the extent to which patients diagnosed with fibromyalgia differ from those with other rheumatic disorders.

Table 2 demonstrates increasingly abnormal illness status variables with increasing levels of PHQ-15. In this table we restricted analyses to patients with RA, as those patients represent a group selected because they had RA, but unselected with respect to the presence of fibromyalgia or fibromyalgia characteristics. All variable were significantly associated with increasing PHQ-15 categories in ordered logit analyses. As noted above, patients with medium (PHQ-15 = 10–14) and high (PHQ-15≥15) somatic symptom severity satisfied the study somatization syndrome criterion. Younger age patients and women were more likely to be in the more severe categories. Measures of fibromyalgia, including the widespread pain index, the polysymptomatic distress score and fibromyalgia research criteria positivity increased with PHQ-15 somatic symptom severity category. PHQ-15 scores ≥10 showed substantial increases in fibromyalgia prevalence and fibromyalgia-associated scores.

In addition, self-reported current "mental illness" was approximately 4 times greater in medium PHQ-15 severity and almost 14 times greater compared with the minimal PHQ-15 severity group. Lifetime mental illness varied little across the first 3 categories, but was approximately double in the severe somatic severity group.

Table 2. Characteristics of rheumatoid arthritis patients according to PHQ-15 category.

Variable	PHQ-15 Category			
	PHQ-15 (0–4) Minimal	PHQ-15 (5–9) Low	PHQ-15 (10–14) Medium	PHQ-15 (10–30) High
N (Total = 4718) (%)	1651 (35.0)	1821 (38.6)	928 (19.7)	318 (6.7)
Age (years)	65.3 (12.2)	64.0 (12.0)	61.2 (12.8)	57.8 (13.2)
Sex (% male)	26.1	17.9	9.5	9.4
Fibromyalgia survey criteria (+) (%)	1.2	11.3	47.6	84.9
Polysymptomatic distress scale	3.7 (3.5)	8.6 (5.0)	14.2 (5.8)	20.3 (6.4)
Widespread pain index	2.0 (2.7)	4.7 (4.2)	8.0 (5.0)	12.1 (5.3)
PHQ-15	2.4 (1.4)	6.8 (1.4)	11.6 (1.4)	17.0 (2.5)
Mental component score (SF-36)	56.0 (7.6)	50.4 (10.0)	43.8 (11.1)	37.4 (11.3)
Mental health (SF-36)	85.2 (12.5)	76.4 (15.8)	66.4 (18.3)	55.1 (22.5)
"Mental illness" now (%)	0.5	0.9	1.9	6.9
"Mental illness" ever (%)	9.2	8.5	10.9	19.5
Psychiatric disorder now (%)	4.1	12.6	26.6	45.6
Psychiatric disorder ever (%)	30.4	46.8	69.1	81.5
Physical component score (SF-36)	45.3 (9.9)	36.8 (10.2)	30.6 (8.6)	27.9 (7.2)
HAQ (0–3)	0.55 (0.62)	0.97 (0.66)	1.39 (0.61)	1.64 (0.54)
VAS Pain (0–10)	1.8 (1.9)	3.5 (2.4)	5.3 (2.4)	6.4 (2.2)
EuroQol EQ-5D (0–1)	0.84 (0.11)	0.75 (0.12)	0.65 (0.15)	0.55 (0.17)
College graduate (%)	46.5	41.6	34.9	28.6
Current smoker (%)	6.7	8.5	10.8	13.8
Body mass index	26.9 (5.8)	28.7 (7.1)	29.8 (7.7)	31.9 (9.1)
Married (%)	74.2	73.2	69.7	68.2
Employed (%)	34.1	31.3	26.9	24.0
Disabled (%)	5.1	11.6	22.0	35.0
Hospitalized in last 6 months (%)	7.6	10.1	13.9	18.2

PHQ-15– Patient Health Questionnaire-15, HAQ – Health assessment questionnaire.
Continuous scales show mean and (standard deviation). Variables in column 1 predict increases/decreases in severity across PHQ-15 categories at $p<0.05$.

When mental illness, depression and substance abuse were combined (psychiatric disorder), substantial increases were noted across the PHQ-15 categories. In those with severe somatic symptom reporting, current reported psychiatric illness was 45.6% and lifetime illness was 81.5%. Using Ware's 42 cut-off for prediction of depressive disorders [38], most such disorders can be seen to occur in those with PHQ-15>10.

PHQ-15 category increases were also associated with substantial increases in pain scores, decreased quality of life and functional ability. These differences are clinically significant and important in the clinical evaluation and care of rheumatoid arthritis. Finally, PHQ-15 increases reflected less education, more cigarette smoking, higher body mass index, more work disability, and an increased rate of hospitalization in the previous six months.

Table 3 approached the relation of somatic symptom severity and clinical variables by classifying RA patients according to the number of symptoms that were "severe, continuous, life-disturbing problems" for the 3 specific symptom variables that are part of the ACR research criteria: fatigue, unrefreshed sleep and cognitive problems. In contrast to the percent of patients in the 4 PHQ categories (35.0%, 38.6%, 19.7%, 6.7%) shown in Table 2, more than 85% of Table 3 patients were in the 0 group. The 4 percentages were 85.2%, 7.1%, 6.3%, and 1.6%. In addition, fibromyalgia criteria positivity was 11.4% in the 0 group, and 56.7%, 75.3%, and 87.1% in the 1, 2 and 3 groups, respectively. Because being >0 indicates a very severe "life-disturbing" symptom, psychological variables were similarly severely abnormal and more so than in the medium and severe categories of PHQ-15 shown in Table 2. Overall, the major change in severity variables in Table 3 occurs between the 0 and 1 group. For most variables in Table 3, categories of 1, 2 and 3 are associated with small, but progressively more abnormal symptoms and characteristics.

Table 4 applies the 0–3 count test of Table 3 to noninflammatory patients who satisfy fibromyalgia criteria, with the goal of trying understand if applying the count variables provides additional information about somatic symptoms and psychological variables, as well as with ordinary clinical variables. The data tend to suggest that once the fibromyalgia criteria are satisfied, the count of very severe symptoms provide only a relatively equal small to moderate step-wise increase in variable severity. Of interest, the increase across the 0–3 categories is associated with small increases in the PHQ-15 of 1.1, 0.9, 1.2; and of 2.1, 1.1 and 1.3 in the longer (0–31) PSD scale.

Table 3. Characteristics of patients with rheumatoid arthritis according the number of severe; continuous, life-disturbing problems with fatigue, unrefreshed sleep or cognition.

Variable	*Count*			
Number of severe; continuous, life-disturbing problems for Fatigue, Unrefreshed sleep or cognitive problems	**0**	**1**	**2**	**3**
N (Total = 4780) (%)	4071 (85.2%)	338 (7.1%)	301 (6.3%)	70 (1.6%)
Age (years)	64.4 (12.3)	60.6 (12.7)	58.0 (12.9)	55.7 (11.8)
Sex (% male)	20.2	11.2	7.6	5.7
FM research criteria (%)	11.4	56.7	75.3	87.1
Polysymptomatic distress scale	7.3 (5.8)	15.3 (5.9)	18.1 (6.4)	21.9 (6.7)
Widespread pain index	4.2 (4.4)	8.0 (5.3)	9.2 (5.9)	11.2 (6.3)
PHQ-15	6.0 (3.9)	10.9 (4.1)	12.4 (4.4)	14.2 (5.4)
Mental component score (SF-36)	52.0 (9.9)	41.7 (11.0)	38.9 (11.7)	34.4 (11.7)
Mental health 5-item (SF-36)	78.8 (16.0)	63.7 (19.7)	59.0 (21.6)	49.9 (24.8)
"Mental illness" now (%)	0.8	3.0	5.0	11.4
"Mental illness" ever (%)	8.8	14.5	16.6	24.3
Psychiatric disorder now (%)	10.5	33.1	38.2	60.0
Psychiatric disorder ever (%)	42.8	71.9	77.4	90.0
Physical component score (SF-36)	39.6 (11.0)	29.8 (8.6)	27.0 (7.9)	28.0 (6.8)
HAQ (0–3)	0.84 (0.69)	1.48 (0.59)	1.66 (0.57)	1.79 (0.60)
VAS Pain (0–10)	3.0 (2.4)	5.6 (2.4)	6.5 (2.2)	7.1 (2.2)
EuroQol EQ-5D (0–1)	0.78 (0.12)	0.62 (0.16)	0.55 (0.17)	0.48 (0.19)
College graduate (%)	42.6	34.0	28.6	30.0
Current smoker (%)	7.7	12.4	15.3	21.4
Body mass index	28.0 (6.8)	30.5 (7.4)	31.4 (8.8)	31.5 (8.8)
Married (%)	73.9	63.0	67.4	57.1
Employed (%)	31.7	26.4	24.9	20.3
Disabled ((%)	9.2	29.7	36.9	43.5
Hospitalized in last 6 months (%)	9.5	14.8	16.3	18.6

PHQ-15– Patient Health Questionnaire-15, HAQ – Health assessment questionnaire.
Continuous scales show mean and (standard deviation).

The Relation of PHQ-15 to PSD, and the Concept of Fibromyalgia as a Somatic Symptom Disorder

When examined across the full length of the PHQ-15 and PSD scales in the RA patients of Table 2 and 3, as well as in patients with non-inflammatory disorders, the Pearson correlation coefficient between PHQ-15 and PSD was 0.74. We also evaluated the ability of the PSD and PHQ-15 scales to predict criteria positive fibromyalgia. The area under the receiver operating curve (AUC-ROC) was 0.97 for PSD and 0.89 for PHQ-15. Using a cutpoint of 10 on the PHQ-15 scale, the sensitivity and specificity of PHQ-15 for fibromyalgia diagnosis was 80.9% and 80.0% (correctly classified = 80.3%) compared with 84.3% and 93.7% (correctly classified = 91.7%) for the PSD scale. The kappa value for agreement in diagnosis was 0.57 (moderate agreement). The relation of PHQ-15 to PSD can be seen graphically in Figure 1. The vertical lines at 5, 10 and 15 show the PHQ-15 groups. The horizontal line at 12 roughly separates fibromyalgia negative patients (<12) from mostly fibromyalgia criteria positive patients (≥12). Patients with fibromyalgia whose PHQ-15 score is <10 (PHQ-15 0–9, PDS ≥12) are misclassified by PHQ-15 because their symptom score is too low; they satisfy ACR research criteria by virtue of a high widespread pain index. In addition, patients with PHQ-15≥10 who do not meet ACR criteria fail because they have too low of a WPI score. These data show that PHQ-15 and PSD are similar in their ability to identify the same type of patients, differing only in the number of painful sites that are required by the ACR research criteria.

Discussion

The data of this study demonstrate the extent to which fibromyalgia can be labeled a somatic symptom disorder or what Kroenke has labeled a "physical symptom disorder:" Such a disorder "would consist of one or more physical symptoms currently present, not fully explainable by another medical or psychiatric disorder (with the exception of functional somatic syndromes), causing functional impairment. Duration must be at least 6 months, and severity could be graded as mild, moderate, or severe using a 15-symptom checklist (PHQ-15). Finally, the type of symptoms or symptom syndromes present in the patient could be specified. Conclusions: PSD should be considered as a simpler and more inclusive diagnosis to replace several somatoform diagnoses currently in use" [15]. When characterized that way 89.9% of those with fibromyalgia have PHQ-15 scores ≥10, the level others have suggested is a requirement for somatic symptom syndromes [28,34]. In addition, as shown in Table 2, patients with this

Table 4. Characteristics of 440 patients with criteria positive 'primary' fibromyalgia according the number of severe; continuous, life-disturbing problems with fatigue, unrefreshed sleep or cognition.

Variable	*Count*			
Number of severe; continuous, life-disturbing problems for Fatigue, Unrefreshed sleep or cognitive problems	**0**	**1**	**2**	**3**
N (Total = 440) (%)	214 (48.6%)	92 (20.9%)	88 (20.0%)	46 (10.5%)
Age (years)*	62.8 (11.8)	61.0 (12.6)	56.5 (12.5)	53.3 (11.2)
Sex (% male)	11.7	9.8	9.1	6.5
FM research criteria (%)	100.0	100.0	100.0	100.0
Polysymptomatic distress scale*	18.1 (4.3)	20.2 (4.6)	21.3 (5.1)	22.6 (6.1)
Widespread pain index	11.6 (4.0)	12.4 (4.2)	11.8 (4.8)	11.8 (5.7)
PHQ-15*	12.1 (3.8)	13.2 (3.7)	14.1 (3.9)	15.3 (5.6)
	(64.0%)	61.4%	55.4%	52.2%
Mental component score (SF-36)*	42.9 (11.0)	40.9 (11.1)	37.3 (11.5)	31.3 (13.2)
Mental health (SF-36)*	65.6 (18.4)	61.8 (20.0)	57.2 (20.8)	42.7 (25.8)
"Mental illness" now (%)*	2.8	6.5	8.0	23.9
"Mental illness" ever (%)	17.8	20.7	19.3	34.8
Psychiatric disorder now (%)*	38.8	35.9	35.2	60.9
Psychiatric disorder ever (%)	77.1	82.6	81.8	89.1
Physical component score (SF-36)*	30.3 (8.5)	28.3 (8.7)	27.9 (6.9)	28.1 (9.1)
HAQ (0–3)*	1.25 (0.61)	1.47 (0.59)	1.35 (0.59)	1.54 (0.67)
Pain (0–10)*	5.8 (2.0)	6.7 (2.2)	7.0 (1.9)	7.3 (2.2)
EQ-5D*	0.65 (0.15)	0.57 (0.17)	0.57 (0.16)	0.47 (0.20)
College graduate (%)	35.0	34.8	36.4	28.3
Current smoker (%)	12.1	15.2	17.0	17.4
Body mass index	31.2 (7.4)	32.0 (9.2)	32.0 (7.4)	30.4 (8.7)
Married (%)	71.5	64.1	67.0	65.2
Employed (%)*	22.4	25.0	34.1	26.1
Disabled (self-reported work status) (%)*	27.1	31.5	23.9	34.8
Hospitalized (%)	11.7	15.2	19.3	13.0

PHQ-15- Patient Health Questionnaire-15, HAQ - Health assessment questionnaire.
Continuous scales show mean and (standard deviation).
* = $p<0.05$.

disorder have substantially abnormal scores for functional status and physical and mental health.

In a previous population based study, we have shown that fibromyalgia can be considered to be a dimensional or continuum disorder rather than a discrete illness, and that the polysymptomatic distress (or fibromyalgianess) scale provides a general, useful measure of the fibromyalgia continuum [32]. The PHQ-15 and the polysymptomatic distress scale tap into the same somatic dimension, and are correlated at 0.74. The essential difference between the scales is that the polysymptomatic distress scale weights pain, as measured by the widespread pain index, more than the PHQ-15 does. In noninflammatory patients satisfying the fibromyalgia criteria, joint and back pain account for a 26% of the total PHQ-15 score, while the WPI accounts for 58% of the polysymptomatic distress score. These differences can be appreciated in the agreements/non-agreements of Figure 1. Overall, these findings fit with the idea that fibromyalgia is a pain-predominant somatic symptom disorder.

Much current thought suggests that, as Wessely put it, "There is only one functional somatic syndrome" [43]. "... a substantial overlap exists between the individual syndromes and that the similarities between them outweigh the differences" "...existing definitions of these syndromes in terms of specific symptoms is of limited value; instead we believe a dimensional classification is likely to be more productive" [44]. This view, nuanced differently by different authors, is reflected in much current thinking [5,15,16,17,45,46]. In addition, the current predominant emphasis on pain extent (severity) in fibromyalgia was new to fibromyalgia/fibrositis, beginning in the 1980s. In fact, the dominant Yunus criteria that preceded the 1990 ACR criteria emphasized symptoms over pain [27,47]. These observations, with respect to the dimensional nature of fibromyalgia-type symptom severity and the dimensional nature of pain/symptom inclusion suggest that fibromyalgia is a more mutable, uncertain concept than often acknowledged. That is, the content of fibromyalgia is somewhat variable and is dimensional. Like the PHQ-15 at low levels of severity (PHQ-15 = 5–9), the polysymptomatic distress scale tracks symptoms to below syndromal levels. We believe that neuroscience investigators who rely on fibromyalgia as a hard diagnosis with specific cut-off, may be tapping instead into a common core of functional syndromes that is essentially dimensional. It may well be that the investigation of neuroscience issues would more appro-

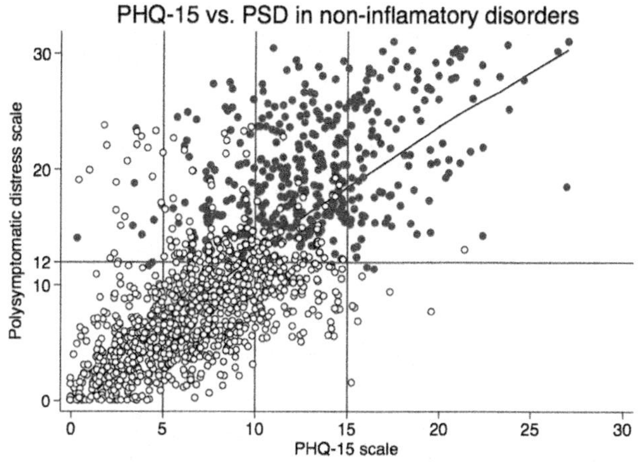

Figure 1. The relation of the PHQ-15 and Polysymptomatic Distress (PSD) scales. The vertical lines at 5, 10 and 15 define the PHQ-15 severity groups (0–4, 5–9, 10–14, ≥15). The horizontal line at 12 roughly separates fibromyalgia negative patients (<12) from mostly fibromyalgia criteria positive patients (≥12). A small amount if random jitter is added to the symbols to make overlapping symbols easier to see.

priately be directed over the range of the polysymptomatic distress and PHQ-15 scales.

The DSM-5 somatic symptom disorder differs in at least one important way from the syndromes described above: it perforce describes a mental disease. Given one severe, persistent somatic symptom, the diagnosis of DSM-5 SSD in patients with rheumatic diseases depends, in all practical cases, in satisfying the mandate of at least one of the following: (1) Disproportionate and persistent thoughts about the seriousness of one's symptoms; (2) Persistently high level of anxiety about health or symptoms; and (3) "Excessive time and energy devoted to these symptoms or health concerns. "Disproportionate," "high levels" and "excessive time" are judgments. They can be determined, according to the DSM, by "clinical experience, training and judgment based on guidance such as that contained in the DSM-5 text to recognize when a patient's thoughts, feelings and behaviors are indicative of a mental disorder" [14]. To test this judgment, the APA committee carried on clinical trials at a single psychiatric clinic site using approximately 420 psychiatric patients who were currently symptomatic for any DSM-IV diagnoses or high-probability symptoms associated with the DSM-5 diagnoses. Forty-two subjects had an SSD-like disorder (Complex somatic symptom disorder) [48,49]. Although the "SSD was found to have very good reliability [10], only previously diagnosed psychiatric patients were studied, no patients had disorders like rheumatoid arthritis or fibromyalgia (to our understanding), and physician examiners were single-center professors and allied psychiatric staff. From this we conclude that the ability to reliably and validly identify SSD patients in rheumatic disorders, including rheumatoid arthritis and fibromyalgia, was not tested; and that available reliability data cannot be extrapolated to such patients.

The data of the current study showed that psychological and psychiatric problems increased with increasing PHQ-15 and polysymptomatic distress scores. We also found that 51.4% of patients with fibromyalgia and 14.8% with RA had fatigue, sleep or cognitive problems that were severe, continuous, and life-disturbing (Tables 3 and 4). Among those with fibromyalgia (Table 4) there was evidence of self-report of severe functional, pain and quality of life disturbances. Whether these findings represent "disproportionate," "high levels" or "excessive time" could be a matter of conjecture, but a strong case can be made that these data suggest that almost all patients with fibromyalgia meet the DSM-5 B criterion, as do a substantial fraction of those with RA.

There are additional reasons to believe that validity and reliability of the DSM SSD may be unsatisfactory in persons with illnesses like fibromyalgia and rheumatoid arthritis. Research and clinical data are split on whether fibromyalgia patients exaggerate [22,23,24,25], including whether rheumatoid arthritis patients with fibromyalgia "over-report." A study of the RA Disease Activity Index concluded that "The DAS28 [50] [a measure of disease activity in RA], as expected, proved to be inappropriate to express disease activity in FM patients. DAS28 values for expressing disease activity in RA patients may be flawed by coexisting FM ..." [51]. Patients indicate that unsympathetic and non-understanding physicians are an important problem for them [52]. It is likely that some assessors would rate rheumatic patients as disproportionate with regard to intensity of symptoms while others would find patients adequately model their predicament. In addition, there is no clear definition of a "serious" illness. So it is possible that the presence of a mental illness may depend more on the examiner than the patient. The 14-item Whitely index [53] has been used (and recommended by DSM authors) as a method to assess disproportionate and excessive features. But it contains questions like "Do you often worry about the possibility that you have got a serious illness? Are you bothered by many aches and pains? Do you find that you are often aware of various things happening in your body? Is it hard for you to believe the doctor when he tells you there is nothing for you to worry about? Do you get the feeling that people are not taking your illness seriously enough?" The questions appear to lack face validity when assessing symptoms in fibromyalgia (and other rheumatic illnesses), and the expected answers should be "yes" Overall, our data suggest that fibromyalgia meets non-DSM criteria for somatization syndromes, and those with fibromyalgia report severe physical and psychological symptoms. But we are dubious that the DSM-5 approach can distinguish validly and reliably which fibromyalgia patients are and which are not mentally ill, particularly in clinical care settings where diagnosis will come most often from generalists.

Author Contributions

Conceived and designed the experiments: FW WH. Performed the experiments: FW. Analyzed the data: FW. Contributed reagents/materials/analysis tools: FW BW WH. Wrote the paper: FW BW RK WH. Developed the ideas behind this study: FW BW RK WH.

References

1. Wolfe F, Smythe HA, Yunus MB, Bennett RM, Bombardier C, et al. (1990) The American College of Rheumatology 1990 Criteria for the Classification of Fibromyalgia. Report of the Multicenter Criteria Committee. Arthritis Rheum 33: 160–172.
2. Wolfe F, Clauw D, Fitzcharles MA, Goldenberg D, Katz RS, et al. (2010) The American College of Rheumatology Preliminary Diagnostic Criteria for Fibromyalgia and Measurement of Symptom Severity. Arthritis Care Res 62: 600–610.

3. Wolfe F, Clauw D, Fitzcharles MA, Goldenberg D, Häuser W, et al. (2011) Fibromyalgia Criteria and Severity Scales for Clinical and Epidemiological Studies: A Modification of the ACR Preliminary Diagnostic Criteria for Fibromyalgia. J Rheumatol 38: 113–122.
4. Lipowski ZJ (1988) Somatization: The concept and its clinical application. AmJPsychiatry 145: 1358–1368.
5. Kroenke K (2007) Somatoform disorders and recent diagnostic controversies. Psychiatric Clinics of North America 30: 593–619.
6. Association AP (1980) Diagnostic and statistical manual of mental disorders (DSM-III): Amer Psychiatric Pub Inc.
7. American Psychiatric Association (1994) Diagnostic and statistical manual of mental disorders: DSM-IV: Amer Psychiatric Pub Inc. 886 p.
8. American Psychiatric Association (2000) Diagnostic and statistical manual of mental disorders: DSM-IV-TR: American Psychiatric Pub.
9. American Psychiatric Association (2013) Diagnostic and statistical manual of mental disorders: DSM-5: Amer Psychiatric Pub Inc. 991 p.
10. Dimsdale JE, Creed F, Escobar J, Sharpe M, Wulsin L, et al. (2013) Somatic Symptom Disorder: An important change in DSM. Journal of psychosomatic research.
11. Grabe H, Meyer C, Hapke U, Rumpf H-J, Juergen Freyberger H, et al. (2003) Specific somatoform disorder in the general population. Psychosomatics 44: 304–311.
12. Fink P, Hansen MS, Søndergaard L (2005) Somatoform disorders among first-time referrals to a neurology service. Psychosomatics 46: 540–548.
13. Fink P, Sørensen L, Engberg M, Holm M, Munk-Jørgensen P (1999) Somatization in Primary Care: Prevalence, Health Care Utilization, and General Practitioner Recognition. Psychosomatics 40: 330–338.
14. American Psychiatric Association (2013) Somatic Symptom Disorder. Available: http://www.psychiatry.org/File%20Library/Practice/DSM/DSM-5/DSM-5-Somatic-Symptom-Disorder.pdf. Accessed 2013 Sep 3.
15. Kroenke K (2006) Physical symptom disorder: a simpler diagnostic category for somatization-spectrum conditions. Journal of psychosomatic research 60: 335–339.
16. Barsky AJ, Borus JF (1999) Functional somatic syndromes. AnnInternMed 130: 910–921.
17. Fink P, Schroder A (2010) One single diagnosis, bodily distress syndrome, succeeded to capture 10 diagnostic categories of functional somatic syndromes and somatoform disorders. J Psychosom Res 68: 415–426.
18. Crombez G, Beirens K, Van Damme S, Eccleston C, Fontaine J (2009) The unbearable lightness of somatisation: A systematic review of the concept of somatisation in empirical studies of pain. Pain 145: 31–35.
19. Frances A, Chapman S (2013) DSM-5 somatic symptom disorder mislabels medical illness as mental disorder. Australian and New Zealand Journal of Psychiatry 47: 483–484.
20. Frances A (2013) The new somatic symptom disorder in DSM-5 risks mislabeling many people as mentally ill. BMJ: British Medical Journal 346.
21. Gross M (2013) Has the manual gone mental? Current biology 23: R295–R298.
22. Houtveen JH, Rietveld S, de Geus EJ (2003) Exaggerated perception of normal physiological responses to stress and hypercapnia in young women with numerous functional somatic symptoms. Journal of psychosomatic research 55: 481–490.
23. Mittenberg W, Patton C, Canyock EM, Condit DC (2002) Base Rates of Malingering and Symptom Exeggeration. Journal of Clinical and Experimental Neuropsychology 24: 1094–1102.
24. Gervais RO, Russell AS, Green P, Allen LM, III, Ferrari R, et al. (2001) Effort testing in patients with fibromyalgia and disability incentives955. JRheumatol 28: 1892–1899.
25. Hidding A, van Santen M, De Klerk E, Gielen X, Boers M, et al. (1994) Comparison between self-report measures and clinical observations of functional disability in ankylosing spondylitis, rheumatoid arthritis and fibromyalgia. J Rheumatol 21: 818–823.
26. Barker KK (2005) The fibromyalgia story: medical authority and women's worlds of pain: Temple Univ Pr.
27. Wolfe F, Walitt B (2013) Culture, science and the changing nature of fibromyalgia. Nature Reviews Rheumatology.
28. Kocalevent R-D, Hinz A, Brähler E (2013) Standardization of a screening instrument (PHQ-15) for somatization syndromes in the general population. BMC Psychiatry 13: 91.
29. Kroenke K, Spitzer RL, Williams JBW (2002) The PHQ-15: validity of a new measure for evaluating the severity of somatic symptoms. Psychosomatic Medicine 64: 258–266.
30. Wolfe F, Michaud K (2011) The National Data Bank for rheumatic diseases: a multi-registry rheumatic disease data bank. Rheumatology (Oxford) 50: 16–24.
31. Wolfe F (2010) New Criteria for fibromyalgia: a twenty year journey. Arthritis Care Res 62: 583–584.
32. Wolfe F, Brähler E, Hinz A, Häuser W (2013) Fibromyalgia prevalence, somatic symptom reporting, and the dimensionality of polysymptomatic distress: results from a survey of the general population. Arthitis Care and Research 65: 777–785.
33. Walitt B, Fitzcharles MA, Hassett AL, Katz RS, H‰user W, et al. (2011) The Longitudinal Outcome of Fibromyalgia: A Study of 1555 Patients. The Journal of rheumatology.
34. Körber S, Frieser D, Steinbrecher N, Hiller W (2011) Classification characteristics of the Patient Health Questionnaire-15 for screening somatoform disorders in a primary care setting. Journal of psychosomatic research 71: 142–147.
35. Van Ravesteijn H, Wittkampf K, Lucassen P, Van De Lisdonk E, Van Den Hoogen H, et al. (2009) Detecting somatoform disorders in primary care with the PHQ-15. The Annals of Family Medicine 7: 232–238.
36. Ware JE, Sherbourne CD (1992) The MOS 36-Item Short-Form Health Survey (SF-36).1. Conceptual Framework and Item Selection. MedCare 30: 473–483.
37. McHorney CA, Ware JE Jr, Lu JF, Sherbourne CD (1994) The MOS 36-item Short-Form Health Survey (SF-36): III. Tests of data quality, scaling assumptions, and reliability across diverse patient groups. MedCare 32: 40–66.
38. Ware Jr JE, Gandek B (1998) Overview of the SF-36 health survey and the international quality of life assessment (IQOLA) project. Journal of Clinical Epidemiology 51: 903–912.
39. Ware JE, Gandek B (1994) The SF-36 health survey: development and use in mental health research and the IQOLA project. International Journal of Mental Health 23: 49–73.
40. Fries JF, Spitz PW, Kraines RG, Holman HR (1980) Measurement of patient outcome in arthritis. Arthritis Rheum 23: 137–145.
41. Obradovic M, Lal A, Liedgens H (2013) Validity and responsiveness of EuroQol-5 dimension (EQ-5D) versus Short Form-6 dimension (SF-6D) questionnaire in chronic pain. Health and Quality of Life Outcomes 11: 110.
42. Landis J, Koch G (1977) The measurement of observer agreement for categorical data. Biometrics 33: 159.
43. Wessely S, White PD (2004) There is only one functional somatic syndrome. The British Journal of Psychiatry 185: 95–96.
44. Wessely S, Nimnuan C, Sharpe M (1999) Functional somatic syndromes: one or many? Lancet 354: 936–939.
45. Creed FH, Davies I, Jackson J, Littlewood A, Chew-Graham C, et al. (2012) The epidemiology of multiple somatic symptoms. Journal of psychosomatic research.
46. Sharpe M, Carson A (2001) ìUnexplainedî Somatic Symptoms, Functional Syndromes, and Somatization: Do We Need a Paradigm Shift? Annals of internal medicine 134: 926.
47. Yunus M, Masi AT, Calabro JJ, Miller KA, Feigenbaum SL (1981) Primary fibromyalgia (fibrositis): clinical study of 50 patients with matched normal controls. Semin Arthritis Rheum 11: 151–171.
48. Regier DA, Narrow WE, Clarke DE, Kraemer HC, Kuramoto SJ, et al. (2013) DSM-5 Field Trials in the United States and Canada, part II: test-retest reliability of selected categorical diagnoses. American journal of psychiatry 170: 59–70.
49. Clarke DE, Narrow WE, Regier DA, Kuramoto SJ, Kupfer DJ, et al. (2013) DSM-5 Field Trials in the United States and Canada, part I: study design, sampling strategy, implementation, and analytic approaches. American journal of psychiatry 170: 43–58.
50. van der Heijde DMFM, van 't Hof M, van Riel PLCM, Theunisse LAM, Lubberts EW, et al. (1990) Judging disease activity in clinical practice in rheumatoid arthritis: first step in the development of a disease activity score. Ann Rheum Dis 49: 916–920.
51. Leeb B, Andel I, Sautner J, Nothnagl T, Rintelen B (2004) The DAS28 in rheumatoid arthritis and fibromyalgia patients. Rheumatology 43: 1504.
52. Barker KK (2011) Listening to Lyrica: contested illnesses and pharmaceutical determinism. Social Science & Medicine.
53. Speckens AEM, Spinhoven P, Sloekers P, Bolk JH, van Hemert AM (1996) A validation study of the Whitely Index, the Illness Attitude Scales, and the Somatosensory Amplification Scale in general medical and general practice patients. Journal of psychosomatic research 40: 95–104.

6

Safety with Ocrelizumab in Rheumatoid Arthritis: Results from the Ocrelizumab Phase III Program

Paul Emery[1,2]*, William Rigby[3], Paul P. Tak[4¤], Thomas Dörner[5], Ewa Olech[6], Carmen Martin[7], Laurie Millar[7], Helen Travers[7], Elena Fisheleva[7]

1 Leeds Institute of Rheumatic and Musculoskeletal Medicine, University of Leeds, Leeds, United Kingdom, **2** NIHR Leeds Musculoskeletal Biomedical Research Unit, Leeds Teaching Hospitals NHS Trust, Leeds, United Kingdom, **3** The Geisel School of Medicine at Darthmouth, Lebanon, New Hampshire, United States of America, **4** Academic Medical Centre, University of Amsterdam, Amsterdam, the Netherlands, **5** Charité University Hospitals and DRFZ, Berlin, Germany, **6** University of Nevada School of Medicine, Las Vegas, Nevada, United States of America, **7** Roche Products, Ltd, Welwyn Garden City, United Kingdom

Abstract

Objective: The objective was to determine the safety of ocrelizumab (OCR) in patients with rheumatoid arthritis (RA).

Methods: This was an analysis of the double-blind, placebo-controlled periods and long-term follow-up of 4 OCR phase III trials in RA (SCRIPT, STAGE, FILM and FEATURE). Safety data per study and the results of a meta-analysis of serious infectious events (SIEs) are presented.

Results: Overall, 868 patients received placebo, 1064 patients OCR 200 mg×2 (or 400 mg×1) (OCR200), and 827 patients OCR 500 mg×2 (OCR500) plus background methotrexate (MTX) at baseline and 24 weeks. During the double-blind, placebo-controlled periods, the incidence of adverse events and serious adverse events was comparable between the OCR+ MTX and placebo +MTX groups. Infusion-related reactions were more common with OCR+MTX and decreased in frequency with subsequent infusions. Serious infusion-related reactions were rare (0.1%). Serious infections occurred more frequently with OCR500+MTX. In the meta-analysis, a statistically significant difference from placebo +MTX in incidence of SIEs per 100 patient-years of 2.4 (95% CI, 0.3–4.5) was observed with OCR500+MTX, but not with OCR200+MTX (0.6; 95% CI, −1.3 to 2.4). Patients recruited in Asia exhibited a higher risk of serious infections (hazard ratio, 1.78; 95% CI, 1.03–3.06). The incidence of human anti-human antibodies was <5%. Long-term follow-up indicated no differences in malignancy rates between the treatment groups. There was no apparent difference in time to B-cell repletion between the OCR dose groups.

Conclusions: In placebo-controlled clinical trials of RA, OCR500+MTX was associated with a higher risk of serious infections compared with placebo +MTX. The safety profile of OCR 200+MTX was comparable with placebo+MTX.

Trial Registration: STAGE Clinical Trials.gov NCT00406419 SCRIPT Clinical Trials.gov NCT00476996 FILM Clinical Trials.gov NCT00485589 FEATURE Clinical Trials.gov NCT00673920

Editor: C. Mary Schooling, CUNY, United States of America

Funding: This study was funded by F. Hoffmann-La Roche, the employer of Carmen Martin, Laurie Millar, Helen Travers, and Elena Fisheleva. EO has received research funding from Abbvie, Genentech, Pfizer, UCB and Vertex. The funders had no role in study design, data collection and analysis, decision to publish, or preparation of the manuscript.

Competing Interests: This study was funded by F. Hoffmann-La Roche, the employer of Carmen Martin, Laurie Millar, Helen Travers, and Elena Fisheleva. Helen Travers holds stock in Roche. PE has provided expert advice and undertaken clinical trials for Pfizer, Merck Sharpe Dome, Abbvie, UCB, Roche, BMS and Novartis. WR has served as a consultant for Roche. PPT has served as a consultant for Roche/Genentech and became an employee of GlaxoSmithKline after completion of this work. TD has served as a consultant for Roche and has received speakers' bureau honoraria from Roche. EO has received research funding from Abbvie, Genentech, Pfizer, UCB and Vertex, consultancy fees from Abbvie, Crescendo, Genentech, Janssen, Pfizer and UCB, and speakers' bureau honoraria from Abbvie, Crescendo and UCB. There are no patents, products in development or marketed products to declare.

* E-mail: p.emery@leeds.ac.uk

¤ Current address: GlaxoSmithKline, Stevenage, United Kingdom

Introduction

Although the immunopathogenesis of rheumatoid arthritis (RA) is not fully understood, accumulating evidence suggests that B cells have multiple potential roles through both antibody-dependent and antibody-independent pathways [1,2]. Rituximab is a chimeric mouse-human monoclonal antibody that depletes CD20+ B cells and has been shown to be an effective therapy in patients with RA [3–7]. Pooled analysis of long-term safety data from patients receiving rituximab within a global clinical trial program indicated that rituximab is well tolerated over time and during multiple courses of treatment [8,9]. However, as with all chimeric antibodies, immunogenicity may be a potential concern. A safety analysis showed that 11% of patients with RA developed a titer positive for human anti-chimeric antibody (HACA) on at least one occasion during treatment with rituximab [8]. The presence of

HACAs was not associated with the development of infusion-related reactions (IRRs) or loss of efficacy on retreatment. Thus, the clinical impact of HACA directed at rituximab remains unclear.

Ocrelizumab (rhuMAb 2H7, [OCR]) is a humanized anti-CD20 monoclonal antibody. In vitro characterization of OCR demonstrated enhanced antibody-dependent cell-mediated cytotoxicity and reduced complement-dependent cytotoxicity compared with rituximab (unpublished data), although the clinical implications of these differences remain unclear. The efficacy and safety of OCR in RA has been evaluated in a robust phase III clinical trial program in a broad spectrum of patients [10–13]. In May 2010, OCR development in RA was terminated as a result of the overall risk-benefit assessment from the 2 pivotal phase III studies STAGE and SCRIPT. The efficacy and safety profiles of the OCR 200 mg (OCR200) and OCR 500 mg (OCR500) dosing regimens led the sponsors to conclude that OCR did not demonstrate an additional benefit over existing therapies, including rituximab for patients with RA, and that an application for regulatory approval of OCR in RA was not warranted. This paper presents the key safety outcomes of the 4 phase III OCR trials in RA to provide an overview of the safety of OCR in patients with RA and background methotrexate (MTX) treatment.

Patients and Methods

The CONSORT checklist is available as supporting information; see Checklist S1.

Ethics Statement

These studies were conducted at 686 sites across more than 20 different countries in accordance with the ethical principles of the Declaration of Helsinki. Ethical approval from the local institutional review board at each study center was obtained before the start of each study and all patients provided written informed consent. All studies included were previously registered with ClinicalTrials.gov (registration nos. NCT00406419, NCT00476996, NCT00485589 and NCT00673920).

Patients

Patients included in the analyses were participants in 1 of 4 OCR phase III trials [10–13]. The analysis population represented a broad spectrum of patients, ranging from patients with early RA who were MTX-naive (FILM [12], registration no. NCT00485589) to patients with advanced RA disease who were refractory to disease-modifying antirheumatic drugs (DMARDs) (FEATURE [13], registration no. NCT00673920 and STAGE [10], registration no. NCT00406419) and/or anti-TNFs (SCRIPT [11], registration no. NCT00476996). The overwhelming majority of patients received background MTX; leflunomide could also be used instead of MTX in SCRIPT.

Study Designs

All 4 trials were phase III international, randomized, and double-blind, placebo-controlled (DBPC); STAGE was conducted at 209 centers in 24 countries, SCRIPT was conducted at 227 centers in 25 countries, FEATURE was conducted at 96 centers in 14 countries and FILM was conducted at 154 centers in 21 countries. The study designs and numbers of patients randomized were reported previously [10–13] and are summarized in Table 1. During the DBPC period of STAGE, SCRIPT and FILM, patients received treatment on Days 1 and 15 followed by a retreatment course at Weeks 24 and 26 (patients in FILM were eligible for 2 additional retreatment courses at Weeks 52 and 54, and Weeks 76 and 78). At the end of the DBPC period in FEATURE (Week 24), all patients were re-randomized to receive either OCR200 ×2+MTX or OCR 400 mg (OCR400) +MTX for a 24-week double-blind (but not placebo-controlled) treatment period. After completion of the double-blind period (48 weeks [SCRIPT, STAGE and FEATURE] and 104 weeks [FILM]), patients entered an open-label extension, where they were treated with OCR500 ×2+MTX (SCRIPT, STAGE and FILM) or OCR400+MTX (FEATURE) at the discretion of the investigator. At the time that FILM was terminated, all patients had completed 52 weeks of DBPC treatment and only a few had completed 104 weeks and entered the open-label extension. Therefore, analysis of the DBPC period for FILM included only the Week 52 data. At the time that FEATURE, SCRIPT and STAGE were terminated, all patients had completed the double-blind 48-week period. Upon withdrawal from treatment, all patients were required to continue in safety follow-up (SFU) for at least 48 weeks from the first infusion of their last course and until their CD19+ B-cell counts either returned to baseline level or the lower limit of normal (80 cells/μl), whichever was lower.

Safety Assessments

In each trial, clinical adverse events (AEs) and serious AEs (SAEs) were recorded, and the intensity of AEs was graded using the National Cancer Institute Common Toxicity Criteria (version 3) and coded according to MedDRA (version 12.1). Malignancies were identified using the wide standard MedDRA query Malignant or Unspecified Tumors. Serious infectious events (SIEs) also included those requiring intravenous antibiotics. IRRs and symptoms were recorded on a specifically designed page of the case report form.

Immunogenicity and Pharmacodynamics

The primary pharmacodynamic (PD) marker for OCR is the presence of CD20+ B cells in the blood. Because the presence of OCR in serum could confound assays of CD20+ cells, CD19 was used to measure the levels of peripheral B cells following treatment (limit of detection, 0.05×10^9 cells/l in conventional flow cytometry). In each trial, serum samples were collected at prespecified time points for the determination of human anti-human antibodies (HAHAs) and B-cell levels (CD19+ cells). A bridging format enzyme-linked immunosorbent assay was used to determine HAHA titers. All positive samples were further confirmed by competitive binding to anti-IgM, followed by implementation of an additional decision tree to confirm or reject true positivity.

Statistical Analysis

Safety and PD analyses were conducted on the safety population, which included all patients in each trial who were randomized, received any part of an infusion of study drug, and underwent at least one assessment of safety. Evaluation of the safety data for each study led to the conduct of a fixed-effects meta-analysis of SIEs. The incidence rate difference in SIEs from placebo (PBO)+MTX during the DBPC period, weighted by study size was calculated for both dose groups using data from all four studies (STAGE, SCRIPT, FEATURE and FILM). An exploratory, hypothesis-generating analysis of risk factors for SIEs was performed on STAGE, SCRIPT and FILM DBPC pooled data sets. The multivariate approach (COX regression models) investigated treatment group as a risk factor, with baseline covariates that included but were not limited to age, body mass index, body surface area, weight, race, region, previous use of biological and nonbiological DMARDs, MTX dose, corticosteroid

Table 1. Summary of 4 Phase III Studies of Ocrelizumab.

Trial Name	Patients Treated, n	RA Characteristics	Treatment Groups+MTX[a]	Duration of PBO-Controlled Period, weeks
STAGE	1006	MTX-IR; 51% to 54% steroid use; Baseline DAS28 ≈6.4	PBO (n = 320); OCR200 (n = 343); OCR500 (n = 343)	48
SCRIPT	836	TNF-IR; 56% to 62% steroid use; Baseline DAS28 ≈6.5	PBO (n = 277); OCR200 (n = 277); OCR500 (n = 282)	48
FEATURE	312	MTX-IR/biological DMARD-IR; 52% to 59% steroid use; Baseline DAS28 ≈6.5	PBO (n = 64); OCR200 (n = 131); OCR400 (n = 117)	24
FILM	605	MTX-naïve; 39% to 42% steroid use; Baseline DAS28 ≈7.0	PBO (n = 207); OCR200 (n = 196); OCR500 (n = 202)	104[b]

Abbreviations: DAS28, disease activity score in 28 joints; DMARD, disease-modifying antirheumatic drug; IR, inadequate responder; MTX, methotrexate; OCR200, ocrelizumab 200 mg×2; OCR500, ocrelizumab 500 mg×2; PBO, placebo; RA, rheumatoid arthritis; TNF, tumor necrosis factor.
[a]All patients in all studies received background MTX 7.5 to 25 mg/week (7.5–20 mg/week in FILM), except for in SCRIPT, in which MTX or leflunomide was permitted. Treatment with corticosteroids (≤10 mg/day prednisolone or equivalent) was permitted in all studies provided the dose was stable 4 weeks prior to baseline.
[b]Study terminated early. Safety evaluation conducted for 52-week data.

use, RA disease duration, presence of selected comorbid conditions and study.

All available malignancy data from baseline to long-term SFU (up to 5 years of follow-up) in the 4 trials were pooled. Immunogenicity results included all data available for the DBPC periods.

PD data were analyzed using Kaplan-Meier methodology and included all data available after each patient completed at least 72 weeks of SFU after the last dose in each study.

In all analyses in which the FEATURE study was included, patients who received OCR200 or OCR400+MTX were grouped together in the OCR200+MTX group.

Results

Patient Population

The safety analysis population comprised 2759 patients (868 patients treated with PBO+MTX, 1064 with OCR200+MTX and 827 with OCR500+MTX; Figure 1). The majority of patients were female and white and had a mean age ranging from approximately 49 to 55 years (Table 2). Disease duration varied because of the different patient populations. Patients in SCRIPT had long-standing RA, with a duration of approximately 11 to 12 years; patients in FILM had a considerably shorter disease duration of approximately 1.2 years. Corticosteroid (<10 mg/d) use varied from 39% to 42% in FILM to 56% to 62% in SCRIPT. In SCRIPT, leflunomide was received by 10.1%, 15.2% and 14.5% of the PBO+MTX, OCR200+MTX and OCR500+MTX groups, respectively, with mean doses of 19.6, 18.3 and 17.4 mg/d, respectively. All other patients in SCRIPT and all patients in the other trials received concomitant MTX.

Overall Safety Profile

In all 4 trials, the incidence of all AEs during the DBPC periods was comparable in the PBO+MTX–treated and OCR+MTX–treated patients (Table 3). Grade 3 AEs were relatively infrequent, occurring in approximately 5% to 10% of patients across the treatment groups, with no clear differences between the PBO+MTX and OCR+MTX groups. The incidence of grade 4 AEs was 0% to 2.5%. AEs leading to patient withdrawal were infrequent; the most common in all 4 trials were IRRs and infections. Patients who received OCR500+MTX in FILM had a higher incidence of AEs leading to withdrawal than did patients who received PBO+MTX (5.9% vs 1.0%). Although the incidence of SAEs varied across the trials, there were no clear differences in general between the PBO+MTX and OCR+MTX groups or between the different dose groups (Table 3); the percentages of patients reporting ≥1 SAE were approximately 8% to 14% (OCR200+MTX) and 11% to 14% (OCR500+MTX), compared with 8% to 12% (PBO+MTX). The most common SAEs overall were infections and infestations. In STAGE and FEATURE, the occurrence of SAEs in other system organ classes was infrequent and comparable across treatment groups. In SCRIPT, serious musculoskeletal and connective tissue disorders were reported more frequently by patients in the PBO+MTX group (4.3%) compared with the OCR200+MTX (2.5%) and OCR500+MTX (2.5%) groups; this difference was mainly driven by an increased reporting of "exacerbation of RA." The occurrence of SAEs in other system organ classes in SCRIPT was infrequent and comparable across treatment groups. In FILM, SAEs classified as respiratory, thoracic, and mediastinal disorders occurred more frequently with OCR500+MTX (2.5%) than with OCR200+MTX (0.5%) and PBO+MTX (0%); the most common SAE in this body system was interstitial lung disease, which was reported in 3 patients in the OCR500+MTX group. The occurrence of other body-system SAEs was infrequent and comparable across treatment groups.

Infusion-Related Reactions

The most common AEs overall were IRRs. The incidence of IRRs was approximately 2 to 3 times higher in the OCR+MTX group relative to the PBO+MTX group (Table 3). The highest incidence of IRRs occurred during and following the first infusion of the first course; the second infusion was tolerated better, and IRRs became less frequent with subsequent infusions. The most common symptoms were pruritus, pyrexia, flushing, laryngeal/throat irritation, headache, nausea, rash, chills/rigors, hypertension, urticaria and dizziness. IRRs were reported slightly more frequently with OCR500+MTX than with OCR200+MTX in both STAGE and SCRIPT but at a similar frequency with both OCR+MTX doses in FILM. Only 2 patients in STAGE and 1 patient in FILM reported a serious IRR. The 2 serious IRRs that occurred in STAGE were recorded for 1 patient in each of the 2 OCR+MTX groups. Both occurred during the first infusion of the first course and resolved following symptomatic treatment. In addition, 1 patient (OCR500+MTX) had an anaphylactoid reaction that began 45 min after the start of the first infusion of the first course. The reaction resolved without sequelae following symptomatic treatment. One patient in the OCR500+MTX group

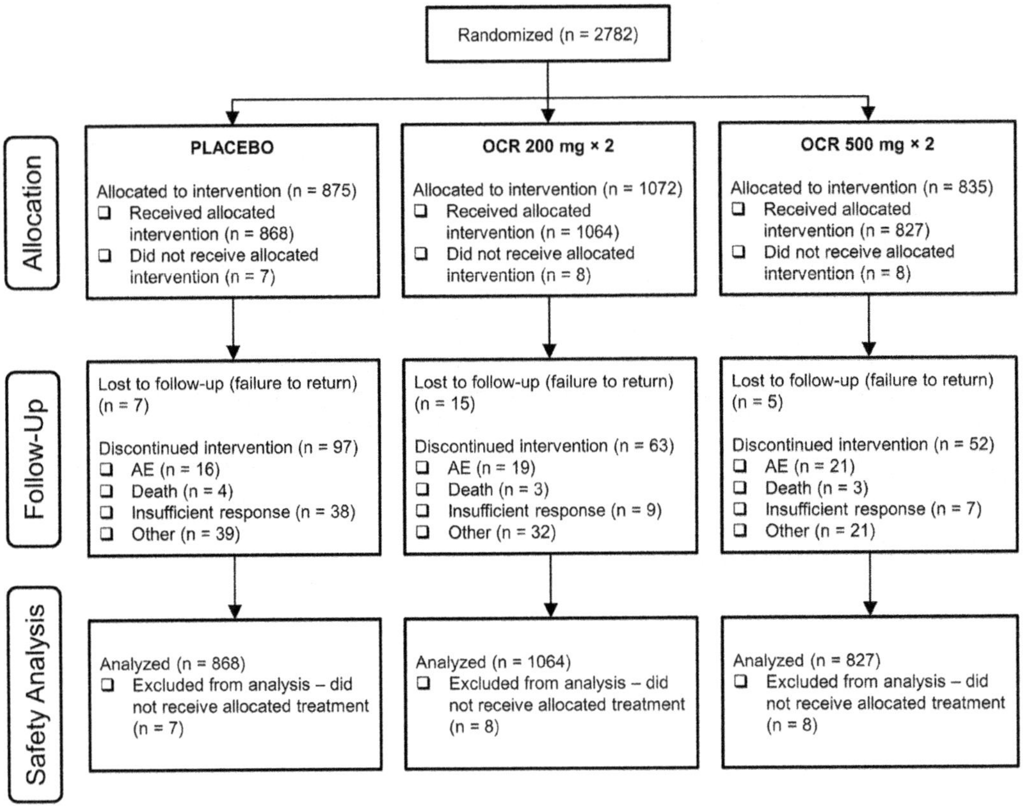

Figure 1. Patient disposition flow diagram of pooled safety population.

Table 2. Baseline Patient Characteristics in Pooled Safety Populations[a].

Characteristic	PBO+MTX[b]	OCR200+MTX[b]	OCR500+MTX[b]
	(n = 868)	**(n = 1064)**	**(n = 827)**
Female, %	74.0 to 87.5	77.3 to 82.5	80.0 to 83.7
White, %	68.8 to 74.4	65.9 to 73.0	67.0 to 75.6
Mean age, years	49.2 to 54.2	50.8 to 54.5	48.6 to 53.8
Mean RA disease duration, years	1.2 to 11.8	1.2 to 12.7	1.2 to 12.3
Serological status, %			
— RF+/ACPA+	83.0 to 87.9	80.2 to 87.8	77.1 to 86.1
— RF+/ACPA−	4.8 to 8.5	6.6 to 9.7	4.5 to 8.5
— RF−/ACPA+	6.3 to 9.4	5.1 to 11.2	to 15.3
— RF−/ACPA−	0 to 1.6	0 to 1.2	0.7 to 1.5
SJC (66 joints), mean	16.6 to 21.1	16.5 to 19.4	17.1 to 19.5
TJC (68 joints), mean	26.0 to 31.6	26.2 to 30.8	26.4 to 30.0
CRP (mg/dl), mean	2.4 to 3.8	1.8 to 3.5	1.9 to 3.4
ESR (mm/h), mean	46.7 to 60.0	44.5 to 55.8	45.5 to 58.1
HAQ-DI, mean	1.5 to 1.8	1.5 to 1.8	1.5 to 1.7
DAS28-ESR, mean	6.4 to 7.0	6.4 to 7.0	6.4 to 6.9
Oral corticosteroid use, %	40 to 62	39 to 58	42 to 56

Abbreviations: ACPA, anti-citrullinated peptide antibody; CRP, C-reactive protein; DAS28, disease activity score in 28 joints; ESR, erythrocyte sedimentation rate; HAQ-DI, Health Assessment Questionnaire Disease Index; MTX, methotrexate; OCR200, ocrelizumab 200 mg×2; OCR500, ocrelizumab 500 mg×2; PBO, placebo; RA, rheumatoid arthritis; RF, rheumatoid factor; SJC, swollen joint count; TJC, tender joint count.

[a]Data shown as ranges (minimum and maximum values) across the 4 trials.

[b]All patients in all studies received background MTX 7.5 to 25 mg/week (7.5 to 20 mg/week in FILM), except for in SCRIPT, in which MTX or leflunomide was permitted.

Table 3. Summary of Safety During the Double-Blind, Placebo-Controlled Periods[a].

Safety Profile	PBO+MTX[b]	OCR200+MTX[b]	OCR500+MTX[b]
STAGE (MTX-IR)			
Patients, n	320	343	343
Any AE, n (%)	254 (79.4)	282 (82.2)	287 (83.7)
— Grade 3, n (%)	25 (7.8)	20 (5.8)	25 (7.3)
— Grade 4, n (%)	2 (<1)	2 (<1)	2 (<1)
— Serious, n (%)	37 (11.6)	26 (7.6)	38 (11.1)
AEs leading to withdrawal, n (%)	5 (1.6)	5 (1.5)	6 (1.7)
Deaths, n (%)	1 (<1)	0 (0.0)	3 (<1)
IRRs, n (%)	31 (9.7)	69 (20.1)	80 (23.3)
— Serious, n (%)	0 (0.0)	1 (<1)	1 (<1)
Infections, n (%)	173 (54.1)	188 (54.8)	194 (56.6)
— Serious, n (%)	10 (3.1)	11 (3.2)	21 (6.1)
Malignancies, n (%)	6 (1.9)	3 (<1)	4 (1.2)
SCRIPT (TNF-IR)			
Patients, n	277	277	282
Any AE, n (%)	227 (81.9)	232 (83.8)	238 (84.4)
— Grade 3, n (%)	28 (10.1)	25 (9.0)	28 (9.9)
— Grade 4, n (%)	1 (<1)	2 (<1)	3 (1.1)
— Serious, n (%)	32 (11.6)	40 (14.4)	32 (11.3)
AEs leading to withdrawal, n (%)	10 (3.6)	11 (4.0)	7 (2.5)
Deaths, n (%)	1 (<1)	0 (0.0)	0 (0.0)
IRRs, n (%)	30 (10.8)	53 (19.1)	67 (23.8)
— Serious, n (%)	0 (0.0)	0 (0.0)	0 (0.0)
Infections, n (%)	143 (51.6)	150 (54.2)	164 (58.2)
— Serious, n (%)	7 (2.5)	14 (5.1)	12 (4.3)
Malignancies, n (%)	5 (1.8)	7 (2.5)	2 (<1)
FEATURE (MTX-IR/biological DMARD-IR)			
Patients, n	64	248	N/A
Any AE, n (%)	40 (62.5)	162 (65.3)	—
— Grade 3, n (%)	4 (6.3)	8 (3.2)	—
— Grade 4, n (%)	0 (0.0)	0 (0.0)	—
— Serious, n (%)	5 (7.8)	5 (2.0)	—
AEs leading to withdrawal, n (%)	2 (3.1)	3 (1.2)	—
Deaths, n (%)	0 (0.0)	0 (0.0)	—
IRRs, n (%)	7 (10.9)	53 (21.4)	—
— Serious, n (%)	0 (0.0)	0 (0.0)	—
Infections, n (%)	24 (37.5)	90 (36.3)	—
— Serious, n (%)	2 (3.1)	5 (2.0)	—
Malignancies, n (%)	0 (0.0)	1 (<1)	—
FILM (MTX-naïve)			
Patients, n	207	196	202
Any AE, n (%)	167 (80.7)	171 (87.2)	167 (82.7)
— Grade 3, n (%)	16 (7.7)	18 (9.2)	24 (11.9)
— Grade 4, n (%)	0 (0.0)	1 (<1)	5 (2.5)
— Serious, n (%)	21 (10.1)	18 (9.2)	28 (13.9)
AEs leading to withdrawal, n (%)	2 (1.0)	3 (1.5)	12 (5.9)
Deaths, n (%)	2 (1.0)	2 (1.0)	1 (<1)
IRRs, n (%)	18 (8.7)	52 (26.5)	54 (26.7)
— Serious, n (%)	0 (0.0)	0 (0.0)	1 (<1)

Table 3. Cont.

Safety Profile	PBO+MTX[b]	OCR200+MTX[b]	OCR500+MTX[b]
Infections, n (%)	106 (51.2)	101 (51.5)	105 (52.0)
— Serious, n (%)	6 (2.9)	5 (2.6)	10 (5.0)
Malignancies, n (%)	2 (1.0)	0 (0.0)	1 (<1)

Abbreviations: AE, adverse event; DMARD, disease-modifying antirheumatic drug; IR, inadequate responder; IRR, infusion-related reaction; MTX, methotrexate; OCR200, ocrelizumab 200 mg×2; OCR500, ocrelizumab 500 mg×2; PBO, placebo; TNF, tumor necrosis factor.
[a]Multiple events in individual patients were only counted once. Serious infections were defined as those requiring intravenous antibiotics and/or hospitalization or classified as serious by the investigator. Any opportunistic infection was classified as a serious infection.
[b]All patients in all studies received background MTX 7.5 to 25 mg/week (7.5 to 20 mg/week in FILM), except for in SCRIPT, in which MTX or leflunomide was permitted.

of FILM reported a serious IRR, which occurred approximately 12 hours after the second infusion of the second course. This patient experienced weakness, headache, elevated blood pressure and increased heart rate. Following hospitalization, the patient received antihypertensive medication and the elevated blood pressure resolved within 24 hours; the results of an electrocardiogram were normal.

Human Anti-Human Antibodies

At baseline, pre-infusion, 0.6% of all patients were HAHA-positive—a result that was expected given the specificity and sensitivity of the assay used. In all 4 trials, the proportion of patients who developed HAHAs during the DBPC periods was low and comparable between the OCR+MTX and PBO+MTX groups. In FILM, the incidence of HAHAs over 52 weeks was 4/202 (2.0%), 2/194 (1.0%), and 8/201 (4.0%) in the PBO+MTX, OCR200+MTX and OCR500+MTX groups, respectively. The corresponding HAHA incidences in SCRIPT over 48 weeks were 5/274 (1.8%), 8/273 (2.9%) and 7/277 (2.5%), respectively, and in STAGE were 9/318 (2.8%), 16/338 (4.7%) and 7/339 (2.1%), respectively. In FEATURE, the HAHA incidence ranged from 0% in patients who received PBO followed by OCR 200 mg×2 to 10.7% (3/28) in patients who received PBO followed by OCR 400 mg×1. Among all patients who were HAHA-positive post-baseline, there was no apparent association between HAHA positivity and corresponding CD19 counts or DAS28 scores in any of the treatment groups across the 4 trials. Of the 3 patients who experienced a serious IRR, none was HAHA-positive at any time point tested; of the patients who were HAHA-positive, 4 experienced IRRs—all grade 1 or 2.

Serious Infections

In the DBPC periods of FILM, SCRIPT and STAGE, the rates of SIEs (events per 100 patient-years) were higher in the OCR500+MTX group than in the PBO+MTX group (Figure 2). SIE rates were comparable between the OCR200+MTX and PBO+MTX groups in these trials, with the exception of SCRIPT. In SCRIPT, there was also a numerically higher rate of SIEs with OCR200+MTX. The most common types of SIEs in all trials were respiratory tract infections (most frequently pneumonia), cellulitis and urinary tract infections.

A meta-analysis of SIEs was conducted. Following pooling of data by treatment group, the weighted difference in incidence rate per 100 patient-years from PBO in patients with SIEs was significantly higher with OCR500+MTX (2.4; 95% CI, 0.3–4.5) but not with OCR200+MTX (0.6; 95% CI, −1.3 to 2.4) (Figure 3, A and B).

SIE rates by region for the individual studies (Asia versus Rest of World) showed that SIE rates were particularly high in patients recruited in Asia treated with OCR500+MTX (Figure 4). To explore this further, individual patient data from the larger studies was pooled (STAGE, SCRIPT and FILM) and an exploratory COX regression analysis of risk factors for SIEs was performed. After adjustment for all risk factors in the final model, the following results were found: prior cardiac disease (hazard ratio [HR], 2.29; 95% CI, 1.37–3.83; p = 0.002); use of oral corticosteroids at baseline (HR, 1.69; 95% CI, 1.08–2.65; p = 0.022); history of diabetes (HR, 1.77; 95% CI, 1.02–3.05; p = 0.041); treatment group (relative to PBO+MTX; OCR200+MTX [HR, 1.30; 95% CI, 0.76–2.24; p = 0.341] and OCR500+MTX [HR, 1.87; 95% CI, 1.13–3.11; p = 0.016]); and body weight (≤47.5 kg [5th percentile] relative to >47.5 kg; HR, 2.02; 95% CI, 1.00–4.67; p = 0.049). In addition, after adjustment for these risk factors, patients recruited in Asia appeared to have a higher risk of SIEs compared with those recruited outside of Asia (HR [Asia vs non-Asia] 1.78; 95% CI, 1.03–3.06; p = 0.039). It was not possible to determine whether this effect was driven by race or region because an overwhelming majority of Asian patients were recruited from

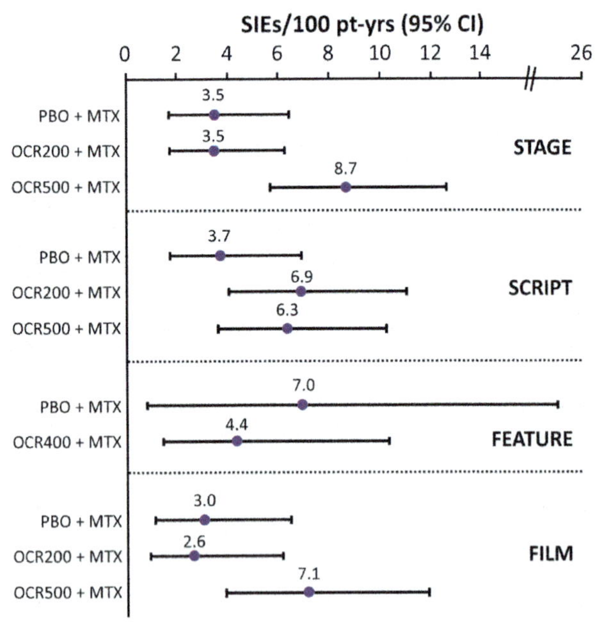

Figure 2. Rates of serious infectious events (SIEs) in the double-blind, placebo-controlled periods. Multiple occurrences of the same event in one individual were counted multiple times. MTX, methotrexate; OCR200, ocrelizumab 200 mg×2; OCR500, ocrelizumab 500 mg×2; PBO, placebo; pt-yrs, patient-years.

A.

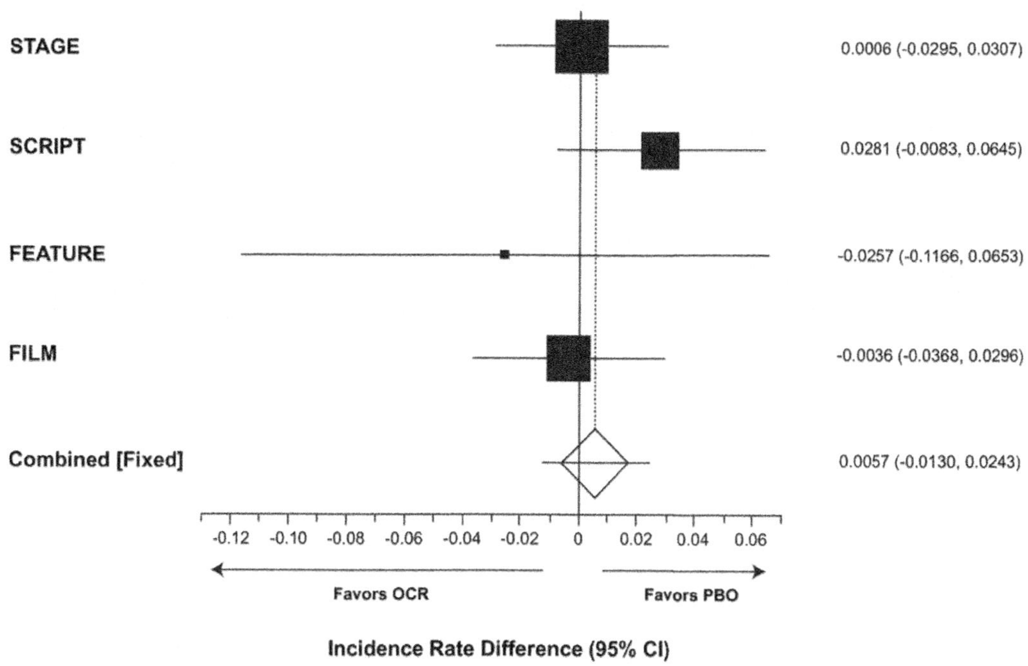

B.

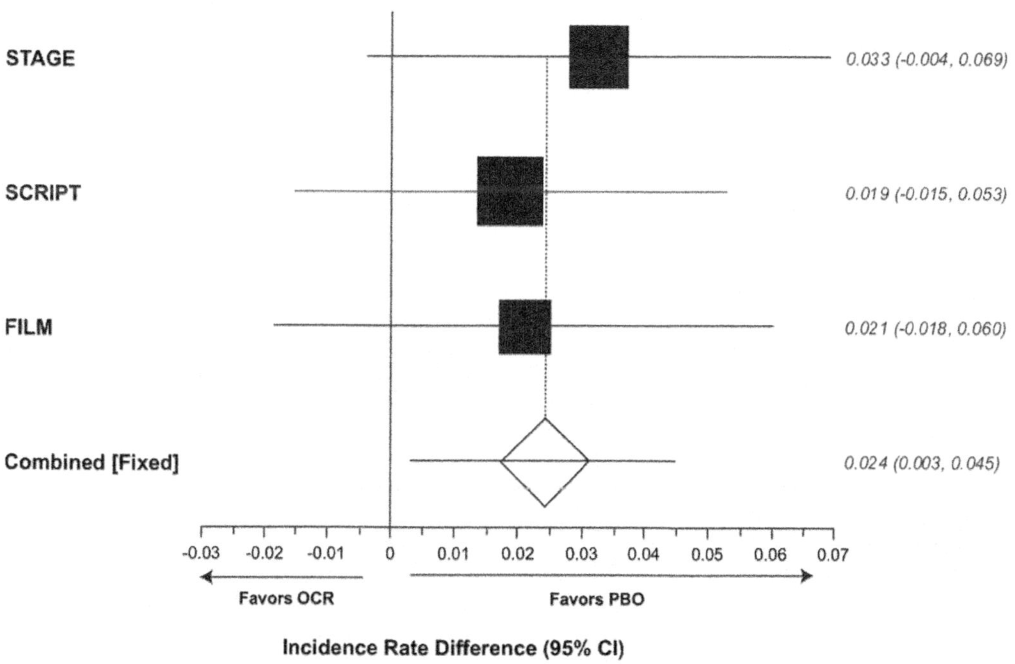

Figure 3. Fixed-effects meta-analysis of incidence rate differences in serious infectious events (SIEs). (A) OCR200+MTX; (B) OCR500+MTX. The pooled rate difference accounts for study and is weighted according to the inverse of the estimated variance. These analyses are based on patients with at least one event (does not count all events). Zero indicates no difference, and a positive value indicates that ocrelizumab (OCR) is worse. MTX, methotrexate; OCR200, ocrelizumab 200 mg×2; OCR500, ocrelizumab 500 mg×2; PBO, placebo.

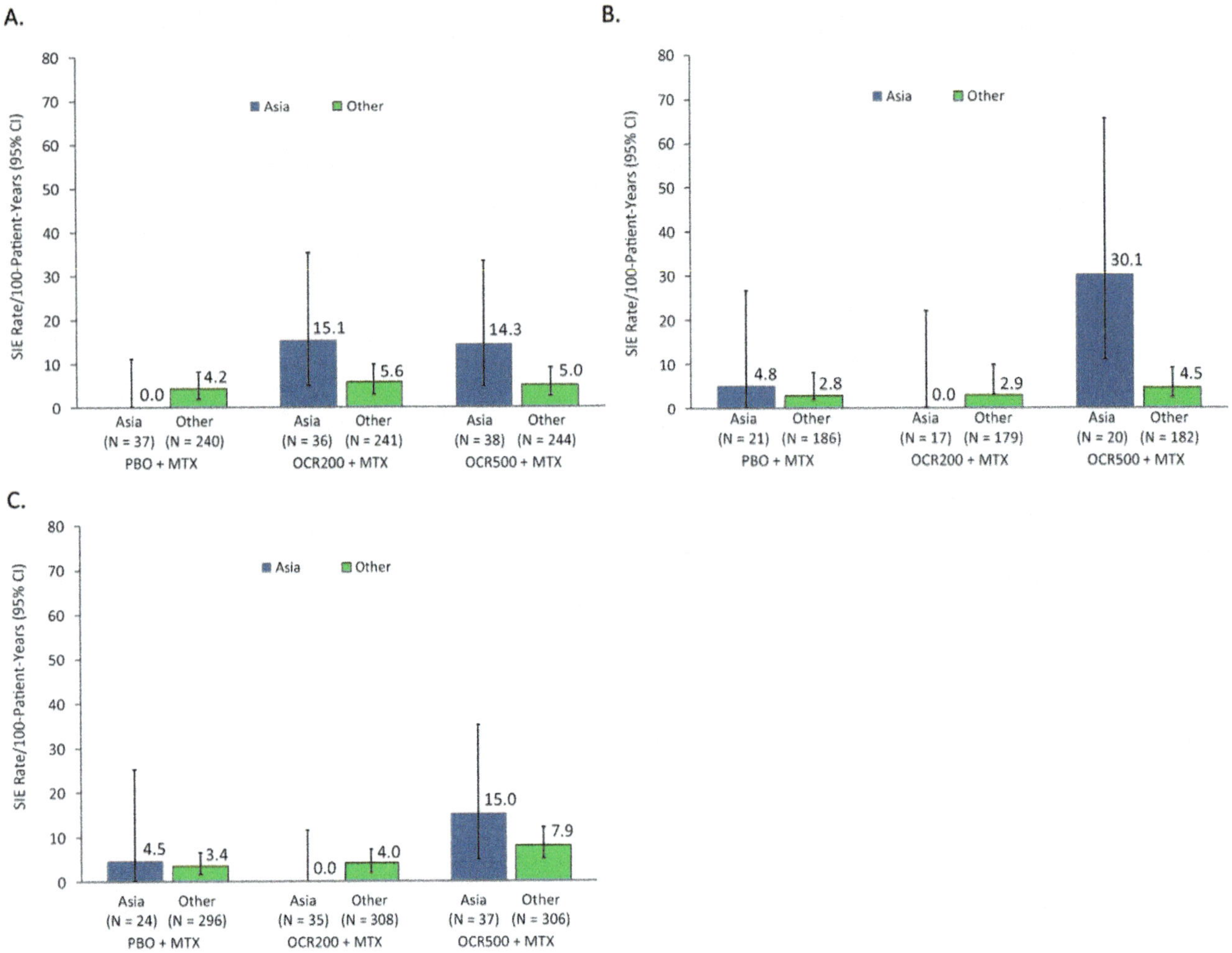

Figure 4. Rates of serious infectious events (SIEs) by region. (A) STAGE; (B) SCRIPT; (C) FILM. MTX, methotrexate; OCR200, ocrelizumab 200 mg×2; OCR500, ocrelizumab 500 mg×2; PBO, placebo. "Asia" includes China, Hong Kong, Indonesia, Malaysia, Philippines, Republic of Korea, Singapore, Taiwan, Thailand and Japan; "Other" includes North and South America, Europe and South Africa.

the Asian region. Study was not significant in the model after adjustment for the risk factors specified. In the exploratory model analyses, there were no statistically significant treatment interactions, including a nonsignificant interaction between Asia and treatment.

Data from the long-term SFU of patients during B-cell depletion post-OCR treatment indicated that the incidence of SIEs decreased over time, and the previously identified imbalance in SIEs in the pivotal studies (STAGE and SCRIPT) in the OCR500+MTX group disappeared. Rates of SIEs in Asian countries also decreased over the long-term follow-up, although it should be noted that the Asian groups consisted of small numbers of patients, and the CIs were wide and overlapped with those of the non-Asian population.

Opportunistic Infections

A total of 10 opportunistic infections were recorded during the DBPC period. One occurred in the PBO+MTX group (*Mycobacterium abscessus* on the thigh in a patient from Thailand), 5 in the OCR200+MTX group (de novo pulmonary tuberculosis [n = 2; Mexico], hepatitis B reactivation [Japan], *Mycobacterium kansasii* infection [Germany] and histoplasmosis [United States]) and 4 in the OCR500+MTX group (*Pneumocystis jiroveci* [Japan], esophageal candidiasis [France], *Varicella* pneumonia [South Korea] and systemic *Candida* infection [South Korea]). No cases of progressive multifocal leukoencephalopathy were recorded, and no fatal outcomes resulted from opportunistic infection. The patient with hepatitis B virus reactivation tested negative for hepatitis B surface antigen, positive for hepatitis B core antibody and negative for hepatitis B virus DNA at the time of enrollment. Approximately 300 patients with this serologic status for hepatitis B virus were enrolled in the RA program, and no other cases of hepatitis B reactivation were observed.

Malignancies

Pooled long-term follow-up data (of up to 5 years) from the four studies showed that the rate of malignancies per 100 patient-years was 1.18 (95% CI, 0.61–2.06) in the PBO+MTX group (n = 865; 1018 patient-years), 1.51 (95% CI, 0.99–2.19) in the OCR200+MTX group (n = 1121; 1792 patient-years) and 1.41 (95% CI, 1.07–1.83) in the OCR 500+MTX group (n = 1849; 4034 patient-years). The rate of all active treatments combined (n = 2434; 5826

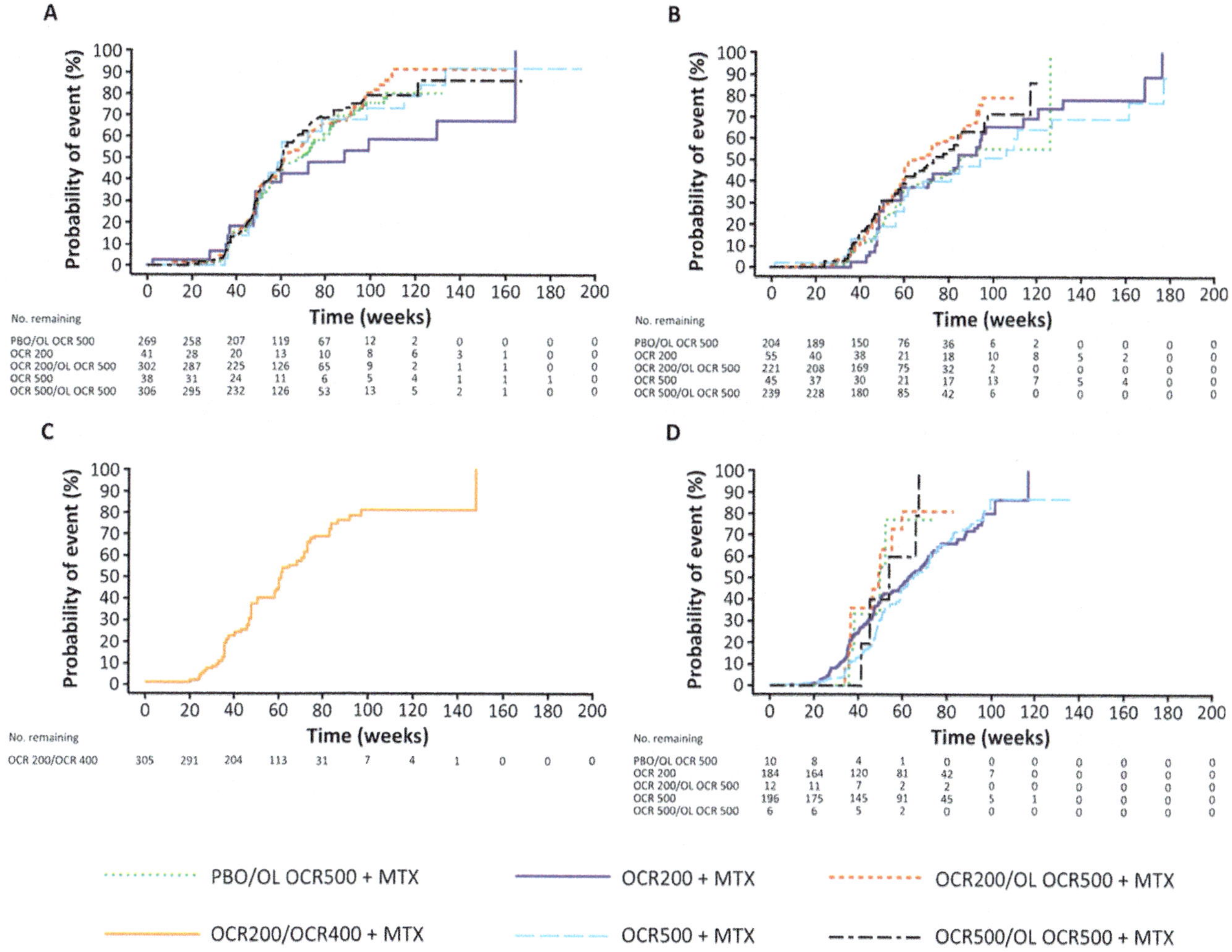

Figure 5. Cumulative probability of B-cell repletion in each clinical trial. (A) STAGE; (B) SCRIPT; (C) FEATURE and (D) FILM. B-cell repletion was defined as a return of CD19+ levels to baseline or 80 cells/µL, whichever was lower. Data summarized under the PBO/OL OCR500+MTX, OCR200/OL OCR500+MTX and OCR500/OL OCR500+MTX treatment groups are OL data only. The x-axis represents the number of weeks since the first infusion of the last course of OCR. MTX, methotrexate; OCR200, ocrelizumab 200 mg×2; OCR500, ocrelizumab 500 mg×2; OL, open-label; PBO, placebo.

patient-years) was 1.44 (95% CI, 1.15–1.78). In summary, these pooled analyses revealed no differences in the rate of malignancies between treatment groups.

Deaths

Overall, 10 deaths occurred during the DBPC periods (Table 3). The 4 deaths in the PBO+MTX groups were due to acute myocardial infarction (n = 2), congestive cardiac failure (n = 1) and rheumatoid vasculitis (n = 1). Of the 6 fatalities among OCR+ MTX-treated patients, 4 occurred in patients receiving the OCR500 dose (1 each due to respiratory failure, sepsis, acute myocardial infarction and ischemic stroke) and 2 in patients receiving the OCR200 dose (1 each due to hemorrhagic stroke and acute respiratory failure).

Pharmacodynamics

In all 4 trials, following the initiation of OCR treatment, a rapid depletion of CD19+ B cells was observed in the OCR200+MTX and OCR500+MTX groups as early as the first post-dose evaluation time point at week 2, in contrast with the PBO+ MTX groups. Kaplan-Meier curves of times to B-cell repletion (return of CD19+ levels to baseline or ≥80 cells/µl, whichever was lower) in each of the 4 studies are shown in Figure 5. Data from FILM allowed evaluation of the potential dose effect (after 2–4 courses) on B-cell repletion. No clinically meaningful difference was observed in the median time to B-cell repletion from the first dose of the last course between the OCR200+MTX (63.6 weeks; 95% CI, 53–72) and OCR500+MTX (66.1 weeks; 95% CI, 60–73) groups. In addition, the median times to B-cell repletion were similar between the OCR200+MTX and OCR500+MTX groups in the DBPC period of FILM and between the OCR200/OL OCR500+MTX and OCR500/OL OCR500+MTX groups in the open-label extension of STAGE, respectively, suggesting that a greater number of OCR re-treatments were not associated with a longer repletion time. A slightly more prolonged B-cell repletion profile was observed in SCRIPT when compared with the other studies; this may be related to this patient population having more severe, long-term disease with multiple previous treatments. There was no indication that the time to B-cell repletion in patients recruited in Asia was different from that in patients recruited outside Asia.

Discussion

This report summarizes the safety results from the 4 phase III trials conducted with OCR in patients with RA. The majority of the population studied included patients with long-standing RA, who had been using numerous immunosuppressive treatments in the past and at least one immunosuppressive agent in combination with OCR during participation in the studies. Approximately one-third of the population studied previously received biological DMARDs and more than one-half of the patients were concomitantly receiving systemic corticosteroids. These factors have to be taken into consideration when interpreting safety data from the OCR clinical trial program in RA.

Although the overall safety profiles were generally comparable between the PBO+MTX and both OCR+MTX dose groups, an imbalance in the incidence of SIEs during the DBPC periods was observed in the OCR500+MTX group. A meta-analysis of SIEs in the DBPC treatment periods indicated a significantly higher rate of SIEs among patients who were treated with OCR500+MTX when compared with PBO+MTX. This was not observed with the lower dose studied. Other factors associated with risk of SIEs were prior cardiac disease, use of oral corticosteroids at baseline, and history of diabetes. Patients recruited in Asia were also at a higher risk of SIEs than were those recruited outside of Asia. Because nearly all Asian patients were recruited in the Asian region, we were unable to distinguish between geographic effects and ethnicity. In addition, the low number of SIEs in the DBPC period meant that we had limited statistical power in the analyses of interactions of risk factors, such as Asian region with treatment.

Confounding factors may have contributed to the higher incidence of opportunistic infections (9 cases across the OCR+MTX groups: 5 cases in the OCR200+MTX group and 4 cases in the OCR500+MTX group compared with a single case in the PBO group) such as endemic areas for histoplasmosis in the United States, tuberculosis in Mexico, and hepatitis B in Japan. In addition, the patient with *Candida* infections was receiving high-dose steroid treatment for concurrent medical conditions.

The clinical development of OCR was initiated in part with the aim of evaluating the potential safety advantage of a humanized molecule over chimeric antibodies. Humanization may be expected to reduce the incidence of anti-drug antibody responses. The incidence of HAHAs was low across the 4 trials (<5%) and, in general, comparable between the pooled OCR+MTX and PBO+MTX groups. There was no association between IRRs and development of HAHAs. In addition, there were no clear differences in the incidence of HAHAs when single-infusion and dual-infusion OCR were compared, although, because the patient numbers in FEATURE were small, the question of whether a difference exists between single- and dual-infusion OCR remains open. In a previous pooled analysis of approximately 2500 patients in the rituximab RA clinical trial program, 11% of those treated with rituximab developed human anti-chimeric antibodies [8].

As expected, both doses of OCR rapidly depleted B cells shortly after infusion. The question was whether the higher rates of serious infections seen in patients treated with OCR500+MTX could have been explained, in part, by differences in B-cell depletion/repletion profiles between the higher and lower doses. It should be noted that evaluation of B-cell levels in clinical trials is limited by measurement of peripheral CD19 counts only; however, the analyses suggested that there was no difference in time to peripheral B-cell repletion between the OCR500 and OCR200 doses. Moreover, the number of repeat treatment courses also did not seem to have a clinically meaningful effect on time to B-cell repletion.

The conclusion that the two doses of OCR, in combination with MTX tested in the RA clinical trials did not demonstrate a superior benefit-risk profile compared with available treatments led to the termination of the clinical development program of OCR in RA. OCR500+MTX demonstrated clinical benefit by improving signs and symptoms of RA and radiographic outcomes [10–13]; however this dose was associated with an increased incidence of SIEs. OCR200+MTX did not show superior efficacy compared with existing therapies, but was safe and well-tolerated.

The clinical development of OCR is continuing in multiple sclerosis, for which there remains an unmet need for more effective therapies and background immunosuppressant therapy is not used. A phase II study in multiple sclerosis reported good efficacy and safety data, with no imbalance in serious infections between PBO and OCR (maximum dose up to 1000 mg×2 for 24 weeks) [14]. Phase III studies are continuing and, because of the low prevalence of multiple sclerosis in Asia, no investigational sites in that region have been included.

Acknowledgments

The authors and sponsors thank all patients and investigators for their contributions to the ocrelizumab RA clinical trials. Support for third party writing assistance was provided by F. Hoffmann-La Roche.

Author Contributions

Conceived and designed the experiments: PE WR PPT CM LM HT EF. Performed the experiments: PE WR CM LM EF. Analyzed the data: PE WR CM LM HT EF. Contributed reagents/materials/analysis tools: PE WR PPT TD EO. Wrote the paper: PE WR PPT TD EO CM LM HT EF.

References

1. Dörner T, Kinnman N, Tak PP (2010) Targeting B cells in immune-mediated inflammatory disease: a comprehensive review of mechanisms of action and identification of biomarkers. Pharmacol Ther 125: 464–475.
2. Silverman GJ, Carson DA (2003) Roles of B cells in rheumatoid arthritis. Arthritis Res Ther 5: S1–6.
3. Cohen SB, Emery P, Greenwald MW, Dougados M, Furie RA, et al. (2006) Rituximab for rheumatoid arthritis refractory to anti-tumor necrosis factor therapy: Results of a multicenter, randomized, double-blind, placebo-controlled, phase III trial evaluating primary efficacy and safety at twenty-four weeks. Arthritis Rheum 54: 2793–2806.
4. Edwards JC, Szczepanski L, Szechinski J, Filipowicz-Sosnowska A, Emery P, et al. (2004) Efficacy of B-cell-targeted therapy with rituximab in patients with rheumatoid arthritis. N Engl J Med 350: 2572–2581.
5. Emery P, Fleischmann R, Filipowicz-Sosnowska A, Schechtman J, Szczepanski L, et al. (2006) The efficacy and safety of rituximab in patients with active rheumatoid arthritis despite methotrexate treatment: Results of a phase IIB randomized, double-blind, placebo-controlled, dose-ranging trial. Arthritis Rheum 54: 1390–1400.
6. Emery P, Deodhar A, Rigby WF, Isaacs JD, Combe B, et al. (2010) Efficacy and safety of different doses and retreatment of rituximab: A randomised, placebo-controlled trial in patients who are biologic naive with active rheumatoid arthritis and an inadequate response to methotrexate (Study Evaluating Rituximab's Efficacy in MTX iNadequate rEsponders (SERENE)). Ann Rheum Dis 69: 1629–1635.
7. Rubbert-Roth A, Tak PP, Zerbini C, Tremblay JL, Carreño L, et al. (2010) Efficacy and safety of various repeat treatment dosing regimens of rituximab in patients with active rheumatoid arthritis: Results of a Phase III randomized study (MIRROR). Rheumatology (Oxford) 49: 1683–1693.

8. van Vollenhoven RF, Emery P, Bingham CO III, Keystone EC, Fleischmann R, et al. (2010) Long term safety of patients receiving rituximab in rheumatoid arthritis clinical trials. J Rheumatol 37: 558–567.
9. van Vollenhoven RF, Emery P, Bingham CO III, Keystone E, Fleischmann R, et al. (2012) Long-term safety of rituximab in rheumatoid arthritis: 9.5-year follow-up of the global clinical trial programme with focus on adverse events of interest in RA patients. Ann Rheum Dis [Epub ahead of print].
10. Rigby W, Tony HP, Oelke K, Combe B, Laster A, et al. (2012) Safety and efficacy of ocrelizumab in patients with rheumatoid arthritis and an inadequate response to methotrexate: Results of a forty-eight-week randomized, double-blind, placebo-controlled, parallel-group phase III trial. Arthritis Rheum 64: 350–359.
11. Tak PP, Mease PJ, Genovese MC, Kremer J, Haraoui B, et al. (2012) Safety and efficacy of ocrelizumab in patients with rheumatoid arthritis and an inadequate response to at least one tumor necrosis factor inhibitor: Results of a forty-eight-week randomized, double-blind, placebo-controlled, parallel-group phase III trial. Arthritis Rheum 64: 360–370.
12. Stohl W, Gomez-Reino J, Olech E, Dudler J, Fleischmann RM, et al. (2012) Safety and efficacy of ocrelizumab in combination with methotrexate in MTX-naive subjects with rheumatoid arthritis: The phase III FILM trial. Ann Rheum Dis 71: 1289–1296.
13. Huffstutter JE, Taylor J, Schechtman J, Leszczynski P, Brzosko M, et al. (2011) Single versus dual infusion of B cell depleting antibody ocrelizumab (humanized aCD20) in rheumatoid arthritis: Results from the Phase III FEATURE trial. Int J Clin Rheumatol 6: 689–696.
14. Kappos L, Li D, Calabresi PA, O'Connor P, Bar-Or A, et al. (2011) Ocrelizumab in relapsing-remitting multiple sclerosis: A phase 2, randomised, placebo-controlled, multicentre trial. Lancet 378: 1779–1787.

7

A Potential Role of Myeloid DAP12-Associating Lectin (MDL)-1 in the Regulation of Inflammation in Rheumatoid Arthritis Patients

Der-Yuan Chen[1,2,3,4,5], Ling Yao[2]ᵠ, Yi-Ming Chen[1,2]ᵠ, Chi-Chen Lin[3], Kui-Chou Huang[6], Szu-Ting Chen[5], Joung-Liang Lan[1,2,7,8]*, Shie-Liang Edmond Hsieh[5,9]*

1 Faculty of Medicine, National Yang-Ming University, Taipei, Taiwan, R.O.C., **2** Division of Allergy, Immunology and Rheumatology, Taichung Veterans General Hospital, Taichung, Taiwan, R.O.C., **3** Institute of Biomedical Science, National Chung-Hsing University, Taichung, Taiwan, R.O.C., **4** Institute of Microbiology and Immunology, Chung Shan Medical University, Taichung, Taiwan, R.O.C., **5** Infection and Immunity Research Center, National Yang-Ming University, Taipei, Taiwan, R.O.C., **6** Department of Orthopedics and Traumatology, Taichung Veterans General Hospital, Taichung, Taiwan, R.O.C., **7** Division of Immunology and Rheumatology, China Medical University Hospital, Taichung, Taiwan, R.O.C., **8** College of Chinese Medicine, China Medical University, Taichung, Taiwan, R.O.C., **9** Institute of Clinical Medicine, National Yang-Ming University, Taipei City, Taiwan

Abstract

The pathogenic roles of myeloid DAP12-associating lectin-1(MDL-1) and DAP12 in human rheumatoid arthritis (RA) remain unknown. Frequencies of MDL-1-expressing monocytes in 22 active RA patients, 16 inactive RA patients, 12 osteoarthritis (OA) patients and 10 healthy controls (HC) were determined by flow-cytometry analysis. The mRNA expression levels of MDL-1 and DAP12 on PBMCs were evaluated by quantitative PCR, and their protein expression levels in the synovium were examined by immunohistochemistry. Significantly higher median percentages of circulating MDL-1-expressing monocytes were observed in active RA patients (53.6%) compared to inactive RA patients (34.1%), OA patients (27.9%), and HC (21.2%). Levels of MDL-1 and DAP12 gene expression in PBMCs and their protein expression in the synovium were significantly higher in active RA patients than in inactive RA or OA patients. MDL-1 levels were positively correlated with parameters of disease activity, articular damage, and levels of proinflammatory cytokines. MDL-1 activator (Dengue virus type 2 antigen) stimulation on PBMCs resulted in significantly enhanced levels of proinflammatory cytokines in RA patients compared to those in OA patients or HC, indicating that MDL-1 activation is functional. Frequencies of MDL-1-expressing monocytes and levels of MDL-1 and DAP12 gene expression significantly decreased after effective therapy. Concordant overexpression of MDL-1 and DAP12 were correlated with increased production of proinflammatory cytokines in RA patients, suggesting their roles in regulating articular inflammation.

Editor: Oliver Frey, University Hospital Jena, Germany

Funding: This work was supported by a grant (TCVGH-YM1000204) from Taichung Veterans General Hospital and National Yang-Ming University. The funders had no role in study design, data collection and analysis, decision to publish, or preparation of the manuscript.

Competing Interests: The authors have declared that no competing interests exist.

* E-mail: dychen@vghtc.gov.tw (JLL); slhsieh@ym.edu.tw (SLEH)

ᵠ These authors contributed equally to this work.

Introduction

Rheumatoid arthritis (RA) is a chronic inflammatory disease characterized by the infiltration of macrophages and T cells into the joints, synovial hyperplasia, and bone erosions associated with excessive osteoclast activity [1–2]. Results of recent studies show that the osteoclastogenesis induced by receptor activator of NF-κB (RANK)-RANK ligand (RANKL) is augmented through the immunoreceptor tyrosine-based activation motif (ITAM)-harboring signaling pathway [3–4]. In addition, macrophage-derived proinflammatory cytokines such as tumor necrosis factor (TNF)-α, interleukin (IL)-1β, and IL-6, are crucial mediators in rheumatoid synovitis and subsequent bone destruction in RA [5–6]. IL-17A can stimulate monocytes to produce proinflammatory cytokines, and thus amplify the inflammatory cascade [7]. Additionally, enhanced expression of IL-17 has been observed in rheumatoid synovium [8]. Accumulating evidence shows that alterations in proinflammatory cytokines are viewed as both a possible important pathogenic factor and a potential target for therapeutic intervention in RA [9–13].

The ITAM-dependent signaling pathway is an important "co-stimulatory" pathway for RANKL-dependent regulation of bone remodeling [14–15]. DNAX activation protein 12 (DAP12), a type I transmembrane homodimer [16], is a novel ITAM-bearing signaling glycoprotein that has been implicated in immune responses and in osteoclast formation [17–18]. DAP12 expression has also been demonstrated to be increased in the synovium of active RA patients [19]. Myeloid DAP12-associated lectin-1 (MDL-1) is a C-type lectin domain family 5-member A (CLEC5A) and contains a charged residue in the transmembrane region that enables it to bind with DAP12 [20–21]. MDL-1 associates non-covalently with adaptor DAP12 to form receptor complexes involved in inflammatory responses [21]. Recent studies show that MDL-1 is highly expressed on TNF-activated monocytes [20] and

Table 1. Clinical characteristics and laboratory findings in patients with active rheumatoid arthritis (RA), inactive RA, patients with knee osteoarthritis (OA) and healthy controls (HC).

	Active RA (n = 22)	Inactive RA (n = 16)	Knee OA (n = 12)	HC (n = 10)
Mean age (years)	50.3±10.4	56.9±17.5	58.3±5.6	52.0±8.3
Female (%)	18 (81.8%)	12 (75.0%)	10 (83.3%)	7 (70.0%)
RF positivity (%)	16 (72.7%)	12 (75.0%)	NA	NA
Anti-CCP positivity (%)	15 (68.2%)	10 (62.5%)	NA	NA
CRP (mg/dl)	2.54±1.91*	0.43±0.25	NA	NA
DAS-28	4.94±0.95*	2.90±0.30	NA	NA
Daily steroid dose (mg)	5.2±2.0*	2.5±1.3	NA	NA
DMARDs used				
Methotrexate	19 (86.4%)	11 (68.8%)	NA	NA
Sulfasalazine	17 (77.3%)	10 (62.5%)	NA	NA
Hydroxychloroquine	16 (72.7%)	8 (50.0%)	NA	NA
Cyclosporine	4 (18.2%)	0 (0.0%)	NA	NA

Data are presented as mean ± SD or number (percentage); NA: not applicable.
RF: rheumatoid factor; Anti-CCP: anti-cyclic citrullinated peptide antibodies; CRP: C-reactive protein; DAS28: disease activity score for 28-joints; DMARDs: disease-modifying anti-rheumatic drugs.
A result was considered positive for RF when the concentration was ≥15 IU/ml; a result was considered positive for anti-CCP antibodies if the titer was ≥20 IU/ml.
*p<0.001, versus inactive RA group, determined using the Mann-Whitney U test.

acts as a key regulator of synovitis and bone erosion in murine arthritis [22]. Cross-linking of MDL-1 receptors induces DAP12-ITAM-dependent calcium mobilization [17,20] and activation of spleen tyrosine kinase (Syk) [4,17].

Recently, the roles of MDL-1 and its associated adaptor-DAP12 were highlighted in a study of murine arthritis [22]. Joyce-Shaikh *et al.* demonstrated that activation of MDL-1 receptors during joint inflammation enhanced myeloid cell infiltration and promoted expression of proinflammatory cytokines including IL-1β, IL-6, IL-17A, and TNF-α, resulting in cartilage damage and bone erosion [22]. In contrast, the functional blockade of MDL-1 receptor via MDL-1 deletion reduced the clinical signs of murine arthritis [22]. Chen *et al.* also observed that the knockdown of MDL-1/CLEC5A suppressed the release of proinflammmatory cytokines by Dengue virus (DV)-infected macrophages [23]. These results suggest that therapeutic targeting of the MDL-1 receptor may inhibit both synovitis and the bone destructive pathway during inflammatory conditions. However, there is no data concerning the role of MDL-1 in the pathogenesis of human RA.

In this study, we investigated the percentages of circulating MDL-1-expressing monocytes using flow-cytometry analysis, and analyzed serum levels of markers for systemic inflammation and proinflammatory cytokines in RA patients, OA patients, and healthy control subjects. The mRNA expression levels of MDL-1 and its associated adaptor-DAP12 on peripheral blood mononuclear cells (PBMCs) were examined by quantitative PCR (qPCR). In addition, the expression levels of MDL-1 and DAP12 in synovial membrane (SM) were determined by immunohistochemistry (IHC). The relationship between MDL-1 expression levels and parameters of disease activity was also evaluated for all RA patients.

Materials and Methods

Subjects

A total of 38 consecutive patients who fulfilled the 2010 RA classification criteria of the American College of Rheumatology (ACR)/European League Against Rheumatism (EULAR) collaborative initiative [24] were enrolled in this study. Early RA was defined as RA with a symptom duration ≦2 years [25]. Disease activity was assessed by the 28-joint disease activity score (DAS28) [26]. Inactive RA, known as RA with low disease activity, is defined as a DAS28 ≦3.2 [27]. Radiographs of both hands and feet were assessed for erosions and joint space narrowing (JSN) using the Genant modified total Sharp score (range 0–290) [28] by two independent readers blinded to laboratory data. Twelve patients who fulfilled the 1986 ACR criteria for knee osteoarthritis (OA) [29] were included as controls. Ten age-matched healthy volunteers, who had no rheumatic disease, were used as normal controls.

Ethics Statement

This study was approved by the Institutional Review Board of Taichung Veterans General Hospital, and written consent was obtained from all participants according to the Declaration of Helsinki.

Quantitation of MDL-1-expressing Cells Using Flow Cytometry Analysis

To quantify expression levels of MDL-1, 1000 µl samples of whole blood were obtained and stained with phycoerythrin (PE)-conjugated anti-MDL-1 mAb (R&D Systems, Minneapolis, MN, USA) and Phycoerythrin-Cyanin 5 (PC5)-conjugated anti-CD14 mAb (Beckman Coulter, Brea, CA, USA) according to protocols of the respective manufacturers. Fluorescent antibodies, mouse IgG2b-PE (R&D Systems, Minneapolis, MN, USA) and IgG2a-PC5 (Beckman Coulter, Brea, CA, USA) were used as isotype controls. After incubation for 20 minutes in the dark at room temperature, cells were reacted with 500 µl of OptiLyse C Lysis Solution (Beckman Coulter, USA) for 10 minutes to lyse red blood cells. Then, 500 µl PBS was added into each tube to stop the reaction prior to flow cytometry (Beckman Coulter, Brea, CA, USA) analysis. Monocytes were gated on the basis of CD14+/side

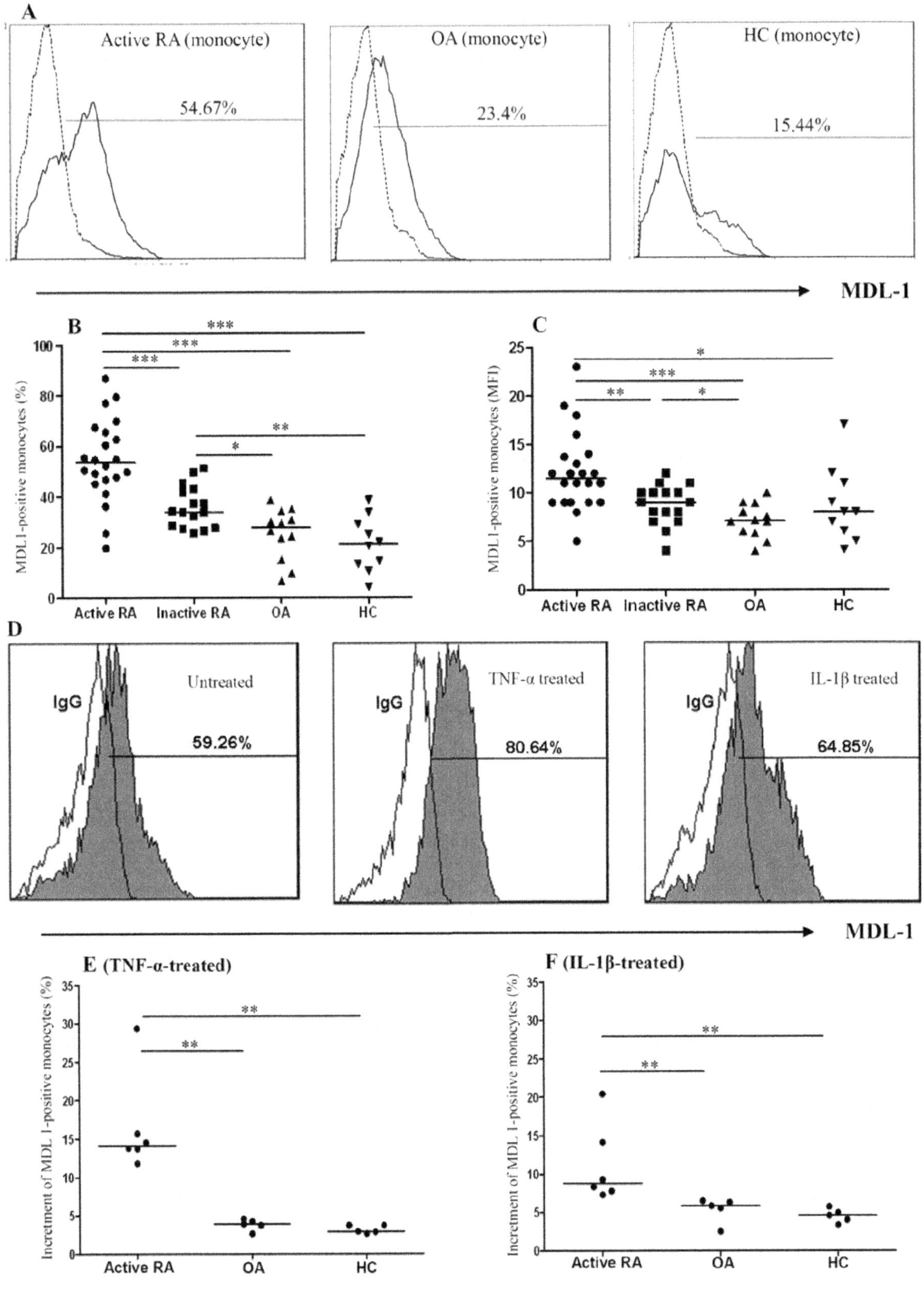

Figure 1. Representative examples of flow cytometric histograms (A) of MDL-1-expressing monocytes obtained from peripheral blood of one active RA patient, one OA patient, and one healthy subject. Comparisons of the percentages and mean fluorescence intensity (MFI) of circulating MDL-1-expressing monocytes are shown for 22 active RA patients, 16 inactive RA patients, 12 OA patients, and 10 healthy control subjects (B and C respectively). To evaluate the effects of TNF-α or IL-1β on MDL-1 expression, we examined changes in the percentages of circulating MDL-1-expressing monocytes in active RA patients, OA patients and healthy subjects. Representative examples of flow cytometric histograms (D) of

MDL-1-expressing monocytes obtained from one active RA patient after stimulation with TNF-α or IL-1β. Comparisons of the increment of the percentages of MDL-1-expressing monocytes after stimulation with TNF-α and IL-1β are shown for 6 active RA patients, 5 OA patients, and 5 healthy subjects (E and F respectively). The middle horizontal line indicates median value for each group. *$p<0.05$, **$p<0.01$, ***$p<0.001$, as determined by Mann-Whitney U test.

scatters (SSC) and at least 2×10^5 total cells from each sample were analyzed.

Quantitative PCR Analysis for mRNA Expression Levels of MDL-1, DAP12, and Proinflammatory Cytokines on PBMCs

PBMCs were immediately isolated from venous blood using Ficoll-Paque^{TM} PLUS (GE Healthcare Biosciences AB, Uppsala, Sweden) density gradient centrifugation. Total cellular RNA was obtained from PBMCs by the guanidinium isothiocyanate method [30]. RNA was quantitated by spectrophotometry at 260 nm. A 2.5 μg RNA aliquot was reverse transcribed with 200U of Moloney murine leukemia virus reverse transcriptase (Fermentas, Thermo Fisher Scientific Inc., MD, USA). The qPCR was performed using the IQ^2 Fast qPCR System (Bio-genesis Technology Inc., Taipei, Taiwan) with a method modified from that described in previous reports [31–32]. The primers utilized in this study were adapted and redesigned based on information published on websites. The following are the oligonucleotide primers used for MDL-1, sense primer 5′-CAATTGTCAA-CACGCCAGAG-3′ and antisense primer 5′-GTC GCA-CAGTTGAAATTCTG-3′; DAP12, sense primer 5′-AGC-GATTGCAGTTGCTC TAC-3′ and antisense primer 5′-GTGATACGCTGTTTCCGGGT-3′; IL-1β, sense primer 5′-GCTGATGGCCCTAAACAGATGAA-3′ and antisense primer 5′-TGA AGCCCTTGCTGTAGTGGTG-3′; IL-6, sense primer 5′-AAGCCAGAGCTGTC AGATGAGTA-3′ and antisense primer 5′-TGT CCTGCAGCCACTGGTTC-3′; IL-17A, sense primer 5′-TGTCCACCATGTGGCCTAAGAG-3′ and antisense primer 5′-GTCCGAAATGAGGCTGTCTTTGA-3′; TNF-α, sense primer 5′-CCACTTCGA AACCTGGGATTC -3′ and antisense primer 5′-TTAGTGGTTGCCAGCACT TCA-3′; the housekeeping gene GAPDH, sense primer 5′-GAAGGT-GAAGGTC GGAGTC-3′ and antisense primer 5′-GAA-GATGGTGATGGGATTTC-3′. PCR was performed in a total volume of 10.0 μL containing 10 ng of cDNA, 5 μL 2x IQ2 Fast qPCR System Master Mix, 0.375 μL of each oligonucleotide primer, and RNase-free water. Amplification cycles were performed at 95°C for 10 min, followed by 40 cycles of denaturation at 95°C for 10 s, annealing and extension at 60 °C for 30 s. The purity of PCR products was assessed by dissociation curve plots. To standardize mRNA expression levels of MDL-1 and DAP12, the expression levels of the housekeeping gene GAPDH were determined in parallel with each sample. The relative expression levels of MDL-1 and DAP12 were calculated using the comparative threshold cycle (Ct) method and evaluated using $2^{-\Delta\Delta Ct}$, where $\Delta\Delta Ct$ = Patent ($Ct_{\text{target gene}}-Ct_{\text{GAPDH}}$)–Mean of controls ($Ct_{\text{target gene}}-Ct_{\text{GAPDH}}$) [33].

Determination of Levels of Proinflammatory Cytokines Using ELISA

Serum levels of TNF-α, IL-6, and IL-17A were determined in 22 active RA patients, 16 inactive RA patients, 12 OA patients and 10 healthy control subjects using ELISA (PeproTech Inc., Rocky Hill, NJ, USA) according to the manufacturer's instructions. IL-1β levels were determined using ELISA (RayBiotech Inc., Norcross, GA, USA). Levels of supernatant cytokine were determined using the aforementioned ELISA.

Ex Vivo Study to Elucidate Factors Affecting the Expression of MDL-1 and DAP12

Joyce-Shaikh [22] reported that TNF-α but not interferon (IFN)-γ promoted MDL-1 expression in murine arthritis. To elucidate probable factors affecting MDL-1 expression in human RA, we examined changes in percentages of circulating MDL-1-expressing monocytes, and changes in mRNA expression levels of MDL-1 and DAP12 on PBMCs treated with TNF-α (5 μg/ml, R&D Systems Inc., Minneapolis, MN, USA) and IL-1β (5 μg/ml, R&D Systems Inc.) using a method modified from previous reports [22].

Ex Vivo Induction of Cytokines on PBMCs Treated with MDL-1 Activator

To explore the functional role of MDL-1 activation which may have a possible link with DAP12 and inflammatory response in human RA; we examined changes in mRNA expression levels and supernatant levels of downstream cytokines on PBMCs treated with MDL-1 activator using a method modified from previous reports [34]. Based on results of a previous study showing Dengue virus is a potent activator of MDL-1 [23], we used Dengue virus type 2 (DV2)-antigen (20 μg/ml, MyBioSource Inc., San Diego, CA, USA) as the MDL-1 activator [35]. PBMCs were obtained from 6 active RA patients, 5 OA patients, and 5 healthy volunteers, and were re-suspended in RPMI 1640 medium (Thermo Fisher Scientific Inc., Waltham, MA, USA) supplemented with 100 units/ml penicillin, 100 μg/ml streptomycin, and 10% fetal blood serum at a final concentration of 1×10^6 cells/well. PBMC samples were incubated at 37°C in a 5% CO_2 humidified atmosphere for 24 h in the absence or presence of the MDL-1 activator, DV2-antigen (20 μg/ml, MyBioSource Inc.). Changes in mRNA expression levels of MDL-1, DAP12, and downstream cytokines, including IL-1β, IL-6, IL-17A, and TNF-α were determined by the aforementioned method. The cell-free supernatant was harvested, and levels of IL-1β, IL-6, IL-17A, and TNF-α were determined by the aforementioned method.

Immunohistochemistry for MDL-1 and DAP12 Expression on SM

Synovial tissue specimens were obtained during joint replacement surgery or arthroscopic synovectomy for knee arthritis. Immunostaining for MDL-1 and DAP12 on SM was performed as previously described [19] with modifications on samples obtained from 15 active RA patients, 14 inactive RA patients, and 12 OA patients. Paraffin-embedded samples were cut into 4-μm sections, incubated to assist binding to slides, and then deparaffinized in xylene for a total of 20 minutes at 56°C, followed by rehydration through a series of descending ethanol concentrations. Peroxidase blocking with 3% hydrogen peroxide for 10 min and protein blocking with 2% horse serum for 20 min at room temperature were performed. The sections were then washed with PBS and overlaid overnight with a goat monoclonal antibodies against MDL-1 (Abcam, Cambridge, UK) and DAP12 (Santa Cruz Biotechnology, CA, USA) at concentrations of 2 μg/ml. To

Table 2. Levels of circulating MDL-1-expressing monocytes, mRNA expression levels of MDL-1 and DAP12 on PBMCs, and levels of serum proinflammatory cytokines in patients with active rheumatoid arthritis (RA), patients with inactive RA, patients with osteoarthritis (OA) and healthy controls (HC).

MDL-1 and cytokines, patient groups	Median (interquartile range)
MDL-1-expressing monocytes (%)	
Active RA	53.6 (46.4–66.1)***###§§§
Inactive RA	34.1 (27.9–42.7)**#
OA	27.9 (17.1–33.5)
HC	21.2 (12.6–30.2)
MDL-1-expressing monocytes (MFI)	
Active RA	11.5 (9.0–13.8)*###§§
Inactive RA	9.0 (7.3–10.0)#
OA	7.1 (5.8–8.7)
HC	8.0 (5.8–11.3)
MDL-1 transcript levels on PBMCs	
Active RA	1.64 (1.31–2.38)***###§§§
Inactive RA	0.89 (0.64–1.36)#
OA	0.71 (0.50–1.24)
HC	0.99 (0.44–1.29)
DAP12 transcript levels on PBMCs	
Active RA	1.53 (1.09–1.74)**##§§
Inactive RA	1.06 (0.92–1.21)#
OA	0.77 (0.54–1.09)
HC	0.90 (0.67–1.26)
Interleukin-1β (pg/ml)	
Active RA	9.28 (7.88–18.49)***##
Inactive RA	8.93 (8.17–12.84)*** ##
OA	7.53 (6.09–7.94)
HC	4.39 (2.54–7.15)
Interleukin-6 (pg/ml)	
Active RA	1530.1 (921.3–2004.0)*** §§
Inactive RA	754.0 (543.7–1333.2)***
OA	920.9 (476.0–1798.2)***
HC	74.7 (52.7–94.4)
Interleukin-17A (pg/ml)	
Active RA	145.79 (101.83–273.34)*
Inactive RA	114.38 (92.46–181.14)
OA	131.70 (86.81–202.85)
HC	86.57 (51.74–181.08)
Tumor necrosis factor-α (pg/ml)	
Active RA	142.37 (80.45–322.80)*** ###
Inactive RA	95.28 (34.40–155.10)** #
OA	39.54 (16.00–66.46)
HC	24.30 (17.70–35.38)

MDL-1: Myeloid DAP12-associated lectin-1; MFI: mean fluorescence intensity; DAP12: DNAX adaptor protein 12; PBMCs: peripheral blood mononuclear cells; *$p<0.05$, **$p<0.01$, ***$p<0.001$, vs. HC; #$p<0.05$, ##$p<0.01$, ###$p<0.001$, vs. OA;
§$p<0.05$, §§$p<0.01$, §§§$p<0.001$, vs. inactive RA group, were determined by Mann-Whitney U test.

identify the cell types that express MDL-1 and DAP12 in synovial membrane, serial sections were stained with mouse monoclonal antibodies against CD68 (Leica Microsystems, Wetziar, Germany) and mouse monoclonal Ab against CD15 (Leica Microsystems). After washing with PBS, binding of the secondary polymer/HRP anti-goat IgG (Nichirei Biosciences, Tokyo, Japan) was detected using an immunodetection kit (Lab Vision Corporation, Fremont, CA, USA). Negative controls were obtained by using the mouse IgG1 isotype control antibody. Appropriate positive controls were used throughout the study. Then, the specimens were counter-stained with Mayer's hematoxylin, and images were captured with a LEICA DMRBE microscopic/Pixera Digital Camera System (Leitz Microsystems, Wetzlar, Germany). The data of positive staining for MDL-1 and DAP12 within the SM were expressed as mean value/SM cross section area.

Determination of Serum Levels of C-reactive Protein (CRP), Rheumatoid Factor (RF)-IgM and Anti-cyclic Citrullinated Peptide (Anti-CCP) Antibody

Serum levels of CRP and RF-IgM were measured by nephelometry (Dade Behring Inc. Newark, DE, USA). Determination of anti-CCP antibody was performed by ELISA using a commercial kit (INOVA Diagnostics Inc., San Diego, CA, USA).

Statistical Analysis

Results are presented as the mean ± standard deviation (SD) or median (interquartile range). The nonparametric Kruskal-Wallis test was used for comparisons between groups. When this test showed a significant difference, the exact P-value was determined using the Mann-Whitney U test. The correlation coefficient was calculated using the nonparametric Spearman's rank correlation test. The Wilcoxon signed rank test was employed to compare levels of circulating MDL-1-expressing monocytes and the mRNA expression levels of MDL-1 as well as DAP12 during follow-up in RA patients after therapy. A P-value <0.05 was considered statistically significant.

Results

Baseline Characteristics of RA Patients and OA Patients

As illustrated in Table 1, RA patients were stratified into active patients (DAS28, mean±SD, 4.94±0.95) and inactive patients (DAS28, 2.90±0.30). As expected, active RA patients had higher levels of serum CRP and daily doses of oral corticosteroids compared to inactive RA patients. There were no significant differences between active RA patients and inactive RA patients regarding baseline demographic data, positive rates of RF and anti-CCP antibodies, or the proportions of DMARDs used. There were no significant differences in demographic data between RA patients and OA patients.

Percentages of Circulating MDL-1-expressing Monocytes

Representative examples of flow cytometric histograms of MDL-1 expression on monocytes obtained from one active RA patient, one OA patient, and one healthy volunteer are shown in Figure 1A. Significantly higher percentages of MDL-1-expressing monocytes were observed in active RA patients compared to inactive RA patients, OA patients, or healthy control subjects (Figure 1B and Table 2). Similarly, significantly higher mean fluorescence intensity (MFI) of MDL-1 staining on monocytes was observed in active RA patients compared to inactive RA patients, OA patients, or healthy control subjects (Figure 1C). The percentages of MDL-1-expressing monocytes were significantly

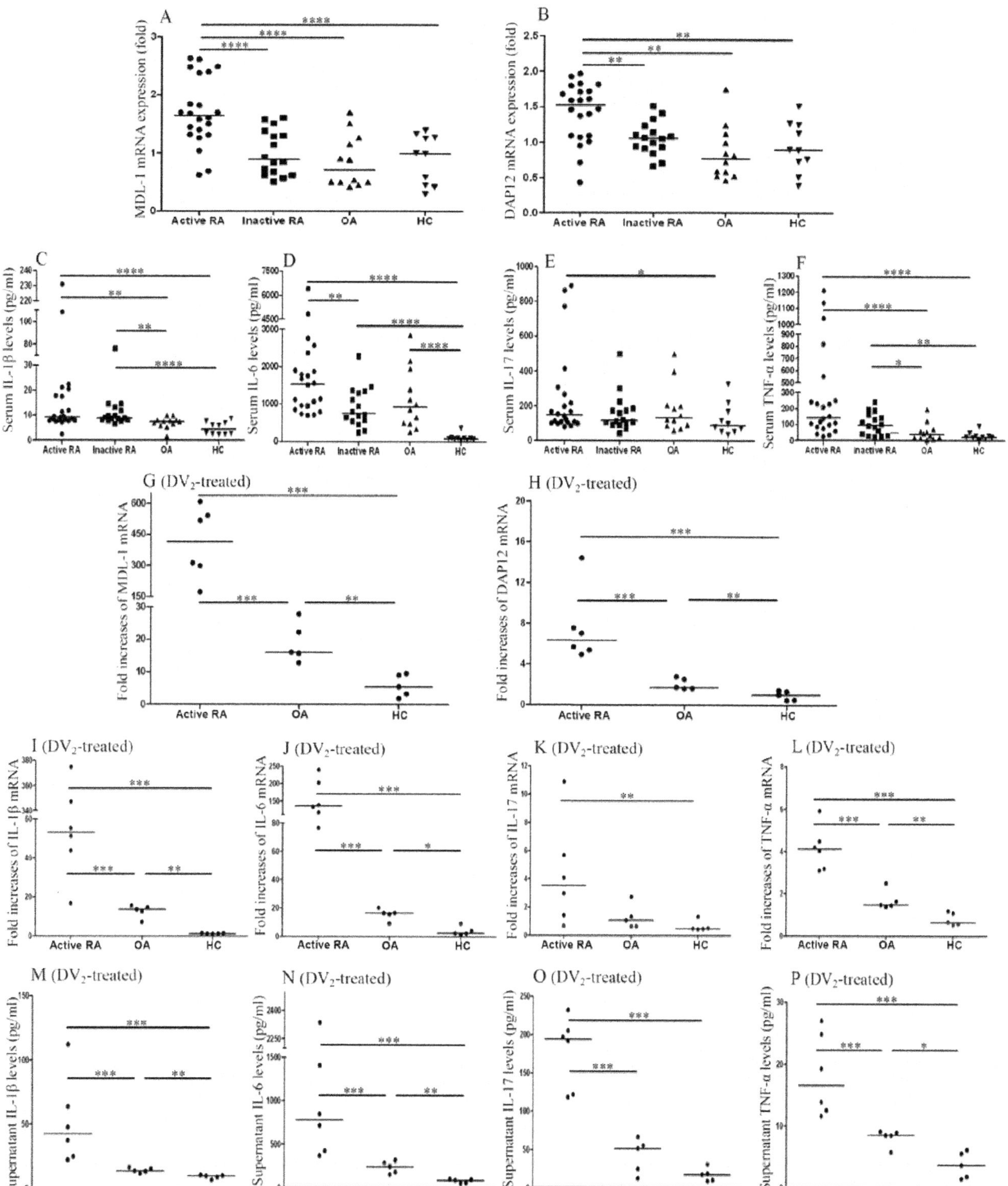

Figure 2. Comparisons of relative expression levels of MDL-1 and DAP12 mRNA on peripheral blood mononuclear cells (A, B; respectively) and serum levels of IL-1β, IL-6, IL-17A, and TNF-α, (C, D, E, F; respectively) are shown for 22 active RA patients, 16 inactive RA patients, 12 OA patients, and 10 healthy subjects. To explore the functional role of MDL-1 activation, we examined the fold-increases of mRNA expression levels of MDL-1 and DAP12 (G, H; respectively), and the fold-increases of mRNA expression levels and supernatant levels of downstream cytokines, including IL-1β, IL-6, IL-17A, and TNF-α (I–P) on PBMCs treated with MDL-1 activator (Dengue virus type 2 [DV2]-antigen) in 6 active RA patients, 5 OA patients, and 5 healthy controls. The horizontal line indicates median value for each group. *$p<0.05$, **$p<0.01$, ***$p<0.005$, ****$p<0.001$, as determined by Mann-Whitney U test.

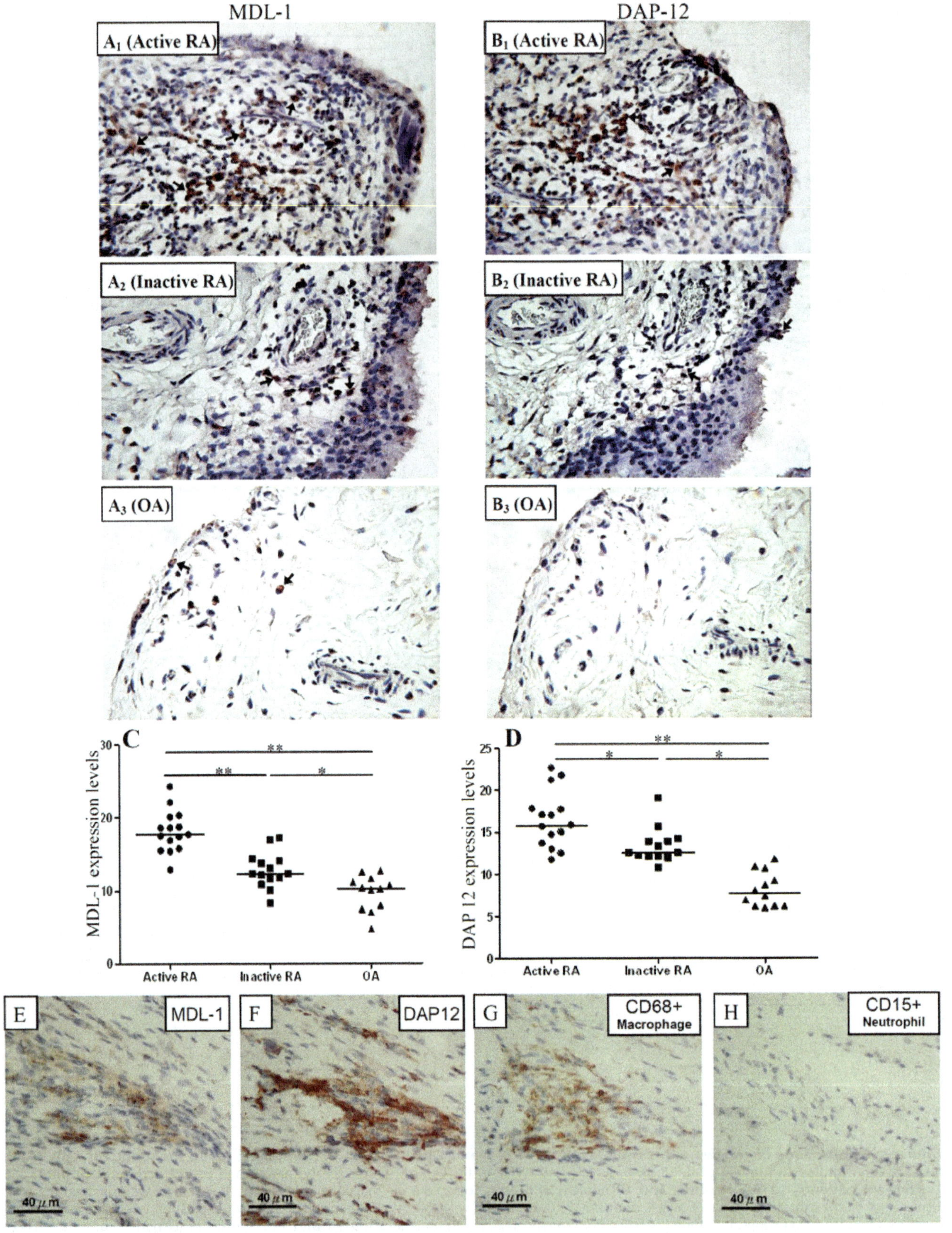

Figure 3. Representative examples of immunostaining with MDL-1 and DAP12 (arrows, original magnification x 200) obtained from synovial membranes of one active RA patient (A1 and B1; respectively), one inactive RA patient (A2 and B2; respectively), one OA patient (A3 and B3; respectively). Comparisons of expression levels of MDL-1 and DAP12 on synovial membranes (C and D; respectively) are

shown for 15 active RA patients, 14 inactive RA patients, and 12 OA patients. The horizontal line indicates median value for each group. *$p<0.005$, **$p<0.001$, as determined by Mann-Whitney U test. We also demonstrated that strongly positive staining of MDL-1 and DAP12 were expressed on CD68+ macrophages, not on CD15+ neutrophils in serial sections of synovial biopsy specimens from one RA patient (Figures 3E–3H).

higher in inactive RA patients than in OA patients, or healthy control subjects. However, there was no significant difference in the percentages or MFI of MDL-1-expressing monocytes between early RA patients (n = 8) and late RA patients (n = 30), or between OA patients and healthy control subjects.

In addition, we examined whether TNF-α or IL-1β could affect MDL-1 expression; our results showed that TNF-α stimulation of PBMCs from RA patients induced a higher increment of MDL-1-expressing monocytes (median 14.1%, interquartile range [IQR] 13.2–19.1%) compared with stimulation of PBMCs from OA patients (median 3.9%, IQR3.2–4.4%, $p<0.01$) or healthy controls (median 2.9%, IQR2.7–3.7%, $p<0.01$; Figure 1E). Similarly, IL-1β stimulation of PBMCs from RA patients induced a higher increment of MDL-1-expressing monocytes (median 8.8%, IQR7.6–15.7%) compared with stimulation of PBMCs from OA patients (median 5.8%, IQR4.0–6.4%, $p<0.01$) or from healthy control subjects (median 4.6%, IQR3.7–5.3%, $p<0.01$; Figure 1F).

mRNA Expression Levels of MDL-1and DAP12 Using qPCR

As shown in Figures 2A–2B and Table 2, significantly higher levels of MDL-1 and DAP12 mRNA expression were found on PBMCs from active RA patients compared to PBMCs from inactive RA patients, OA patients, or healthy controls. However, there was no significant difference in mRNA expression levels of MDL-1 or DAP12 between early RA patients and late RA patients, between inactive RA patients and OA patients, or between OA patients and healthy control subjects.

Serum Levels of Proinflammatory Cytokines

As shown in Figures 2C–2F and Table 2, levels of serum IL-1β, IL-6, IL-17A, and TNF-α were significantly higher in active RA patients compared to healthy subjects. Active RA patients had significantly higher IL-6 levels than those in inactive RA patients, and also had higher levels of IL-1β and TNF-α compared to OA patients. Inactive RA patients had significantly higher levels of IL-1β, IL-6, and TNF-α compared to healthy controls, and higher levels of IL-1β and TNF-α compared to OA patients. OA patients had significantly higher levels of IL-6 compared to healthy controls. However, there was no significant difference in serum levels of IL-1β, IL-17A, and TNF-α between OA patients and healthy control subjects.

Functionality of MDL-1-mediated Production of Proinflammatory Cytokines

We examined whether the enhanced MDL-1expression was functional in terms of DAP12 expression and proinflammatory cytokine production. Our results showed that DV2-antigen stimulation of PBMCs from active RA patients induced greater folds increases of MDL-1 (median, 414.8, IQR 267.0–557.6), DAP12 (median, 6.4, IQR 5.3–9.3), IL-1β (median, 53.3, IQR 37.0–354.1), IL-6 (median, 135.4, IQR 106.7–211.5), IL-17A (median, 3.5, IQR 1.2–7.0), and TNF-α (median, 4.1, IQR 3.1–4.8) compared to stimulation of PBMCs from OA patients (median, 16.0, IQR 14.2–25.0, $p<0.005$; 1.7, IQR 1.6–2.7, $p<0.005$; 13.6, IQR 9.8–15.1, $p<0.005$; 16.4, IQR 12.3–18.3, $p<0.005$; 1.1, IQR 0.6–2.0, $p=0.052$; and 1.5, IQR 1.4–2.1, $p<0.005$; respectively) or from healthy control subjects (median, 5.5, IQR 2.6–9.3, $p<0.005$; 1.0, IQR 0.5–1.4, $p<0.005$; 1.1, IQR 1.0–1.4, $p<0.005$; 2.3, IQR 1.7–6.5, $p<0.005$; 0.5, IQR 0.5–0.9, $p<0.01$; and 0.6, IQR 0.6–1.1, $p<0.005$; respectively, Figures 2G–2L). Similarly, we demonstrated that DV2-antigen stimulation of PBMCs from active RA patients induced higher levels of supernatant IL-1β (median, 42.5 pg/ml, IQR 24.2–75.8 pg/ml), IL-6 (median, 779.6 pg/ml, IQR 408.9–1637.9 pg/ml), IL-17A (median, 194.5 pg/ml, IQR 121.0–211.9 pg/ml), and TNF-α (median, 16.6 pg/ml, IQR 12.3–25.4 pg/ml) compared to stimulation of PBMCs from OA patients (median, 13.6 pg/ml, IQR

Table 3. Correlation between expression levels of MDL-1 and disease activity parameters as well as cytokine levels in 38 patients with rheumatoid arthritis.

Parameters	MDL-1 expression on monocytes	MDL-1 mRNA levels on PBMCs	MDL-1 protein levels on SM
DAS28	0.392*	0.428**	0.613***
CRP, mg/dl	0.289*	0.395*	0.596**
Erosion score	0.569**	0.641***	0.546**
JSN score	0.476**	0.484**	0.393*
IL-1β, pg/ml	0.437**	0.274*	0.389*
IL-6, pg/ml	0.468**	0.387*	0.410*
IL-17A, pg/ml	0.262*	0.280*	0.135
TNF-α, pg/ml	0.605***	0.459**	0.321
DAP12 mRNA levels on PBMCs	0.656***	0.702***	0.447*
DAP12 protein levels on SM	0.119	0.207	0.462**

MDL-1: Myeloid DAP12-associated lectin-1; DAP12: DNAX adaptor protein 12; PBMCs: peripheral blood mononuclear cells; SM: synovial membranes; DAS28: disease activity score for 28-joints; CRP: C-reactive protein; JSN score: joint space narrowing score; IL-1β: interleukin-1β; IL-6: interleukin-6; IL-17A: interleukin-17A; TNF-α: tumor necrosis factor-α.

*$p<0.05$, **$p<0.005$, ***$p<0.001$ were obtained by the nonparametric Spearman's correlation test.

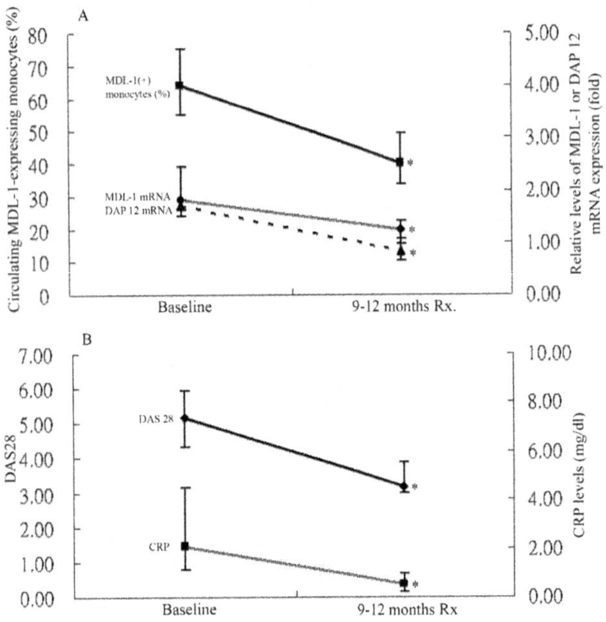

Figure 4. Changes in (A) percentages of circulating MDL-1-expressing monocytes and mRNA expresison levels of MDL-1 and DAP12, and changes in (B) disease activity score for 28-joints (DAS28) and C-reactive protein (CRP) levels in 12 RA patients at active phase (at baseline) and after 9–12 months of therapy. Data are presented as mean ± SEM. *p<0.005, versus active phase, determined by the Wilcoxon signed rank test.

12.6–15.7 pg/ml, p<0.005; 241.5 pg/ml, IQR 168.2–303.9 pg/ml, p<0.005; 51.8 pg/ml, IQR 19.1–61.1 pg/ml, p<0.005; and 8.5 pg/ml, IQR 7.1–9.0 pg/ml, p<0.005; respectively) or from healthy control subjects (median, 9.9 pg/ml, IQR 7.9–10.3 pg/ml, p<0.005; 88.5 pg/ml, IQR 58.7–98.9 pg/ml, p<0.005; 17.8 pg/ml, IQR 9.9–25.3 pg/ml, p<0.005; and 3.7 pg/ml, IQR 1.7–5.9 pg/ml, p<0.005; respectively, Figures 2M–2P).

Expression Levels of MDL-1 and DAP12 on Synovial Membranes Using IHC

Representative examples of immunostaining for MDL-1 and DAP12 on synovial biopsy specimens from one active RA patient, one inactive RA patient, and one OA patient are shown in Figure 3. There were higher expression levels of MDL-1 and DAS12 protein in synovial membranes from active RA patients (median 17.70, IQR 15.80–20.10 and 15.80, IQR 13.70–17.80; respectively) compared to levels in SMs from inactive RA patients (12.30, IQR 11.40–14.18, p<0.05 and 12.55, IQR 12.10–13.98, p<0.05; respectively) or from OA patients (10.25, IQR 7.53–11.48, p<0.005 and 7.75, IQR 6.20–10.33, p<0.001; respectively). We also observed significantly higher expression levels of MDL-1 and DAS12 protein in SMs from inactive RA patients compared to those from OA patients (p<0.05 and p<0.005; respectively). In addition, we found that strongly positive staining of MDL-1 and DAP12 were expressed on CD68+ macrophages, not on CD15+ neutrophils in serial sections of SMs (Figures 3E–3H). However, there are limitations of protein staining assessment when using this approach, such as accounting for nonspecific staining and identifying cell associated staining and vascular staining.

Correlations of MDL-1 Expression Levels with Disease Activity Parameters, Erosion Scores, Joint Space Narrowing Scores, and DAP12 Expression Levels in RA Patients

As illustrated in Table 3, MDL-1 expression levels were positively correlated with DAS28, CRP levels, erosion scores, and JSN scores in RA patients. The percentages of circulating MDL-1-expressing monocytes and mRNA expression levels of MDL-1 were positively correlated with serum levels of IL-1β, IL-6, IL-17A, and TNF-α in RA patient. Moreover, MDL-1 expression levels were positively correlated with DAP12 expression levels in synovial membranes from RA patients.

Changes in Percentages of Circulating MDL-1-expressing Monocytes and mRNA Expression Levels of MDL-1 and DAP12 on PBMCs from RA Patients after Therapy

Twelve active RA patients were available for examination of their expression levels of MDL-1 and DAP12 in the active phase (baseline time-point) and after 9–12 months of therapy with triple DMARDs, including methotrexate, hydroxychloroquine, and sulfasalazine. As shown in Figure 4, the percentages of MDL-1-expressing monocytes significantly decreased (mean ± standard error of the mean; 65.22±3.35% vs. 40.83±2.38%, p<0.005), paralleling the decreases in DAS28 (5.15±0.27 vs. 3.35±0.24, p<0.005) and CRP (2.93±0.64 mg/dl vs. 0.70±0.19 mg/dl, p<0.005). Similarly, the relative expression levels of MDL-1 and DAP12 mRNA also significantly declined (1.98±0.13 vs. 1.20±0.08; 1.65±0.07 vs. 0.85±0.06, both p<0.005), paralleling the decreases in DAS28 and CRP.

Discussion

MDL-1, a novel member of the C-type lectin family, has been shown to be involved in murine joint inflammation [22]. However, the role of MDL-1 in the pathogenesis of human RA remains unclear. The present study is the first attempt to characterize the expression of MDL-1 and its associated adaptor-DAP12 in RA patients. Our results show that MDL-1 is highly expressed on circulating monocytes in active RA patients, consistent with the findings of an increased expression of MDL-1 on murine bone marrow macrophages [22], and the involvement of MDL-1 in the activation of myeloid cells [20] in other recent studies. In addition, our data demonstrated significantly higher percentages and MFI of circulating MDL-1-expressing monocytes in active RA patients compared to inactive RA patients and OA patients. The results are similar to those of another study showing enhanced percentages of MDL-1-expressing monocytes following arthritis induction [22]. We also showed that the percentages of circulating MDL-1-expressing monocytes were positively correlated with DAS28, erosion scores, and JSN scores in RA patients, supporting the previous findings of that MDL-1 is a key regulator of synovitis and bone erosion during progression of autoimmune arthritis [22]. Moreover, the percentages of MDL-1-expressing monocytes significantly decreased after effective therapy in our RA patients. These observations strongly suggest that MDL-1 overexpression plays a major role in the pathogenesis of human RA.

Since Joyce-Shaikh observed that TNF-α could promote MDL-1 expression in murine arthritis [22], we examined the role of TNF-α or IL-1β in the regulation of MDL-1 expression. The *ex vivo* study demonstrated that TNF-α or IL-1β stimulation on PBMCs from our active RA patients resulted in significantly enhanced levels of MDL-1 expression when compared to those from OA patients or from healthy control subjects. Therefore, there still exists the possibility that MDL-1 upregulation may represent an epiphenomenon of rheumatoid inflammation rather than serve as a primary event in the pathogenesis of human RA.

To verify MDL-1 expression at the mRNA level in human RA, qPCR for MDL-1 gene expression on PBMCs was performed for our RA patients and control groups. We demonstrated that relative gene expression levels of MDL-1 were significantly higher in active RA patients when compared to inactive RA patients, OA patients, or healthy controls. Moreover, the gene expression levels of MDL-1 were positively correlated with DAS28, CRP levels, erosion scores, and JSN scores in RA patients. Such results provide robust evidence of MDL-1 overexpression in active RA patients. However, studies with large cohorts of RA patients should be conducted to confirm our findings.

To confirm the production of MDL-1 in inflamed joint tissues, we investigated MDL-1 expression levels in SMs from RA patients and OA patients by IHC. The results showed significantly higher levels of MDL-1 protein in SMs from active RA patients in comparison to levels in SMs from inactive RA patients or OA patients; this was consistent with previous findings of that MDL-1 was expressed on inflamed joints in collagen-induced arthritis [22]. Besides, as revealed in another study that MDL-1 expression co-localizes with a subset of CD68+ macrophages [16], we found strongly positive staining of MDL-1 and DAP12 expressed on CD68+ macrophages, not on CD15+ neutrophils (Figure 3E–3H). Moreover, we demonstrated that MDL-1 expression levels in SMs from RA patients were positively correlated with DAS28, erosion scores, and JSN scores. Our data support the previous findings of that mice treated with MDL-1 agonist had higher arthritis scores than the isotype controls, whereas MDL-1 blockade markedly reduced arthritis and bone erosion [22]. These observations imply that MDL-1 overexpression might be a novel biomarker for disease activity and a potential therapeutic target.

MDL-1 interacts with the ITAM-bearing adaptor protein DAP12 [21], which activate the Syk-signaling pathway, leading to synovial inflammation and bone erosion [4]. Our results provide the first evidence that both MDL-1 and DAP12 were highly expressed on PBMCs at the gene expression level, and also in SMs at the protein level in active RA patients, indicating the potential involvement of MDL-1/DAP12 in RA pathogenesis. Similarly, DAP12 expression levels in synovial tissue have been found to be significantly higher in active RA patients than those in inactive RA patients or OA patients [19]. Moreover, we demonstrated a positive correlation not only between mRNA expression levels of MDL-1 and those of DAP12 on PBMCs, but also between the protein expression levels of MDL-1 and those of DAP12 in the SMs from RA patients. Such results support the findings that MDL-1 expression is coupled with expression of DAP12, which acts as a signaling molecule for the MDL-1 receptor [21]. In the *ex vivo* study, we also demonstrated a six-fold increase of DAP12 mRNA expression levels on PBMCs treated with MDL-1 activator. These observations support the recent finding that DAP12 gene expression levels on myeloid cells were elevated in MDL-1 agonist-treated mice, whereas MDL-1 blockade suppressed DAP12 expression [22]. In addition, MDL-1 has been shown to associate with DAP12 to form receptor complexes involved in monocytic activation and inflammatory responses [36–37]. These findings suggest potential links between MDL-1 and DAP12, and support the observations of a critical role of MDL-1/DAP12 complex in the pathogenesis of arthritis and osteoclastogenesis [22,38]. Involvement of the MDL-1/DAP12 signaling pathway in RA pathogenesis was reinforced by the finding that the severity of arthritis was markedly lower in both DAP12$^{-/-}$ and MDL-1$^{-/-}$ mice when compared to wild-type mice [22]. However, in our study, MDL-1 mRNA expression levels on PBMCs were not in parallel with DAP12 protein expression levels in the SMs from RA patients. Probable reasons for this result include the small sample size and that MDL-1/DAP12 coupling signaling occurs mainly in inflamed tissues.

In agreement with the recent finding that MDL-1 cross-linking could trigger the secretion of proinflammatory cytokines [22], we found that the elevated levels of serum IL-1β, IL-6, IL-17A, and TNF-α were positively correlated with MDL-1 expression levels in RA patients. Moreover, we investigated the functional relation between MDL-1 activation and the downstream proinflammatory cytokines. The results show that MDL-1 activator (DV2-antigen) stimulation on PBMCs induced greater-fold increases of mRNA expression levels of IL-1β (up to ~53-fold), IL-6 (up to ~135-fold), IL-17A (up to ~3.5-fold), and TNF-α (up to ~4-fold) in active RA patients compared to those in OA patients or healthy subjects, indicating that MDL-1 activation is functional. Such results support another study showing that treatment with MDL-1 agonist enhanced the expression of IL-1β, IL-6, IL-17A and TNF-α; whereas MDL-1 blockade suppressed cytokine gene expression [22]. Up-regulated expression of MDL-1 together with elevated levels of proinflammatory cytokines may have pathogenic relevance by representing a potential mechanism of amplification of synovial inflammation in active RA patients.

There are some limitations of our study. This was a preliminary study that enrolled a limited number of active RA patients. In addition, we did not investigate the role of DAP10 in the pathogenesis of human RA because of the different associated receptors, signaling kinase, and intracellular domain [36,39]. Because most of patients enrolled in our study were not in early RA stage, our results might not be directly applicable to early RA patients. Therefore, a long-term study enrolling a larger group of patients, including an early RA population, is required for validation of our findings.

Conclusion

Our results show that MDL-1 and its associated adaptor-DAP12 were concordantly overexpressed on PBMCs and the inflamed synovium in active RA patients. We also provide the first evidence that MDL-1 upregulation may have a possible link with DAP12 and inflammatory responses in human RA. The preliminary results might partly explain the role of MDL-1-linked signaling in the inflammatory cascade of RA. Such studies may be of translational interest because they may provide further evidence that can be used to develop potentially therapeutic modalities for RA, including the use of MDL-1 and Syk kinase inhibitors [22,40–41].

Acknowledgments

The authors thank the Biostatistics Task Force of Taichung Veterans General Hospital, Taichung, Taiwan.

Author Contributions

Conceived and designed the experiments: DYC JLL. Performed the experiments: LY YMC. Analyzed the data: LY YMC CCL KCH STC SLEH DYC JLL. Contributed reagents/materials/analysis tools: STC SLEH. Wrote the paper: DYC JLL.

References

1. Choy EH, Panayi GS (2001) Cytokine pathways and joint inflammation in rheumatoid arthritis. N Engl J Med 344: 907–916.
2. Goldring SR, Gravallese EM (2000) Pathogenesis of bone erosions in rheumatoid arthritis. Curr Opin Rheumatol 12: 195–199.
3. Koga T, Inui M, Inoue K, Kim S, Suematsu A, et al. (2004) Costimulatory signals mediated by the ITAM motif cooperate with RANKL for bone homeostasis. Nature 428: 758–763.
4. Mócsai A, Humphrey MB, Van Ziffle JA, Hu Y, Burghardt A, et al. (2004) The immunomodulatory adapter proteins DAP12 and Fc receptor gamma-chain (FcRgamma) regulate development of functional osteoclasts through the Syk tyrosine kinase. Proc Natl Acad Sci U S A. 101: 6158–6163.
5. Firestein GS (2003) Evolving concepts of rheumatoid arthritis. Nature 423: 356–361.
6. McInnes IB, Schett G (2007) Cytokines in the pathogenesis of rheumatoid arthritis. Nat Rev Immunol. 7: 429–442.
7. Van Bezooijen RL, Van Der Wee-Pals L, Papapoulos SE, Lowik CW (2002) Interleukin 17 synergies with tumor necrosis factor alpha to induce cartilage destruction in vitro. Ann Rheum Dis. 61: 870–876.
8. Chabaud M, Lubberts E, Joosten L, van den Berg W, Miossec P (2001) IL-17 derived from juxta-articular bone and synovium contributes to joint degradation in rheumatoid arthritis. Arthritis Res Ther. 3: 168–177.
9. Cohen SB, Moreland LW, Cush JJ, Greenwald MW, Block S, et al. (2004) A multicentre, double blind, randomised, placebo controlled trial of anakinra (Kineret), a recombinant interleukin 1 receptor antagonist, in patients with rheumatoid arthritis treated with background methotrexate. Ann Rheum Dis. 63: 1062–1068.
10. Yazici Y, Curtis JR, Ince A, Baraf H, Malamet RL, et al. (2012) Efficacy of tocilizumab in patients with moderate to severe active rheumatoid arthritis and a previous inadequate response to disease-modifying antirheumatic drugs: the ROSE study. Ann Rheum Dis. 71: 198–205.
11. van der Heijde D, Klareskog L, Rodriguez-Valverde V, Codreanu C, Bolosiu H, et al. (2006) Comparison of etanercept and methotrexate, alone and combined, in the treatment of rheumatoid arthritis: Two-year clinical and radiographic results from the TEMPO study, a double-blind, randomized trial. Arthritis Rheum. 54 1063–1074.
12. Kievit W, Fransen J, Adang EM, den Broeder AA, Bernelot HJ, et al. (2011) Long-term effectiveness and safety of TNF-blocking agents in daily clinical practice: results from the Dutch rheumatoid arthritis monitoring register. Rheumatology 50: 196–203.
13. Genovese MC, Van den Bosch F, Roberson SA, Bojin S, Biagini IM et al. (2010) A humanized anti-IL-17 monoclonal antibody, in the treatment of patients with rheumatoid arthritis: a phase 1 randomized double-blind, placebo-controlled, proof of concept study. Arthritis Rheum 62: 929–939.
14. Mao D, Epple H, Uthgenannt B, Novack DV, Faccio R (2006) PLCgamma2 regulates osteoclastogenesis via its interaction with ITAM proteins and GAB2. J Clin Invest 116: 2869–2879.
15. Takayanagi H (2005) Mechanistic insight into osteoclast differentiation in osteoimmunology. J Mol Med 83: 170–179.
16. Olcese L, Cambiaggi A, Semenzato G, Bottino C, Moretta A, et al. (1997) Human killer cell activatory receptors for MHC class I molecules are included in a multimeric complex expressed by natural killer cells. J Immunol. 158: 5083–5086.
17. Lanier LL, Corliss BC, Wu J, Leong C, Phillips JH (1998) Immunoreceptor DAP12 bearing a tyrosine-based activation motif is involved in activating NK cells. Nature 391: 703–707.
18. Humphrey MB, Ogasawara K, Yao W, Spusta SC, Daws MR, et al. (2004) The signaling adapter protein DAP12 regulates multinucleation during osteoclast development. J Bone Miner Res 19: 224–234.
19. Crotti TN, Dharmapatni AA, Alias E, Zannettino ACW, Smith MD, et al. (2012) The immunoreceptor tyrosine-based activation motif (ITAM)-related factors are increased in synovial tissue and vasculature of rheumatoid joints. Arthritis Res Ther 14: R245.
20. Bakker AB, Baker E, Sutherland GR, Phillips JH, Lanier LL (1999) Myeloid DAP12-associated lectin (MDL)-1 is a cell surface receptor involved in the activation of myeloid cells. Proc Natl Acad Sci USA. 96: 9792–9796.
21. Aoki N, Kimura Y, Kimura S, Nagato T, Azumi M, et al. (2009) Expression and functional role of MDL-1 (CLEC5A) in mouse myeloid lineage cells. J Leukoc Biol. 85: 508–517.
22. Joyce-Shaikh B, Bigler ME, Chao CC, Murphy EE, Blumenschein WM, et al. (2010) Myeloid DAP12-associating lectin (MDL)-1 regulates synovial inflammation and bone erosion associated with autoimmune arthritis. J Exp Med. 207: 579–589.
23. Chen ST, Lin YL, Huang MT, Wu MF, Cheng SC, et al. (2008) Lei HY, Lee CK, Chiou TW, Wong CH, Hsieh SL. CLEC5A is critical for dengue-virus-induced lethal disease. Nature 453: 672–678.
24. Aletaha D, Neogi T, Silman AJ, Funovits J, Felson DT, et al. (2010) The 2010 rheumatoid arthritis classification criteria: an American College of Rheumatology/European League Against Rheumatism collaborative initiative. Ann Rheum Dis 69: 1580–8.
25. Heimans L, Wevers-de Boer KV, Visser K, Goekoop RJ, van Oosterhout M, et al. (2013) A two-step treatment strategy trial in patients with early arthritis aimed at achieving remission: the IMPROVED study. Ann Rheum Dis May 28.
26. Prevoo MLL, van't Hof MA, Kuper HH, van Leeuwen MA, van de Putte LBA, et al. (1995) Modified disease activity scores that include twenty-eight-joint counts: development and validation in a prospective longitudinal study of patients with rheumatoid arthritis. Arthritis Rheum. 38: 44–48.
27. Smolen JS, Aletaha D, Bijlsma JW, Breedveld FC, Boumpas D, et al. (2011) Treating rheumatoid arthritis to target: recommendations of an international task force. Ann Rheum Dis. 70: 631–637.
28. Genant HK, Jiang Y, Peterfy C, Lu Y, Redei J, et al. (1998) Assessment of rheumatoid arthritis using a modified scoring method on digitized and original radiographs. Arthritis Rheum. 41: 1583–1590.
29. Altman R, Asch E, Bloch D, Bole G, Borenstein D, et al. (1986) Development of criteria for the classification and reporting of osteoarthritis. Classification of osteoarthritis of the knee. Diagnostic and Therapeutic Criteria Committee of the American Rheumatism Association. Arthritis Rheum. 29: 1039–1049.
30. Chomczynski P, Sacchi N (1987) Single-step method of RNA isolation by acid guanidium thiocyanate-phenol-chloroform extraction. Anal Biochem. 162: 156–159.
31. Gibson UEM, Heid CA, Williams PM (1996) A novel method for real time quantitative PCR. Genome Res. 6: 995–1001.
32. Gingras MC, Lapillonne H, Margolin JF (2001) TREM-1, MDL-1, and DAP12 expression is associated with a mature stage of myeloid development. Mol Immunol. 38: 817–824.
33. Livak KJ, Schmittgen TD (2001) Analysis of relative gene expression data using real-time quantitative PCR and the 2(-Delta Delta C(T)) Method. Methods (2001) 25: 402–408.
34. Chen DY, Lin CC, Chen YM, Lan JL, Hung WT, et al. (2013) Involvement of TLR7 MyD88-dependent signaling pathway in the pathogenesis of adult-onset Still's disease. Arthritis Res Ther 15: R39.
35. Yang XM, Jiang LF, Tang YX, Yin Y, Liu WQ, et al. (2010) Establishment and characterization of dengue virus type 2 nonstructural protein 1 specific T cell lines. Comp Immunol Microbiol Infect Dis 33: e75–80.
36. Wu J, Cherwinski H, Spies T, Phillips JH, Lanier LL, et al. (2000) DAP10 and DAP12 form distinct, but functionally cooperative, receptor complexes in natural killer cells. J Exp Med 192: 1059–1067.
37. Tomasello E, Cant C, Buhring HJ, Vely F, Andre P, et al. (2000) Association of signal-regulatory proteins beta with KARAP/DAP-12. Eur J Immunol 30: 2147–2156.
38. Inui M, Kikuchi Y, Aoki N, Endo S, Maeda T, et al. (1999) Signal adaptor DAP10 associates with MDL-1 and triggers osteoclastogenesis in cooperation with DAP12. Proc Natl Acad Sci USA. 106: 4816–4821.
39. Wu J, Song Y, Bakker AB, Bauer S, Spies T, et al. (1999) An activating receptor complex on natural killer and T cells formed by NKG2D and DAP10. Science 285: 730–732.
40. Weinblatt ME, Kavanaugh A, Genovese MC, Musser TK, Grossbard EB, et al. (2010) An oral spleen tyrosine kinase (Syk) inhibitor for rheumatoid arthritis. N Engl J Med. 363: 1303–1312.
41. Genovese MC, Kavanaugh A, Weinblatt ME, Peterfy C, DiCarlo J, et al. (2011) An oral Syk kinase inhibitor in the treatment of rheumatoid arthritis: a three-month randomized, placebo-controlled, phase II study in patients with active rheumatoid arthritis that did not respond to biologic agents. Arthritis Rheum. 63: 337–345.

8

IFNα Serum Levels Are Associated with Endothelial Progenitor Cells Imbalance and Disease Features in Rheumatoid Arthritis Patients

Javier Rodríguez-Carrio[1], Banesa de Paz[1], Patricia López[1], Catuxa Prado[1], Mercedes Alperi-López[2], Francisco Javier Ballina-García[2], Ana Suárez[1]*

1 Area Of Immunology, Department Of Functional Biology, Faculty Of Medicine, University Of Oviedo, Oviedo, Spain, 2 Department Of Rheumatology, Hospital Universitario Central De Asturias, Oviedo, Spain

Abstract

Introduction: IFNα has been largely implicated in the ethiopathogenesis of autoimmune diseases but only recently it has been linked to endothelial damage and accelerated atherosclerosis in autoimmunity. In addition, proinflammatory conditions are supposed to be implicated in the cardiovascular status of these patients. Since a role for IFNα in endothelial damage and impaired Endothelial Progenitor Cell (EPC) number and function has been reported in other diseases, we aimed to evaluate the potential associations of IFNα serum levels on EPC populations and cytokine profiles in Rheumatoid Arthritis (RA) patients.

Methods: pre-EPC, EPC and mature EPC (mEPC) populations were quantified by flow cytometry analyzing their differential CD34, CD133 and VEGFR2 expression in blood samples from 120 RA patients, 52 healthy controls (HC), and 83 systemic lupus erythematosus (SLE) patients as disease control. Cytokine serum levels were measured by immunoassays and clinical and immunological data, including cardiovascular (CV) events and CV risk factors, were retrospectively obtained by reviewing clinical records.

Results: Long-standing, but not recent onset RA patients displayed a significant depletion of all endothelial progenitor populations, unless high IFNα levels were present. In fact, the IFN^{high} RA patient group (n = 40, 33%), showed increased EPC levels, comparable to SLE patients. In addition, high IFNα serum levels were associated with higher disease activity (DAS28), presence of autoantibodies, higher levels of IL-1β, IL-6, IL-10 and MIP-1α, lower amounts of TGF-β, and increased mEPC/EPC ratio, thus suggesting higher rates of endothelial damage and an endothelial repair failure. Finally, the relationship between high IFNα levels and occurrence of CV events observed in RA patients seems to support this hypothesis.

Conclusions: IFNα serum marker could be used to identify a group of RA patients with increased disease activity, EPC imbalance, enhanced proinflammatory profile and higher cardiovascular risk, probably due, at least in part, to an impaired endothelial repair.

Editor: Peter Szodoray, Institute of Immunology, Rikshospitalet, Norway

Funding: This work was supported by European Union FEDER funds and the Fondo de Investigación Sanitaria (FIS, PI08/0570 and PI12/0053). JRC is a recipient of a FPU grant from the Ministerio de Educación. CP was supported by a fellowship from FIS and BdP was supported by a fellowship from FICYT. The funders had no role in study design, data collection and analysis, decision to publish, or preparation of the manuscript.

Competing Interests: The authors have declared that no competing interests exist.

* E-mail: Anasua@Uniovi.Es

Introduction

Rheumatoid Arthritis (RA) is associated with increased cardiovascular (CV) disease morbidity and mortality rates that cannot be explained by traditional risk factors [1,2]. Moreover, endothelial dysfunction, the main cause of premature atherosclerosis, has been found even in young RA patients without traditional CV risk factors [3], thus suggesting the involvement of disease-related pathways.

Endothelial damage leads to denuded sites at the endothelial wall that must be repaired. In this sense, bone marrow-derived Endothelial Progenitor Cells (EPCs) carry out vasculogenesis and endothelial repair functions, contributing to vascular homeostasis [4]. Although there is no consensus on their precise phenotypic definition, functional EPC are characterized by the expression of Vascular Endothelial Growth Factor Receptor-2 (VEGFR-2 or CD309), CD34 and CD133 [5,6]; whereas those lacking CD34 expression are considered a pre-EPC subpopulation [7]. During EPC differentiation, CD133 expression is lost and they begin to express mature endothelial-specific markers, becoming mature EPC (mEPC) with lower vasculogenic functionality [6]. As endothelial status depends on injury and repair, the balance between EPC populations could be a surrogate marker which may be used as a potential CV risk factor. In fact, some studies have shown that circulating EPC could serve as a predictor of CV events in several conditions [8,9]. EPC studies in RA patients, however, are contradictory.

On the other hand, disease-related risk factors have been identified [10,11], suggesting that immune dysregulation could play a role in RA endothelial damage. Although the specific pathways remains unclear, a number of inflammatory and immune mediators seem to have a role, including C-reactive protein (CRP), cytokines, chemokines and growth factors [12,13], most of them dysregulated in RA patients and implicated in the pathogenesis of autoimmune diseases. Among these mediators, it is worth noting the case of IFNα, since type-I interferons play a role in the pathogenesis of SLE and probably other autoimmune diseases [14], and recent evidence suggests their involvement in endothelial damage and EPC dysfunction. It has been reported that IFNα impair EPC function *in vitro* as well as *in vivo* and, as a consequence, endothelial repair [15–18]. Moreover, type I IFNs have been linked to atherothrombosis by acting on platelets and foam cells [19]. In addition, IFNα-signature has been linked to vasculopathy in systemic sclerosis patients [20].

Since previous studies suggest that circulating EPC populations and type I IFNs could be involved in increasing cardiovascular risk in autoimmune diseases, the main aim of this study is to determine EPCs frequency in RA patients' peripheral blood and evaluate the potential associations with IFNα serum levels and clinical and immunological features.

Patients and Methods

Patients and Controls

Our study involved 120 RA patients fulfilling the 1987 revised criteria of the American College of Rheumatology, recruited from the Rheumatology outpatient clinic of the Hospital Universitario Central de Asturias, and 52 sex- and age-matched unrelated healthy controls (47 women, age (mean±SD): 44.74±11.04 years). Eighty-three SLE patients (79 women, age: 48.28±16.30 years, disease duration: 12.3±8.9 years, SLEDAI: 4.02±4.11) were included as disease controls. Routine clinical examination, information on clinical and immunological manifestations, therapies received in the previous three months and 28-joint disease activity score (DAS28) were obtained at the time of sampling. Clinical response to anti-TNFα therapy, in a six-month period, was analyzed using EULAR response criteria [21]. Patients were classified on having a "good" "moderate" or "no response" according to DAS28 change from baseline (6-month previous clinical visit). Patients' clinical records were exhaustively revised in order to register the history of CV events and traditional CV risk factors (diabetes mellitus, hypercholesterolemia, hypertension and smoking habits). A CV event was considered if the patient suffered from heart failure, ischemic heart disease, cerebrovascular accident or peripheral arteriopathy from their RA diagnosis. Clinical definition of CV events and risk factors was performed as previously stated [22,23].

Ethics Statement

Approval for the study was obtained from the Regional Ethics Committee for Clinical Investigation (Servicio de Salud del Principado de Asturias, Hospital Universitario Central de Asturias), according to the Declaration of Helsinki. All procedures were performed with an informed written consent from all individuals.

Flow Cytometry EPCs Quantification

Blood samples were immediately transported to the laboratory and processed. EPC were analyzed by FACS as described previously [24], following EUSTAR recommendations [25] with few modifications. Briefly, 100 µl of peripheral blood were preincubated with 10 µl of FcR Blocking Reagent (Miltenyi Biotech) for 20 minutes, followed by 30-minutes triple-labelling with anti-VEGFR2-phycoerythrin (PE, R&D Systems), anti-CD34-fluorescein isothiocyanate (FITC, BD Pharmigen) and anti-CD133-allophycocyanin (APC, Miltenyi Biotech) or with identical isotype antibodies (BD Pharmigen). Labelled cells were lysed with 2 ml BD Lysing Solution (BD Biosciences) for 5 minutes and washed twice with PBS. Finally, samples were analyzed in a BD FACSCanto II flow cytometer. After gating the lymphocyte population, CD34-positive events were selected and analyzed in a CD133 *vs.* VEGFR2 dot plot, thus considering CD34/VEGFR2/CD133 triple-positive cells as EPCs while $CD34^{+}VEGFR2^{+}CD133^{-}$ cells were identified as mature EPCs (mEPCs) [24] (Figure 1A). On the other hand, VEGFR2-positive events within the lymphocyte gate were analyzed for CD34/CD133 expression and $CD34^{-}VEGFR2^{+}CD133^{+}$ cells were considered as pre-EPCs. At least 100,000 events in the lymphocyte gate and more than 100 $CD34^{+}$ cells were acquired per sample. Cell counts were expressed as the number of positive cells per 100,000 events in the lymphocyte gate.

Cytokine Serum Levels Quantifications

Serum aliquots were stored at −80°C until cytokine immunoassay measurement. Levels of IL-1β, IL-6, IL-8, IL-10, IFNα, MIP-1α (CCL3) and $VEGF\text{-}A_{165}$were quantified using a Cytometric Bead Array Flex Set (BD) and analyzed in a BD FACS Canto II flow cytometer using FCAP Array v.1.0.1. For IL-1β, IL-6 and IL-10, an Enhanced Sensitivity Flex Set was needed. Technical detection limits were 48.4 fg/ml for IL-1β, 68.4 fg/ml for IL-6, 1.2 pg/ml for IL-8, 13.7 fg/ml for IL-10, 1.5 pg/ml for IFNα, 0.2 pg/ml for MIP-1α and 4.0 pg/ml for $VEGF\text{-}A_{165}$. TGF-β1 and TNFα serum levels were quantified using ELISA kits (OptEIA, BD Bioscience), in accordance with the manufacturer's instructions. Detection limits for these cytokines were 5 ng/ml and 0.48 pg/ml, respectively.

Statistical Analysis

All data are presented as median (Interquartile Range) unless otherwise stated. Comparisons were performed by non-parametric tests (Mann-Whitney U, Kruskal-Wallis tests and Spearman's rank) as data were not normally distributed. Categorical variables were compared with a chi-squared test. The association between categorical variables and the CV events was assessed and adjusted for other factors (sex, age, traditional CV risk factors and disease activity) using multiple logistic regression analysis. Adjusted odds ratios (OR) and 95% confidence intervals (95% CI) were calculated so as to evaluate the strength of the associations. A p-value <0.05 was considered statistically significant. All data were analyzed with SPSS v.15.0 software.

Results

Circulating EPC Populations and IFNα Serum Levels in RA Patients

We aimed to investigate the possible relationship between EPC populations and IFNα levels in RA patients. To this end, IFNα serum levels and circulating pre-EPC, EPC and mEPC populations were quantified in 52 healthy controls (HC) and 120 RA patients with different disease duration (range 0–219 months) (Table 1). No significant differences in any endothelial progenitor population were found between patients and HC. However, disease duration was negatively correlated with EPC ($r = -0.316$, $p<0.001$) and mEPC ($r = -0.342$, $p<0.001$), suggesting an EPC

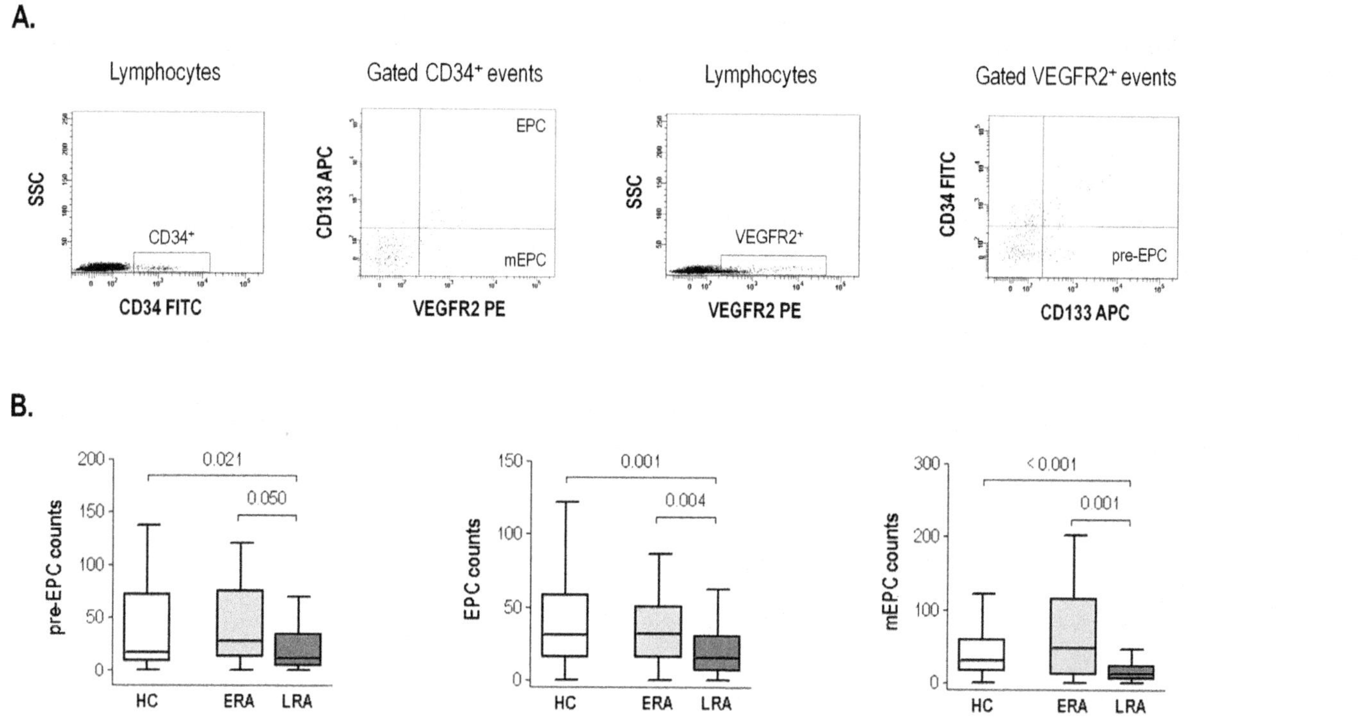

Figure 1. EPC analyses in RA patients by flow cytometry. (A) Gating strategy of EPC, mEPC and pre-EPC analysis by flow cytometry in peripheral blood samples. Representative dot plots of a HC are shown. (B) The size of endothelial precursor populations is influenced by disease duration. Pre-EPC, EPC and mEPC counts in early (ERA, disease duration <1 year, n = 36) and long-standing (LRA, n = 84) Rheumatoid Arthritis patients and healthy controls (HC, n = 52). Differences were measured by Mann-Withney U-test.

depletion associated with disease progression. In fact, patients at recent onset (less than one year, n = 36, early RA, ERA) showed similar levels of these populations than HC, whereas those with longer disease duration (n = 84, long-standing RA, LRA) exhibited a significant depletion of all EPC populations (Figure 1B). Neither associations with age at sampling, age at diagnosis, nor autoantibodies status were found.

On the other hand, IFNα serum levels were increased in RA patients compared with HC (20.25±47.61 vs. 1.76±3.08 pg/ml, $p = 0.001$), and positively correlated with all endothelial progenitor populations in patients (EPC: $r = 0.294$, $p<0.001$; mEPC $r = 0.265$, $p<0.001$, pre-EPC $r = 0.367$, $p<0.001$) but not in controls. Of note, this cytokine was associated with DAS-28 score ($r = 0.253$, $p = 0.023$) but unrelated to disease duration ($r = 0.055$, $p = 0.547$). In fact, ERA and LRA patients showed similar IFNα levels (14.43±31.16 vs. 22.74±53.10, $p = 0.718$).

In spite of the IFNα increase in RA, Figure 2 evidences that only a fraction of patients showed high levels of this molecule, whereas the other group presented low levels, similar to HC. Thus, we classified RA patients in IFN^{low} and IFN^{high} using the HC 90th percentile ($P90^{th} = 4.092$ pg/ml) as cut off. As shown in Table 1, these RA groups did not differ in age, disease duration or treatment followed, but IFN^{high} patients (n = 40, 33%) exhibited higher disease activity (DAS28) and ESR as well as increased positivity for autoantibodies. Other clinical markers such as Tender Joint Count, Patient Global Assessment or CRP were slightly augmented.

EPC Populations Differ According to IFNα Levels

In view of these results, we analyzed EPC populations in RA patients according to IFNα levels and disease duration, using as controls healthy donors (HC) and patients with SLE, a disease presenting altered levels of IFNα and EPCs [24]. Figure 3 shows that among ERA patients, those with normal IFNα levels (IFN^{low}) displayed similar pre-EPC, EPC and mEPC counts to HC, whereas IFN^{high} ERA patients exhibited higher levels of these populations compared with both HC and IFN^{low}, but similar to SLE patients. However, the most remarkable results were detected in LRA patients, since those with normal IFNα levels showed significantly lower pre-EPC and EPC counts than HC, thus highlighting a significant depletion that was missing in IFN^{high} patients. Therefore, EPC depletion seems to be a characteristic of RA patients unless the presence of high IFNα levels hides this effect. In fact, no significant differences in EPC populations were present between SLE and IFN^{high} RA patients, independently of disease duration. In any case, it is important to note that although IFN^{high} RA patients displayed enhanced EPC populations, the mEPC/EPC ratio, indicative of the endothelial repair capability [5,6], was increased in this group compared with their IFN^{low} counterparts (1.22(1.40) vs. 0.56(1.71), $p = 0.013$), thus suggesting an endothelial repair failure in these patients. Interestingly, no significant differences in mEPC/EPC ratio were found between ERA and LRA patients ($p = 0.090$), neither by treatments (all $p>0.050$), so there is no evidence that disease duration or longer exposure to treatment drugs could modify the mEPC/EPC ratio in RA patients.

IFNα is Associated with a Higher Rate of Cardiovascular Events

Taking into account the reported role of IFNα in endothelial damage and vascular repair, we aimed to evaluate the relevance of IFNα serum levels as a CV risk factor for RA patients. To this end,

Table 1. Demographic, immunological and clinical parameters of the RA patients.

	RA patients	IFNα	
	(n = 120)	IFN^{low} (n = 80)	IFN^{high} (n = 40)
Sex (female/male)	101/19	70/10	31/9
Age at sampling, years	55.33±15.23	55.24±15.04	55.56±16.00
Age at diagnosis, years	53.09±18.00	52.78±14.97	53.77±16.23
Disease duration, months	21.02±20.50	23.33±20.83	16.00±19.26
Clinical features			
Number of tender joints	5.24±5.25	4.29±5.59	6.86±7.00
Number of swollen joints	2.50±3.31	1.83±3.15	3.64±3.38
Patient global assessment (0–100)	32.05±23.63	28.13±25.20	38.79±19.69
Pain of patient's assessment (0–10)	3.21±2.42	2.71±2.40	4.07±2.30
Duration of morning stiffness, min	48.42±70.93	46.25±78.30	52.14±58.72
DAS28	3.81±1.61	3.35±1.52	4.59±1.49*
HAQ	0.77±0.70	0.68±0.70	0.95±0.67
CRP, mg/dl	0.39±0.63	0.28±0.45	0.59±0.83
ESR, mm/h	23.47±19.94	16.87±10.64	34.78±26.71*
RF positivity, n (%)	68 (56.7)	36 (45.0)	32 (80.0)***
Anti-CCP positivity, n (%)	69 (57.5)	36 (45.0)	33 (82.5)***
ANA positivity, n (%)	46 (38.3)	25 (31.2)	21 (52.5)*
Smoking habit, n (%)	49 (40.8)	32 (40.0)	17 (42.5)
Hypertension, n (%)	30 (25.0)	19 (23.7)	11 (27.5)
Hypercholesterolemia, n (%)	11 (9.1)	8 (6.6)	3 (2.5)
Diabetes mellitus, n (%)	15 (12.5)	8 (10.0)	7 (17.5)
Treatments *n (%)*			
None or NSAIDs	19 (15.8)	10 (10.1)	9 (22.5)
Glucocorticoids	58 (48.3)	40 (50.0)	18 (45.0)
Methotrexate	79 (65.8)	57 (71.3)	22 (55.0)
Leflunomide	16 (13.3)	11 (13.7)	5 (12.5)
TNF-α blockers	26 (21.6)	14 (17.5)	12 (30.0)
Cardiovascular events, *n(%)*			
Cardiovascular events	27 (22.5)	12 (15.0)	15 (37.5)**
Ischemic heart disease	10 (8.33)	4 (5.0)	6 (15.0)
Cerebrovascular accidents	4 (3.33)	2 (2.5)	2 (5.0)
Heart failure	12 (10.0)	6 (7.5)	6 (15.0)
Peripheral arteriopathy	1 (0.83)	0 (0.0)	1 (2.5)

Data of the whole RA patients group and classified according to IFNα serum levels. Data are expressed as (mean ± SD) unless otherwise was stated. Differences between categorical variables were evaluated by chi-square test, whereas Mann-Withney U test was used for continuous ones. *p<0.05, **p<0.01, ***p<0.001. IFN^{low}: serum levels <90th percentile in HC (4.092 pg/ml); IFN^{high}: serum levels ≥90th percentile in HC.

we analyzed the CV events suffered by RA patients in relation to both IFNα groups, demographic and clinical variables. The frequency of RA patients who had suffered CV events was higher in the IFN^{high} than in the IFN^{low} group (37.5 vs 15.0%, p = 0.005), although no significant differences between groups were detected in traditional CV risk factors (Table 1), thus supporting the role of IFNα as an independent CV risk factor. Univariate logistic regression analysis (Table 2) revealed that high IFNα levels, male sex, age at diagnosis, hypertension and diabetes were associated with the risk of CV events. After multivariate analysis by logistic regression adjusted by age at diagnosis, sex, disease activity (DAS28) and traditional CV risk factors, only the association with IFNα and age at diagnosis remained significant.

On the other hand, patients who had suffered CV events showed an increased mEPC/EPC ratio compared to those who had not experienced such complications (1.27(3.21) vs. 1.00(2.04), p = 0.010), as well as lower VEGF levels (55.84(90.69) vs. 122.34(150.39) pg/ml, p = 0.044), thus supporting the relevance of angiogenic cytokines and EPC balance in the endothelial repair maintenance. All these results support that high IFNα serum levels in RA patients could be associated with a higher rate of CV events, maybe by increasing the mEPC/EPC ratio and impairing endothelial repair.

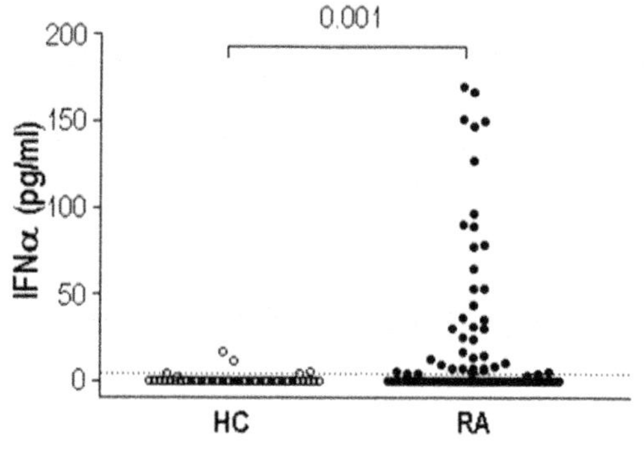

Figure 2. IFNα serum levels are increased in a subgroup of RA patients. IFNα was quantified in 52 HC and 120 RA patients by CBA immunoassay. Dotted line represents HC 90th Percentile (4.092 pg/ml), used to classify RA patients in IFN^{low} (n = 80, 66%) or IFN^{high} (n = 40, 33%). Differences were measured by Mann-Withney U-test.

$IFN^{low/high}$ Groups Differ in their Cytokine Profiles

Finally, to analyze whether IFNα serum marker may influence cytokine profiles in RA patients, we studied IL-1β, IL-6, IL-8, IL-10, MIP-1α, VEGF-A_{165}, TNFα and TGF-β levels in patients and controls. The whole RA population was characterized by increased levels of IL-6 (1.05(3.41) vs. 0.32(1.15) pg/ml, p = 0.004), IL-8 (17.12(18.08) vs. 10.18(14.06) pg/ml, p = 0.008), IL-10 (0.37(0.68) vs. 0.10(0.18) pg/ml), and TNFα (5.76(4.01) vs. 3.26(1.93) pg/ml, p = 0.015), whereas TGF-β was decreased (14.47(4.60) vs. 19.42(6.71) ng/ml, p<0.001). Regarding to disease duration, we observed that LRA patients showed lower amounts of IL-1β (p = 0.002), IL-6 (p = 0.001) and IL-10 (p = 0.028) and slightly higher of TGF-β (p = 0.060) than ERA, whereas TNFα levels were strikingly higher in the LRA group (p<0.001). Restoration of cytokine levels in LRA could probably be due to a successful response to the therapy, since almost all LRA patients were under treatment while half of the ERA patients were untreated. In fact, striking differences were observed between treated and untreated patients in IL-1β (p<0.001), IL-6 (p = 0.002) and IL-10 (p = 0.004), but not in TNFα.

Interestingly, it is remarkable that IFN^{high} patients showed a cytokine profile more similar to SLE patients than those IFN^{low}, except for IL-1β (Figure 4A). In fact, IFN^{high} RA patients displayed higher levels of IL-1β (0.47(1.48) vs. 0.13(0.06) pg/ml, p<0.001), IL-6 (1.93(13.76) vs. 0.75(2.27) pg/ml, p = 0.004), IL-10 (0.65(1.15) vs. 0.26(0.46) pg/ml, p<0.001), MIP-1α (3.29(4.47) vs. 0.00(4.28) pg/ml, p = 0.001) and lower of TGF-β (12.86(4.01) vs. (14.98(5.45) ng/ml, p = 0.025) than IFN^{low} patients. In addition, although no association between IFNα and TNFα levels was detected in the whole RA group (r = −0.028, p = 0.766), a positive correlation was found in the IFN^{high} group (r = 0.407, p = 0.011). All these results indicate that both IFNα and treatment influence cytokine levels. In fact, Figure 4B shows that treatments seem to restore IL-1β, IL-6, IL-8, IL-10 and TGF-β levels to a greater extent in IFN^{low} patients than in IFN^{high} ones. Moreover, several clinical markers suggest a better outcome of IFN^{low}-treated patients than in their IFN^{high} counterparts (Figure 4C), thus suggesting a potential IFNα role in therapy outcomes.

Finally, we analyzed the clinical response to anti-TNF therapy among a 6-month period, since it has been proposed a role of the IFN/TNF cross-regulation in the response to this treatment [26–27]. Of note, within the IFN^{low} group (n = 14), 35% of the patients (n = 5) reached a good response, and a similar percentage was found for those with a moderate response. In contrast, any patient

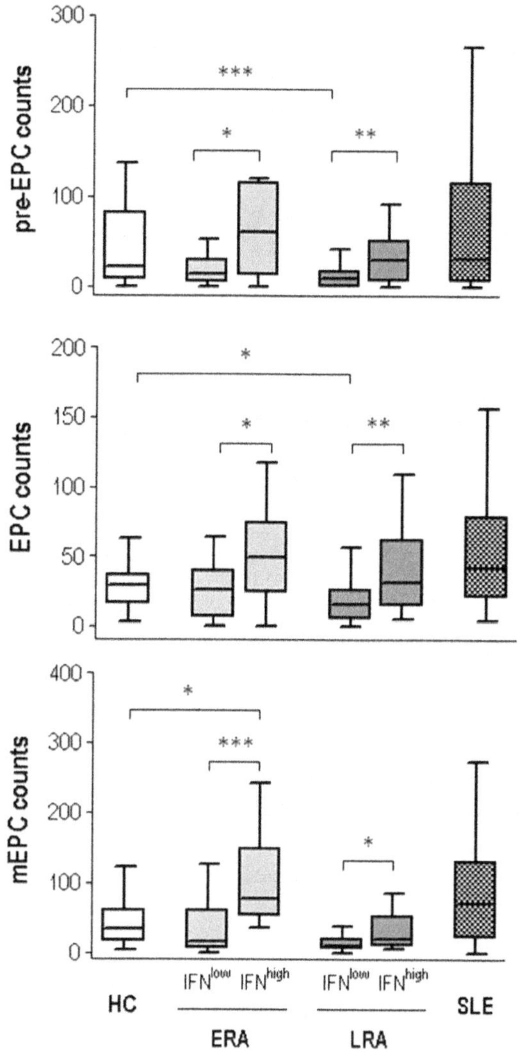

Figure 3. Long-standing RA patients with low IFNα levels exhibited a depletion of all endothelial progenitor populations. Pre-EPC, EPC and mEPC counts in early (ERA) and long-standing (LRA) Rheumatoid Arthritis patients were analyzed according to their IFNα serum levels. Healthy donors (HC) and SLE patients were included as both healthy and disease controls. Differences were assessed by Kruskal-Wallis test and Dunn's multiple comparisons post hoc test. *p<0.05, **p<0.01.

of the IFN^{high} group (n = 12) reached a good response, whereas only 41.6% (n = 5) fulfilled the criteria for a moderate one and more than a half (n = 7) exhibited no response to anti-TNF treatment.

Discussion

Recent evidence suggests a role of type I IFNs in vascular damage and EPC disbalance, mainly in SLE patients [15–18,24], probably due to the central involvement of IFNα in the SLE pathogenesis [14,28–30]. However, whether IFNα levels could play a major role in the clinical outcome and/or vascular damage in RA patients remains unknown.

Although most of the previous works reported an EPC depletion in RA patients that could be associated with disease activity [31–33], recent studies show contradictory results [34–36]. Our data

Table 2. Association between presence of IFNα serum marker and CV events in RA patients.

	Cardiovascular events		Univariate Analysis		Multivariate Analysis*	
	Absent (n = 93)	**Present (n = 27)**	**OR [95% CI]**	***p***	**OR [95% CI]**	***p***
IFNα						
IFN^{low}	68 (73.1)	12 (44.4)	**1**		**1**	
IFN^{high}	25 (26.9)	15 (55.6)	**3.400 [1.401–8.253]**	**0.007**	**4.816 [1.254–18.488]**	**0.022**
Sex						
Women	83 (89.2)	18 (66.6)	**1**			
Men	10 (10.8)	9 (33.6)	**4.150 [1.475–11.680]**	**0.007**		
Age at diagnosis	51.00 (17.00)	56.00 (23.00)	**1.050 [1.008–1.093]**	**0.019**	**1.038 [1.015–1.084]**	**0.021**
DAS28 score	3.94 (2.66)	3.26 (2.09)	0.814 [0.580–1.143]	0.235		
HTA						
Normotensive	72 (77.4)	15 (55.5)	**1**			
Hypertensive	21 (22.6)	12 (44.4)	**3.032 [1.218–7.547]**	**0.017**		
DM						
Non-diabetic	84 (91.3)	20 (74.1)	**1**			
Diabetic	9 (8.7)	7 (25.9)	**3.675 [1.192–11.326]**	**0.023**		
Smoking habit						
Non-smoker	50 (53.7)	19 (70.3)	1			
Smoker	43 (46.3)	8 (29.6)	1.947 [0.773–4.904]	0.157		
Hypercholesterolemia						
Normocholesterolemic	83 (89.2)	26 (96.2)	1			
Hypercholesterolemic	10 (10.7)	1 (3.70)	0.311 [0.038–2.559]	0.278		
RF						
Negative	34 (36.5)	8 (30.8)	1			
Positive	60 (64.5)	19 (69.2)	1.530 [0.598–3.916]	0.375		
Anti-CCP						
Negative	33 (35.4)	7 (25.9)	1			
Positive	50 (53.7)	20 (74.1)	1.791 [0.678–4.734]	0.415		
ANA						
Negative	56 (60.2)	18 (66.6)	1			
Positive	37 (47.3)	9 (33.3)	0.730 [0.296–1.800]	0.499		

Associations were evaluated by logistic regression analysis using the presence of CV events (ischemic heart disease, n = 10; cerebrovascular accidents, n = 4; heart failure, n = 14; peripheral arteriopathy, n = 1) as dependent variable. Associations that reached statistic significance in multivariate analyses are highlighted in bold.
*Multivariate analysis adjusted by sex, age at diagnosis, disease activity, smoking habits and presence or absence of HTA, DM and hypercholesterolemia. Accuracy of prediction of the final model was 76.7%.

may explain these conflicting data, since we demonstrated that only a group of RA patients exhibited a significant EPC depletion. We have previously confirmed that EPC population decreases with disease duration, whereas at disease onset it was similar to healthy subjects [24]. This finding is in line with previous studies where CV risk in RA patients has been reported to be associated with disease duration, probably due to disease-specific factors [37]. In addition, we reported for the first time, that EPC and pre-EPC populations were significantly reduced in patients with low IFNα serum levels, whereas higher levels of this cytokine were associated with higher counts of EPC populations, which leads to an increase in the mEPC/EPC ratio, in a similar way to the results observed in SLE [24]. Moreover, IFN^{high} patients displayed higher disease activity and an elevated prevalence of autoantibodies, as was reported in IFN^{high} SLE patients [38]. Thus, we think that IFNα serum levels could be an important bias in EPC studies in autoimmune diseases and it could be taken into account in future works.

Recent genomic studies have reported the presence of type I IFN signature in around 25–50% of RA patients [28–30,39], which is according to our IFN^{high} subset size (30%) and using similar criteria as cut off (90th percentile), but no correlations had been detected between IFN signature and clinical or immunological disease parameters. However, in this study, we showed that serum IFNα is correlated with clinical parameters, in the same way that has been previously reported in SLE patients [40], thus supporting the feasibility of IFNα serum marker in autoimmunity.

Although EPC depletion has been linked to higher rates of CV disease, our data show that IFN^{high} patients, with increased EPC counts, exhibit a higher occurrence of CV events, thus highlighting the role of IFNα levels as an independent CV risk biomarker. In fact, these results are in accordance with the reported role of IFNα in vascular damage and EPC dysfunction [15,17,18], and with the

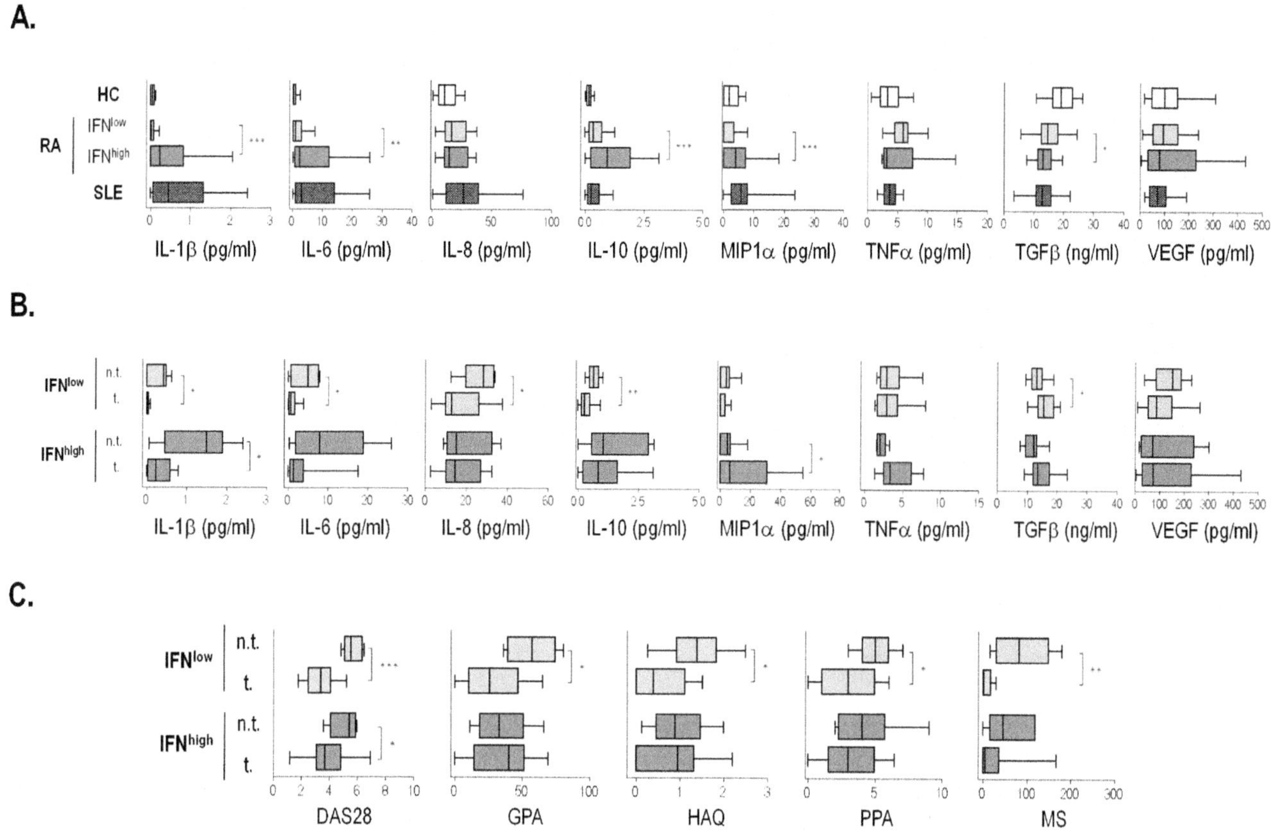

Figure 4. Cytokine profiles and disease features in RA patients are dependent on IFNα serum levels. (A) Proinflammatory cytokines are increased in IFN^{high} patients compared with both HC and IFN^{low} patients. (B) Serum cytokines levels are restored in IFN^{low}-treated patients but not in IFN^{high} ones. (C) Improvement in clinical parameters in IFN^{low}-treated patients compared with IFN^{high} group. Differences between groups were assessed by Mann-Withney U-test. n. t.: non-treated; t.: treated. *p<0.05, **p<0.01, ***p<0.001.

increased mEPC/EPC ratio found in these patients, suggestive of an impaired EPC function. Actually, recent studies have linked endothelial repair failure in autoimmunity with the IFNα pathway, probably by altering the balance between endothelial cell apoptosis and vascular repair mediated by EPC [15]. This effect has been proposed to be mediated, at least in part, through VEGF repression in EPC [16]. Accordingly, IFN signature in EPC-treated cultures has been associated with impaired functionality and endothelial dysfunction [18]. Moreover, type I IFNs have been linked to atherosclerosis progression and vascular damage in both murine models [17] and human patients [41–43], thus proposing a type I IFN-mediated pathogenic role in CV disease in autoimmune patients. In addition, IFNα pharmacological treatment in non-RA subjects has been associated with CV disease [44,45]. The increased rate of CV events in IFN^{high} patients reported in our study support these findings. Accordingly, Somers *et al.* [42] reported that type I IFNs were independently associated with atherosclerotic development after adjusting for Framingham (traditional) risk factors. Similarly, in SLE, high disease activity is considered a better CV disease predictor than traditional risk factors [46].

In view of our results, we hypothesize that a potential mechanism by which IFNα could increase CV risk may be by promoting a premature EPC differentiation, generating mEPC (CD133$^-$) with little or no vasculogenic and/or repair capability [6], probably similar to the "non-angiogenic phenotype" reported in murine SLE models [16], consequently resulting in a defective EPC-mediated endothelial repair. That is, although counterintuitive, higher EPC counts are not associated with cardioprotection, but endothelial repair failure, because of the high IFNα levels, which are causing a shift towards the mEPC phenotype. In addition, we showed that patients who had experienced CV events exhibited a higher mEPC/EPC ratio, thus linking IFNα, EPC maturation and impaired EPC functionality.

Another interesting finding was the differences in the cytokine patterns of RA patients, which seem to be related to treatment and IFNα levels. In fact, IFN^{high} RA patients showed cytokine disturbances closer to SLE patients, characterized by a proinflammatory profile and higher IL-10 levels, which are associated with disease activity and poor prognosis markers, suggesting that this cytokine could be acting as a proinflammatory mediator in these conditions, as some authors have reported [47,48]. Moreover, the IFN^{high} group exhibited a positive correlation between IFNα and TNFα serum levels, similar to previously reported in SLE patients [49,50]. Although Palucka *et al.* [26] have been proposed a negative cross-regulation between these cytokines, many other associations have been published thereafter, highlighting the relevance of the disease, the experimental model, the sample origin and the characteristics of the patients. It seems that, in some autoimmune disorders, the negative TNF/IFN cross-regulation loop is missed, leading to high serum levels of both cytokines in patients in which they may exert a pathological effect [39,49]. Moreover, different associations of these two mediators have been reported even in a single disease [51], as seen in our study.Actually, we think that IFN^{high} RA patients might display an impaired endothelial repair partly due to their proinflammatory cytokine network, mainly represented by higher serum levels of IL-1β and IL-6 (a Th17 inducer cytokines) and low TGF-β, compared to their IFN^{low} counterparts. In fact, reported *in vitro* experiments showed that proinflammatory conditions are enough to impair EPC functionality [33,52,53]. Moreover, Mälarstig *et al.* [13] have showed that raised IL-10 levels are associated with poor outcomes and enhanced systemic inflammation in acute coronary syndrome, supporting, at least in part, our findings.

Finally, differences in cytokine levels between treated and untreated patients among IFN^{low} and IFN^{high} groups suggest that IFNα could be a predictive factor for treatment outcomes, being IFN^{high} patients associated with a poor response. This was especially clear for anti-TNF therapy, since clinical response among the previous 6 months was higher in those patients within the IFN^{low} group. Similar conclusions were published by other authors [29,54]. Therefore, this result makes us hypothesize that the IFN^{high} group could benefit from an anti-IFNα therapy [55] rather than traditional DMARDs. However, relatively short follow-up period, differences in treatment duration and the low numbers of patients included do not lead us to achieve consistent conclusions in this issue.

Conclusions

In summary, we show that high IFNα serum levels could identify a group of RA patients with increased disease activity, EPC imbalance, enhanced proinflammatory profile and higher cardiovascular risk, probably due, at least in part, to an impaired endothelial repair. In addition, IFNα could be not only a marker of poor prognosis, but also of poor response to therapy, thus highlighting the relevance of this cytokine as a potential therapeutic target in RA.

Author Contributions

Conceived and designed the experiments: AS. Performed the experiments: JRC BdP PL CP. Analyzed the data: JRC AS. Contributed reagents/materials/analysis tools: MAL FJBG AS. Wrote the paper: JRC AS.

References

1. Avina-Zubieta JA, Thomas J, Sadatsafavi M, Lehman AJ, Lacaille D (2012) Risk of incident cardiovascular events in patients with rheumatoid arthritis: a meta-analysis of observational studies. Ann Rheum Dis. annrheumdis-2011-200726 [pii];10.1136/annrheumdis-2011-200726 [doi].
2. Wolfe F, Mitchell DM, Sibley JT, Fries JF, Bloch DA, et al. (1994) The mortality of rheumatoid arthritis. Arthritis Rheum 37: 481–494.
3. Hansel S, Lassig G, Pistrosch F, Passauer J (2003) Endothelial dysfunction in young patients with long-term rheumatoid arthritis and low disease activity. Atherosclerosis 170: 177–180. S0021915003002818 [pii].
4. Pompilio G, Capogrossi MC, Pesce M, Alamanni F, DiCampli C, et al. (2009) Endothelial progenitor cells and cardiovascular homeostasis: clinical implications. Int J Cardiol 131: 156–167. S0167-5273(08)00949-2 [pii];10.1016/j.ijcard.2008.08.033 [doi].
5. Gehling UM, Ergun S, Schumacher U, Wagener C, Pantel K, et al. (2000) In vitro differentiation of endothelial cells from AC133-positive progenitor cells. Blood 95: 3106–3112.
6. Peichev M, Naiyer AJ, Pereira D, Zhu Z, Lane WJ, et al. (2000) Expression of VEGFR-2 and AC133 by circulating human CD34(+) cells identifies a population of functional endothelial precursors. Blood 95: 952–958.
7. Friedrich EB, Walenta K, Scharlau J, Nickenig G, Werner N (2006) CD34−/CD133+/VEGFR-2+ endothelial progenitor cell subpopulation with potent vasoregenerative capacities. Circ Res 98: e20–e25. 01.RES.0000205765.28940.93 [pii];10.1161/01.RES.0000205765.28940.93 [doi].
8. Hill JM, Zalos G, Halcox JP, Schenke WH, Waclawiw MA, et al. (2003) Circulating endothelial progenitor cells, vascular function, and cardiovascular risk. N Engl J Med 348: 593–600. 10.1056/NEJMoa022287 [doi];348/7/593 [pii].
9. Werner N, Kosiol S, Schiegl T, Ahlers P, Walenta K, et al. (2005) Circulating endothelial progenitor cells and cardiovascular outcomes. N Engl J Med 353: 999–1007. 353/10/999 [pii];10.1056/NEJMoa043814 [doi].
10. Full LE, Ruisanchez C, Monaco C (2009) The inextricable link between atherosclerosis and prototypical inflammatory diseases rheumatoid arthritis and systemic lupus erythematosus. Arthritis Res Ther 11: 217. ar2631 [pii];10.1186/ar2631 [doi].
11. Sattar N, McCarey DW, Capell H, McInnes IB (2003) Explaining how "high-grade" systemic inflammation accelerates vascular risk in rheumatoid arthritis. Circulation 108: 2957–2963. 10.1161/01.CIR.0000099844.31524.05 [doi];108/24/2957 [pii].
12. Dessein PH, Joffe BI, Singh S (2005) Biomarkers of endothelial dysfunction, cardiovascular risk factors and atherosclerosis in rheumatoid arthritis. Arthritis Res Ther 7: R634-R643. ar1717 [pii];10.1186/ar1717 [doi].
13. Malarstig A, Eriksson P, Hamsten A, Lindahl B, Wallentin L, et al. (2008) Raised interleukin-10 is an indicator of poor outcome and enhanced systemic inflammation in patients with acute coronary syndrome. Heart 94: 724–729. hrt.2007.119271 [pii];10.1136/hrt.2007.119271 [doi].
14. Ronnblom L (2011) The type I interferon system in the etiopathogenesis of autoimmune diseases. Ups J Med Sci 116: 227–237. 10.3109/03009734.2011.624649 [doi].
15. Denny MF, Thacker S, Mehta H, Somers EC, Dodick T, et al. (2007) Interferon-alpha promotes abnormal vasculogenesis in lupus: a potential pathway for premature atherosclerosis. Blood 110: 2907–2915. blood-2007-05-089086 [pii];10.1182/blood-2007-05-089086 [doi].
16. Thacker SG, Berthier CC, Mattinzoli D, Rastaldi MP, Kretzler M, et al. (2010) The detrimental effects of IFN-alpha on vasculogenesis in lupus are mediated by repression of IL-1 pathways: potential role in atherogenesis and renal vascular rarefaction. J Immunol 185: 4457–4469. jimmunol.1001782 [pii];10.4049/jimmunol.1001782 [doi].
17. Thacker SG, Zhao W, Smith CK, Luo W, Wang H, et al. (2012) Type I interferons modulate vascular function, repair, thrombosis, and plaque progression in murine models of lupus and atherosclerosis. Arthritis Rheum 64: 2975–2985. 10.1002/art.34504 [doi].
18. Lee PY, Li Y, Richards HB, Chan FS, Zhuang H, et al. (2007) Type I interferon as a novel risk factor for endothelial progenitor cell depletion and endothelial dysfunction in systemic lupus erythematosus. Arthritis Rheum 56: 3759–3769. 10.1002/art.23035 [doi].
19. Kaplan MJ, Salmon JE (2011) How does interferon-alpha insult the vasculature? Let me count the ways. Arthritis Rheum 63: 334–336. 10.1002/art.30161 [doi].
20. Tan FK, Zhou X, Mayes MD, Gourh P, Guo X, et al. (2006) Signatures of differentially regulated interferon gene expression and vasculotrophism in the peripheral blood cells of systemic sclerosis patients. Rheumatology (Oxford) 45: 694–702. kei244 [pii];10.1093/rheumatology/kei244 [doi].
21. van Gestel AM, Anderson JJ, van Riel PL, Boers M, Haagsma CJ, et al. (1999) ACR and EULAR improvement criteria have comparable validity in rheumatoid arthritis trials. American College of Rheumatology European League of Associations for Rheumatology. J Rheumatol 26: 705–711.
22. Ho KK, Pinsky JL, Kannel WB, Levy D (1993) The epidemiology of heart failure: the Framingham Study. J Am Coll Cardiol 22: 6A–13A.
23. Rodriguez-Rodriguez L, Gonzalez-Juanatey C, Palomino-Morales R, Vazquez-Rodriguez TR, Miranda-Filloy JA, et al. (2011) TNFA -308 (rs1800629) polymorphism is associated with a higher risk of cardiovascular disease in patients with rheumatoid arthritis. Atherosclerosis 216: 125–130. S0021-9150(11)00192-4 [pii];10.1016/j.atherosclerosis.2010.10.052 [doi].
24. Rodriguez-Carrio J, Prado C, de PB, Lopez P, Gomez J, et al. (2012) Circulating endothelial cells and their progenitors in systemic lupus erythematosus and early rheumatoid arthritis patients. Rheumatology (Oxford) 51: 1775–1784. kes152 [pii];10.1093/rheumatology/kes152 [doi].
25. Distler JH, Allanore Y, Avouac J, Giacomelli R, Guiducci S, et al. (2009) EULAR Scleroderma Trials and Research group statement and recommendations on endothelial precursor cells. Ann Rheum Dis 68: 163–168. ard.2008.091918 [pii];10.1136/ard.2008.091918 [doi].
26. Palucka AK, Blanck JP, Bennett L, Pascual V, Banchereau J (2005) Cross-regulation of TNF and IFN-alpha in autoimmune diseases. Proc Natl Acad Sci U S A 102: 3372–3377. 0408506102 [pii];10.1073/pnas.0408506102 [doi].
27. Cantaert T, Baeten D, Tak PP, van Baarsen LG (2010) Type I IFN and TNFalpha cross-regulation in immune-mediated inflammatory disease: basic concepts and clinical relevance. Arthritis Res Ther 12: 219. ar3150 [pii];10.1186/ar3150 [doi].
28. Higgs BW, Liu Z, White B, Zhu W, White WI, et al. (2011) Patients with systemic lupus erythematosus, myositis, rheumatoid arthritis and scleroderma share activation of a common type I interferon pathway. Ann Rheum Dis 70: 2029–2036. ard.2011.150326 [pii];10.1136/ard.2011.150326 [doi].
29. Reynier F, Petit F, Paye M, Turrel-Davin F, Imbert PE, et al. (2011) Importance of correlation between gene expression levels: application to the type I interferon signature in rheumatoid arthritis. PLoS One 6: e24828. 10.1371/journal.pone.0024828 [doi];PONE-D-11-05657 [pii].

30. van der Pouw Kraan TC, Wijbrandts CA, van Baarsen LG, Voskuyl AE, Rustenburg F, et al. (2007) Rheumatoid arthritis subtypes identified by genomic profiling of peripheral blood cells: assignment of a type I interferon signature in a subpopulation of patients. Ann Rheum Dis 66: 1008–1014. ard.2006.063412 [pii];10.1136/ard.2006.063412 [doi].
31. Egan CG, Caporali F, Garcia-Gonzalez E, Galeazzi M, Sorrentino V (2008) Endothelial progenitor cells and colony-forming units in rheumatoid arthritis: association with clinical characteristics. Rheumatology (Oxford) 47: 1484–1488. ken299 [pii];10.1093/rheumatology/ken299 [doi].
32. Grisar J, Aletaha D, Steiner CW, Kapral T, Steiner S, et al. (2005) Depletion of endothelial progenitor cells in the peripheral blood of patients with rheumatoid arthritis. Circulation 111: 204–211. 01.CIR.0000151875.21836.AE [pii];10.1161/01.CIR.0000151875.21836.AE [doi].
33. Herbrig K, Haensel S, Oelschlaegel U, Pistrosch F, Foerster S, et al. (2006) Endothelial dysfunction in patients with rheumatoid arthritis is associated with a reduced number and impaired function of endothelial progenitor cells. Ann Rheum Dis 65: 157–163. ard.2005.035378 [pii];10.1136/ard.2005.035378 [doi].
34. Allanore Y, Batteux F, Avouac J, Assous N, Weill B, et al. (2007) Levels of circulating endothelial progenitor cells in systemic sclerosis. Clin Exp Rheumatol 25: 60–66. 1982 [pii].
35. Jodon dV, V, Avouac J, Ponceau A, Ruiz B, Kahan A, et al. (2010) Enhanced late-outgrowth circulating endothelial progenitor cell levels in rheumatoid arthritis and correlation with disease activity. Arthritis Res Ther 12: R27. ar2934 [pii];10.1186/ar2934 [doi].
36. Yiu KH, Wang S, Mok MY, Ooi GC, Khong PL, et al. (2010) Role of circulating endothelial progenitor cells in patients with rheumatoid arthritis with coronary calcification. J Rheumatol 37: 529–535. jrheum.090782 [pii];10.3899/jrheum.090782 [doi].
37. Kerola AM, Kauppi MJ, Kerola T, Nieminen TV (2012) How early in the course of rheumatoid arthritis does the excess cardiovascular risk appear? Ann Rheum Dis 71: 1606–1615. annrheumdis-2012-201334 [pii];10.1136/annrheumdis-2012-201334 [doi].
38. Kirou KA, Lee C, George S, Louca K, Peterson MG, et al. (2005) Activation of the interferon-alpha pathway identifies a subgroup of systemic lupus erythematosus patients with distinct serologic features and active disease. Arthritis Rheum 52: 1491–1503. 10.1002/art.21031 [doi].
39. Cantaert T, van Baarsen LG, Wijbrandts CA, Thurlings RM, van de Sande MG, et al. (2010) Type I interferons have no major influence on humoral autoimmunity in rheumatoid arthritis. Rheumatology (Oxford) 49: 156–166. kep345 [pii];10.1093/rheumatology/kep345 [doi].
40. Bauer JW, Baechler EC, Petri M, Batliwalla FM, Crawford D, et al. (2006) Elevated serum levels of interferon-regulated chemokines are biomarkers for active human systemic lupus erythematosus. PLoS Med 3: e491. 05-PLME-RA-0506R3 [pii];10.1371/journal.pmed.0030491 [doi].
41. Kirou KA, Cole P, Salmon JE, Roman MJ, Crow MK (2013) Identification of molecular pathways associated with progression of carotid atherosclerosis in systemic lupus erythematosus [abstract]. Arthritis Rheum 54: suppl:S807.
42. Somers EC, Zhao W, Lewis EE, Wang L, Wing JJ, et al. (2012) Type I interferons are associated with subclinical markers of cardiovascular disease in a cohort of systemic lupus erythematosus patients. PLoS One 7: e37000. 10.1371/journal.pone.0037000 [doi];PONE-D-12-02237 [pii].
43. Zhao W, Somers EC, McCune WJ, Kaplan MJ (2009) Type I Interferon gene signatures are associated with vascular risk and atherosclerosis in systemic lupus erythematosus [abstract]. Arthritis Rheum 60: suppl 10: 582.
44. Kobayashi T, Sato Y, Hasegawa Y, Nagasawa T, Yoda Y, et al. (1992) Multiple myeloma complicated by congestive heart failure following first administration of recombinant alpha-interferon. Intern Med 31: 936–940.
45. Kuwata A, Ohashi M, Sugiyama M, Ueda R, Dohi Y (2002) A case of reversible dilated cardiomyopathy after alpha-interferon therapy in a patient with renal cell carcinoma. Am J Med Sci 324: 331–334.
46. Esdaile JM, Abrahamowicz M, Grodzicky T, Li Y, Panaritis C, et al. (2001) Traditional Framingham risk factors fail to fully account for accelerated atherosclerosis in systemic lupus erythematosus. Arthritis Rheum 44: 2331–2337.
47. Cush JJ, Splawski JB, Thomas R, McFarlin JE, Schulze-Koops H, et al. (1995) Elevated interleukin-10 levels in patients with rheumatoid arthritis. Arthritis Rheum 38: 96–104.
48. Lacki JK, Samborski W, Mackiewicz SH (1997) Interleukin-10 and interleukin-6 in lupus erythematosus and rheumatoid arthritis, correlations with acute phase proteins. Clin Rheumatol 16: 275–278.
49. Lopez P, Gomez J, Prado C, Gutierrez C, Suarez A (2008) Influence of functional interleukin 10/tumor necrosis factor-alpha polymorphisms on interferon-alpha, IL-10, and regulatory T cell population in patients with systemic lupus erythematosus receiving antimalarial treatment. J Rheumatol 35: 1559–1566. 08/13/0621 [pii].
50. Weckerle CE, Mangale D, Franek BS, Kelly JA, Kumabe M, et al. (2012) Large-scale analysis of tumor necrosis factor alpha levels in systemic lupus erythematosus. Arthritis Rheum 64: 2947–2952. 10.1002/art.34483 [doi].
51. Kariuki SN, Crow MK, Niewold TB (2008) The PTPN22 C1858T polymorphism is associated with skewing of cytokine profiles toward high interferon-alpha activity and low tumor necrosis factor alpha levels in patients with lupus. Arthritis Rheum 58: 2818–2823. 10.1002/art.23728 [doi].
52. Deng XL, Li XX, Liu XY, Sun L, Liu R (2010) Comparative study on circulating endothelial progenitor cells in systemic lupus erythematosus patients at active stage. Rheumatol Int 30: 1429–1436. 10.1007/s00296-009-1156-4 [doi].
53. Grisar J, Steiner CW, Bonelli M, Karonitsch T, Schwarzinger I, et al. (2008) Systemic lupus erythematosus patients exhibit functional deficiencies of endothelial progenitor cells. Rheumatology (Oxford) 47: 1476–1483. ken286 [pii];10.1093/rheumatology/ken286 [doi].
54. van Baarsen LG, Wijbrandts CA, Rustenburg F, Cantaert T, van der Pouw Kraan TC, et al. (2010) Regulation of IFN response gene activity during infliximab treatment in rheumatoid arthritis is associated with clinical response to treatment. Arthritis Res Ther 12: R11. ar2912 [pii];10.1186/ar2912 [doi].
55. Yao Y, Richman L, Higgs BW, Morehouse CA, de los RM, et al. (2009) Neutralization of interferon-alpha/beta-inducible genes and downstream effect in a phase I trial of an anti-interferon-alpha monoclonal antibody in systemic lupus erythematosus. Arthritis Rheum 60: 1785–1796. 10.1002/art.24557 [doi].

9

Myeloid Deletion of SIRT1 Aggravates Serum Transfer Arthritis in Mice via Nuclear Factor-κB Activation

Young-Sool Hah[1]◔, Yun-Hong Cheon[2]◔, Hye Song Lim[2], Hee Young Cho[1], Byung-Hyun Park[3], Sun-O Ka[3], Young-Rae Lee[4], Dong-Won Jeong[1], Hyun-Ok Kim[2], Myung-Kwan Han[5]*, Sang-Il Lee[2]*

1 Clinical Research Institute, Gyeongsang National University Hospital, Jinju, Republic of Korea, **2** Department of Internal Medicine and Institute of Health Science, Gyeongsang National University School of Medicine, Jinju, Republic of Korea, **3** Department of Biochemistry, Chonbuk National University Medical School, Jeonju, Republic of Korea, **4** Department of Oral biochmistry, Wonkwang University School of Dentistry, Iksan, Republic of Korea, **5** Department of Microbiology, Chonbuk National University Medical School, Republic of Korea

Abstract

Objective: SIRT1 modulates the acetylation of the p65 subunit of nuclear factor-κB (NF-κB) and plays a pivotal role in the inflammatory response. This study sought to assess the role of SIRT1 in rheumatoid arthritis (RA) using a myeloid cell-specific SIRT1 knockout (mSIRT1 KO) mouse.

Methods: mSIRT1 KO mice were generated using the loxP/Cre recombinase system. K/BxN serum transfer arthritis was induced in mSIRT1 KO mice and age-matched littermate loxP control mice. Arthritis severity was assessed by clinical and pathological scoring. The levels of inflammatory cytokines in the serum and joints were measured by ELISA. Migration, M1 polarization, cytokine production, osteoclastogenesis, and p65 acetylation were assessed in bone marrow-derived monocytes/macrophages (BMMs).

Results: mSIRT1 KO mice showed more severe inflammatory arthritis and aggravated pathological findings than control mice. These effects were paralleled by increases in IL-1, TNF-α, TRAP-positive osteoclasts, and F4/80$^+$ macrophages in the ankles of mSIRT1 KO mice. In addition, BMMs from mSIRT1 KO mice displayed hyperacetylated p65 and increased NF-κB binding activity when compared to control mice, which resulted in increased M1 polarization, migration, pro-inflammatory cytokine production, and osteoclastogenesis.

Conclusion: Our study provides *in vivo* evidence that myeloid cell-specific deletion of SIRT1 exacerbates inflammatory arthritis via the hyperactivation of NF-κB signaling, which suggests that SIRT1 activation may be beneficial in the treatment of inflammatory arthritis.

Editor: Deyu Fang, Northwestern University Feinberg School of Medicine, United States of America

Funding: This work was supported by the National Research Foundation of Korea Grant funded by the Korean Government (NRF-2011-013-E00020). The funders had no role in study design, data collection and analysis, decision to publish, or preparation of the manuscript.

Competing Interests: The authors have declared that no competing interests exist.

* E-mail: iamtom@chonbuk.ac.kr (MKH); goldgu@gnu.ac.kr (SIL)

◔ These authors contributed equally to this work.

Introduction

The mammalian sirtuin members, named SIRT1 to SIRT7, are class III histone deacetylases that regulate senescence, stress resistance, metabolism, and inflammation [1,2]. In particular, SIRT1 has been demonstrated to be a pivotal molecule in the modulation of inflammation through the deacetylation of histones and non-histone proteins [3]. However, there are limited and controversial data regarding the roles of SIRTs in rheumatoid arthritis (RA). Niederer *et al.* showed that TNF-α-induced over-expression of SIRT1 contributes to chronic inflammation by increasing proinflammatory cytokines and inhibiting apoptosis in RA synovial cells [4]. Subsequently, the same authors reported that SIRT6 attenuates cigarette smoke- and TNF-α-induced matrix metalloproteinase-1 (MMP1) production in RA fibroblast-like synoviocytes (RA-FLS) [5]. More recently, we showed that SIRT6 over-expression effectively reduces the inflammatory response in RA-FLS and the arthritis severity in collagen-induced arthritis (CIA) [6]. However, the protective or pro-inflammatory roles of SIRT1 in *in vivo* models of RA have not been analyzed.

Activated myeloid cells, such as monocytes/macrophages, neutrophils, myeloid dendritic cells, and osteoclasts, are known to be prominent participants in inflammatory arthritis such as RA [7]. The activation of nuclear factor-κB (NF-κB) in macrophages results in the transactivation of many pro-inflammatory cytokines and chemokines and leads to RA-FLS activation and the infiltration of large numbers of immune cells into the synovium [8]. Thus, the essential role of NF-κB has been well recognized in the pathogenesis of RA [8,9]. In a recent report, using a myeloid cell-specific SIRT1 knockout (mSIRT1 KO) mouse model, the deletion of SIRT1 in macrophages led to hyperactive NF-κB signaling, which resulted in enhanced inflammatory signaling in response to environmental stress [10]. However, to our knowledge, no report has assessed the role of myeloid cell-derived SIRT1 in animal models of RA. Thus, to investigate the *in vivo* function of SIRT1 in RA, we generated mSIRT1 KO mice and explored the specific contribution of myeloid cell-derived SIRT1 using the K/BxN serum transfer arthritis model.

Materials and Methods

Generation of mSIRT1 KO mice

SIRT1$^{loxP/loxP}$ mice (B6.129-Sirt1^{tm1Ygu}/J) and LysM-Cre mice (B6.129P2-lyz2$^{tm1(cre)Ifo}$/J) were purchased from Jackson Laboratory (Bar Harbor, ME, USA). SirT1$^{loxP/loxP}$ and LysM-Cre mice were crossed to obtain mSIRT1 KO mice. To avoid potential variations that could be contributed by gender and genetic background, male mice from the F2 generation, SIRT1$^{loxP/loxP}$LysM-Cre$^{+/+}$ (mSIRT1 KO) and SIRT1$^{loxP/loxP}$LysM-Cre$^{-/-}$ (WT), were used for the studies. All of the experimental animals used in this study were maintained under the protocol approved by the Institutional Animal Care and Use Committee of the Gyeongsang National University (GLA-100917-M0092).

K/BxN serum transfer arthritis and clinical evaluation

KRN TCR-transgenic mice were a gift from D. Mathis and C. Benoist (Harvard Medical School, Boston, Massachusetts) and from the Institut de Genetique et de Biologie Moleculaire et Cellulaire and were maintained on a B6 background (K/B). To induce K/BxN serum transfer arthritis [11], serum samples were pooled from arthritic adult K/BxN mice. mSIRT1 KO and WT mice were injected with K/BxN serum (50 μL) intraperitoneally on days 0 and 2, and the severity of arthritis was defined as previously described [12]. Clinical arthritis scores were evaluated using a scale of 0–4 for each paw for a total score of 16. Ankle thickness was measured with a caliper placed across the ankle joint at the widest point.

Histopathological and biochemical analysis

Decalcified and paraffin-embedded joint sections were stained with hematoxylin and eosin for morphological analysis or with a tartrate-resistant acid phosphatase (TRAP) staining kit (Sigma-Aldrich, Hempstead, NY USA) for osteoclast analysis. The joint sections were scored using a semi-quantitative scoring system [12], according to synovial inflammation and bone erosion. The number of TRAP-positive multi-nucleated cells that contained 3 or more nuclei were counted in 10 areas of each ankle (200×, n = 10 mice for each group). The F4/80$^+$ cells were immunohistochemically detected with a rat monoclonal antibody directed against F4/80 (Santa Cruz Biotechnology Inc., Santa Cruz, CA, USA). The number of F4/80$^+$ cells was counted in 8 randomly selected high-power fields (400×) for each ankle joint (n = 10 mice for each group). The joint tissue concentrations of IL-1β, TNF-α, and IL-6 were measured by ELISA (R&D Systems, Minneapolis, MN, USA).

Bone marrow-derived macrophage (BMM) culture and differentiation

For the BMM cultures, bone marrow was isolated from the femurs and tibias of WT and mSIRT1 KO mice and cultured in minimum essential medium alpha (α-MEM) supplemented with 10% fetal bovine serum (FBS). The cells were plated and cultured overnight in the presence of macrophage colony-stimulating factor (M-CSF, 10 ng/ml). The non-adherent cells were collected and cultured for 3 days in the presence of M-CSF (10 ng/ml). The floating cells were removed, and the adherent cells were used as BMMs. To assess inflammatory cytokine production, BMMs were pretreated with TNF-α (10 ng/ml) for 24 h. The culture supernatants were collected, and the secreted IL-1β level was quantified by ELISA (R&D Systems). For M1 and M2 differentiation, BMMs were treated with IFN-γ (50 U/ml, Invitrogen) and IL-4 (10 ng/ml; Invitrogen, Carlsbad, CA), respectively.

Assessment of osteoclast formation

BMMs (5×10^5) were seeded into 24-well culture plates and maintained in α-MEM-containing recombinant mouse M-CSF (10 ng/ml) and RANKL (10 or 30 ng/ml). After 7 days in culture, the cells were cytochemically stained for TRAP using a commercially available kit (Sigma-Aldrich, Hempstead, NY, USA). The BMMs were rinsed promptly in PBS buffer, fixed with formalin (10% in PBS) for 10 min, and rinsed in distilled water. TRAP was histochemically revealed by a simultaneous coupling reaction using Naphthol AS-BI-phosphate as the substrate and Fast violet B as the diazonium salt. The cells were then incubated for 90 min at 37°C in the dark and rinsed 3 times in distilled water. The residual activity was inhibited by incubation with 4% NaF for 30 min. TRAP-positive cells demonstrating more than 3 nuclei were considered osteoclasts. The number of newly generated osteoclasts was assessed by light microscopic examination.

BMM migration assay

Murine BMMs (5×10^5) were plated onto 8-μm pore chemotaxis membranes (Corning, Acton, MA, USA) within Boyden chamber inserts in FBS-free α-MEM. After attachment, MCP-1 (R&D Systems, Minneapolis, MN, USA) was added to the lower chamber, and the cells were incubated at 37°C in 5% CO_2 for 2 h. The cells that remained on the upper section of the filters were removed mechanically. The cells that migrated to the lower section of the filters were fixed with 4% paraformaldehyde in PBS, stained with DAPI (Invitrogen-Molecular Probes, Eugene, OR, USA), and counted in 10 random fields/filter using an optical microscope (Nikon Co., Tokyo, Japan).

Western blot analysis

Cells were lysed in RIPA buffer (50 mM Tris, pH 7.2, 150 mM NaCl, 1% NP40, 0.1% SDS) supplemented with a protease inhibitor cocktail (Calbiochem, Cambridge, MA, USA). The cells were then sonicated and centrifuged at 12,000 g for 10 min at 4°C to remove insoluble debris. The protein concentration was determined using the BCA assay (Thermo Scientific, Waltham, MA, USA). Total proteins (30 μg) were resolved on a SDS-polyacrylamide gel, and the gels were then electroblotted onto a nitrocellulose membrane. After blocking with a 5% skim milk solution, the membranes were incubated with specific antibodies against acetylated p65 (1:1,000; Cell Signaling Technology, Beverly, MA, USA) or β-actin (1:5,000; Sigma-Aldrich, Hempstead, NY, USA), and the proteins were identified with the ECL detection system.

Immunofluorescence assay

BMMs were plated onto a glass coverslip in RPMI 1640 supplemented with 10% FBS and incubated overnight at 37°C. The following day, the cells were treated with TNF-α (10 ng/ml) for 1 h. At the end of the treatments, the cells were washed with PBS, fixed in PBS containing 4% paraformaldehyde, and permeabilized with 0.1% Triton X-100 in PBS for 10 min at room temperature. Then, the cells were blocked with 2% bovine serum albumin (BSA) in PBS for 1 h and incubated with primary monoclonal antibodies against acetylated p65 overnight at 4°C. After washing in PBS, the cells were further incubated with TRITC-conjugated secondary anti-mouse IgG for 1 h. The nuclei were stained with DAPI (0.5 μg/mL; Invitrogen-Molecular Probes). The cover slips were mounted and stored in the dark at 4°C. Fluorescent images were obtained from analyses using the FV-1000 confocal microscope system (Olympus, Tokyo, Japan).

Electrophoretic mobility shift assay (EMSA)

Nuclear extract preparation and EMSAs were performed as described previously [9]. Nuclear extracts prepared from WT and mSIRT1 KO primary macrophage cells were incubated with a proteinase inhibitor cocktail (Calbiochem, Cambridge, MA, USA) to inhibit endogenous protease activity. An oligonucleotide containing the κ-chain binding site (κB, 5′-CCGGTTAACAGAGGGGGCTTTCCGAG-3′) was synthesized and used as a probe for the gel retardation assay. The 2 complementary strands were then annealed and labeled with [α-^{32}P]dCTP. Next, labeled oligonucleotides (10,000 cpm), 10 μg of nuclear extracts, and binding buffer (10 mM Tris-HCl, pH 7.6, 500 mM KCl, 10 mM EDTA, 50% glycerol, 100 ng poly(dI•dC), 1 mM dithiothreitol) were then incubated for 30 min at room temperature in a final volume of 20 μl. The reaction mixtures were analyzed by electrophoresis on 4% polyacrylamide gels in a 0.5× Tris-borate buffer, and the gels were dried and examined by autoradiography. Specificity of the DNA-protein interactions for NF-κB was demonstrated by competition assays using a 50-fold excess of unlabeled oligonucleotide.

Statistical analysis

Data are expressed as the mean ± SE. Statistical comparisons were performed using 2-tailed Student's t-tests. *P* values less than 0.05 were considered statistically significant.

Results

Myeloid SIRT1 deletion leads to the exacerbation of K/BxN serum transfer arthritis

To ascertain the role of the myeloid cell-specific SIRT1 deletion in inflammatory arthritis, we generated mSIRT1 KO mice (Fig. 1) and induced passive K/BxN arthritis in mSIRT1 KO mice and matched littermate control (WT) mice. In the K/BxN serum transfer model, the arthritis severity and change in ankle thickness were significantly increased in mSIRT1 KO mice as compared to WT mice (Fig. 2A). There was no difference in arthritis severity between SIRT1$^{+/+}$LysM-Cre$^{+/+}$ and SIRT1$^{+/+}$LysM-Cre$^{-/-}$ mice (data not shown). It is well known that pro-inflammatory cytokines, such as IL-1β and TNF-α, play key roles in the pathogenesis of RA. Therefore, we measured cytokine levels in the synovial tissues on day 10 using ELISA. The levels of TNF-α and IL-1β were higher in the ankle lysates of mSIRT1 KO mice than WT mice, although the IL-6 levels were not increased (Fig. 2B). Histopathological analysis further revealed that mSIRT1 KO mice demonstrated more severe synovial inflammation and bone erosions than WT mice (Fig. 2C left panel, 2D). Because macrophages are important mediators of innate immunity and are critical in the pathogenesis of inflammatory arthritis, we next examined macrophage infiltration into the synovial tissue. mSIRT1 mice showed increased F4/80$^+$ macrophage infiltration in the synovial tissues when compared to WT mice (Fig. 2C middle panel, 2E). We next counted TRAT-positive cells to confirm the relationship between bone erosion and the number of osteoclasts, and TRAP-positive osteoclasts were markedly increased in the joints of mSIRT1 KO mice (Fig. 2C right panel, 2F).

Myeloid SIRT1 deletion increases the activation of macrophages and osteoclastogenesis

In RA, activated macrophages play a central role, and the imbalance of pro-inflammatory and anti-inflammatory macrophages is often observed. The macrophage polarization state can

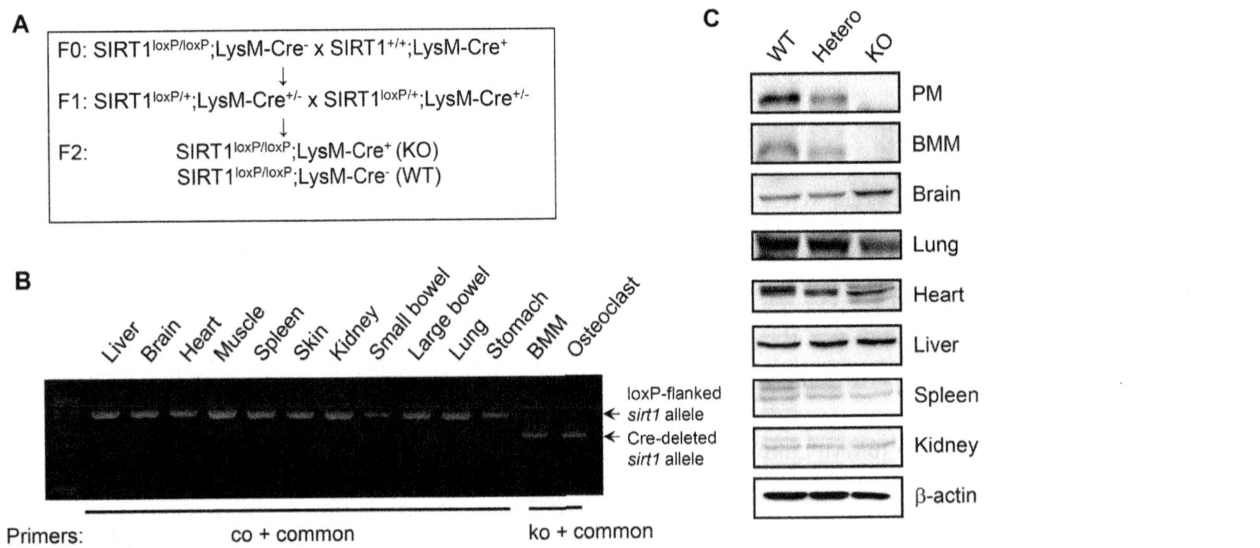

Figure 1. Myeloid cell-specific deletion of SIRT1. (A) Breeding strategy. (B) PCR genotyping. PCR analysis of several tissues from a SIRT1$^{loxP/loxP}$;LysM-Cre$^{+/+}$ mouse was performed using 3 primers designed against sequences upstream and downstream of the loxP-flanked *sirt1* exon 4: 5′ KO primer, 5′-GGTTGACTTAGGTCTTGTCTG; 5′ KO primer, 5′-AGGCGGATTTCTGAGTTCGA; and 3′ common primer, 5′-CGTCCCTTGTAATGTTTCCC. The use of these primers enabled discrimination between the loxP-flanked (upper band) and the Cre-deleted (lower band) *Sirt1* alleles. (C) Western blot analysis for SIRT1 in peritoneal macrophages (PM), BMMs, osteoclasts, and various tissues from SIRT1$^{loxP/loxP}$; LysM-Cre$^{+/+}$ mice.

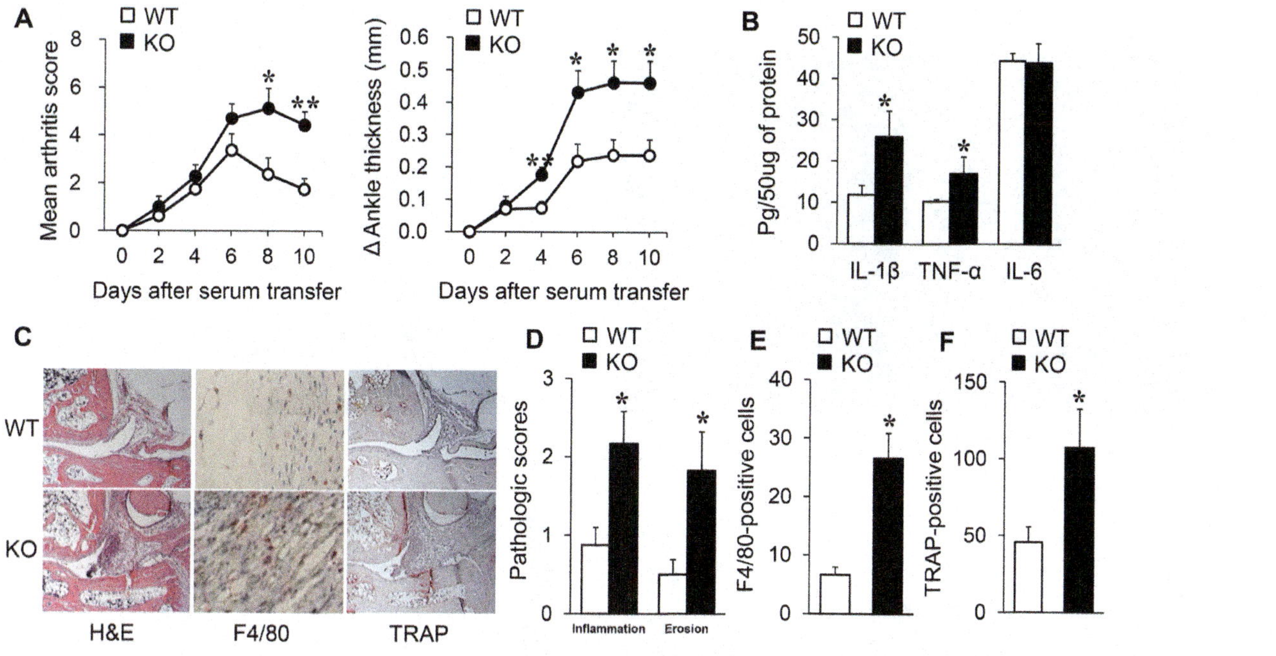

Figure 2. Myeloid cell-specific SIRT1 deficiency aggravates synovial inflammation and bone destruction in K/BxN serum transfer arthritis. Male (8- to 10-week-old) mSIRT1 KO and WT mice were injected with K/BxN serum (50 μL) intraperitoneally on days 0 and 2. (A) The severity of arthritis was defined according to semi-quantitative clinical scoring and the change in ankle thickness. (B) ELISA results for inflammatory cytokines levels in tissue extracts from mouse ankles. (C) Representative sections of the ankle joints stained with H&E, TRAP, and F4/80. The original magnifications are ×100, ×400, and ×100, respectively. (D) Mean pathologic scores for synovial inflammation and bone erosion. (E) F4/80$^+$ macrophages in ankle joints and (F) the numbers of TRAP-positive cells. The results of two independent experiments with 10 mice per group are expressed as mean ± SEM, *$p<0.05$, **$p<0.01$ vs. WT.

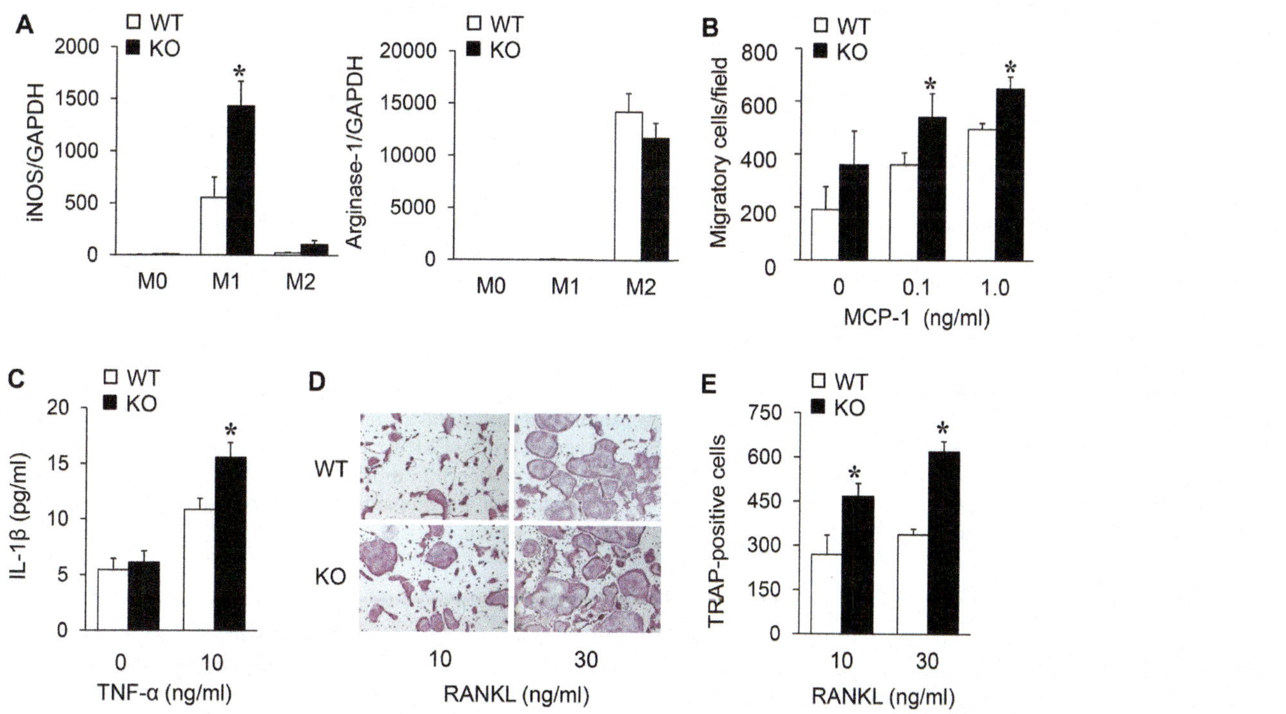

Figure 3. SIRT1 deficiency increases the migration, cytokine release, and osteoclastogenesis of BMMs. (A) Regulation of macrophage polarization by SIRT1. SIRT1-deficient or WT BMMs were treated with either 50 U/ml of IFN-γ (for M1 polarization) or 10 ng/ml of IL-4 (for M2 polarization) for 48 h. (B) Effect of recombinant MCP-1 on the migration of BMMs. (C) Increased release of IL-1β from SIRT1-deficient BMMs following 12-h TNF-α treatment. (D) Microscopic view of TRAP-positive cells from BMM precursors cultured with M-CSF and RANKL. Original magnification, ×100 (E) The TRAP-positive multinucleated osteoclasts in each well were counted. Values = mean ± SE, n=4–5 mice for each group, *$p<0.05$ and **$p<0.01$ vs. WT.

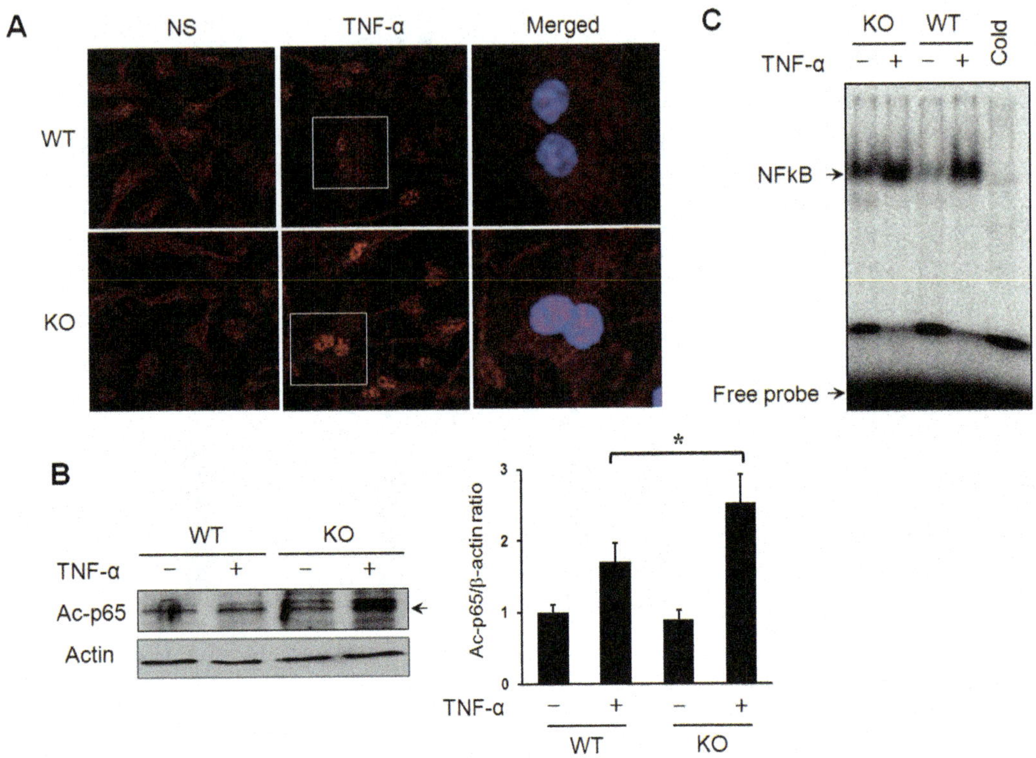

Figure 4. SIRT1 deficiency induces hyperactivation of NF-κB in BMMs. BMMs were cultured from mSIRT1 or WT mice and stimulated with TNF-α (10 ng/ml) for 1 h. (A) Immunostaining for acetylated p65 showed that loss of SIRT1 resulted in higher and sustained levels of acetylated p65 in the nuclei of macrophages following TNF-α treatment. (B) The levels of acetylated p65 were analyzed by Western blotting. Representative blot shown is from one of the three independent experiments with similar results. Values = mean ± SE, *p<0.05 vs. WT. (C) The DNA binding activity of NF-κB was analyzed by EMSA.

be defined by specific markers, such as iNOS and arginase-1 for cells of the M1 and M2 phenotypes, respectively. Thus, to examine the effect of SIRT1 on macrophage polarization, BMMs from mSIRT1 KO and WT mice were treated with IFN-γ for M1 polarization or IL-4 for M2 polarization. In the M1 polarization condition, iNOS expression was significantly increased in BMMs from mSIRT1 KO mice, whereas the levels of arginase-1 were unaltered in the M2 polarization condition (Fig. 3A). These findings suggest that SIRT1-deleted macrophages display increased M1 polarization. Next, we examined the effect of SIRT1 deletion on macrophage migration. Consistent with the increased number of macrophages in the synovium of arthritic mice, the loss of SIRT1 significantly enhanced MCP-1-induced macrophage migration in a dose-dependent manner (Fig. 3B). We also investigated whether SIRT1 deletion affects cytokine production by macrophages by measuring the IL-1β levels in culture media from TNF-α-stimulated mSIRT1 KO and WT macrophages. The results indicated that SIRT1 deletion increased IL-1β secretion 1.5-fold over control macrophages (Fig. 3C). Furthermore, we assessed osteoclastic differentiation from BMMs in medium supplemented with M-CSF and RANKL to investigate the process leading to increased bone resorption in mSIRT1 KO mice. The absence of SIRT1 resulted in the formation of greater numbers of multinucleated TRAP-positive cells (Fig. 3D, E).

Myeloid SIRT1 deletion induces the hyperacetylation of p65 and the hyperactivation of NF-κB

SIRT1 is known to regulate the transcriptional activity of NF-κB through the direct deacetylation of its p65 subunit at lysine 310 [13]. To determine whether loss of SIRT1 in macrophages alters the acetylation status of p65, BMMs from mSIRT1 KO and WT mice were stimulated with TNF-α and analyzed by immunofluorescent staining and Western blotting using an anti-Ac-K310 antibody. BMMs from both mSIRT1 KO and WT mice displayed low basal levels of Ac-p65, and TNF-α treatment induced the acetylation of p65 in both mSIRT1 KO and WT BMMs. However, mSIRT1 KO BMMs displayed significantly higher levels of Ac-p65 and increased p65 levels in their nuclei (Fig. 4A, B). To test whether this increased acetylation of p65 influenced NF-κB binding activity, mSIRT1 KO and WT BMMs were stimulated with TNF-α, and the nuclear fractions of the cell lysates were analyzed by EMSA. The DNA binding activity to an NF-κB consensus sequence in mSIRT1 KO BMMs was increased before and after TNF-α stimulation as compared to that observed in WT BMMs (Fig. 4C).

Discussion

In this study, we used mSIRT1 KO mice to investigate the role of SIRT1 in the K/BxN serum transfer model of inflammatory arthritis. Our results provide *in vivo* evidence that myeloid cell-specific deletion of SIRT1 exacerbates inflammation and bone erosion in K/BxN serum transfer arthritis. Furthermore, our *in vitro* results showed that SIRT1-deleted macrophages display increased M1 polarization, migration, pro-inflammatory cytokine production, and osteoclastogenesis through the hyperacetylation and consequent hyperactivation of NF-κB. Together, our findings suggest that SIRT1 plays a protective role against inflammatory arthritis such as RA.

Several animal studies have demonstrated that SIRT1 exhibits pronounced anti-inflammatory properties. Hepatocyte-specific SIRT1-deleted mice challenged with a high-fat diet developed hepatic inflammation and hepatic steatosis [14], and SIRT1-null mice were shown to accumulate deposits of immune complexes in the liver and kidney and develop an autoimmune-like condition [15]. Furthermore, Schug *et al.* showed that ablation of SIRT1 in macrophages not only increased the inflammatory response but also predisposed mice to the development of insulin resistance and metabolic disorders [10], and our data demonstrated that myeloid cell-specific SIRT1 deletion led to enhanced inflammation and bone destruction in K/BxN serum transfer arthritic mice. These findings suggest that myeloid cell-derived SIRT1 may be a negative regulator of the inflammatory response in RA.

The roles of monocytes/macrophages in RA are characterized by their migration, maturation, activation, cytokine production, and interactions with other synovial cells [7]. Here, we demonstrated that macrophages from mSIRT1 KO mice displayed increased migration in both *in vitro* and *in vivo* experiments. It is widely known that TNF-α, IL-l, and IL-6 released by M1 macrophages are abundant in RA, whereas IL-10 activity, which is characteristic of M2 macrophages, is somewhat diminished [7]. Accordingly, we also found that SIRT1-deficient macrophages exhibited increased M1 polarization and increased proinflammatory cytokine production. Zainabadi previously reported that SIRT1-knockout mice displayed significant bone deficiencies associated with increased osteoclastogenesis [16]. Consistent with this finding, we found that the differentiation and infiltration of osteoclasts were increased in SirT1-deficient BMMs *in vitro* as well as K/BxN serum-induced arthritic M-SIRT1 KO mice *in vivo.* Together, these findings indicate that myeloid cell-derived SIRT1 plays a critical role in the control of macrophage migration and activation as well as osteoclastogenesis.

Previous reports have shown that SIRT1 deacetylates p65 and interferes with the NF-κB signaling pathway, thereby acting as an anti-inflammatory factor [10,17]. Because NF-κB is a molecular target for both the inflammatory response and deacetylation by SIRT1, we investigated changes in the NF-κB signaling pathway in SIRT1-deleted BMMs, and our results showed that the loss of SIRT1 resulted in higher and sustained acetylation of p65 following TNF-α stimulation. We further demonstrated that the DNA binding of NF-κB was increased in M-SIRT1 KO nuclear lysates compared to controls following TNF-α stimulation. Collectively, these data indicate that the absence of SIRT1 leads to hyperacetylation and hyperactivation of NF-κB, which results in the exacerbation of inflammatory arthritis.

In summary, our study provides *in vivo* evidence that myeloid cell-specific deletion of SIRT1 exacerbates inflammatory arthritis. Contrary to previous reports showing a pro-inflammatory role of SIRT1 in synovial cells, our data suggest an anti-inflammatory property of SIRT1 in RA. Recent studies has suggested that, in addition to myeloid cells, suppression of SIRT1 in other immune cells such as in T cells and dendritic cells plays different roles in inflammation [18,19]. In addition, SIRT1 activators may have therapeutic effects in inflammatory autoimmune disease by blocking macrophage trafficking [20]. Thus, further investigation using chronic CIA model and other cell-specific KO mice will be needed to delineate the protective or harmful effect of SIRT1 on RA pathogenesis as well as potential future therapeutic application in RA.

Acknowledgments

The KRN TCR transgenic mice were a gift from D. Mathis and C. Benoist (Harvard Medical School, Boston, Massachusetts) and from the Institut de Genetique et de Biologie Moleculaire et Cellulaire.

Author Contributions

Conceived and designed the experiments: SIL MKH. Performed the experiments: YSH YHC HSL HYC DWJ HOK SOK. Analyzed the data: MKH SIL BHP. Contributed reagents/materials/analysis tools: YRL. Wrote the paper: YSH YHC.

References

1. Michan S, Sinclair D (2007) Sirtuins in mammals: insights into their biological function. Biochem J 404:1–13.
2. Han MK, Song EK, Guo Y, Ou X, Mantel C, et al. (2008) SIRT1 regulates apoptosis and Nanog expression in mouse embryonic stem cells by controlling p53 subcellular localization. Cell Stem Cell 2:241–251.
3. Xie J, Zhang X, Zhang L (2013) Negative regulation of inflammation by SIRT1. Pharmacol Res 67:60–67.
4. Niederer F, Ospelt C, Brentano F, Hottiger MO, Gay RE, et al. (2011) SIRT1 overexpression in the rheumatoid arthritis synovium contributes to proinflammatory cytokine production and apoptosis resistance. Ann Rheum Dis 70:1866–1873.
5. Engler A, Gay RE, Michel BA, Gay S, Ospelt C (2012) SIRT6 Regulates Cigarette Smoke Induced MMP1 Expression in Rheumatoid Arthritis Synovial Fibroblasts. ACR 2012 Abstract #437, S189–S190.
6. Lee HS, Ka SO, Lee SM, Lee SI, Park JW, et al. (2013) Overexpression of sirtuin 6 suppresses inflammatory responses and bone destruction in mice with collagen-induced arthritis. Arthritis Rheum. 65:1776–1785.
7. Kennedy A, Fearon U, Veale DJ, Godson C (2011) Macrophages in synovial inflammation. Front Immunol 2:52.
8. Tak PP, Firestein GS (2001) NF-kappaB: a key role in inflammatory diseases. J Clin Invest 107:7–11.
9. Hah YS, Lee YR, Jun JS, Lim HS, Kim HO, et al. (2010) A20 suppresses inflammatory responses and bone destruction in human fibroblast-like synoviocytes and in mice with collagen-induced arthritis. Arthritis Rheum 62:2313–2321.
10. Schug TT, Xu Q, Gao H, Peres-da-Silva A, Draper DW, et al. (2010) Myeloid deletion of sirt1 induces inflammatory signaling in response to environmental stress. Mol Cell Biol 30:4712–4721.
11. Kouskoff V, Korganow AS, Duchatelle V, Degott C, Benoist C, et al.(1996) Organ-specific disease provoked by systemic autoimmunity. Cell 87:811–822.
12. Lee SI, Boyle DL, Berdeja A, Firestein GS (2012) Regulation of inflammatory arthritis by the upstream kinase mitogen activated protein kinase kinase 7 in the c-Jun N-terminal kinase pathway. Arthritis Res Ther 14:R38.
13. Yeung F, Hoberg JE, Ramsey CS, Keller MD, Jones DR, et al.(2004) Modulation of NF-κB-dependent transcription and cell survival by the SIRT1 deacetylase. EMBO J 23:2369–2380.
14. Purushotham A, Schug TT, Xu Q, Surapureddi S, Guo X, et al. (2009) Hepatocyte specific deletion of sirt1 alters fatty acid metabolism and results in hepatic steatosis and inflammation. Cell Metabolism 9:327–338.
15. Sequeira J, Boily G, Bazinet S, Saliba S, He X, et al. (2008) Sirt1-null mice develop an autoimmune-like condition. Exp Cell Res 314:3069–3074.
16. Zainabadi K (2009) SirT1 regulates bone mass in vivo through regulation of osteoblast and osteoclast differentiation Thesis (Ph. D.)–Massachusetts Institute of Technology, Dept. of Biology.
17. Lee JH, Song MY, Song EK, Kim EK, Moon WS (2009) Overexpression of SIRT1 protects pancreatic beta-cells against cytokine toxicity by suppressing the nuclear factor-kappaB signaling pathway. Diabetes 58:344–351.
18. Zhang J, Lee SM, Shannon S, Gao B, Chen W, et al. (2009) The type III histone deacetylase Sirt1 is essential for maintenance of T cell tolerance in mice. J Clin Invest 119:3048–3058.
19. Yang H, Lee SM, Gao B, Zhang J, Fang D (2013) The histone deacetylase Sirtuin 1 deacetylates IRF1 and programs dendritic cells to control Th17 differentiation during autoimmune inflammation. J Biol Chem. in press.
20. Lee SM, Yang H, Tartar DM, Gao B, Luo X, et al. (2011) Prevention and treatment of diabetes with resveratrol in a non-obese mouse model of type 1 diabetes. Diabetologia 54:1136–1146.

10

Integration of Sequence Data from a Consanguineous Family with Genetic Data from an Outbred Population Identifies *PLB1* as a Candidate Rheumatoid Arthritis Risk Gene

Yukinori Okada[1,2,3,4,5], Dorothee Diogo[1,2,3], Jeffrey D. Greenberg[6], Faten Mouassess[7], Walid A. L. Achkar[7], Robert S. Fulton[8], Joshua C. Denny[9], Namrata Gupta[3], Daniel Mirel[3], Stacy Gabriel[3], Gang Li[1], Joel M. Kremer[10], Dimitrios A. Pappas[11], Robert J. Carroll[9], Anne E. Eyler[12], Gosia Trynka[1,2,3], Eli A. Stahl[13], Jing Cui[1], Richa Saxena[14], Marieke J. H. Coenen[15], Henk-Jan Guchelaar[16], Tom W. J. Huizinga[17], Philippe Dieudé[18,19], Xavier Mariette[20], Anne Barton[21], Helena Canhão[22,23], João E. Fonseca[22,23], Niek de Vries[24], Paul P. Tak[25,26], Larry W. Moreland[27], S. Louis Bridges, Jr.[28], Corinne Miceli-Richard[20], Hyon K. Choi[29,30,31], Yoichiro Kamatani[5,32], Pilar Galan[33], Mark Lathrop[34], Towfique Raj[2,3,35], Philip L. De Jager[2,3,35], Soumya Raychaudhuri[1,2,3,36], Jane Worthington[21,37], Leonid Padyukov[38], Lars Klareskog[38], Katherine A. Siminovitch[39,40,41], Peter K. Gregersen[42], Elaine R. Mardis[8], Thurayya Arayssi[43], Layla A. Kazkaz[44,45], Robert M. Plenge[1,2,3]*

1 Division of Rheumatology, Immunology, and Allergy, Brigham and Women's Hospital, Harvard Medical School, Boston, Massachusetts, United States of America, **2** Division of Genetics, Brigham and Women's Hospital, Harvard Medical School, Boston, Massachusetts, United States of America, **3** Program in Medical and Population Genetics, Broad Institute, Cambridge, Massachusetts, United States of America, **4** Department of Human Genetics and Disease Diversity, Tokyo Medical and Dental University Graduate School of Medical and Dental Sciences, Tokyo, Japan, **5** Laboratory for Statistical Analysis, Center for Integrative Medical Sciences, RIKEN, Yokohama, Japan, **6** New York University Hospital for Joint Diseases, New York, New York, United States of America, **7** Molecular Biology and Biotechnology Department, Human Genetics Division, Damascus, Syria, **8** The Genome Institute, Washington University School of Medicine, St. Louis, Missouri, United States of America, **9** Department of Biomedical Informatics, Vanderbilt University School of Medicine, Nashville, Tennessee, United States of America, **10** Department of Medicine, Albany Medical Center and The Center for Rheumatology, Albany, New York, United States of America, **11** Division of Rheumatology, Department of Medicine, New York, Presbyterian Hospital, College of Physicians and Surgeons, Columbia University, New York, New York, United States of America, **12** Department of Medicine, Vanderbilt University School of Medicine, Nashville, Tennessee, United States of America, **13** The Department of Psychiatry at Mount Sinai School of Medicine, New York, New York, United States of America, **14** Center for Human Genetics Research, Massachusetts General Hospital, Harvard Medical School, Boston, Massachusetts, United States of America, **15** Department of Human Genetics, Radboud University Medical Centre, Nijmegen, The Netherlands, **16** Department of Clinical Pharmacy and Toxicology, Leiden University Medical Center, Leiden, The Netherlands, **17** Department of Rheumatology, Leiden University Medical Centre, Leiden, The Netherlands, **18** Service de Rhumatologie et INSERM U699 Hôpital Bichat Claude Bernard, Assistance Publique des Hôpitaux de Paris, Paris, France, **19** Université Paris 7-Diderot, Paris, France, **20** Institut National de la Santé et de la Recherche Médicale (INSERM) U1012, Université Paris-Sud, Rhumatologie, Hôpitaux Universitaires Paris-Sud, Assistance Publique-Hôpitaux de Paris (AP-HP), Le Kremlin Bicêtre, France, **21** Arthritis Research UK Epidemiology Unit, Centre for Musculoskeletal Research, University of Manchester, Manchester Academic Health Science Centre, Manchester, United Kingdom, **22** Rheumatology Research Unit, Instituto de Medicina Molecular, Faculdade de Medicina da Universidade de Lisboa, Lisbon, Portugal, **23** Rheumatology Department, Santa Maria Hospital–CHLN, Lisbon, Portugal, **24** Department of Clinical Immunology and Rheumatology & Department of Genome Analysis, Academic Medical Center/University of Amsterdam, Amsterdam, The Netherlands, **25** Department of Clinical Immunology and Rheumatology, Academic Medical Center/University of Amsterdam, Amsterdam, The Netherlands, **26** GlaxoSmithKline, Stevenage, United Kingdom, **27** Division of Rheumatology and Clinical Immunology, University of Pittsburgh, Pittsburgh, Pennsylvania, United States of America, **28** Division of Clinical Immunology and Rheumatology, Department of Medicine, University of Alabama at Birmingham, Birmingham, Alabama, United States of America, **29** Channing Laboratory, Department of Medicine, Brigham and Women's Hospital, Harvard Medical School, Boston, Massachusetts, United States of America, **30** Section of Rheumatology, Boston University School of Medicine, Boston, Massachusetts, United States of America, **31** Clinical Epidemiology Research and Training Unit, Boston University School of Medicine, Boston, Massachusetts, United States of America, **32** Centre d'Etude du Polymorphisme Humain (CEPH), Paris, France, **33** Université Paris 13 Sorbonne Paris Cité, UREN (Nutritional Epidemiology Research Unit), Inserm (U557), Inra (U1125), Cnam, Bobigny, France, **34** McGill University and Génome Québec Innovation Centre, Montréal, Canada, **35** Program in Translational NeuroPsychiatric Genomics, Institute for the Neurosciences, Department of Neurology, Brigham and Women's Hospital, Boston, Massachusetts, United States of America, **36** NIHR Manchester Musculoskeletal Biomedical, Research Unit, Central Manchester NHS Foundation Trust, Manchester Academic Health Sciences Centre, Manchester, United Kingdom, **37** National Institute for Health Research, Manchester Musculoskeletal Biomedical Research Unit, Central Manchester University Hospitals National Health Service Foundation Trust, Manchester Academic Health Sciences Centre, Manchester, United Kingdom, **38** Rheumatology Unit, Department of Medicine (Solna), Karolinska Institutet, Stockholm, Sweden, **39** Lunenfeld-Tanenbaum Research Institute, Mount Sinai Hospital, Toronto, Canada, **40** Toronto General Research Institute, Toronto, Canada, **41** Department of Medicine, University of Toronto, Toronto, Canada, **42** The Feinstein Institute for Medical Research, North Shore–Long Island Jewish Health System, Manhasset, New York, United States of America, **43** Weill Cornell Medical College-Qatar, Education City, Doha, Qatar, **44** Tishreen Hospital, Damascus, Syria, **45** Syrian Association for Rheumatology, Damascus, Syria

Abstract

Integrating genetic data from families with highly penetrant forms of disease together with genetic data from outbred populations represents a promising strategy to uncover the complete frequency spectrum of risk alleles for complex traits such as rheumatoid arthritis (RA). Here, we demonstrate that rare, low-frequency and common alleles at one gene locus, *phospholipase B1* (*PLB1*), might contribute to risk of RA in a 4-generation consanguineous pedigree (Middle Eastern ancestry) and also in unrelated individuals from the general population (European ancestry). Through identity-by-descent (IBD) mapping and whole-exome sequencing, we identified a non-synonymous c.2263G>C (p.G755R) mutation at the *PLB1* gene on 2q23, which significantly co-segregated with RA in family members with a dominant mode of inheritance ($P = 0.009$). We further evaluated *PLB1* variants and risk of RA using a GWAS meta-analysis of 8,875 RA cases and 29,367 controls of European ancestry. We identified significant contributions of two independent non-coding variants near *PLB1* with risk of RA (rs116018341 [MAF = 0.042] and rs116541814 [MAF = 0.021], combined $P = 3.2 \times 10^{-6}$). Finally, we performed deep exon sequencing of *PLB1* in 1,088 RA cases and 1,088 controls (European ancestry), and identified suggestive dispersion of rare protein-coding variant frequencies between cases and controls ($P = 0.049$ for C-alpha test and $P = 0.055$ for SKAT). Together, these data suggest that *PLB1* is a candidate risk gene for RA. Future studies to characterize the full spectrum of genetic risk in the *PLB1* genetic locus are warranted.

Editor: Amr H. Sawalha, University of Michigan, United States of America

Funding: R.M.P. is supported by National Institutes of Health (NIH) grants R01-AR057108, R01-AR056768, U01-GM092691, and R01-AR059648 and holds a Career Award for Medical Scientists from the Burroughs Wellcome Fund. Y.O. is supported by grants from the Japan Society of the Promotion of Science (JSPS) and the Japan Science and Technology Agency (JST). G.T. is supported by the Rubicon grant from the Netherlands Organization for Scientific Research (NOW). H.K.C. is supported by NIH (NIAMS) grants R01-AR056291, R01-AR065944, P60 AR047785, and R21 AR056042. S.R. is supported by NIH grants R01AR063759-01A1 and K08-KAR055688A. L.P. and L.K. are supported by a senior investigator grant from the European Research Council (ERC). K.A.S is supported by a Canada Research Chair, the Sherman Family Chair in Genomic Medicine and by grants from the Ontario Research Fund (RE01-061) and the Canadian Institutes of Health Research (MOP79321). This research was generously supported by the Qatar National Research Fund (QNRF), NPRP # 4-344-3-105. The funders had no role in study design, data collection and analysis, decision to publish, or preparation of the manuscript.

Competing Interests: Dr. Paul P. Tak is currently an employee of GlaxoSmithKline (Stevenage, U.K.). The other authors have declared that no competing interests exist.

* E-mail: robert.plenge@merck.com

Introduction

Rheumatoid arthritis (RA [MIM 180300]) is a chronic autoimmune disease with destruction of synovial joints affecting up to 1% of the population worldwide [1]. RA is a heritable disease, and recent genome-wide association studies (GWAS) and related approaches have identified more than 50 RA susceptibility loci [2–4]. However, as is true for most complex traits, a substantial proportion of genetic heritability of RA remains unexplained [5,6]. Simulated data based on GWAS [6] and empirical data from direct sequencing [7] indicate that a mixture of common, low-frequency and rare variants contribute to risk of RA. Indeed, there are now examples of several gene loci that harbor multiple RA risk alleles (from common to rare) [7]. These data suggest that other gene loci also contain multiple RA risk alleles, and integrating deep-sequencing data with dense genotyping data in large patient collections may be a useful strategy to uncover new RA risk loci.

Whole-exome sequencing and identity-by-descent (IBD) mapping of ancestral haplotypes is emerging as a powerful approach to identify rare causal mutations in families with highly penetrant forms of disease [8,9]. In some instances, the same genes that harbor rare mutations that cause disease in families also harbor other risk variants that influence risk of the same or related diseases in outbred populations [10]. Jordan *et al.* identified causal mutations in *CARD14* through the exome sequencing study of a pedigree affected with a Mendelian form of psoriasis [11], and they also reported both rare and common risk variants of *CARD14* in the general psoriasis case-control cohort [12]. Furthermore, a recent GWAS meta-analysis validated *CARD14* as a psoriasis risk locus [13]. Al-Mayouf *et al.* identified a loss-of-function variant in *DNASE1L3* responsible for a familial form of systemic lupus erythematosus (SLE) [14]. *DNASE1L3* was also identified as a gene in an SLE risk locus from GWAS [15]. Contributions of the variants in the maturity-onset diabetes of the young (MODY) genes on type 2 diabetes susceptibility, or the familial hypercholesterolemia (FH) genes on cardiovascular diseases are also well known [16,17].

There are few previous reports of highly penetrant forms of familial RA [18]. Here, we report a consanguineous pedigree with a Mendelian form of RA. Through the integration of IBD mapping and whole-exome sequencing, we identify a rare mutation associated with risk of RA in the *phospholipase B1* (*PLB1*) gene at chromosome 2p23. Our study also demonstrates significant contributions of coding and non-coding variants in *PLB1* on the risk of RA in an outbred population of European ancestry.

Results

The consanguineous pedigree with a Mendelian form of RA

We report a newly identified, 4-generation, consanguineous pedigree from the Middle East in which 8 of 49 individuals are affected with RA (Figure 1, Figure 2, and Table S1). No other family members were found. Each affected case has symmetrical polyarthritis and is positive for anti-citrullinated protein antibodies (ACPA), a key component of the RA classification criteria related to higher disease severity [19]. The proportion of affected cases in the pedigree members (16.3%) was much higher than the population prevalence of RA in the Middle East (~1%). The average age of onset (35.4 years) was also younger compared to those observed in the general European or Middle East populations [1,20]. Together, these observations suggested contribution of pedigree-specific risk factors of RA not explained by known genetic or environmental factors, including *HLA-DRB1* shared epitope (SE) alleles (odds ratio [OR] = 2.47 in the Syrian population [20]). Among the living unaffected subjects of the pedigree, one subject was strongly positive for ACPA (≥60 units; Table S1). Considering the high specificity of ACPA to RA (>95%) and that ACPA can be found in RA case sera over 10 years prior to the diagnosis of the disease [19,21], we classified this one ACPA-positive unaffected subject into the "affected" case group. (We note that results from the IBD mapping and the validation genotyping did not change substantially when we excluded this ACPA-positive unaffected subject from the analysis.)

Whole-genome SNP genotyping and IBD mapping

We anchored our overall study design (Figure 1) based on a model in which a rare mutation was responsible for RA risk in the consanguineous family. Based on the segregation of RA (Figure 2), we initially posited an autosomal recessive mode of inheritance (Figure 1A). Among the 24 family members available to study (5 ACPA-positive RA cases, 1 ACPA-positive unaffected subject, and 18 ACPA-negative unaffected subjects), we used GWAS data to conduct homozygosity mapping. However, we did not observe any IBD regions shared among all 5 ACPA-positive RA cases and 1 ACPA-positive unaffected subject. This result suggested that a different genetic model (e.g., autosomal dominant mode with incomplete penetrance) may be responsible for RA risk in this family.

To search for a genetic mutation that may confer risk of RA under a different mode of inheritance, we developed and applied a newly investigated non-parametric linkage analysis (Figure 3A). This method, which is based on the "SNP streak" approach to assess homogeneity of the adjacent SNP genotypes on the ancestral haplotype [22,23], is applicable to any type of inheritance mode without prior estimation of mutation penetrance. We further extended the method to utilize genotype information from unaffected pedigree members as well as affected cases. The principle of our method is that affected cases should carry at least one copy of the mutation which resides on a single ancestral haplotype in IBD, but never homozygous for the non-mutated allele [22,23]. Therefore, genetic markers adjacent to the causal mutation lose homozygous genotypes for at least one of the alleles (Figure 3A). We used genome-wide SNP data to search the regional IBD stretches that lose one or both homozygous genotypes in affected cases, which serve as candidate regions harboring causal rare mutations. Our method identified 14 IBD stretches spanning 115.9 Mbp (3.7% of human genome) shared in at least one copy of the haplotype among 5 RA cases and 1 ACPA-positive unaffected subject (Figure 3B left panel and Table S2).

To further narrow the number of critical regions as well as the size of each region, we applied our IBD mapping method to use GWAS data in ACPA-negative unaffected subjects to test the presence of each of the 14 IBD stretches. We hypothesized that the

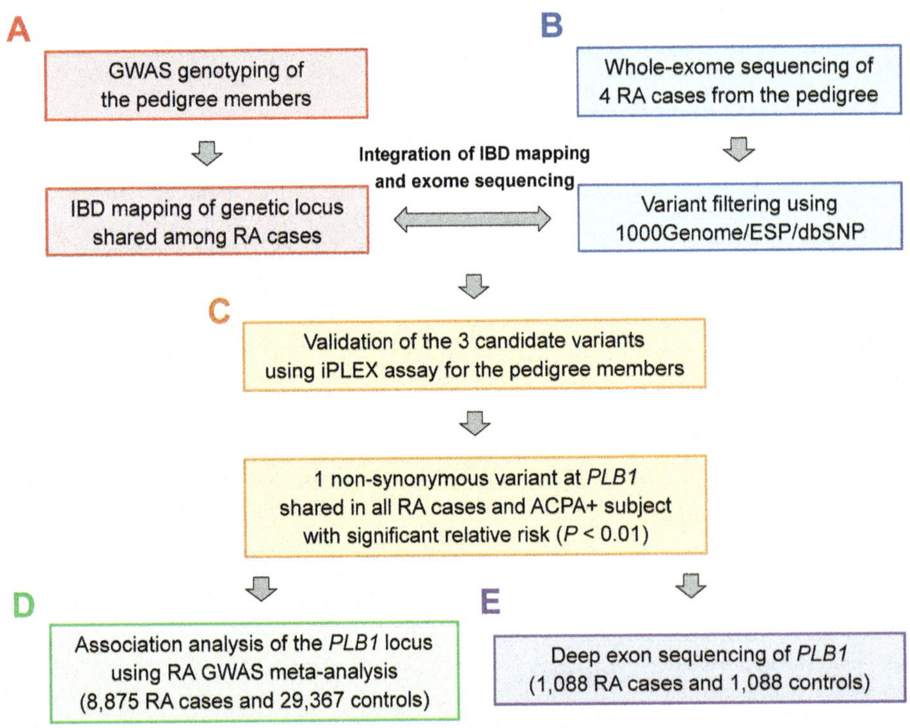

Figure 1. Description of the study design. Our study consists of analysis on three sources of data: (1) rare risk variant detection in the consanguineous pedigree with Mendelian form of RA (A–C), (2) regional association analysis using RA GWAS meta-analysis of European populations (D), and (3) target deep exon sequencing of the European RA case-control cohort (E). (A) We conducted IBD mapping of the pedigree using genome-wide SNP genotype data. (B) Whole-exome sequencing was performed for the 4 affected RA cases of the pedigree. (C) By integrating the results of IBD mapping and whole-exome sequencing, and subsequently conducting the validation assay, we identified a non-synonymous mutation of *PLB1* associated with RA segregation. (D) We evaluated the regional association of the *PLB1* locus using RA GWAS meta-analysis including 8,875 RA cases and 29,367 controls. (E) Deep exon sequencing of *PLB1* and gene-based rare variant test was conducted for 1,088 RA cases and 1,088 controls.

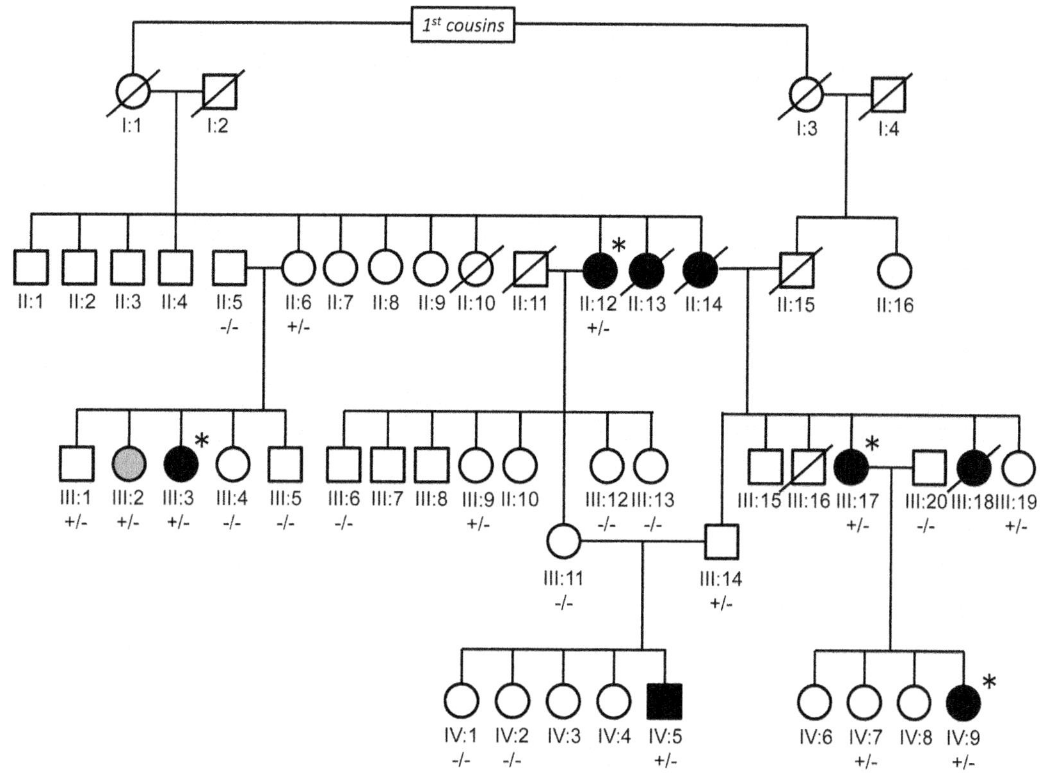

Figure 2. The consanguineous pedigree with Mendelian form of RA. The consanguineous pedigree consists of 49 individuals from 4 generations. The pedigree included 8 individuals affected with RA (colored in black) and 1 ACPA-positive unaffected subject subject (colored in gray). Four RA cases for whom whole-exome sequencing was conducted were indicated with asterisks. Genotypes of the identified *PLB1* p.G755R mutation was indicated by the combination of "+" (mutated allele) and "-" (reference allele).

IBD region containing a causal mutation in this family would be shared by a smaller number of the ACPA-negative unaffected subjects compared to the other IBD regions not containing the mutation. We confined the IBD regions by consecutively restricting the number of the ACPA-negative unaffected subjects harboring the IBD region (see detailed process in Table S2). By this approach, we narrowed the mapped IBD regions into a single stretch with 2.4 Mb length (0.08% of the genome) at 2p23 (from 27.2–29.5 Mb), which was shared among 5 RA cases and 1 ACPA-positive unaffected subject but ≤6 of 18 ACPA-negative unaffected subjects (Figure 3B right panel). We note that the probability to observe at least one IBD region in ≤6 of 18 unaffected subjects was not significant in this pedigree (permutation $P = 0.38$).

Variant filtering in the whole-exome sequencing and overlap with the IBD stretches

To identify the causal mutation in the 2.4 Mb region at 2p23 (which contains 56 protein-coding genes), we performed whole exome sequencing in 4 of the ACPA-positive RA cases (Figure 1B). We did not sequence the rest of one ACPA-positive RA case, since genomic DNA of this subject was not available at the time of sequencing. After whole-exome sequencing, read alignment, and variant calling, we isolated 65,524 variants genome-wide, with average depth of ×290.1 and Ti/Tv ratio of 2.74. On average, 94.0% of the targeted regions (~45 Mbp) yielded ≥10X coverage. Genotype concordance rates of the identified variants commonly included in the whole-genome SNP genotyping results were as high as 99.56% (range = 99.47% to 99.61% for each sample).

Within the 2.4 Mb critical region on 2p23, we identified 168 variants with 99.4% coverage of coding exons at ≥10X coverage. We did not find any copy number variant (CNV) shared among RA cases in this region.

We applied stringent filtering criteria to select for rare pathogenic variants present in this family but not in any public database with non-reference allele frequency ≥0.01 (dbSNP v132, 1000 Genomes Project Phase I data [24], and NHLBI Grand Opportunity Exome Sequencing Project [ESP] 5400 [25]). Of the 168 protein-coding variants within the critical region on 2p23, only one variant was identified by our filtering approach, a missense mutation in the *phospholipase B1* (*PLB1*) gene (Figure 3B right panel). For completeness, we also evaluated the other 13 IBD stretches shared in at least one copy among all 5 RA cases and 1 ACPA-positive unaffected subject, and found one additional missense single-nucleotide variant (SNV) and 1 insertion-deletion (Indel) included in the IBD stretches (Table 1). While we considered all 3 variants to be possibly causal in this family, we considered the one missense mutation in the IBD stretch at 2p23 to be the most promising candidate causal mutation. A full list of the filtered variants from whole exome sequencing is provided in Table S3.

RA risk mutation of *PLB1* in the consanguineous pedigree

To technically confirm the variants identified by whole exome-sequencing, and also to evaluate the segregation pattern of the variants in this family (with an emphasis on the 2p23 variant), we genotyped each of the 3 candidate variants in all available 22 family members (Figure 1C). As expected based on the initial

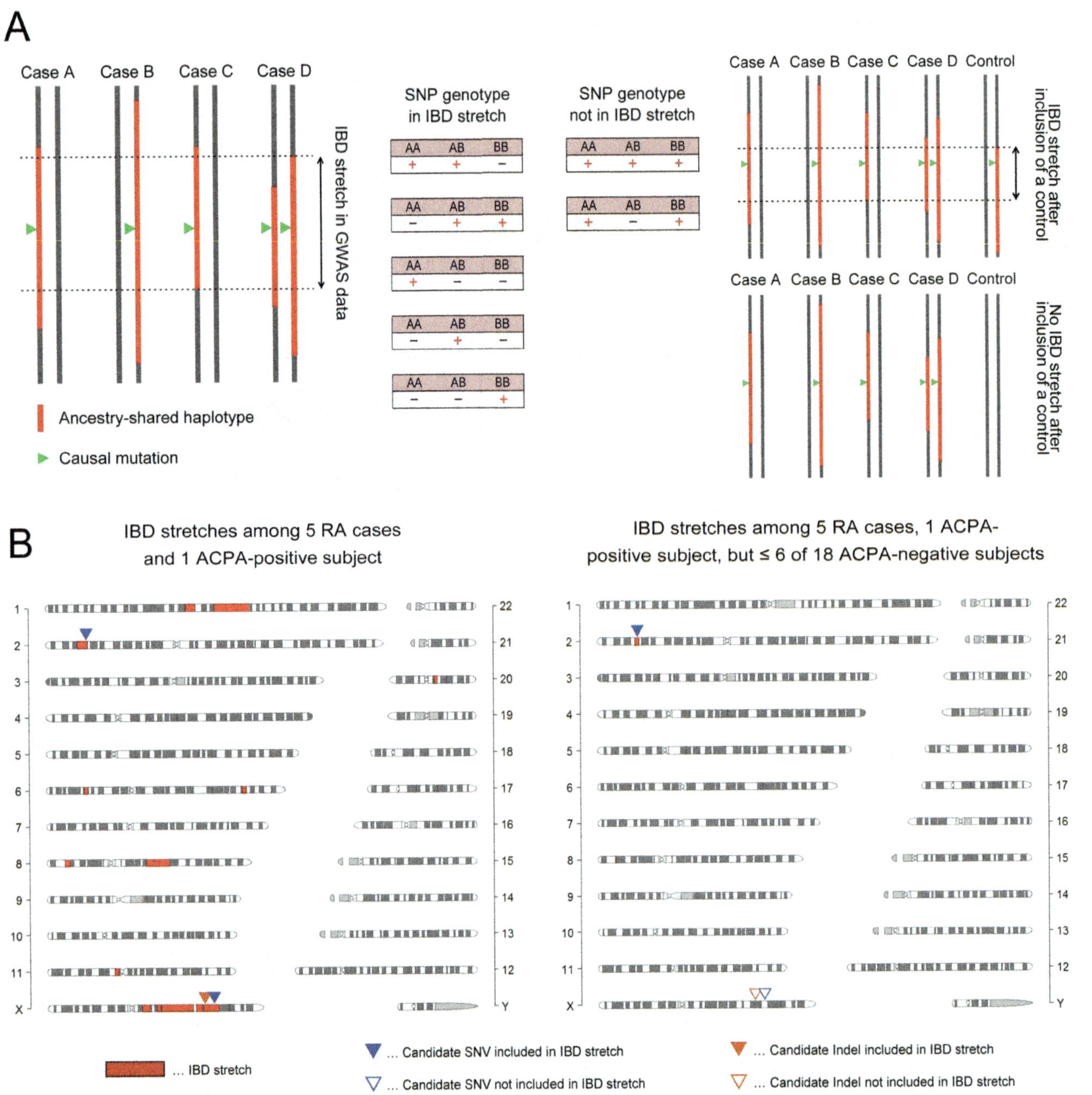

Figure 3. IBD mapping of the pedigree with RA. (A) We investigated the novel non-parametric linkage analysis method which enabled the IBD mapping for the disease with any types of inheritance modes. Affected cases should carry one or two copy of the mutation which resides on a single ancestral haplotype in IBD, thus, SNPs adjacent to the causal mutation lose homozygous genotypes for at least one of the alleles. Our method searched the regional IBD stretches where SNP genotypes of the affected cases followed this rule, and then imputed presence or absence of the ancestral haplotype in the other unaffected subjects separately. (B) Results of the IBD mapping in the consanguineous pedigree with RA. Mapped IBD stretches are indicated as the bands colored in red. As the pedigree members used for the IBD mapping increased (left panel; 5 RA cases and 1 ACPA-positive unaffected subject, right panel; all available subjects), IBD stretches narrowed down (see detailed process in Table S2). Candidate causal SNVs and Indels obtained after whole-genome exome sequencing were indicated as the triangles colored in blue and orange, respectively. The variants included and not included in the IBD stretches of each stages are indicated with filled and non-filled colors. Finally, only one SNV at 2p23 was included in the defined IBD stretch (right panel).

GWAS data and IBD mapping, we found that only the *PLB1* missense mutation co-segregated with RA in the pedigree without Mendelian error. The mutation was observed in all the 5 ACPA-positive RA cases and 1 ACPA-positive unaffected subject while only 6 of 16 ACPA-negative unaffected subjects inherited the *PLB1* mutation ($P = 0.009$; Figure 2 and Table 1). None of the family members was homozygous for this mutation. These observations are consistent with a dominant inheritance mode with a penetrance of 0.50.

PLB1 consists of 58 exons (NM_153021), and the mutation was identified at exon 33 (c.2263G>C [p.G755R]; Figure 4). This mutation was highly conserved (GERP score [26] =4.02), and

Table 1. Results of the validation assay for candidate variants derived from exome sequencing.

Gene[a]	Chr	Position (bp)[b]	Allele Ref/Alt	Amino acid change	Possession of the variant in family members: 5 RA cases and 1 ACPA+ unaffected subject	16 ACPA- unaffected subjects	P^c
PLB1	2	28,816,563	G/C	G755R	6/6	6/16	0.0090
ANKRD58	X	118,893,513	G/A	G295S	6/6	9/16	0.087
AMOT	X	112,022,297	C/CAGG	P1028PL	6/6	14/16	0.74

[a]Genes of which variants were shared among 5 RA cases and 1 ACPA+ unaffected subject are indicated.
[b]Based on NCBI Build 37/hg19.
[c]Mid-P value of Fisher's exact test for RA cases and unaffected subjects are indicated.
RA; rheumatoid arthritis, ACPA; anti-citrullinated protein antibodies.

predicted to be "tolerated" by SIFT [27] but "probably damaging" by PolyPhen-2.0 [28]. This mutation was not registered at any of the databases (dbSNP v132, 1000 Genomes Phase I [24], or ESP5400 [25]), and not present in the result of deep exon sequencing of *PLB1* in the European RA case-control cohort (see below).

GWAS meta-analysis of the *PLB1* locus and RA risk of non-coding variants

To provide additional support for the role of *PLB1* in risk of RA, we evaluated common (minor allele frequency [MAF] >5%) and low-frequency variants (MAF 1–5%) near the *PLB1* gene locus in an outbred population of European ancestry (Figure 1D). We used a GWAS of 8,875 seropositive RA cases and 29,367 controls from 11 studies (Table S4). Five of the GWAS datasets were previously unpublished (3,427 cases and 6,837 controls from ReAct, Dutch, anti-TNF response to therapy collection [ACR-REF], CORRONA, and Vanderbilt) [29–33], which increased the power of our published dataset (Figure 4 and Table 2) [2,4,7]. We observed no evidence of systematic bias genome-wide (inflation factor $\lambda_{GC} = 1.034$; Table S4). We applied genotype imputation using the 1000 Genome Project reference panel [24], and assessed the *PLB1* locus with a set of densely fine-mapped SNPs (919 SNPs for ±50 kbp of *PLB1*; average SNP interval = 0.27 kbp). We considered a value of $P<9.0\times10^{-4}$ as statistically significant based on permutation analysis of all SNPs in the region.

The most strongly-associated signal was observed at a low-frequency intronic SNP in *PLB1*, rs116018341 (MAF = 0.041, OR = 1.18, $P=5.1\times10^{-4}$; Figure 4B upper panel), which surpassed our permutation-based threshold of significance. To determine if additional variants also contributed to risk of RA, we performed forward-type step-wise logistic regression analysis. We found evidence for a second, independent association of a low-frequency *PLB1* intronic SNP, rs116541814 (MAF = 0.020, OR = 1.34, $P=6.5\times10^{-4}$; Figure 4B lower panel). After conditioning on these two variants, no significant regional association was observed ($P>0.01$ for all remaining SNPs).

We built haplotypes containing these two SNPs to test a combined genetic model. The common haplotype including either of the risk alleles for these 2 SNPs demonstrated a significant association with RA risk (MAF = 0.062, OR = 1.21, $P=3.2\times10^{-6}$). These two intronic SNPs were not in linkage disequilibrium (LD) with any of the protein-coding variants of *PLB1* ($r^2<0.3$ for common variants [MAF ≥0.05] and $r^2<0.1$ for low-frequency or rare variants [MAF<0.05]), suggesting that observed RA risk was primarily derived from non-coding variants of *PLB1*.

In order to assess the functional contribution of the non-coding variants, we evaluated overlap of the RA risk SNPs with trimethylation of histone H3 at lysine 4 (H3K4me3) peak of primary CD4$^+$ regulatory T cells (T_{reg} cells). The H3K4me3 mark is particularly informative for cell-type specific overlap with trait-associated variants, and RA risk variants showed significant enrichment in T_{reg} primary cells [34]. The RA risk SNP of rs116018341 (and the SNPs in absolute LD with it; $r^2 = 1.00$), was within one of the H3K4me3 peaks of T_{reg} primary cells ($P=0.043$), while the other risk SNP, rs116541814, was not (Figure 4C). In a search of public eQTL databases (eQTL Browser and Blood eQTL Browser [35], see URL), we found no evidence that either SNP (or SNPs in LD with them, $r^2>0.8$) influenced *PLB1* gene expression.

Deep exon sequencing of *PLB1* and RA risk of protein-coding variants

Finally, we sequenced the coding exons of *PLB1* to search for independent rare variants that may contribute to risk of RA in an outbred population of European ancestry (Figure 1E). Deep exon sequencing was performed in 1,088 RA cases and 1,088 genetically-matched controls from the European populations, as a part of the Pharmacogenomics Research Network (PGRN) sequencing project [Diogo D. et al. Manuscript in preparation]. Overall, 96% of the targeted regions were sequenced with ≥20X coverage. We obtained 102 coding variants (i.e. variants annotated as synonymous, missense, or nonsense) in *PLB1*, of which 92 had MAF<0.01 in controls.

To test for significance, we applied gene-based tests (the burden test, variable threshold test [36], frequency-weighted test [37], C-alpha test [38], and sequence kernel association test [SKAT] [39]) for all rare coding variants with MAF<0.01 (Table 3 and Table S5). We observed suggestive enrichment of rare variants in the protein-coding region of *PLB1* ($P=0.049$ for C-alpha test [38], and $P=0.055$ for SKAT [39]). Both of these gene-based tests allow for opposite directional effects of the variants (two-sided test). In contrast, the gene-based tests which assume same directionality of effects of the variants (one-sided test) did not show significant results ($P>0.30$ for the burden test, variable threshold test [36], and frequency-weighted test [37]). Association signals in two-sided tests were more apparent for synonymous variants ($n=30$, $P<0.022$), but not significant for non-synonymous variants ($n=62$, $P>0.30$).

Discussion

Three lines of evidence suggest that coding and non-coding alleles at *PLB1* contribute to risk of RA. First, IBD mapping and

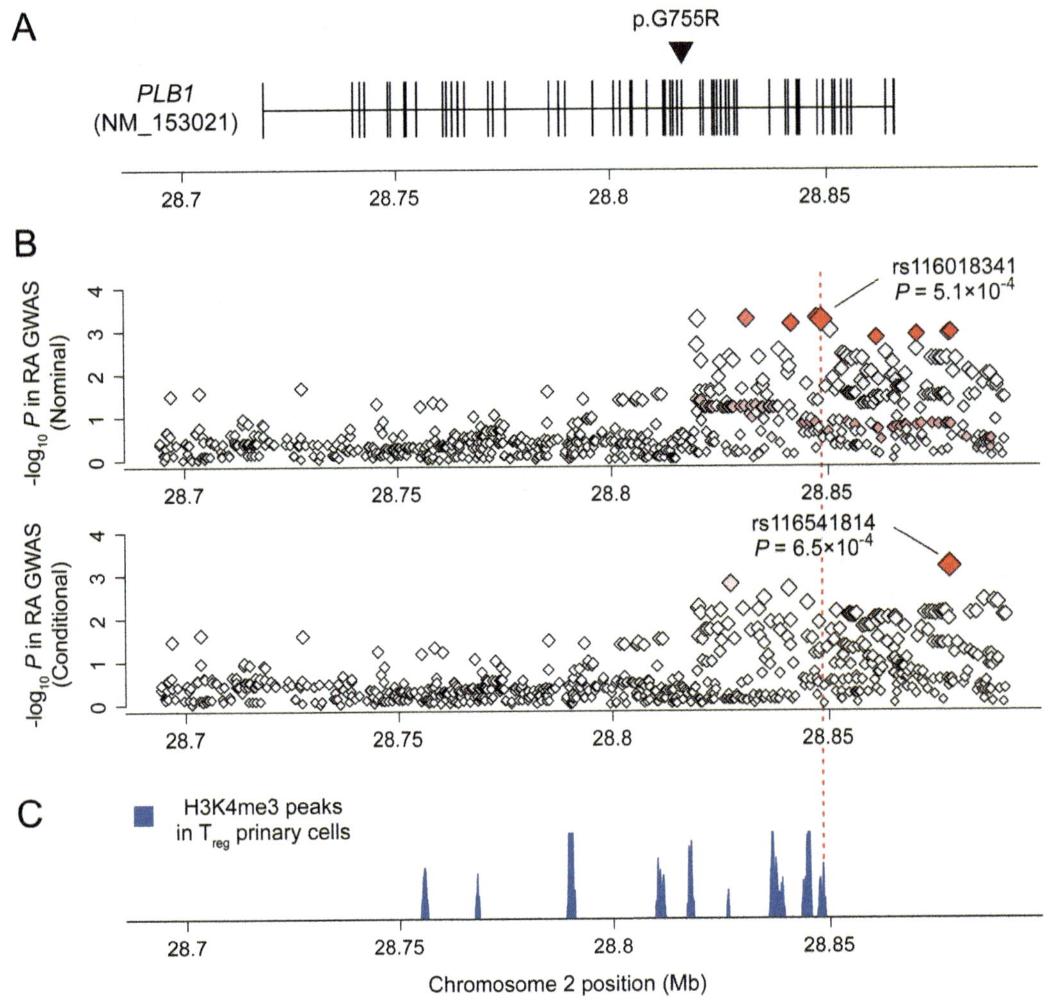

Figure 4. Association of the *PLB1* locus in RA GWAS meta-analysis. (A) Coding regions of *PLB1* and p.G755R mutation identified in the consanguineous RA pedigree. *PLB1* consists of 58 exons (NM_153021), and p.G755R (c.2263G>C) mutation was located at exon 33 (the black triangle). (B) Regional association of *PLB1* in RA GWAS meta-analysis including 8,875 RA cases and 29,367 controls from the European populations. Upper panel showed the results of nominal association, and the lower panel showed the results of conditional analysis with rs116018341, the top SNP in the nominal associations. The red diamond-shaped dots represent P-values of the SNPs in the GWAS meta-analysis, and the intensity of the red color in the dots represents the r^2 value with the most significantly associated SNP. Stepwise logistic regression analysis demonstrated multiple independent signals driven by non-coding variants. (C) H3K4me3 peak of T_{reg} primary cells in the *PLB1* locus. Non-coding RA risk SNP of rs116018341 overlapped with one of the H3K4me3 peaks as the SNP located in the most vicinity of the peak summit (a vertical dashed red line).

Table 2. Results of the GWAS meta-analysis of European RA case-control cohorts in the *PLB1* locus.

rsID	Chr	Position (bp)[a]	A1/A2	A1 Freq. RA cases (n=8,875)	A1 Freq. Controls (n=29,367)	OR (95%CI)	*P*
rs116018341	2	28,848,761	A/C	0.045	0.041	1.18 (1.07–1.29)	5.1×10^{-4}
rs116541814[b]	2	28,877,974	A/G	0.022	0.020	1.34 (1.13–1.59)	6.5×10^{-4}
rs116018341-rs116541814 haplotype[c]	2	-	AG or CA/CG	0.067	0.062	1.21 (1.12–1.32)	3.2×10^{-6}

[a]Based on NCBI Build 37/hg19.
[b]Conditioned with rs116018341.
[c]AA risk haplotype was not observed in the imputation reference panel.
RA; rheumatoid arthritis, ACPA; anti-citrullinated protein antibodies.

Table 3. Results of rare variant tests for *PLB1* coding variants in the European RA case-control cohort.

	Association analysis				
	One-sided test			Two-sided test	
No. variants[a]	BURDEN	VT	FRQWGT	CALPHA	SKAT
92	0.33	0.64	0.60	0.049	0.055

[a]Low-frequency rare coding variant (MAF≤0.01) obtained from deep sequencing of 1,088 RA cases and 1,088 controls were selected.
RA; rheumatoid arthritis, ACPA; anti-citrullinated protein antibodies.
BURDEN; burden test, VT; variable threshold test, FRQWGT; frequency-weighted test, CALPHA; C-alpha test, SKAT; sequence kernel association test.

whole-exome sequencing of a consanguineous Mendelian pedigree from the Middle East identified a rare non-synonymous mutation in *PLB1* (p.G755R). The mutation co-segregated with RA in dominant inheritance with incomplete penetrance but significant relative risk ($P = 0.009$). Second, large-scale RA GWAS meta-analysis in Europeans identified two independent non-coding variants near *PLB1*, which constitute a common risk haplotype associated with risk of RA ($P = 3.2 \times 10^{-6}$). Third, targeted exon sequencing of *PLB1* in Europeans demonstrated suggestive association of rare coding variants with risk of RA ($P < 0.05$). Together, contributions of rare, low-frequency, and common alleles of *PLB1* observed in inbred and outbred populations of different ancestry provide supportive evidence that *PLB1* is a RA risk gene.

Identification of rare causal variants that contribute to complex disease etiology is an important issue in human genetics. Given the expected effect size of rare variants, extremely large sample sizes are required to identify disease-associated rare variants in studies of complex traits in outbred populations alone [40]. Alternatively, assessment of rare causal mutations in pedigrees with Mendelian forms of common disease, and validation of the identified gene in the outbred patient populations, could be an efficient approach. Our study provides support for this approach in RA, thereby complementing findings from previous studies in other diseases [10–17].

PLB1 is an enzyme that has both phospholipase A1 and A2 enzymatic activities. The PLB1 protein contains 3 GDSL-like lipase (acylhydrolase) domains (Figure S1) [41,42]. The p.G755R mutation identified in the consanguineous RA pedigree was located within the second GDSL-like lipase domain (amino acid positions 741 to 1015). GDSL-like lipase domain has essential biological roles of PLB1 protein as lysophopholipase [42], and localizations of the RA risk variant on it might imply their functional impact on the enzymatic activity of PLB1.

The functional etiology of *PLB1* in human disease pathogenesis has not been well investigated. There exist a few reports suggesting contribution of *PLB1* and other phospholipase family genes on human autoimmune disease. The *PLB1* locus has suggestive evidence as a type 1 diabetes risk locus ($P < 10^{-6}$ for the SNP located 70 kbp upstream of *PLB1*) [43]. Duan *et al.* reported that expression of *PLB1* is upregulated in peripheral blood mononuclear cells (PBMCs) of patients with ankylosing spondylitis (an autoimmune disease that shares clinical features with RA) compared to healthy controls [44]. Recently, whole-exome sequencing analysis on a pedigree with a dominantly inherited immunodeficiency and autoimmunity identified a causal mutation in a gene related to *PLB1*, the phospholipase Cγ2 (*PLCG2*) gene [45]. Further studies assessing functional impacts of the *PLB1* mutations on RA pathogenesis are required.

Beyond the novel finding of *PLB1* as a candidate RA risk gene, our study developed and applied novel statistical methodologies. We developed a non-parametric linkage analysis method that enables IBD mapping in a pedigree with any mode of inheritance. Our method utilized genotype information of both affected and unaffected subjects without requiring prior estimation of penetrance. Due to its simple nature, our method is applicable to pedigrees with complex structure, in which classical parametric linkage methods have difficulty in handling inheritance vectors. While exome-sequencing has demonstrated success in pedigrees with typical Mendelian inheritance and complete penetrance, additional approaches, such as we describe, are required for more complex patterns of disease segregation [8].

There are important limitations of our study. First, our search for rare mutations was performed in a single pedigree and not validated in other pedigrees. While we identified independent *PLB1* alleles associated with risk of RA in an outbred European population using a large-scaled GWAS meta-analysis, it would not directly support the risk of *PLB1* p.G755R mutation on RA. As additional families with familial forms of RA (or related conditions) are identified, it will be important to apply similar unbiased approaches to search for mutations in *PLB1* or *PLB1*-like genes. Second, no single genetic variant achieved a genome-wide level of significance in the GWAS meta-analysis and targeted sequencing in outbred populations. However, whether the same conservative significance thresholds should be applied to our study design is a matter of debate. While we found genetic evidence across the three stages of our study, future genetic studies are required to confirm that *PLB1* alleles definitively contribute to risk of RA. Especially, considering the recent studies reporting that large sample size would be necessary for rare variants analysis in the complex diseases [46], additional accumulation of the subjects in *PLB1* target exon sequencing would be desirable. Finally, we did not perform any functional studies of the variants we identified. Future functional studies will be important to determine if these are gain-of-function or loss-of-function alleles.

In conclusion, our study demonstrates significant contributions of rare, low-frequency, and common alleles of *PLB1* to risk of RA by coordinately assessing a consanguineous pedigree with RA and outbred RA cases-control cohorts. We also introduced novel statistical methodologies to assess rare variants in complex pedigrees with uncertain patterns of inheritance. Our study should contribute to our understanding of the causal variants in the pathogenesis of complex diseases.

Materials and Methods

Ethics statement

Our study was approved by the Institutional Review Board of Brigham & Women's Hospital and Tishreen Hospital. All the enrolled subjects provided written informed consent for the participation of the study. For the patients from Syria, written informed consent was provided in Arabic and the study was approved by the Syrian Ministry of Health. Blood samples were collected according to protocols approved by local institutional review boards.

Samples

We report a 4-generation, consanguineous pedigree in which 8 of 49 individuals are affected with RA (Figure 2 and Table S1). The pedigree members were recruited by a board-certified rheumatologist from Tishreen Hospital, Damascus, Syria. All

RA cases fulfilled the revised criteria of the American Rheumatism Association for RA [47]. ACPA titer was determined by by direct assay using QUANTA Lite™ CCP3 IgG ELISA (INOVA Diagnostics, San Diego, CA). In this study, we enrolled 24 living pedigree members including 5 affected cases (II:12, III:3, III:17, IV:5, IV:9), 1 ACPA-positive unaffected subject (III:2), and 18 ACPA-negative unaffected subjects (II:5, II:6, III:1, III:4, III:5, III:6, III:9, III:11, III:12, III:13, III:14, III:19, III:20, IV:1, IV:2, IV:3, IV:4, IV:7; Figure 2).

For the case-control association analysis of RA in the European populations, we studied 8,875 RA cases and 29,367 matched controls for GWAS meta-analysis (Table S4). Six GWAS data has been previously published [2]; additional five GWAS datasets are previously unpublished [29,32,33], as described in more detail below. The 1,088 RA cases and 1,088 matched controls for exon sequencing of *PLB1* represent a subset of patients with GWAS data (Table S4). All the subjects were confirmed to be of European origins using both self-reported ethnicities and the results of principal component analysis (PCA). Part of the subjects in the GWAS and exon sequencing were included in previous studies with detailed descriptions of the cohorts [2,4,7,29,32,33]. There was an overlap of the RA cases involved in the GWAS meta-analysis and exon sequencing ($n = 342$).

Whole-genome SNP genotyping and quality control of the consanguineous pedigree with RA

Whole-genome SNP genotyping was conducted for all the available 24 pedigree members using Illumina HumanOmniExpress Genotyping BeadChip (Illumina, San Diego, CA; Figure 1A). We applied call-rate cutoff thresholds of ≥0.98 for samples and 0.99≥ for SNPs, and filtered out subjects with excess heterozygosity. We used GWAS data to confirm the relationships among all pedigree members using "–genome" option implemented in PLINK v1.07. We excluded monomorphic SNPs in the genotyped pedigree members.

IBD mapping of the consanguineous pedigree with RA

To find the region harboring the ancestral haplotype that co-segregates with affected cases, we conducted IBD mapping of the consanguineous pedigree using whole-genome SNP genotyping data (Figure 1A). After applying LD pruning of the SNPs with $r^2 \geq 0.9$ using LD information obtained from HapMap Phase II CEU subjects, we applied homozygosity mapping of the affected RA cases and the ACPA-positive unaffected subject using "–homozyg" option implemented in PLINK v1.07, a classical non-parametric linkage analysis assuming a recessive mode of disease inheritance [48].

We developed a novel IBD mapping method which extends homozygosity mapping to include any type of inheritance mode. This method, which is based on the "SNP streak" approach to assess homogeneity of the adjacent SNP genotypes on the ancestral haplotype [22,23], is applicable without prior estimation of inheritance mode and mutation penetrance. Our method uses genome-wide SNP data to search the regional IBD stretches that lose one or both homozygous genotypes in affected cases using a sliding window approach (Figure 3A). The window spanning 1 Mbp bin was defined as IBD when all the SNP genotypes in this bin followed the rule mentioned above with exception of no more than 1 SNP, and the IBD stretch was defined when the IBD window continued beyond ≥2 Mbp length.

We further extended the method to utilize genotype data from unaffected pedigree members as well as affected cases. Within the identified IBD stretches shared among affected cases, our method is able to impute presence or absence of the ancestral haplotype in the other unaffected subjects, by checking whether IBD stretch remains or not after inclusion of each of the unaffected subjects separately. We assessed significance of the probability to observe the IBD stretch shared among 5 ACPA-positive RA cases and 1 ACPA-positive unaffected subject while only 6 of 16 ACPA-negative unaffected subjects by a permutation procedure (×10,000 iterations). For each of the iteration steps, we randomly selected 6 members from the pedigree as "affected" subjects, and assessed whether at least one of the IBD stretches observed among these 6 "affected" subjects were observed in ≤6/18 of the other "unaffected" subjects. Java™ software for this novel IBD mapping method is available at http://plaza.umin.ac.jp/~yokada/datasource/software.htm.

We did not apply parametric linkage analysis methods for SNP genotype data such as Merlin [49], since the software did not work properly due to the complex pedigree structure including multiple loops.

Whole-exome sequencing of the RA cases in the consanguineous pedigree

To search for the causal risk mutation in the pedigree, we performed whole-exome sequencing for 4 affected RA cases in the pedigree (II:12, III:3, III:17, IV:9; Figure 1B). DNA library preparation and target exome capture were conducted using the Agilent SureSelect All Exon kit v2 (Agilent Technologies, Santa Clara, CA), which covers 44.9 Mbp of human exon regions. Sequencing was run on Illumina HiSeq2000 (Illumina, San Diego, CA) at the Broad Institute of MIT and Harvard (Cambridge, MA). Sequencing reads were aligned to the Human Reference Genome (UCSC hg19) using Burrows-Wheeler Aligner (BWA) algorithm [50]. Sequence read filtering and variant calling was done using the GATK pipeline as described elsewhere [51,52], and snpEff was used for variant annotation [53]. Calling of CNV was conducted by using the ExomeDepth software version 0.9.7 [54]. Whole-exome sequencing data of the pedigree is available to other researchers upon request.

Filtering of the identified variants was conducted according to the following processes: (i) variants likely to be pathogenic (missense, nonsense, frameshift Indels, or splice-site acceptor/donor); (ii) variants not registered in the databases (dbSNP v132, 1000 Genomes Project Phase I data [24], and ESP5400 [25]) with non-reference allele frequency ≥0.01; (iii) for Indels, ones not located ±5 bp of known variants; and (iv) variants of which ≥1 non-reference alleles were observed in all the exome sequenced 4 RA cases.

Validation iPLEX™ assay of the exome-driven variants

To efficiently validate the results of whole-exome sequencing, we selected the 3 candidate causal variants that were included in the IBD stretches defined using SNP genotype data from 5 ACPA-positive RA cases and 1 ACPA-positive unaffected subject (Figure 1C). We conducted iPLEX™ validation assay (Montréal, Canada) for these selected variants using the available 22 pedigree members except for the 2 ACPA-negative unaffected subjects (IV:3 and IV:4), due to genomic DNA degradation. Relative risk of each validated variant was evaluated using mid-P value of Fisher's exact test, which has more unbiased type I error and higher statistical power compared to original Fisher's exact test [55]. Java™ software for mid-P value of Fisher's exact test is available at http://plaza.umin.ac.jp/~yokada/datasource/software.htm.

Association analysis of the *PLB1* locus using European RA GWAS meta-analysis

To evaluate RA genetic risk of the *PLB1* locus in the general populations, we referred to the results of the currently conducted RA GWAS meta-analysis of the European populations enrolling 8,875 RA cases and 29,367 controls from 11 studies (Figure 1D and Table S4). Five new unpublished GWAS datasets ($n = 3{,}427$ cases and 6,837 controls) from ReAct [29], Dutch (including AMC, BeSt, LUMC, and DREAM) [29], anti-TNF response to therapy collection (ACR-REF: BRAGGSS, BRAGGSS2, ERA, KI, and TEAR) [29-31], the Consortium of Rheumatology Researchers of North America (CORRONA) [32], and Vanderbilt RA case-control cohorts [33] were included along with 6 previously published GWAS datasets ($n = 5{,}448$ cases and 22,530 controls) [2,29]. All GWAS data was filtered using the same criteria as described elsewhere [2–4], including sample and SNP call-rate cutoffs, exclusion of closely-related or outlier subjects, and MAF and Hardy-Weinberg equilibrium cutoffs for SNPs.

After applying QC criteria to each GWAS, whole-genome genotype imputation was performed by minimac [56] using 1000 Genome Project Phase I (α) European data as a reference [24]. We excluded imputed SNPs with MAF<0.005 or imputation score of $Rsq<0.5$ from each GWAS. Associations of the SNPs with RA were evaluated by logistic regression models assuming additive effects of the allele dosages, including top 5 principal components as covariates using mach2dat v1.0.16 (see URL). Meta-analysis was performed for the SNPs available in ≥50% of the studies, by an inverse-variance method assuming a fixed-effects model on the effect sizes of the alleles dosages using the Java^{TM} source code implemented by the authors [57]. Double genomic control (GC) correction was carried out using the inflation factor (λ_{GC}) obtained from the results of each GWAS and the GWAS meta-analysis.

The regional significance threshold was determined by a permutation procedure (permutation $P = 0.05$ with ×10,000 iterations). Case-control phenotype labels were shuffled for each GWAS dataset separately, and the distribution of the smallest *P*-values of the SNPs from respective iteration steps was evaluated. Conditional analysis was conducted by consecutively including the allele dosages of the top-associated SNPs in the *PLB1* locus as covariates in a forward-type stepwise logistic regression approach until no significant regional association was observed after conditioning ($\alpha = 0.01$). Haplotype analysis was conducted by incorporating estimated haplotype dosages consisting of the two non-coding SNPs in *PLB1* (rs116018341 and rs116541814) as independent variables, as described elsewhere [58].

We obtained chromatin immunoprecipitation followed by sequencing (ChIP-seq) assay peaks of H3K4me3 from NIH Roadmap Epigenomics Mapping Consortium [59], and assessed overlap of the SNPs in the *PLB1* locus with H3K4me3 peaks in primary T_{reg} cells, as described elsewhere [60]. Peak overlap enrichment of the SNPs (and SNPs in absolute LD with it; $r^2 = 1.00$) were compared to the neighboring SNPs (±2 Mbp). We physically slid H3K4me3 peak positions by 100 bp bins within ±2 Mbp regions of the SNPs, and assessed overlap with H3K4me3 peaks for each sliding step. Significance of overlap in the original peak positions was evaluated by one-sided exact test assuming enrichment of overlap.

Deep exon sequencing of *PLB1* in European RA case-control cohort

To evaluate contribution of *PLB1* protein-coding variants on the risk of general RA cases, we conducted deep exon sequencing of *PLB1* using genetically matched 1,088 RA cases and 1,088 controls from the European populations (Figure 1E and Table S4). These subjects were collected as a part of the PGRN sequencing project, as described elsewhere [Diogo D. et al. Manuscript in preparation]. All subjects were determined as European ancestry based on PCA conducted along with HapMap Phase III samples as reference populations. RA cases and controls were matched based on the Euclidean distances in all case-control pairs along 10 eigenvalue-weighted PCs. DNA library preparation and target exon capture was conducted using NimbleGen Sequence Capture technology (Roche NimbleGen, Madison, WI), along with another ~850 genes related to autoimmune diseases as a part of the PGRN sequencing project. Sequencing was run on Illumina HiSeq2000 (Illumina, San Diego, CA) at the Genome Institute at Washington University in St. Louis. Sequencing reads were aligned to the Human Reference Genome (UCSC hg19) using the BWA algorithm [50], and duplicated reads were excluded using Picard (see URL). Sequence read filtering and variant calling was done using SAMtools v1.16 and VarScan v2.2.9 [61,62]. Variants were annotated based on *PLB1* transcript (NM_153021) using ANNOVAR [63]. We selected rare protein-coding variants of *PLB1* (MAF<0.01) and evaluated gene-based association signal on RA risk by sets of widely-used rare variants tests, including the burden test, variable threshold test [36], frequency-weighted test [37], C-alpha test [38], and SKAT [39], using PLINKQ-SEQ (with ×100,000 iterations) and SKAT [39] software. PLB1 protein domains were obtained from the Pfam protein families database for UniProt entry Q6P1J6 [41]. Deep exon sequencing data of *PLB1* is available to other researchers upon request.

Web resources

The URLs for data presented herein are as follows:

Java^{TM} software for the IBD mapping and mid-P value of Fisher's exact test, http://plaza.umin.ac.jp/~yokada/datasource/software.htm

Online Mendelian Inheritance in Man (OMIM), http://omim.org/

PLINK, http://pngu.mgh.harvard.edu/~purcell/plink/

GATK, http://www.broadinstitute.org/gatk/

dbSNP, http://www.ncbi.nlm.nih.gov/snp/

1000 Genomes Project, http://www.1000genomes.org/

NHLBI Grand Opportunity Exome Sequencing Project, https://esp.gs.washington.edu/drupal/

minimac, http://genome.sph.umich.edu/wiki/Minimac

mach2dat, http://www.sph.umich.edu/csg/abecasis/MACH/index.html

NIH Roadmap Epigenomics Mapping Consortium, http://www.roadmapepigenomics.org/

Picard, http://picard.sourceforge.net/index.shtml

Annovar, http://www.openbioinformatics.org/annovar/

ExomeDepth, http://cran.r-project.org/web/packages/ExomeDepth/index.html

PLINK-SEQ, http://atgu.mgh.harvard.edu/plinkseq/

SKAT, http://www.hsph.harvard.edu/skat/

Pfam protein families database, http://pfam.sanger.ac.uk/

eQTL Browser, http://eqtl.uchicago.edu/Home.html

Blood eQTL Browser, http://genenetwork.nl/bloodeqtlbrowser/

Supporting Information

Figure S1 Protein structure of *PLB1* and RA risk variant. *PLB1* protein has three GDSL-like lipase domains which have essential biological roles in lysophopholipase activity of the protein. The second GDSL-like lipase domain included p.G755R mutation identified in the consanguineous RA pedigree (the black triangle).

Table S1 Characteristics of RA cases and a ACPA-positive unaffected subject in the consanguineous pedigree with RA.

Table S2 Results of IBD mapping for the consanguineous pedigree with RA.

Table S3 A list of the filtered variants from whole exome sequencing.

Table S4 Characteristics of the subjects in European RA case-control cohorts.

Table S5 Rare variants obtained from deep exon sequencing of *PLB1* in the European RA case-control cohort.

Acknowledgments

We thank Dr. Sara Pulit for her kind supports on exome sequencing analysis, and the members of Arthritis Consortium International (RACI) consortium for supporting the study.

Author Contributions

Conceived and designed the experiments: YO TA LAK RMP. Performed the experiments: RSF NG DM SG GL ERM. Analyzed the data: YO DD RSF GT. Contributed reagents/materials/analysis tools: JDG FM WAA JCD JMK DAP RJC AEE EAS JC RS MJC HG TWH PD XM AB HC JEF ND PPT LWM SB CM HKC YK PG ML TR PLD SR JW LP LK KAS PKG TA LAK. Wrote the paper: YO RMP.

References

1. Alamanos Y, Voulgari PV, Drosos AA (2006) Incidence and prevalence of rheumatoid arthritis, based on the 1987 American College of Rheumatology criteria: a systematic review. Semin Arthritis Rheum 36: 182–188.
2. Stahl EA, Raychaudhuri S, Remmers EF, Xie G, Eyre S, et al. (2010) Genome-wide association study meta-analysis identifies seven new rheumatoid arthritis risk loci. Nat Genet 42: 508–514.
3. Okada Y, Terao C, Ikari K, Kochi Y, Ohmura K, et al. (2012) Meta-analysis identifies nine new loci associated with rheumatoid arthritis in the Japanese population. Nat Genet 44: 511–516.
4. Eyre S, Bowes J, Diogo D, Lee A, Barton A, et al. (2012) High-density genetic mapping identifies new susceptibility loci for rheumatoid arthritis. Nat Genet 44: 1336–1340.
5. Park JH, Wacholder S, Gail MH, Peters U, Jacobs KB, et al. (2010) Estimation of effect size distribution from genome-wide association studies and implications for future discoveries. Nat Genet 42: 570–575.
6. Stahl EA, Wegmann D, Trynka G, Gutierrez-Achury J, Do R, et al. (2012) Bayesian inference analyses of the polygenic architecture of rheumatoid arthritis. Nat Genet 44: 483–489.
7. Diogo D, Kurreeman F, Stahl EA, Liao KP, Gupta N, et al. (2013) Rare, low-frequency, and common variants in the protein-coding sequence of biological candidate genes from GWASs contribute to risk of rheumatoid arthritis. Am J Hum Genet 92: 15–27.
8. Stitziel NO, Kiezun A, Sunyaev S (2011) Computational and statistical approaches to analyzing variants identified by exome sequencing. Genome Biol 12: 227.
9. Raychaudhuri S, Iartchouk O, Chin K, Tan PL, Tai AK, et al. (2011) A rare penetrant mutation in CFH confers high risk of age-related macular degeneration. Nat Genet 43: 1232–1236.
10. Okada Y, Plenge RM (2013) Entering the age of whole-exome sequencing in rheumatic diseases: novel insights into disease pathogenicity. Arthritis Rheum 65: 1975–1979.
11. Jordan CT, Cao L, Roberson ED, Pierson KC, Yang CF, et al. (2012) PSORS2 is due to mutations in CARD14. Am J Hum Genet 90: 784–795.
12. Jordan CT, Cao L, Roberson ED, Duan S, Helms CA, et al. (2012) Rare and common variants in CARD14, encoding an epidermal regulator of NF-kappaB, in psoriasis. Am J Hum Genet 90: 796–808.
13. Tsoi LC, Spain SL, Knight J, Ellinghaus E, Stuart PE, et al. (2012) Identification of 15 new psoriasis susceptibility loci highlights the role of innate immunity. Nat Genet 44: 1341–1348.
14. Al-Mayouf SM, Sunker A, Abdwani R, Abrawi SA, Almurshedi F, et al. (2011) Loss-of-function variant in DNASE1L3 causes a familial form of systemic lupus erythematosus. Nat Genet 43: 1186–1188.
15. Harley JB, Alarcon-Riquelme ME, Criswell LA, Jacob CO, Kimberly RP, et al. (2008) Genome-wide association scan in women with systemic lupus erythematosus identifies susceptibility variants in ITGAM, PXK, KIAA1542 and other loci. Nat Genet 40: 204–210.
16. Vaxillaire M, Froguel P (2008) Monogenic diabetes in the young, pharmacogenetics and relevance to multifactorial forms of type 2 diabetes. Endocr Rev 29: 254–264.
17. Willer CJ, Sanna S, Jackson AU, Scuteri A, Bonnycastle LL, et al. (2008) Newly identified loci that influence lipid concentrations and risk of coronary artery disease. Nat Genet 40: 161–169.
18. Teitsson I, Thorsteinsson J, Arnason A, Valdimarsson H (1985) Rheumatic diseases in an Icelandic family. Clinical and immunological survey. Scand J Rheumatol 14: 109–118.
19. Neogi T, Aletaha D, Silman AJ, Naden RL, Felson DT, et al. (2010) The 2010 American College of Rheumatology/European League Against Rheumatism classification criteria for rheumatoid arthritis: Phase 2 methodological report. Arthritis Rheum 62: 2582–2591.
20. Kazkaz L, Marotte H, Hamwi M, Angelique Cazalis M, Roy P, et al. (2007) Rheumatoid arthritis and genetic markers in Syrian and French populations: different effect of the shared epitope. Ann Rheum Dis 66: 195–201.
21. Chibnik LB, Mandl LA, Costenbader KH, Schur PH, Karlson EW (2009) Comparison of threshold cutpoints and continuous measures of anti-cyclic citrullinated peptide antibodies in predicting future rheumatoid arthritis. J Rheumatol 36: 706–711.
22. Leibon G, Rockmore DN, Pollak MR (2008) A SNP streak model for the identification of genetic regions identical-by-descent. Stat Appl Genet Mol Biol 7: Article16.
23. Thomas A (2010) Assessment of SNP streak statistics using gene drop simulation with linkage disequilibrium. Genet Epidemiol 34: 119–124.
24. Genomes Project Consortium, Abecasis GR, Auton A, Brooks LD, DePristo MA, et al. (2012) An integrated map of genetic variation from 1,092 human genomes. Nature 491: 56–65.
25. Tennessen JA, Bigham AW, O'Connor TD, Fu W, Kenny EE, et al. (2012) Evolution and functional impact of rare coding variation from deep sequencing of human exomes. Science 337: 64–69.
26. Davydov EV, Goode DL, Sirota M, Cooper GM, Sidow A, et al. (2010) Identifying a high fraction of the human genome to be under selective constraint using GERP++. PLoS Comput Biol 6: e1001025.
27. Kumar P, Henikoff S, Ng PC (2009) Predicting the effects of coding non-synonymous variants on protein function using the SIFT algorithm. Nat Protoc 4: 1073–1081.
28. Adzhubei IA, Schmidt S, Peshkin L, Ramensky VE, Gerasimova A, et al. (2010) A method and server for predicting damaging missense mutations. Nat Methods 7: 248–249.
29. Cui J, Stahl EA, Saevarsdottir S, Miceli C, Diogo D, et al. (2013) Genome-Wide Association Study and Gene Expression Analysis Identifies CD84 as a Predictor of Response to Etanercept Therapy in Rheumatoid Arthritis. PLoS Genet 9: e1003394.
30. Bathon JM, Martin RW, Fleischmann RM, Tesser JR, Schiff MH, et al. (2000) A comparison of etanercept and methotrexate in patients with early rheumatoid arthritis. N Engl J Med 343: 1586–1593.
31. Moreland LW, O'Dell JR, Paulus HE, Curtis JR, Bathon JM, et al. (2012) A randomized comparative effectiveness study of oral triple therapy versus etanercept plus methotrexate in early aggressive rheumatoid arthritis: the treatment of Early Aggressive Rheumatoid Arthritis Trial. Arthritis Rheum 64: 2824–2835.
32. Fisher MC, Hochberg MC, El-Taha M, Kremer JM, Peng C, et al. (2012) Smoking, smoking cessation, and disease activity in a large cohort of patients with rheumatoid arthritis. J Rheumatol 39: 904–909.
33. Carroll RJ, Eyler AE, Denny JC (2011) Naive Electronic Health Record phenotype identification for Rheumatoid arthritis. AMIA Annu Symp Proc 2011: 189–196.
34. Trynka G, Sandor C, Han B, Xu H, Stranger BE, et al. (2013) Chromatin marks identify critical cell types for fine mapping complex trait variants. Nat Genet 45: 124–130.
35. Westra HJ, Peters MJ, Esko T, Yaghootkar H, Schurmann C, et al. (2013) Systematic identification of trans eQTLs as putative drivers of known disease associations. Nat Genet 45: 1238–1243.

36. Price AL, Kryukov GV, de Bakker PI, Purcell SM, Staples J, et al. (2010) Pooled association tests for rare variants in exon-resequencing studies. Am J Hum Genet 86: 832–838.
37. Madsen BE, Browning SR (2009) A groupwise association test for rare mutations using a weighted sum statistic. PLoS Genet 5: e1000384.
38. Neale BM, Rivas MA, Voight BF, Altshuler D, Devlin B, et al. (2011) Testing for an unusual distribution of rare variants. PLoS Genet 7: e1001322.
39. Wu MC, Lee S, Cai T, Li Y, Boehnke M, et al. (2011) Rare-variant association testing for sequencing data with the sequence kernel association test. Am J Hum Genet 89: 82–93.
40. Kiezun A, Garimella K, Do R, Stitziel NO, Neale BM, et al. (2012) Exome sequencing and the genetic basis of complex traits. Nat Genet 44: 623–630.
41. Punta M, Coggill PC, Eberhardt RY, Mistry J, Tate J, et al. (2012) The Pfam protein families database. Nucleic Acids Res 40: D290–D301.
42. Akoh CC, Lee GC, Liaw YC, Huang TH, Shaw JF (2004) GDSL family of serine esterases/lipases. Prog Lipid Res 43: 534–552.
43. Bradfield JP, Qu HQ, Wang K, Zhang H, Sleiman PM, et al. (2011) A genome-wide meta-analysis of six type 1 diabetes cohorts identifies multiple associated loci. PLoS Genet 7: e1002293.
44. Duan R, Leo P, Bradbury L, Brown MA, Thomas G (2010) Gene expression profiling reveals a downregulation in immune-associated genes in patients with AS. Ann Rheum Dis 69: 1724–1729.
45. Ombrello MJ, Remmers EF, Sun G, Freeman AF, Datta S, et al. (2012) Cold urticaria, immunodeficiency, and autoimmunity related to PLCG2 deletions. N Engl J Med 366: 330–338.
46. Hunt KA, Mistry V, Bockett NA, Ahmad T, Ban M, et al. (2013) Negligible impact of rare autoimmune-locus coding-region variants on missing heritability. Nature 498: 232–235.
47. Arnett FC, Edworthy SM, Bloch DA, McShane DJ, Fries JF, et al. (1988) The American Rheumatism Association 1987 revised criteria for the classification of rheumatoid arthritis. Arthritis Rheum 31: 315–324.
48. Lander ES, Botstein D (1987) Homozygosity mapping: a way to map human recessive traits with the DNA of inbred children. Science 236: 1567–1570.
49. Abecasis GR, Cherny SS, Cookson WO, Cardon LR (2002) Merlin–rapid analysis of dense genetic maps using sparse gene flow trees. Nat Genet 30: 97–101.
50. Li H, Durbin R (2010) Fast and accurate long-read alignment with Burrows-Wheeler transform. Bioinformatics 26: 589–595.
51. McKenna A, Hanna M, Banks E, Sivachenko A, Cibulskis K, et al. (2010) The Genome Analysis Toolkit: a MapReduce framework for analyzing next-generation DNA sequencing data. Genome Res 20: 1297–1303.
52. DePristo MA, Banks E, Poplin R, Garimella KV, Maguire JR, et al. (2011) A framework for variation discovery and genotyping using next-generation DNA sequencing data. Nat Genet 43: 491–498.
53. Cingolani P, Platts A, Wang le L, Coon M, Nguyen T, et al. (2012) A program for annotating and predicting the effects of single nucleotide polymorphisms, SnpEff: SNPs in the genome of Drosophila melanogaster strain w1118; iso-2; iso-3. Fly (Austin) 6: 80–92.
54. Plagnol V, Curtis J, Epstein M, Mok KY, Stebbings E, et al. (2012) A robust model for read count data in exome sequencing experiments and implications for copy number variant calling. Bioinformatics 28: 2747–2754.
55. Andres M, Quevedo S, Mato S (1998) Fisher's Mid-P-value arrangement in 2x2 Comparative trials. Computational Statistics & Data Analysis 29: 107–115.
56. Howie B, Fuchsberger C, Stephens M, Marchini J, Abecasis GR (2012) Fast and accurate genotype imputation in genome-wide association studies through pre-phasing. Nat Genet 44: 955–959.
57. Okada Y, Sim X, Go MJ, Wu JY, Gu D, et al. (2012) Meta-analysis identifies multiple loci associated with kidney function-related traits in east Asian populations. Nat Genet 44: 904–909.
58. Okada Y, Yamazaki K, Umeno J, Takahashi A, Kumasaka N, et al. (2011) HLA-Cw*1202-B*5201-DRB1*1502 Haplotype Increases Risk for Ulcerative Colitis but Reduces Risk for Crohn's Disease. Gastroenterology 141: 864–871.
59. Bernstein BE, Stamatoyannopoulos JA, Costello JF, Ren B, Milosavljevic A, et al. (2010) The NIH Roadmap Epigenomics Mapping Consortium. Nat Biotechnol 28: 1045–1048.
60. Okada Y, Wu D, Trynka G, Raj T, Terao C, et al. (2013) Genetics of rheumatoid arthritis contributes to biology and drug discovery. Nature doi:10.1038/nature12873.
61. Li H, Handsaker B, Wysoker A, Fennell T, Ruan J, et al. (2009) The Sequence Alignment/Map format and SAMtools. Bioinformatics 25: 2078–2079.
62. Koboldt DC, Chen K, Wylie T, Larson DE, McLellan MD, et al. (2009) VarScan: variant detection in massively parallel sequencing of individual and pooled samples. Bioinformatics 25: 2283–2285.
63. Wang K, Li M, Hakonarson H (2010) ANNOVAR: functional annotation of genetic variants from high-throughput sequencing data. Nucleic Acids Res 38: e164.

11

Ultrasonographic Assessment of Enthesitis in HLA-B27 Positive Patients with Rheumatoid Arthritis, a Matched Case-Only Study

Antonio Mera-Varela[1,2], Aida Ferreiro-Iglesias[1], Eva Perez-Pampin[1], Marisol Porto-Silva[1], Juan J. Gómez-Reino[1,2], Antonio Gonzalez[1]*

1 Research Laboratory 10 and Rheumatology Unit, Instituto de Investigacion Sanitaria – Hospital Clinico Universitario de Santiago, Santiago de Compostela, Spain, **2** Department of Medicine, University of Santiago de Compostela, Santiago de Compostela, Spain

Abstract

Introduction: HLA-B27 has a modifier effect on the phenotype of multiple diseases, both associated and non-associated with it. Among these effects, an increased frequency of clinical enthesitis in patients with Rheumatoid Arthritis (RA) has been reported but never explored again. We aimed to replicate this study with a sensitive and quantitative assessment of enthesitis by using standardized ultrasonography (US).

Methods: The Madrid Sonography Enthesitis Index (MASEI) was applied to the US assessment of 41 HLA-B27 positive and 41 matched HLA-B27 negative patients with longstanding RA. Clinical characteristics including explorations aimed to evaluate spondyloarthrtitis and laboratory tests were also done.

Results: A significant degree of abnormalities in the entheses of the patients with RA were found, but the MASEI values, and each of its components including the Doppler signal, were similar in HLA-B27 positive and negative patients. An increase of the MASEI scores with age was identified. Differences in two clinical features were found: a lower prevalence of rheumatoid factor and a more common story of low back pain in the HLA-B27 positive patients than in the negative. The latter was accompanied by radiographic sacroiliitis in two HLA-B27 positive patients. No other differences were detected.

Conclusion: We have found that HLA-B27 positive patients with RA do not have more enthesitis as assessed with US than the patients lacking this HLA allele. However, HLA-B27 could be shaping the RA phenotype towards RF seronegativity and axial involvement.

Editor: Chi Zhang, University of Texas Southwestern Medical Center, United States of America

Funding: The study was supported by grants 10CSA918040PR from the Xunta de Galicia (http://www.sergas.e/MostrarContidos_N3_T01.aspx?IdPaxina = 10142) and PI08/0744 of the Instituto de Salud Carlos III (http://www.isciii.es/) that are partially financed by the European Regional Development Fund of the European Union. The funders had no role in study design, data collection and analysis, decision to publish, or preparation of the manuscript.

Competing Interests: The authors have declared that no competing interests exist.

* E-mail: antonio.gonzalez.martinez-pedrayo@sergas.es

Introduction

Research in the genetic component of RA etiology has experienced a marked progress in recent years with the identification of a large number of susceptibility loci [1,2]. However, there are still many unsolved questions. Among them the relative to genotype-phenotype relationships are very prominent. It is expected that genotypes will have an important role in shaping the RA phenotype and that identification of these relationships will help manage patients in a personalized manner. The most established relationship has been the observed between a large number of RA susceptibility factors and the production of anti-citrullinated protein antibodies (ACPA). The earlier discovered association of the shared epitope (SE) with severe RA, including progression of erosive arthritis, seems to be explained by SE association with ACPA production. Other lines of active research in this field include the search for genetic factors modifying progression of erosions [3,4], or response to treatment [5,6] and of loci associated with ACPA negative patients [7,8]. Some of these studies are focused in RA susceptibility loci [4,6,8], which are good candidates because of their involvement in the disease mechanisms. Additional candidates are the genetic factors associated with related diseases. These loci are also of known functional relevance and they have the potential of being involved in subgroups of RA patients sharing clinical characteristics with the disease where the loci were identified.

One of these candidates is HLA-B27 [9,10,11,12,13]. It is strongly associated with ankylosing spondylitis (AS) and with other spondyloarthritis (SpA), but not with RA [14,15]. HLA-B27 has also modifier effects on the phenotype that have been observed in its associated diseases and in some non-HLA-B27 associated diseases. Among the HLA-B27 associated diseases, there are multiple reports showing earlier disease onset, more involvement of sacroiliac and spine joints, a higher tendency to chronicity and more prevalence of back pain in HLA-B27 positive than in negative patients [16,17,18,19,20,21]. In addition, non-HLA-B27 associated diseases can be modified to show higher prevalence of archetypical AS clinical features. For example, HLA-B27 positive patients with inflammatory bowel disease show an increased prevalence of sacroiliitis, spondylitis and enthesitis [22,23]. HLA-B27 also increases the prevalence of sacroiliitis in patients with familial Mediterranean fever [24]; and of sacroiliitis, inflammatory back pain and enthesitis in children with Juvenile Idiopatic Arthritis [25,26]. Therefore, it is not surprising that some researchers have thought the presence of HLA-B27 could modify the phenotypes of patients with RA towards resembling SpA. There have been some reports in this direction [9,10,11,12,13], but all these studies were done more than a decade ago and none of their findings have become established. One of these studies reported an increased prevalence of clinical enthesitis in patients with early arthritis fulfilling RA criteria [9].

Enthesitis, the inflammation of the entheses, is very prevalent and relatively specific of all forms of SpA motivating its inclusion as part of the disease classification criteria [15,27]. Enthesitis is present in early SpA and, occasionally, it is the unique disease manifestation for some time. This has lead some authors to consider enthesitis the primary lesion in this group of diseases [28]. Now we have the possibility to identify early enthesitis when it is not yet clinically apparent either to patients or to physical exploration thanks to magnetic resonance imaging and ultrasonography (US) [29,30,31,32,33]. This property of US has been applied to a variety of clinical situations demanding sensitive evaluation. Examples include SpA with subclinical enthesopathy [34], recurrent acute anterior uveitis without SpA [35], long term dialysis [36], and patients with psoriasis without psoriatic arthritis [36,37], showing in all these cases an increased frequency of abnormalities. US evaluation has also shown an increased frequency of abnormalities in patients with RA relative to healthy controls in spite of the complete absence of clinical enthesitis [38,39]. Only one of these studies assessed HLA-B27, concerning recurrent anterior uveitis, and it found that enthesitis was associated with this HLA allele [35].

Therefore, we have now the opportunity to analyze the prevalence of enthesitis in RA patients stratified for HLA-B27 status with the sensitivity and accuracy allowed by US. With this aim, we have selected all available RA patients positive for HLA-B27 in our hospital and matched RA patients negative for HLA-B27. The two groups were compared with the Madrid Sonography Enthesitis Index (MASEI) [31], focused anamnesis and physical exploration. No differences in the MASEI or any of its components were detected. This result excludes a role of HLA-B27 in the enthesal abnormalities of these patients. However, a modifier effect of HLA-B27 on the phenotype of the patients with RA was suggested by its association with RF negative status and a more frequent story of low back pain.

Materials and Methods

Ethics statement

All patients gave their written informed consent to participate. Sample collection and the study protocol were approved by the Comite de Investigacion Clinica de Galicia (Spain).

Selection of patients

DNA and serum samples from patients with RA according to ACR classification criteria were used [40]. All patients were of Spanish ancestry and were attending the Rheumatology Unit of the Hospital Clinico Universitario de Santiago. HLA-B27 positive patients were selected. Gender, age at disease onset and current age of these patients was used to select matched HLA-B27 negative patients at a 1:1 ratio. Patients were invited to participate in the study and they gave their written informed consent. The rheumatologist and the nurse involved in recruitment and evaluation of the patients were blind to their HLA-B27 status.

Laboratory studies

Two complementary genotyping reactions were used to determine the HLA-B27 status (available from the authors upon request). The first PCR was based on the method of Bon et al. [41]. It amplifies HLA-B*2701-*2706 alleles, which are the most common in the Caucasian population and the most associated with AS. The second PCR used a combination of 3 primers described by Faner et al. [42]. It amplifies a larger number of alleles than the first, from HLA-B*2701 to *2724 except for HLA-B*2718 and HLA-B*2723. PCR amplification was done with a multiplex PCR system (KAPA2G fast HotStart, Kapa Biosystems, Woburn, MA). Detection of the PCR products was performed with single-base extension (SNaPshot Multiplex Kit from Applied Biosystems, Foster City, CA) using probes targeting a non polymorphic base. In this way, the most frequents alleles of HLA-B27 were covered by two PCR. Four samples were positive only in the second amplification, which is consistent with the low frequency of the rare alleles in Spain [43].They were excluded from analysis because of their more uncertain status.

HLA-DBR1 alleles were determined by a sequencing based typing method (SBT) using the AlleleSEQR HLA-DRB1 Typing kit (Abbott Diagnostics, Abbott Park, Germany), which includes bidirectional sequencing of the second exon of DRB1. Ambiguous samples were additionally sequenced with group-specific primers (AlleleSEQR HLA-DRB1 GSSP, Abbott). The anti-CCP status of the patients was determined using the EDIA ACPA Kit (Euro-Diagnostica, Arnhem, The Netherlands). Quantification and setting of the cut-off level at 5 units/ml were done according to the manufacturer's instructions. RF status was determined by rate nephelometry with the IMMAGE Immunochemistry Systems (Beckman Coulter, Ireland), which covers all Ig isotypes.

Clinical and Ultrasound evaluation

Patient history was reviewed and a specific anamnesis of symptoms and signs characteristic of HLA-B27 associated diseases was conducted. Physical exploration was done looking for signs of axial involvement with instruments developed for SpA as the Schober test, BASDAI and BASFI scores and assessment of the lateral trunk flexion. A modified Schober test according with Moll and Wright was used[44]. Inflammatory back pain was defined as lumbar pain at night or with morning stiffness that does not improve with rest or that improves with exercise and that persists for more than a month. Plain antero-posterior pelvic radiographs were evaluated for the presence of sacroiliitis. This assessment was independently done by two rheumatologists in a blind form.

In addition, the presence of enthesitis was evaluated by a rheumatologist experienced in US focused on articular and periarticular locations and blind to the HLA-B27 status of patients. A General Electric LogiqQ7 US machine with a 10–14 MHz linear array transducer was used. The power Doppler setting was standardized with a pulse repetition frequency (PRF) of 500 Hz with a low wall filter and 35–40 dB of gain. The Madrid Sonography Enthesitis Index (MASEI) was used for quantitative and standardized assessment [31]. This index evaluates 6 features in 6 entheses. A value $\geq$ 18 has been defined as characteristic of SpA. The 6 features are enthesis thickness, structure, calcifications, erosions, bursae and power Doppler signal. The 6 bilaterally assessed locations are proximal plantar fascia, distal Achilles tendon, distal and proximal patellar tendon insertion, distal quadriceps tendon and brachial triceps tendon.

Statistical analysis

HLA-B27 positive patients with RA were considered cases and the matched HLA-B27 negative patients were controls. Demographic, clinical, laboratory, radiographic and ultrasound characteristics were compared between the two groups using Student T test or the Fisher exact test for contingency tables depending on the quantitative or qualitative nature of the variables, respectively. Detailed US results were compared with the Man-Whitney U test and non-parametric statistics because they showed many zero values. All analyses were done with Statistica 7.0 (StatSoft, Tulsa, OK). Differences with P<0.05 were considered statistically significant.

Results

Analysis of 672 patients with RA identified 65 that were HLA-B27+, the remaining 607 were HLA-B27- (11 additional patients showed an uncertain HLA-B27 status and were not included). The HLA-B27 positive subgroup of patients showed less RF positive subjects, 50.0 %, than the HLA-B27 negative subgroup 64.6 % (P = 0.025). Also the ACPA status showed a trend to decreased prevalence in this subgroup (Table 1). However, there were not more patients with low titers of ACPA (between 5 and 45 units) in the HLA-B27 positive (33.3 %) than in the HLA-B27 negative subgroup (32.8 %). The other characteristics, gender, age at disease onset, erosive arthritis and carrier status of the SE, were similar in the two subgroups of patients (Table 1).

A total of 41 HLA-B27 positive patients were available and willing to participate in the study. One HLA-B27- patient was selected for each HLA-B27+ patient trying to match them for gender, age at disease onset and current age. The resulting groups were very similar not only in the selected variables but also in other characteristics as height, weight, serology and SE status (Table 2). During the visit for evaluation one of the patients in the HLA-B27 positive subgroup was found to have SpA in spite of his previous classification as RA and was excluded from further analysis. Specific anamnesis and physical evaluation of the patients were done blind to their HLA-B27 status. They disclosed a higher prevalence of low back pain, mechanical or inflammatory, in the HLA-B27 positive subgroup, 27.5 %, than in the HLA-B27 negative subgroup, 7.5 %, P = 0.037. This difference was similarly distributed between inflammatory and mechanical pain (Table 3). No other symptom or evaluation showed differences between the two patient groups. Specifically there were not differences in modified Schober's test, BASDAI or BASFI scores or in the lateral flexion of the spine (Table 3). A few patients reported a story of past skin lesions that could correspond to psoriasis but without differences between the two subgroups.

Two rheumatologists that were blind to the HLA-B27 status of the patients evaluated plain pelvic radiographs for the presence of sacroiliitis. Their assessment was fully concordant identifying 2 patients with sacroiliitis. The two were positive for HLA-B27. This was not significantly different from the result in the HLA-B27 negative subgroup, but we investigated it further. A review of the two patients with sacroiliitis did not challenge their classification as RA: the two showed erosive RA and one of them was positive for ACPA and homozygous for the SE. The two patients had a story of inflammatory low back pain.

Systematic evaluation of the entheses following the MASEI procedure (representative images in Figure 1) yielded no differences between the two subgroups of patients (Table 4). Mean MASEI values were even nominally lower in the HLA-B27 positive subgroup. Also, the threshold score of 18 proposed as specific of AS [31], was not discriminating between the two subgroups: there were 13 patients above this value in the HLA-B27 positive subgroup and 10 in the HLA-B27 negative subgroup. In addition, no difference was detected with any of the components of the index (Table 4). This is specially relevant for the power Doppler signal (Figure 2) because it has been differentially associated with SpA relative to other diseases including RA [39]. But no difference was detected comparing the whole distribution of values (Table 4), or the percentage of

Table 1. Characteristics of the patients with RA in function of the HLA-B27 subgroup.

	HLA-B27-	HLA-B27+	*P* value
Women %	77.6 (471/607)[a]	72.3 (47/65)	0.3
Age of disease onset, mean (SD)	46.3 (14.8)	44.9 (16.7)	0.5
Rheumatoid Factor % [b]	64.6 (369/571)	50.0 (30/60)	0.025
Anti-CCP %	63.0 (376/597)	50.8 (33/65)	0.05
Anti-CCP median (IQR) [c]	93.3 (32.8−198.0)	67.4 (18.7−141.3)	0.3
Carrier SE %	53.3 (286/537)	56.4 (31/55)	0.7
Erosive arthritis %	65.8 (369/561)	61.7 (37/60)	0.5

[a]Number with the feature/total number of patients with available information.
[b]Median and IQR were 122 (61−445) in the HLA-B27- subgroup and 235 (128−366) in the HLA-B27+ subgroup (*P* = 0.8). This information was available only for 127 RF+ patients.
[c]Median and interquartile range of the anti-CCP positive patients.

Table 2. Characteristics of the patients recruited for detailed analysis in function of the HLA-B27 subgroup.

	HLA-B27-	HLA-B27+	*P* value
Women %	73.2 (30/41)[a]	80.5 (33/41)	0.6
Age of disease onset, mean (SD)	41.9 (15.7)	43.9 (17.3)	0.6
Current age, mean (SD)	64.8 (15.2)	64.4 (14.7)	0.9
Weight, mean (SD)	68.8 (12.2)	68.3 (13.7)	0.8
Height, mean (SD)	159.5 (7.8)	158.3 (8.7)	0.5
Ever smoking %	24.4 (10/41)	24.4 (10/41)	1
Rheumatoid factor %	55.0 (22/40)	50.0 (20/40)	0.8
Anti-CCP %	40.0 (16/40)	51.2 (21/41)	0.4
Carrier of SE %	55.0 (22/40)	57.9 (22/38)	0.8
Erosive arthritis %	65.0 (26/40)	53.9 (21/39)	0.4
Biologics %	50.0 (20/40)	60.0 (24/40)	0.5
Anti-TNF [b]	60.0 (12/20)	45.8 (11/24)	0.4
Rituximab	15.0 (3/20)	16.7 (4/24)	1.0
Abatacept	10.0 (2/20)	20.8 (5/24)	0.4
Tocilizumab	15.0 (3/20)	16.7 (4/24)	1.0
Methotrexate	65.0 (13/20)	83.3 (20/24)	0.2
Leflunomide	20.0 (4/20)	0.0 (0/24)	0.04

[a]Number with the feature/total number of patients with available information.
[b]Including Etanercept, Adalimumab and Infliximab.

Table 3. Results of the anamnesis and exploration of recruited patients in function of the HLA-B27 subgroup.

	HLA-B27-	HLA-B27+	*P* value
Back pain %	7.5 (3/40)	27.5 (11/40)	0.037
Inflammatory back pain %	2.5 (1/40)	12.5 (5/40)	0.2
Non-inflammatory back pain %	5.0 (2/40)	15.5(6/40)	0. 3
Story of 'psoriatic' lesions %	7.3 (3/40)	5.0 (2/40)	1.0
Schober's test, mean (SD)	3.7 (1.0)	3.8 (1.0)	0.9
Right lateral flexion, mean (SD)	13.2 (4.0)	12.7 (4.4)	0.6
Left lateral flexion, mean (SD)	13.4 (4.3)	11.8 (3.6)	0.1
BASDAI, mean (SD)	4.3 (2.5)	4.6 (2.4)	0.6
BASFI, mean (SD)	2.9 (2.4)	3.4 (2.2)	0.4
Sacroiliitis Rx %	0.0 (0/34)[a]	5.7 (2/35)	0.3

[a]Number with the feature/total number of patients with available information.

positive signals (9/40 in HLA-B-27 positive patients *vs.* 13/41 in HLA-B27 negative patients) or the mean values in the patients showing Doppler signals (4.7 *vs.* 4.6, in the HLA-B27 positive and negative patients, respectively). The only associations we identified were unrelated with the HLA-B27 status: a significant increase of the MASEI value in men relative to women (not shown), and an increase of the score with age due to calcifications (not shown). The two patients with sacroiliitis lacked signs of enthesitis (MASEI values of 4 and 8).

Discussion

Our analyses have not shown any specific enthesal abnormality in the HLA-B27 positive patients with RA. The sensitive and quantitative evaluation allows us to exclude a significant HLA-B27 modifier effect towards enthesitis in the RA patients. However, an excess of patients in the HLA-B27 positive group referred a story of low back pain that in two of the patients was associated with radiographic sacroiliitis. These findings together with a lower prevalence of RF keep open the possibility of a modifier effect of the HLA-B27 allele on the phenotype of RA patients, but excluding the presence of enthesitis.

Our primary aim was to compare the frequency of enthesitis between HLA-B27 positive and negative patients with RA using systematic US examination. This imaging technology has shown sensitivity for detecting a high percentage of SpA patients with subclinical enthesitis [15,29,30,31,32,33,34,39]. It is applied with scoring protocols that help differentiate SpA patients from controls, from subjects that have suffered mechanical injury and from other forms of inflammatory arthritis [31,32,33]. Specifically, the MASEI protocol used here has shown high sensitivity and specificity and it is very comprehensive because it includes assessment of 6 features in 6 enthesal sites and both grey scales and power Doppler [31,33]. The assessment of power Doppler is a distinct advantage of this method over the most commonly used GUESS procedure for our study because the Doppler signal is the most specific feature distinguishing SpA from mechanical and RA enthesal abnormalities [39].

We have found significant abnormalities in the entheses of patients with RA confirming findings of previous US studies [38,39,45]. However, no differences were found between HLA-B27 positive and negative patients, even for components of the index that are more specific for SpA like the Doppler signal. Therefore, it is clear that the presence of HLA-B27 does not induce enthesal pathology in RA patients and that all the abnormalities found in these patients are produced with independence of this genetic factor.

Other interesting aspect of our MASEI results is that only patients older than 50 years of age showed values over the threshold identifying patients with AS or SpA [31,33]. Therefore, our results do not question the specificity of this threshold for early SpA, which starts most often below this age. An increase of enthesal abnormalities with age was already shown more than a decade ago [46]. It was described as independent of the underlying disease and, as in our study, to be mostly due to calcification.

Two of the other clinical features we have analyzed were different between HLA-B27 positive and negative patients with RA. The first was the prevalence of RF, which was less common in HLA-B27 positive patients. It was accompanied by a trend to lower prevalence of ACPA. This result could imply either association of HLA-B27 with RF seronegative RA or misclassification of patients. The latter possibility can be reasonably excluded because we only found a patient with SpA among the 41 that were specifically revised. In addition, the HLA-B27+ RF- patients were not different in any respect from the HLA-B27- RF- subgroup. For example, the HLA-B27+RF- and B27-RF- patients were comparable at percentage of ACPA+, 26.7 % vs. 25.6 %, erosive arthritis, 51.7 % vs. 45.7 %, or percentage of carriers of SE, 44.4 % vs. 43.1 %, respectively. This leaves us with the possibility that HLA-B27 could be a susceptibility factor for RF seronegative RA. Only studies in additional sample collections will be needed to clarify this matter.

An increased prevalence of low back pain was also associated with HLA-B27 in the patients with RA. This outcome from the anamnesis was combined with the identification of two patients

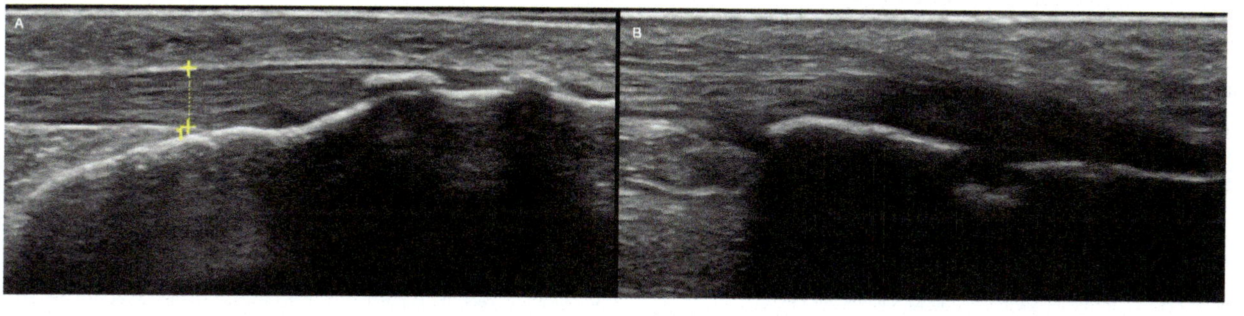

Figure 1. Representative images of features detected with US exploration. A) Example of analysis of the Achilles tendon thickness measured between the two yellow crosses in one patient, and B) Erosion detected in the superior pole of the calcaneous in a different patient.

Table 4. Ultrasonographic evaluation of the entheses following the MASEI procedure.

	HLA-B27-	HLA-B27+	*P* value
MASEI, mean (SD)	14.2 (9.3)	13.6 (8.8)	0.7
MASEI, median ($_{10-90}$R)*	11.0 (5−24)	11.5 (4−27)	0.7
MASEI >18, %	24.4 (10/41)	32.5 (13/40)	0.5
- structure, median ($_{10-90}$R)	0 (0−1)	0 (0−1.5)	0.8
- thickness, median ($_{10-90}$R)	2 (0−5)	2 (0−5)	0.08
- erosion, median ($_{10-90}$R)	3 (0−6)	0 (0−10.5)	0.8
- calcification, median ($_{10-90}$R)	7 (2−13)	5 (2.5−14)	0.7
- Doppler, median ($_{10-90}$R)	0 (0−6)	0 (0−3)	0.3
- bursitis, median ($_{10-90}$R)	0 (0−1)	0 (0−1)	0.8

*The range between percentiles 10 and 90.

with radiographic sacroiliitis among the patients with inflammatory low back pain. The two results are in agreement with the idea that HLA-B27 could modify RA towards the axial joints. This idea is supported by previous studies showing association between sacroiliitis and HLA-B27, both in HLA-27-associated diseases [17,19,20,21], and in some non-associated diseases [22,23,24,26] including RA [10,12,13]. In fact, this is the unique association with HLA-B27 that has been replicated in different RA studies. However, two previous studies did not found differences in the sacroiliac joints between HLA-B27 positive and negative patients with RA [47,48]. These findings should motivate new studies directed to the analysis of low back pain and to the identification of sacroiliitis. MRI will be the technology of choice for these studies because it is very sensitive for incipient changes in the sacroiliac joints [29], and it could provide more definitive results than radiography given the small size of the HLA-B27 positive subgroup.

In relation with the low back pain association, it could be argued that its presence questions the classification of the patients as RA. However, this type of reasoning is incompatible with the aim of our study. When the aim is to identify patients with RA

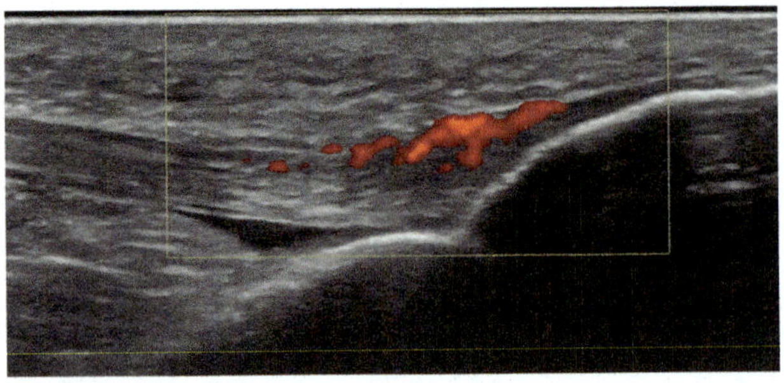

Figure 2. Positive power Doppler signal identifying tibial tuberosity enthesitis. The signal (in red) is detected in the tibial insertion of the patellar ligament in one of the studied patients.

showing phenotypes resembling SpA, we need to consider classification of RA before doing any extra analysis and keep this classification constant along the study.

Conclusions

We have found that HLA-B27 positive patients with RA do not have more enthesitis as assessed with US than those lacking this allele. However, these patients referred a more prevalent story of low back pain and were more often seronegative for RF than the HLA-B27 negative patients indicating that HLA-B27 could be shaping the RA phenotype in other directions deserving further and more focused analysis.

Acknowledgments

Authors acknowledge the patients with RA participating in this study by their availability and generosity. AF-I has a pre-doctoral bursary from the Instituto de Salud Carlos III (Spain).

Author Contributions

Conceived and designed the experiments: AM-V AG. Performed the experiments: AM-V AF-I EP-P MP-S JJG-R. Analyzed the data: AM-V AF-I AG. Wrote the paper: AM-V AF-I AG.

References

1. Gregersen PK (2010) Susceptibility genes for rheumatoid arthritis - a rapidly expanding harvest. Bull NYU Hosp Jt Dis 68: 179–182.
2. Plenge RM, Raychaudhuri S (2010) Leveraging human genetics to develop future therapeutic strategies in rheumatoid arthritis. Rheum Dis Clin North Am 36: 259–270.
3. Knevel R, Krabben A, Brouwer E, Posthumus MD, Wilson AG, et al. (2012) Genetic variants in IL15 associate with progression of joint destruction in rheumatoid arthritis: a multicohort study. Ann Rheum Dis.
4. van der Linden MP, Feitsma AL, le Cessie S, Kern M, Olsson LM, et al. (2009) Association of a single-nucleotide polymorphism in CD40 with the rate of joint destruction in rheumatoid arthritis. Arthritis Rheum 60: 2242–2247.
5. Plant D, Bowes J, Potter C, Hyrich KL, Morgan AW, et al. (2011) Genome-wide association study of genetic predictors of anti-tumor necrosis factor treatment efficacy in rheumatoid arthritis identifies associations with polymorphisms at seven loci. Arthritis Rheum 63: 645–653.
6. Cui J, Saevarsdottir S, Thomson B, Padyukov L, van der Helm-van Mil AH, et al. (2010) Rheumatoid arthritis risk allele PTPRC is also associated with response to anti-tumor necrosis factor alpha therapy. Arthritis Rheum 62: 1849–1861.
7. Padyukov L, Seielstad M, Ong RT, Ding B, Ronnelid J, et al. (2011) A genome-wide association study suggests contrasting associations in ACPA-positive versus ACPA-negative rheumatoid arthritis. Ann Rheum Dis 70: 259–265.
8. Seddighzadeh M, Gonzalez A, Ding B, Ferreiro-Iglesias A, Gomez-Reino JJ, et al. (2012) Variants Within STAT Genes Reveal Association with Anticitrullinated Protein Antibody-negative Rheumatoid Arthritis in 2 European Populations. J Rheumatol 39: 1509–1516.
9. El-Gabalawy HS, Goldbach-Mansky R, Smith D, 2nd, Arayssi T, Bale S, et al. (1999) Association of HLA alleles and clinical features in patients with synovitis of recent onset. Arthritis Rheum 42: 1696–1705.
10. Jajic Z, Jajic I (1991) HLA-B27 antigen and rheumatoid arthritis. Acta Med Iugosl 45: 195–202.
11. Jaraquemada D, Ollier W, Awad J, Young A, Silman A, et al. (1986) HLA and rheumatoid arthritis: a combined analysis of 440 British patients. Ann Rheum Dis 45: 627–636.
12. Rantapaa Dahlqvist S, Nordmark LG, Bjelle A (1984) HLA-B27 and involvement of sacroiliac joints in rheumatoid arthritis. J Rheumatol 11: 27–32.
13. Rundback JH, Rosenberg ZS, Solomon G (1993) The radiographic features of rheumatoid arthritis in HLA-B27-positive patients. Skeletal Radiol 22: 263–267.
14. Reveille JD, Maganti RM (2009) Subtypes of HLA-B27: history and implications in the pathogenesis of ankylosing spondylitis. Adv Exp Med Biol 649: 159–176.
15. Dougados M, Baeten D (2011) Spondyloarthritis. Lancet 377: 2127–2137.
16. Feldtkeller E, Khan MA, van der Heijde D, van der Linden S, Braun J (2003) Age at disease onset and diagnosis delay in HLA-B27 negative vs. positive patients with ankylosing spondylitis. Rheumatol Int 23: 61–66.
17. Skare TL, Leite N, Bortoluzzo AB, Goncalves CR, Da Silva JA, et al. (2012) Effect of age at disease onset in the clinical profile of spondyloarthritis: a study of 1424 Brazilian patients. Clin Exp Rheumatol 30: 351–357.
18. Queiro R, Torre JC, Gonzalez S, Lopez-Larrea C, Tinture T, et al. (2003) HLA antigens may influence the age of onset of psoriasis and psoriatic arthritis. J Rheumatol 30: 505–507.
19. Chung HY, Machado P, van der Heijde D, D'Agostino MA, Dougados M (2011) HLA-B27 positive patients differ from HLA-B27 negative patients in

clinical presentation and imaging: results from the DESIR cohort of patients with recent onset axial spondyloarthritis. Ann Rheum Dis 70: 1930–1936.

20. Kaarela K, Jantti JK, Kotaniemi KM (2009) Similarity between chronic reactive arthritis and ankylosing spondylitis.A 32-35-year follow-up study. Clin Exp Rheumatol 27: 325–328.
21. Queiro R, Sarasqueta C, Belzunegui J, Gonzalez C, Figueroa M, et al. (2002) Psoriatic spondyloarthropathy: a comparative study between HLA-B27 positive and HLA-B27 negative disease. Semin Arthritis Rheum 31: 413–418.
22. Rodriguez-Reyna TS, Martinez-Reyes C, Yamamoto-Furusho JK (2009) Rheumatic manifestations of inflammatory bowel disease. World J Gastroenterol 15: 5517–5524.
23. Orchard TR, Holt H, Bradbury L, Hammersma J, McNally E, et al. (2009) The prevalence, clinical features and association of HLA-B27 in sacroiliitis associated with established Crohn's disease. Aliment Pharmacol Ther 29: 193–197.
24. Kasifoglu T, Calisir C, Cansu DU, Korkmaz C (2009) The frequency of sacroiliitis in familial Mediterranean fever and the role of HLA-B27 and MEFV mutations in the development of sacroiliitis. Clin Rheumatol 28: 41–46.
25. Berntson L, Damgard M, Andersson-Gare B, Herlin T, Nielsen S, et al. (2008) HLA-B27 predicts a more extended disease with increasing age at onset in boys with juvenile idiopathic arthritis. J Rheumatol 35: 2055–2061.
26. Flato B, Smerdel A, Johnston V, Lien G, Dale K, et al. (2002) The influence of patient characteristics, disease variables, and HLA alleles on the development of radiographically evident sacroiliitis in juvenile idiopathic arthritis. Arthritis Rheum 46: 986–994.
27. Rudwaleit M, van der Heijde D, Landewe R, Akkoc N, Brandt J, et al. (2011) The Assessment of SpondyloArthritis International Society classification criteria for peripheral spondyloarthritis and for spondyloarthritis in general. Ann Rheum Dis 70: 25–31.
28. McGonagle D, Gibbon W, Emery P (1998) Classification of inflammatory arthritis by enthesitis. Lancet 352: 1137–1140.
29. Maksymowych WP (2009) Progress in spondylarthritis. Spondyloarthritis: lessons from imaging. Arthritis Res Ther 11: 222.
30. D'Agostino MA, Aegerter P, Bechara K, Salliot C, Judet O, et al. (2011) How to diagnose spondyloarthritis early? Accuracy of peripheral enthesitis detection by power Doppler ultrasonography. Ann Rheum Dis 70: 1433–1440.
31. de Miguel E, Cobo T, Munoz-Fernandez S, Naredo E, Uson J, et al. (2009) Validity of enthesis ultrasound assessment in spondyloarthropathy. Ann Rheum Dis 68: 169–174.
32. Balint PV, Kane D, Wilson H, McInnes IB, Sturrock RD (2002) Ultrasonography of entheseal insertions in the lower limb in spondyloarthropathy. Ann Rheum Dis 61: 905–910.
33. de Miguel E, Munoz-Fernandez S, Castillo C, Cobo-Ibanez T, Martin-Mola E (2011) Diagnostic accuracy of enthesis ultrasound in the diagnosis of early spondyloarthritis. Ann Rheum Dis 70: 434–439.
34. Ruta S, Gutierrez M, Pena C, Garcia M, Arturi A, et al. (2011) Prevalence of subclinical enthesopathy in patients with spondyloarthropathy: an ultrasound study. J Clin Rheumatol 17: 18–22.
35. Munoz-Fernandez S, de Miguel E, Cobo-Ibanez T, Madero R, Ferreira A, et al. (2009) Enthesis inflammation in recurrent acute anterior uveitis without spondylarthritis. Arthritis Rheum 60: 1985–1990.
36. Gutierrez M, Zeiler M, Filippucci E, Salaffi F, Becciolini A, et al. (2011) Sonographic subclinical entheseal involvement in dialysis patients. Clin Rheumatol 30: 907–913.
37. Naredo E, Moller I, de Miguel E, Batlle-Gualda E, Acebes C, et al. (2011) High prevalence of ultrasonographic synovitis and enthesopathy in patients with psoriasis without psoriatic arthritis: a prospective case-control study. Rheumatology (Oxford) 50: 1838–1848.
38. Genc H, Cakit BD, Tuncbilek I, Erdem HR (2005) Ultrasonographic evaluation of tendons and enthesal sites in rheumatoid arthritis: comparison with ankylosing spondylitis and healthy subjects. Clin Rheumatol 24: 272–277.
39. D'Agostino MA, Said-Nahal R, Hacquard-Bouder C, Brasseur JL, Dougados M, et al. (2003) Assessment of peripheral enthesitis in the spondylarthropathies by ultrasonography combined with power Doppler: a cross-sectional study. Arthritis Rheum 48: 523–533.
40. Arnett FC, Edworthy SM, Bloch DA, McShane DJ, Fries JF, et al. (1988) The American Rheumatism Association 1987 revised criteria for the classification of rheumatoid arthritis. Arthritis Rheum 31: 315–324.
41. Bon MA, van Oeveren-Dybicz A, van den Bergh FA (2000) Genotyping of HLA-B27 by real-time PCR without hybridization probes. Clin Chem 46: 1000–1002.
42. Faner R, Casamitjana N, Colobran R, Ribera A, Pujol-Borrell R, et al. (2004) HLA-B27 genotyping by fluorescent resonance emission transfer (FRET) probes in real-time PCR. Hum Immunol 65: 826–838.
43. Mathieu A, Paladini F, Vacca A, Cauli A, Fiorillo MT, et al. (2009) The interplay between the geographic distribution of HLA-B27 alleles and their role in infectious and autoimmune diseases: a unifying hypothesis. Autoimmun Rev 8: 420–425.
44. Moll JM, Wright V (1971) Normal range of spinal mobility. An objective clinical study. Ann Rheum Dis 30: 381–386.
45. Falsetti P, Frediani B, Fioravanti A, Acciai C, Baldi F, et al. (2003) Sonographic study of calcaneal entheses in erosive osteoarthritis, nodal osteoarthritis, rheumatoid arthritis and psoriatic arthritis. Scand J Rheumatol 32: 229–234.
46. Shaibani A, Workman R, Rothschild BM (1993) The significance of enthesopathy as a skeletal phenomenon. Clin Exp Rheumatol 11: 399–403.
47. Saraux A, Guedes C, Allain J, Valls I, Baron D, et al. (1997) HLA-B27 in French patients with rheumatoid arthritis. Scand J Rheumatol 26: 269–271.
48. Jurik AG, de Carvalho A, Graudal H (1987) Radiographic visualisation of seropositive rheumatoid arthritis in carriers of HLA-B27. RöFo - Fortschritte auf dem Gebiet der R 147: 14–20.

12

Prevalence of Anti-Citrullinated Protein Antibodies (ACPA) in Patients with Diffuse Large B-Cell Lymphoma (DLBCL): A Case-Control Study

Gunter Assmann[1]*, Klara Shihadeh[2], Viola Poeschel[1], Niels Murawski[1], Jutta Conigliarou[1], Mei Fang Ong[3], Michael Pfreundschuh[1]

1 Department of Internal Medicine I, José-Carreras-Centre for Immuno- and Gene Therapy, University Medical School of Saarland, Homburg/Saar, Germany, **2** Department of Internal Medicine, General Hospital of Herrenberg, Esslingen-Herrenberg, Germany, **3** Institute of Medical Biometry, Epidemiology and Medical Informatics, Saarland University, Homburg/Saar, Germany

Abstract

Background: Antibodies against citrullinated proteins (ACPA) have been recognised as the most specific serum marker for rheumatoid arthritis. However, serum autoantibodies such as anti-nuclear antibodies have also been detected in the sera of different lymphatic malignancies without accompanying rheumatologic disease. Therefore, we conducted a study to evaluate the prevalence of ACPA in diffuse large B-cell non-Hodgkin lymphoma (DLBCL).

Methods: Sera of 395 DLBCL patients and 258 age-matched healthy controls were investigated to evaluate the prevalence of ACPA and RF. ACPA-positive data were stratified into subgroups of RF positivity and established prognostic parameters for DLBCL, including overall survival. In addition, the ACPA serum concentrations levels were compared to an ACPA-positive RA cohort (n = 175). The statistics were performed with $\chi 2$ test and Mann- Whitney-U test; Kaplan-Meyer curves (log rank test) were used to analyse the overall survival. P-value <0.05 was statistically significant.

Results: ACPA, but not RF, occurred significantly more frequently in the sera of DLBCL patients than in healthy controls (3.5% versus 0.8%, p = 0.030). However, the ACPA serum concentration levels were significantly lower than in RA patients (median 10.4 versus 124.1 U/ml, p = 0.0001). After subgroup stratification, ACPA positivity in DLBCL was significantly associated with male gender (4.4% versus 0%, p = 0.022; odds ratio 1.046, CI 1.014–1.079) and with RF-IgM seropositivity (1.77% versus 0%, p = 0.043), but not with prognostic parameters for DLBCL.

Conclusions: DLBCL is associated with a significantly higher prevalence of ACPA, with an increased prevalence in male patients, and simultaneous RF-IgM positivity. However, ACPA is not prognostic for DLBCL. The prevalence of RF-IgM, -IgA, or -IgG did not differ from healthy controls.

Editor: Massimo Pietropaolo, University of Michigan Medical School, United States of America

Funding: The authors have no support or funding to report.

Competing Interests: The authors have declared that no competing interests exist.

* E-mail: gunter.assmann@uks.eu

Introduction

Patients with rheumatoid arthritis (RA) are at an increased risk of lymphoproliferative diseases such as myeloma and high-grade B-cell non-Hodgkin lymphoma (B-NHL) compared with the healthy population [1,2,3]. The severity and duration as well as anti-rheumatic treatment of RA might further increase this risk [2,3,4]. The diminished apoptotic activity as well as the chronic B cell activation mediated through the tumour necrosis factor (TNF) superfamily, such as BAFF (B cell activating factor belonging to the TNF family), is supposed to be the pathogenetic background for this phenomenon [5,6]. On the other hand, there are no existing data to prove that lymphoma patients are at a higher risk of developing RA. However, serum biomarkers which are established in the diagnostic procedure and prognostic evaluation in RA such as rheumatoid factor (RF) or antinuclear antibodies (ANA) could also be observed in the sera of patients suffering from different forms of lymphatic malignancy.

The rheumatoid factor IgM (of the immunoglobulin M class) is 60–80% positive in RA, but is also positive in up to 50% of non-RA patients suffering from B-lymphocytic leukaemia [7] and additional B-NHL subgroups, such as diffuse-large-B-cell lymphoma (DLBCL), as shown in relatively small cohorts of patients [8]. The antinuclear antibody (ANA) titre also occurs in up to one third of sera derived from RA patients, predicting a severe course of disease and extra-articular manifestations [9]. Several studies have shown that elevated ANA titres are also found in patients with lymphoma [10,11,12]. Anti-citrullinated protein antibodies (ACPA) have been reported to be the best diagnostic serum marker with a 99% specificity for RA [13,14]. Furthermore, numerous longitudinal studies have confirmed that ACPA positivity is associated with a more severe course of RA, particularly concerning the occurrence of bone erosions, compared with ACPA-negative RA patients [15,16,17]. Moreover, the study of Nielen et al., investigating serial measurements in healthy blood donors, could show that ACPA is positive in less than 2% of healthy individuals, but, remarkably, ACPA-positive healthy individuals have to be considered to have an evident predisposition for developing RA in the future [18,19,20]. Klareskog et al. explained this phenomenon with the hypothesis of an extra-articular "immunisation" of B- and T-lymphocytes being reactive to citrullination, which occurs many years prior to RA manifestation. After that, a "second hit" such as trauma or infection could finally trigger the development of RA [21]. Underlining the predictive capacity of ACPA, a large cohort of primary Sjögren syndrome patients was tested, and 9% of the patients were shown to be ACPA-positive, with more than half of them subsequently developing RA in the following 5 years [22]. Whereas citrullination is basically an ubiquitous process in human cells due to inflammation, previously published experimental models hypothesised that citrullination can also play a role in the regulation of apoptosis through the p53-PAD14 network [14,23,24].

The development of ACPA seems to show a link between inflammation and citrullination on one side and autoimmunity and B-cell activation on the other side [18]. Therefore, we conducted a retrospective study analysing the sera of a large cohort of DLBCL patients from the NHLB1/2 study, to evaluate the prevalence of ACPA together with RF-IgM, -IgG, and -IgA in comparison with healthy controls.

Materials and Methods

Study Participants

The department of Medicine I at the University Medical School of Saarland is the study centre of the DSNHL German group (Deutsche Studiengruppe Hochmaligne Non-Hodgkin-Lymphome) and conducted the NHLB1 and NHLB2 studies, which recruited 866 and 831 DLBCL patients, respectively [25,26]. The sera of 395 patients were collected in the laboratory of Medicine I prior to treatment initiation, according to the respective study protocols. Sera from 258 age-matched healthy controls were collected in the Department of Haemostaseology/blood bank and in the Department of Orthopaedics at the University of Saarland; all blood donors were seen by an orthopaedic doctor or rheumatologist to exclude a rheumatologic disorder. Furthermore, 175 ACPA-positive RA patients from the previously published RA study of Assmann et al. were tested for ACPA serum concentrations to compare values with the DLBCL cohort [27]. The study was conducted according to the Helsinki declaration, and was approved by the regional ethics committee (Ethikkommission der Ärztekammer des Saarlandes). All study participants gave their written informed consent. The study population of lymphoma patients was well characterised with respect to all relevant clinical parameters, including previous medical history, stage of lymphoma disease, elevation of serum lactate dehydrogenase (LDH), patients performance status ECOG (eastern cooperative oncology group) and overall survival (an average [mean] observation period of 6.6 years) using datasheets submitted to the biostatistics institution of Leipzig University. All patients as well as healthy controls suffering from any rheumatic disease or under immunosuppressive treatment or cytostatic medication were excluded from the study. The sera of nine out of 258 healthy controls were not tested for ACPA, but were tested for RF. The sera were collected and stored frozen at −56°C.

Enzyme Linked Immunosorbent Assay (ELISA) Tests

All serum tests for antibodies against RF-IgM, RF-IgA, RF-IgG, and ACPA-IgG were performed by standard protocols using EUROIMMUN ELISA test sets (EUROIMMUN, Luebeck, Germany). Positive results of ACPA-IgG ranged from 5 to 200 U/ml. All sera were tested twice, and only sera with two positive tests were considered to be positive. RF-IgM results were additionally stratified into subgroups of negative (<50 IU/ml), positive (50–100 IU/ml), and highly positive results (>100 IU/ml).

Statistics

Differences in age between DLBCL patients and healthy controls were tested by Mann-Whitney test. Differences in gender as well as differences in the frequencies of ACPA and three types of RF between DLBCL and healthy controls were evaluated using χ^2 test. The ACPA concentration levels were compared by Mann-Whitney-U test. Differences with a p-value of <0.05 were considered significant. All results were corrected by Fisher's test if required. The overall survival of DLBCL patients stratified into ACPA-positive and ACPA-negative subgroups was tested by Kaplan-Meyer test (log rank test).

Results

Table 1 shows a summary of the participants' clinical characteristics. Significantly more male DLBCL patients than male healthy controls compared with female participants required a gender-separated evaluation of the investigated seromarkers. In addition, the sera of 65 DLBCL patients were not determined due to gender.

DLBCL patients showed a significantly higher prevalence of ACPA compared to healthy controls (3.5% versus 0.8%, p = 0.030; odds ratio [OR] 1.028, confidence interval [CI] 1.005–1.051), whereas all subtypes of RF such as IgM, IgA, and IgG, were equally prevalent in DLBCL patients and healthy controls: RF-IgM 22.8% versus 21.1%; RF-IgA 15.1% versus 12.6%; and RF-IgG 2.8% versus 1.8%. Table 2 shows the serostatus for RF and ACPA in DLBCL patients and healthy controls after stratification by gender. It is evident that the significant difference between DLBCL patients and healthy controls only occurred only in males, but not in females: 4.4% versus 0% (p = 0.022; OR 1.046, CI 1.017–1.079).

Fourteen out of 395 DLBCL patients versus only two out of 249 healthy controls were ACPA-positive. Table 3 outlines the clinical characteristics of ACPA-positive DLBCL patients (n = 14) compared with ACPA-negative DLBCL patients (n = 381). There was no significant difference in any of the clinical characteristics.

Table 1. Age and gender distribution of DLBCL patients and healthy controls.

	Number	Median age (years)	Gender (%)	
			Male	Female
DLBCL*	395	61	55.2**	44.8
HC	258	57	46.5	53.5

*p = 0.0192 (difference in age of HC versus DLBCL).
**p = 0.038 (difference in gender distribution of HC versus DLBCL).
DLBCL = diffuse large B-cell non-Hodgkin lymphoma patients.
HC = healthy controls.

Table 2. Serostatus for RF and ACPA autoantibodies in DLBCL patients and healthy controls stratified by gender.

		DLBCL			HC				
	M/F	Total number	pos. test	(%)	Total number	pos. test	(%)	p-value	
RF-IgM pos.									
(≥50 U/ml)	M	182	40	22	120	26	21.7	0.949	n.s. 1
	F	148	37	25	138	31	22.5	0.615	n.s. 1
RF-IgM low-pos.									
(50–100 U/ml)	M	182	9	4.9	120	4	3.3		
RF-IgM highly-pos.									
(>100–200 U/ml)	M	182	31	17.0	120	22	18.3	0.776	n.s. 1
RF-IgM low-pos.									
(50–100 U/ml)	F	148	14	9.5	138	12	8.7		
RF-IgM highly-pos.									
(>100–200 U/ml)	F	148	23	15.5	138	19	13.8	0.879	n.s. 1
RF-IgA pos.									
(≥20 U/ml)	M	180	31	17.2	109	12	11.9	0.150	n.s. 1
	F	148	21	14.2	114	16	14.0	0.972	n.s. 1
RF-IgG pos.									
(≥20 U/ml)	M	180	7	3.9	109	1	0.9	0.129	n.s. 1
	F	148	3	2.0	114	3	2.6	0.529	n.s. 1
ACPA-IgG pos.									
(>5–200 U/ml)	M	182	8	4.4	116	0	0.0	0.022	s. 2*
	F	148	6	3.4	133	2	1.5	0.203	n.s. 1

DLBCL = diffuse large B-cell non-Hodgkin lymphoma patients.
HC = healthy controls.
M = male; F = female.
RF = rheumatoid factor; IgM = immunoglobulin M; ACPA = anti-citrullinated cyclic peptide; pos. = positive;
n.s[1]. = not significant; s. = significant;
*s.[2] = confidence interval 1.017–1.079; odds ratio = 1.046.

Figure 1 shows the subgroup analysis of the study population (DLBCL patients and healthy controls) stratified into RF IgM-positive versus -negative participants. Statistical evaluation of the RF IgM-positive participants (DLBCL patients and healthy controls) showed a significantly higher frequency of ACPA-positive DLBCL patients than healthy controls (1.77% versus 0%, p = 0.043). Among the RF IgM-negative participants, the distribution of ACPA positivity was not significantly different (1.77% versus 0.80%, p = 0.493). Figure 2 shows boxplots presenting the significantly different ACPA concentration levels of DLBCL patients and the RA cohort: median 10.4 (range from 5.7 to 153.4) versus 124.1 (5.9–200); p = 0.0001.

Based on the results shown in table 2 and figure 1, the higher frequency of ACPA positivity in DLBCL patients is associated with male gender and RF-IgM seropositivity. To evaluate the impact of ACPA on overall survival in DLBCL patients, a Kaplan-Meier curve was generated for ACPA+and ACPA - DLBCL patients. There was no significant difference in 6-year overall survival: ACPA +66.79 versus 60.26%, p = 0.837 (log rank, Mantel-Cox, Table 3).

Table 3. Clinical characteristics of ACPA positive and negative DLBCL patients.

	ACPA (+)	ACPA (−)	p-value
Age at diagnosis(1)	59.4	59.1	0.657
stage III/IV(1)	35.5%	40.4%	0.724
gender (female)(1)	28.6%	45.1%	0.220
ECOG >1(1)	7.1%	11.8%	0.593
ESR elevated(1)	21.4%	38.3%	0.200
LDH elevated(1)	14.3%	24.2%	0.384
overall survival(2) **(6 years)**	66.79%	60.26%	0.837

(1)Mann-Whitney U Test.
(2)Log rank/Mantel-Cox tests. ACPA = anti-citrullinated cyclic peptide.
ECOG = index of life quality according to the European Cooperative Oncology Group. ESR = erythrocyte sedimentation rate. LDH = lactate dehydrogenase.

Discussion

To the best of our knowledge, our study has proved for the first time the higher prevalence of ACPA in DLBCL patients compared to healthy controls. Our results indicate that DLBCL seems to be a lymphatic malignancy with a small subgroup of ACPA-seropositive patients. Next to our study, there has only been one lymphoma study published, in 2010, which has investigated the prevalence of ACPA in B-cell chronic lymphocytic leukaemia, but this showed no ACPA serum positivity [7]. Cambridge et al. reported positive ACPA serum in 10.4% of the 144 patients with coronary heart disease compared to 3.8% of the 288 healthy

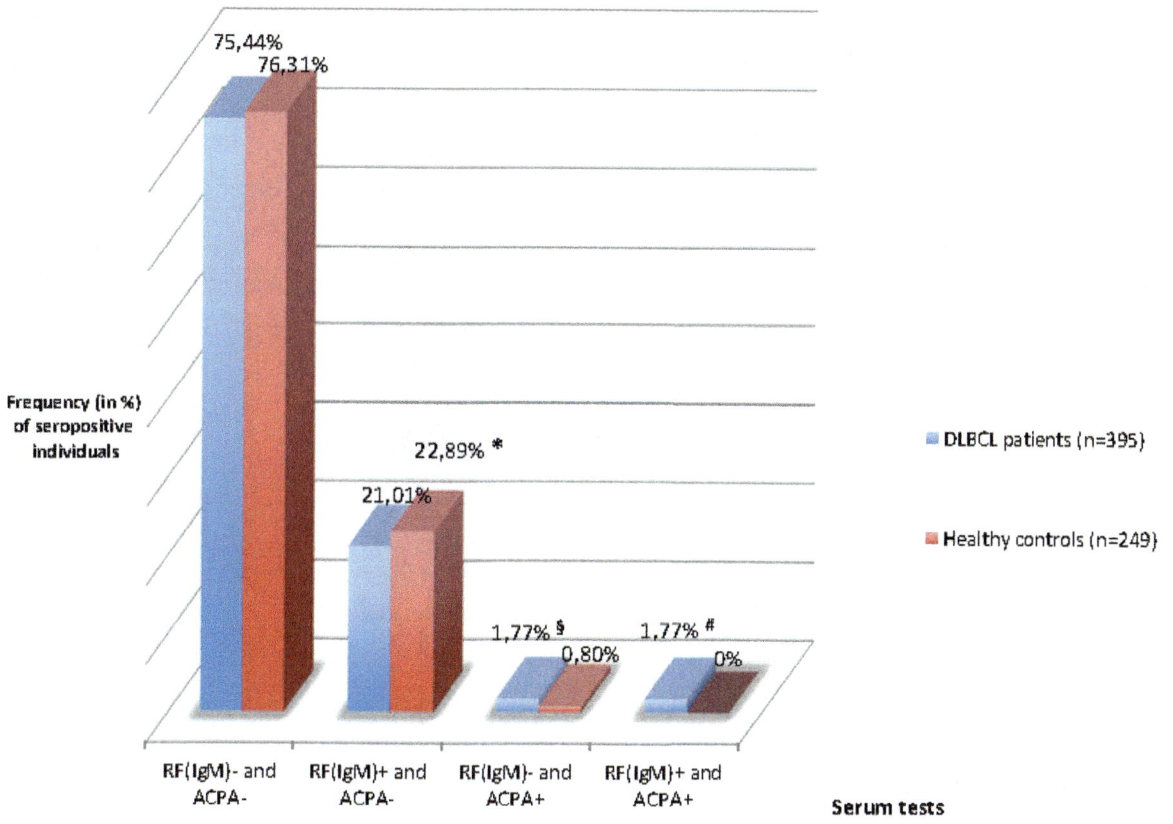

Figure 1. ACPA-positive and -negative DLBCL patients and healthy controls stratified by RF (IgM)-negative and -positive serostatus. DLBCL = diffuse large B-cell non-Hodgkin lymphoma patients. RF−/+ = rheumatoid factor IgM-negative/positive; ACPA−/+ = anti-citrullinated cyclic peptide positive/negative. *no significant difference, p = 0.802. §No significant difference, p = 0.493. #Significantly higher frequency of ACPA in RF (IgM)+DLBCL than in RF(IgM)+HC (p = 0.043).

controls [28]. The study did not investigate a rheumatological or lymphoma patient population, but the authors outlined that the measured ACPA values were relatively lower than those seen in patients with established RA; these results correspond to our data concerning significantly lower ACPA serum concentration levels in DLBCL than in RA. However, Cambridge et al reported a significantly higher prevalence of ACPA in healthy controls compared to most previous studies dealing with the ACPA prevalence e.g. Nielen et al. or Rantapaa-Dahlqvist et al. [19,20]. The data presented here also showed the commonly low prevalence of ACPA in less than 2% of healthy controls. However, the significance of ACPA in DLBCL remains unclear to date. In particular, ACPA-positive lymphoma patients did not differ in all relevant subgroups, such as ECOG, LDH, stage, and the presence or absence of extranodal lymphoma manifestations, representing the prognostic index. Furthermore, the analysis of overall survival of the DLBCL cohort did not demonstrate a significant difference between ACPA-positive and -negative patients.

Surprisingly, subgroup analysis of ACPA serostatus, stratifying the study population according to the presence of RF-IgM, revealed that ACPA positivity occurred significantly more frequently in RF IgM-positive DLBCL patients than in RF-IgM negative patients. Stratified in this way, the frequency of ACPA positivity in the RF-IgM-negative DLBCL cohort did not differ significantly from RF-IgM-negative healthy controls. These results raise the question whether the development of ACPA in DLBCL could be simply due to a non-specific autoantibody production (of more than one serum autoantibody), as a consequence of malignancy-induced uncontrolled B-cell proliferation in lymphoma. In particular, this hypothesis of unspecific autoantibody proliferation could be supported by the fact that the sera of ACPA-positive DLBCL patients were tested and showed significantly lower ACPA concentrations compared to RA patients.

Performing a further subgroup analysis, we have shown that ACPA-positivity has a significant gender bias, with more male DLBCL patients being positive. To the best of our knowledge, there have been no studies published explicitly investigating the gender distribution of ACPA in RA populations, but large epidemiologic studies, as previously published, have led to the conclusion that no relevant gender-related differences in ACPA positivity exist [29,30]. In general, several autoimmune diseases such as RA or lupus erythematodes occur significantly more frequently in females than in males [31]. Therefore, our data of lymphoma, showing a preference of male gender in the frequency of RA-related serum markers such as ACPA, would not correspond to previous data of female preference in RA. The general predisposition of female individuals for developing autoimmune diseases was previously discussed in an animal model, demonstrating the higher rate of increased toll-like receptor 7-driven accumulation of CD11+ B lymphocytes in female than in male mice [32]. However, from this point of view, the observation of the accumulation of those subtypes of B lymphocytes in this experimental model appears unsuited to explain, in general, the autoreactivity against citrullinated proteins in DLBCL and, in particular, the preference of male gender, so far.

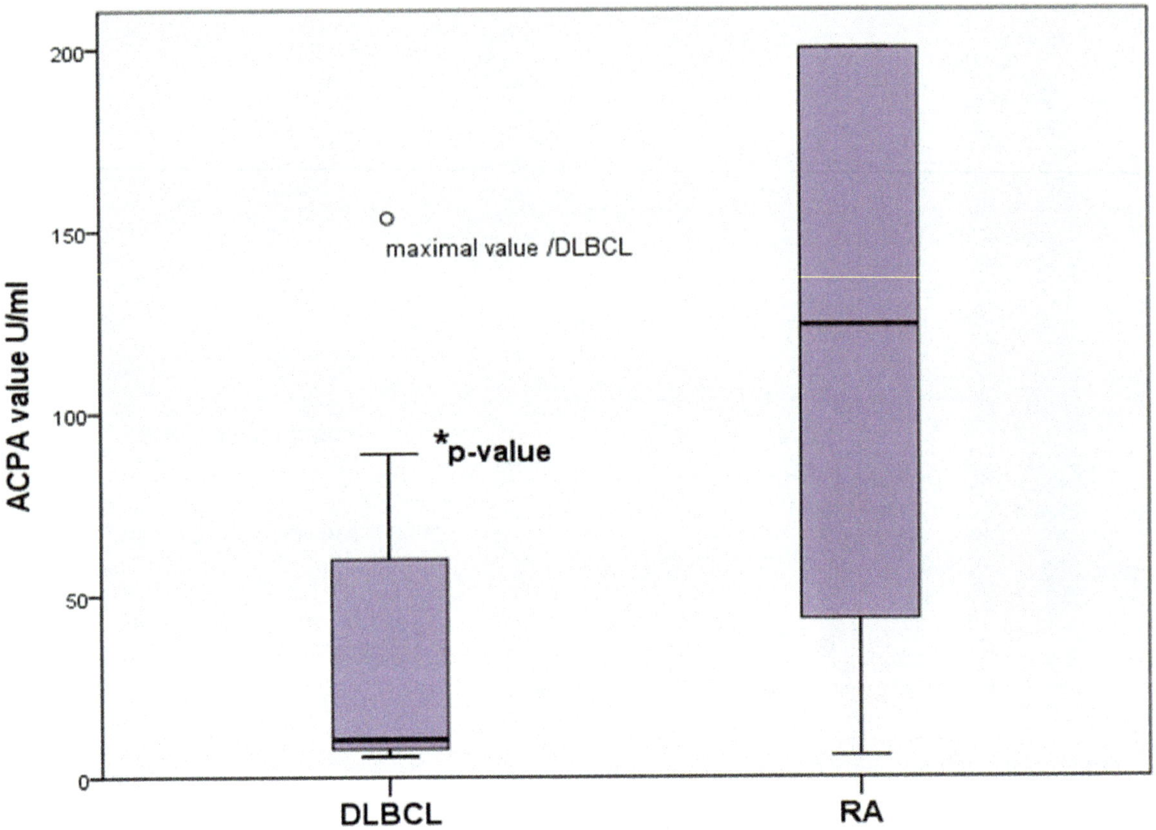

Figure 2. Boxplots presenting results of ACPA serum concentration levels in DLBCL (n = 14) and RA (n = 175). Boxplots with median (10.4 versus 124.1) and first/third quartile, respectively. ACPA−/+ = anti-citrullinated cyclic peptide positive/negative. DLBCL = diffuse large B-cell non-Hodgkin lymphoma patients. *p-value = 0.0001.

Regarding citrullination of proteins and development of ACPA, Ireland et al. previously reported an experimental *in vitro* cell culture model including lymphoma cells, where the antigen presentation of citrullinated peptides was not observed in normal B lymphocytes or B lymphoma cells; however, the serum starvation during *in vitro* experiments using B-cell lymphoma cell lines induced the presentation of citrullinated peptides by B lymphoma cells [33], indicating a possible involvement of citrullinated proteins in the autoreactive activity of B lymphoma cells.

Altogether, no convincing link could been found to explain the occurrence of ACPA in DLBCL, so we assumed that the development of ACPA in DLBCL to be preferentially a non-specific immunological phenomenon.

In this situation, one more aspect of ACPA in DLBCL would remain to be elucidated: whether ACPA has the same predictive significance for the development of future RA in the analogy of healthy individuals.

However, despite the relatively large number of DLBCL patients (n = 395) and healthy controls (n = 258), the cohort of only 16 ACPA-positive participants is small. In addition, the follow-up of about six years, as presented here, has to be considered too short for a representative result.

Moreover, the study analysis could been hampered by administered cytostatic treatment including high dosage prednisolone and cyclophosphamide as a possible rheumatic disease-modifying drug, although high dosage cytostatic short-term treatment has been investigated to have no long-term effects on RA in [34,35].

In conclusion, our study demonstrated a higher prevalence of ACPA in DLBCL patients compared with healthy controls, but our results do not suggest that the targeted clinical application of ACPA evaluation in DLBCL would be useful. With regard to RF-IgM, here we present, to the best of our knowledge, the largest study including gender stratification of DLBCL patients compared with healthy controls, showing no evidence for a higher prevalence of RF-IgM positivity in DLBCL, in contrast to previously published studies. The serum values of RF-IgM which were documented here for healthy controls were higher than in a previously published cohort, but the median age of 57 years in our cohort was higher than in comparable cohorts; furthermore, an inter-assay coefficient of variation for RF-IgM between 4.4% and 16.8% could be previously documented [8,20].

Acknowledgments

We thank Astrid Bonaventure and Natalie Fadle from the Jose Carreras Research Centre for preparing the serum aliquots derived from lymphoma patients. We thank Dr Sandra Grass, Medicine I, University Hospital of Saarland, and Marina Ziepert, Biostatistic Institution of Leipzig University, for preparing the tables containing the clinical parameters of the investigated lymphoma patients. We further thank Dieter Kohn and H. Eichler for their support with the collection of healthy blood donors.

Author Contributions

Conceived and designed the experiments: GA VP NM MFO MP. Performed the experiments: JC VP GA KS. Analyzed the data: GA KS VP MFO NM MP. Contributed reagents/materials/analysis tools: GA MP JC. Wrote the paper: GA MP.

References

1. Goldin LR, Landgren O (2009) Autoimmunity and lymphomagenesis. Int J Cancer 124: 1497–1502.
2. Ehrenfeld M, Abu-Shakra M, Buskila D, Shoenfeld Y (2001) The dual association between lymphoma and autoimmunity. Blood Cells Mol Dis 27: 750–756.
3. Smedby KE, Askling J, Mariette X, Baecklund E (2008) Autoimmune and inflammatory disorders and risk of malignant lymphomas-an update. J Intern Med 264: 514–527.
4. Baecklund E, Iliadou A, Askling J, Ekbom A, Backlin C et al. (2006) Association of chronic inflammation, not its treatment, with increased lymphoma risk in rheumatoid arthritis. Arthritis Rheum 54: 692–701.
5. Rifkin IR, Channavajhala PL, Kiefer HL, Carmack AJ, Landesman-Bollag E et al. (1998) Acceleration of lpr lymphoproliferative and autoimmune disease by transgenic protein kinase CK2 alpha. J Immunol 161: 5164–5170.
6. Mackay F, Tangye SG (2004) The role of the BAFF/APRIL system in B cell homeostasis and lymphoid cancers. Curr Opin Pharmacol 4: 347–354.
7. Brickmann K, Brezinschek RI, Yazdani-Biuki B, Graninger WB, Brezinschek HP (2010) Superior specificity of anti-citrullinated peptide antibodies in patients with chronic lymphocytic leukemia and arthritis. Clin Exp Rheumatol 28: 888–891.
8. Bilici A, Yapici HS, Ercan S, Seker M, Ustaalioglu BB et al. (2012) The prevalence and significance of autoantibodies in patients with non-Hodgkin's lymphoma: are they correlated with clinicopathological features? J BUON 17: 502–507.
9. Nishimura S, Nishiya K, Hisakawa N, Chikazawa H, Ookubo S et al. (1996) Positivity for antinuclear antibody in patients with advanced rheumatoid arthritis. Acta Med Okayama 50: 261–265.
10. Chloraki-Bobota A, Megalakaki C, Repousis P, Chalkiopoulou I, Lalaki I et al. (2006) Prevalence of autoantibodies (ANA, anti ds-DNA, ENA, IMF) and rheumatic syndromes in patients with lymphoproliferative diseases. J BUON 11: 485–489.
11. Guyomard S, Salles G, Coudurier M, Rousset H, Coiffier B et al. (2003) Prevalence and pattern of antinuclear autoantibodies in 347 patients with non-Hodgkin's lymphoma. Br J Haematol 123: 90–99.
12. Altintas A, Cil T, Pasa S, Danis R, Kilinc I et al. (2008) Clinical significance of elevated antinuclear antibody test in patients with Hodgkin's and Non-Hodgkin's lymphoma: a single center experience. Minerva Med 99: 7–14.
13. Schellekens GA, Visser H, de Jong BA, van den Hoogen FH, Hazes JM et al. (2000) The diagnostic properties of rheumatoid arthritis antibodies recognizing a cyclic citrullinated peptide. Arthritis Rheum 43: 155–163.
14. György B, Tóth E, Tarcsa E, Falus A, Buzás EI (2006) Citrullination: a posttranslational modification in health and disease. Int J Biochem Cell Biol 38: 1662–1677.
15. Sebbag M, Chapuy-Regaud S, Auger I, Petit-Texeira E, Clavel C et al. (2004) Clinical and pathophysiological significance of the autoimmune response to citrullinated proteins in rheumatoid arthritis. Joint Bone Spine 71: 493–502.
16. Meyer O, Labarre C, Dougados M, Goupille P, Cantagrel A et al. (2003) Anticitrullinated protein/peptide antibody assays in early rheumatoid arthritis for predicting five year radiographic damage. Ann Rheum Dis 62: 120–6.
17. De Rycke L, Peene I, Hoffman IE, Kruithof E, Union A et al. (2004) Rheumatoid factor and anticitrullinated protein antibodies in rheumatoid arthritis: diagnostic value, associations with radiological progression rate, and extra-articular manifestations., Ann Rheum Dis 63: 1587–1593.
18. Trouw LA, Huizinga TW, Toes RE (2013) Autoimmunity in rheumatoid arthritis: different antigens–common principles. Ann Rheum Dis 72: 132–136.
19. Nielen MM, van Schaardenburg D, Reesink HW, van de Stadt RJ, van der Horst-Bruinsma IE et al. (2004) Specific autoantibodies precede the symptoms of rheumatoid arthritis: a study of serial measurements in blood donors. Arthritis Rheum 50: 380–386.
20. Rantapää-Dahlqvist S, de Jong BA, Berglin E, Hallmans G, Wadell G et al. (2003) Antibodies against cyclic citrullinated peptide and IgA rheumatoid factor predict the development of rheumatoid arthritis. Arthritis Rheum 48: 2741–2749.
21. Klareskog L, Malmström V, Lundberg K, Padyukov L, Alfredsson L (2011) Smoking, citrullination and genetic variability in the immunopathogenesis of rheumatoid arthritis. Semin Immunol 23: 92–98.
22. Ryu YS, Park SH, Lee J, Kwok SK, Ju JH et al. (2013) Follow-up of primary Sjogren's syndrome patients presenting positive anti-cyclic citrullinated peptides antibody. Rheumatol Int 33: 1443–1446.
23. Tanikawa C, Ueda K, Nakagawa H, Yoshida N, Nakamura Y et al. (2009) Regulation of protein Citrullination through p53/PADI4 network in DNA damage response. Cancer Res 69: 8761–8769.
24. Klareskog L, Wedrén S, Alfredsson L (2009) On the origins of complex immune-mediated disease: the example of rheumatoid arthritis. J Mol Med 87: 357–362.
25. Pfreundschuh M, Trümper L, Kloess M, Schmits R, Feller AC et al. (2004) Two-weekly or 3-weekly CHOP chemotherapy with or without etoposide for the treatment of young patients with good-prognosis (normal LDH) aggressive lymphomas: results of the NHL-B1 trial of the DSHNHL. Blood 104: 626–633.
26. Pfreundschuh M, Trumper L, Kloess M, Schmits R, Feller AC et al. (2004) Two-weekly or 3-weekly CHOP chemotherapy with or without etoposide for the treatment of elderly patients with aggressive lymphomas: results of the NHL-B2 trial of the DSHNHL. Blood 104: 634–641.
27. Assmann G, Koenig J, Pfreundschuh M, Epplen JT, Kekow J et al. (2010) Genetic variations in genes encoding RANK, RANKL, and OPG in rheumatoid arthritis: a case-control study. J Rheumatol 37: 900–904.
28. Cambridge G, Acharya J, Cooper JA, Edwards JC, Humphries SE (2013) Antibodies to citrullinated peptides and risk of coronary heart disease. Atherosclerosis 228: 243–246.
29. Wesley A, Bengtsson C, Elkan AC, Klareskog L, Alfredsson L et al. (2013) Epidemiological Investigation of Rheumatoid Arthritis Study Group. Association between body mass index and anti-citrullinated protein antibody-positive and anti-citrullinated protein antibody-negative rheumatoid arthritis: results from a population-based case-control study. Arthritis Care Res (Hoboken) 65: 107–112.
30. Frisell T, Holmqvist M, Källberg H, Klareskog L, Alfredsson L (2013) Familial risks and heritability of rheumatoid arthritis: role of rheumatoid factor/anti-citrullinated protein antibody status, number and type of affected relatives, sex, and age. Arthritis Rheum 65: 2773–2782.
31. Amur S, Parekh A, Mummaneni P (2012) Sex differences and genomics in autoimmune diseases. J Autoimmun 38: 254–625.
32. Rubtsov AV, Rubtsova K, Fischer A, Meehan RT, Gillis JZ et al. (2011) Toll-like receptor 7 (TLR7)-driven accumulation of a novel CD11c^{+} B-cell population is important for the development of autoimmunity. Blood 118: 1305–1315.
33. Ireland JM, Unanue ER (2011) Autophagy in antigen-presenting cells results in presentation of citrullinated peptides to CD4 T cells. J Exp Med 208: 2625–2632.
34. Verburg Ro, Toes RE, Fibbe WE, Breedveld FC, van Laar JM (2002) High dose chemotherapy and autologous hematopoietic stem cell transplantation for rheumatoid arthritis: a review. Hum Immunol 63: 627–637.
35. Verburg RJ, Kruize AA, van den Hoogen FH, Fibbe WE, Petersen EJ et al. (2001) High-dose chemotherapy and autologous hematopoietic stem cell transplantation in patients with rheumatoid arthritis: results of an open study to assess feasibility, safety, and efficacy. Arthritis Rheum 44: 754–760.

13

Construction of Drug Network Based on Side Effects and Its Application for Drug Repositioning

Hao Ye[1], Qi Liu[2], Jia Wei[1]*

1 R&D Information, AstraZeneca, Shanghai, China, 2 School of Life Sciences and Technology, Tongji University, Shanghai, China

Abstract

Drugs with similar side-effect profiles may share similar therapeutic properties through related mechanisms of action. In this study, a drug-drug network was constructed based on the similarities between their clinical side effects. The indications of a drug may be inferred by the enriched FDA-approved functions of its neighbouring drugs in the network. We systematically screened new indications for 1234 drugs with more than 2 network neighbours, 36.87% of the drugs achieved a performance score of **N**ormalized **D**iscounted **C**umulative **G**ain in the top **5** positions (NDCG@5)≥0.7, which means most of the known FDA-approved indications were well predicted at the top 5 positions. In particular, drugs for diabetes, obesity, laxatives and antimycobacterials had extremely high performance with more than 80% of them achieving NDCG@5≥0.7. Additionally, by manually checking the predicted 1858 drug-indication pairs with **E**xpression **A**nalysis **S**ystematic **E**xplorer (EASE) score≤10^{-5} (EASE score is a rigorously modified Fisher exact test p value), we found that 80.73% of such pairs could be verified by preclinical/clinical studies or scientific literature. Furthermore, our method could be extended to predict drugs not covered in the network. We took 98 external drugs not covered in the network as the test sample set. Based on our similarity criteria using side effects, we identified 41 drugs with significant similarities to other drugs in the network. Among them, 36.59% of the drugs achieved NDCG@5≥0.7. In all of the 106 drug-indication pairs with an EASE score≤0.05, 50.94% of them are supported by FDA approval or preclinical/clinical studies. In summary, our method which is based on the indications enriched by network neighbors may provide new clues for drug repositioning using side effects.

Editor: Ozlem Keskin, Koç University, Turkey

Funding: The authors have no support or funding to report.

Competing Interests: One or more of the authors are employed by a commercial company (AstraZeneca R&D China).

* E-mail: jenny.wei@astrazeneca.com

Introduction

The inefficiency of pharmaceutical drug development with high expenditure but low productivity has been widely discussed [1,2,3,4]. Drug repositioning is considered to be a promising strategy to revitalize the slowing drug discovery pipeline due to shorter development timelines and lower risk of unexpected toxicity [5,6,7]. Traditionally, most of the successful examples mainly relied on serendipity or 'happy accidents' (eg, Viagra, Dapoxetine, Duloxetine) [6,8], which made repositioning very unpredictable. In 2006, Lamb et al [9] proposed the connectivity map based on the gene expression profiles of drugs for repositioning, which is the first computational method in this field. Then a group of investigators utilized structural features of compounds/proteins to predict new targets of drugs, such as molecular docking [10,11], QSAR modelling [12]. In addition, the association between diseases/drugs in genetic activity was suggested to facilitate repositioning, such as genome-wide association [13], pathway profiles [14,15], and transcriptional responses [16]. Furthermore, several integrative methods which combined chemical or genetic features were proposed to predict the drug targets or indications, for example, PREDICT [17], TMFS [11]. Obviously, most of these methods focus on the molecular mechanism of action (MOA) from a genotypic perspective. Nevertheless, the pre-clinical outcomes based on MOA often do not correlate well with therapeutic efficacy in drug development. It is estimated that of all the compounds effective in cell assays, only 30% of them could work in animals. Even worse, only 5% of them could work in humans [18].

The gap between MOA and the physiological responses of drugs may limit the usefulness of the methods mentioned above. Side effects are generated when the drugs bind to off-targets, which perturb unexpected metabolic or signaling pathways [19]. Therefore, side effects from clinical patients may be seen as valuable read-outs of drug effects on human bodies, which may also serve as a promising perspective for drug repositioning. Up to now, only a few of the repositioning efforts focus on physiological responses. Most of them are developed using the side effect data in SIDER [20], which was constructed by the Bork' group in 2010. The latest version of SIDER contains 996 drugs and 4192 side effects. Lun proposed *DRoSEf* [21],where the basic hypothesis is that if the side effects associated with a drug are also induced by many drugs treating a disease, then this drug should be evaluated as a candidate to treat that disease. Initially, they constructed side effect profiles of diseases based on drug-indication data and drug-side effect data. The QSAR models were trained to build associations between structures and side effects. Then indications of the drug could be predicted by combining the side effect profiles of diseases with structure and side effect associations. Lun's work pioneered an approach to drug repositioning using side effects and achieved good performance. Up to now, side effects are still the best data available to reflect disease characteristics even if they are not equivalent to pathological symptoms of diseases (for example, side effects may be generated by off-targets, which are not the accompanying disorders of the disease). In addition, the limited quantities of drugs in SIDER may impact the QSAR training processes in *DRoSEF*, which has only worked well in 145 diseases. With expanded coverage of the drugs, *DRoSEF* could achieve more promising performance.

In this study, we intend to propose a network based method for drug repositioning by exploring the entire existing catalog of side effect data. Instead of directly building the relationship between side effects and diseases, we would like to construct drug-drug relationships through side effect similarities. Our basic hypothesis is that drugs with similar side-effect profiles may also share similar therapeutic properties [22]. A drug network could be constructed based on the similarities of side effects. In this way, the indications of a drug may be predicted by the functional distribution of its neighbouring drugs. Since we have already investigated chemical structures [23] and pathway profiles [14,15] for drug repositioning, side effect based repositioning could enhance our computational repositioning platform and provide complementary evidence.

Materials and Methods

Drug side effects

In this study, side effects were extracted from *Meyler's Side Effects of Drugs 15th edition* [24]. Additional drug sides effects, especially for the drugs launched after 2006, were collected from *Side Effects of Drugs Annuals* (2007–2012) [25] and the FDA drug approval package (see **Table 1**). Specifically, each electronic book was converted from PDF to text format by Acrobat professional v10.1. Then, a Java program was implemented to parse the drug information and side effects. Considering the side effects in *Meyler's Side Effects of Drugs 15th edition* and *Side Effects of Drugs Annuals* (2007–2012) were organised using MedDRA vocabularies version 15.1, the *preferred items* (PT level) in MedDRA were utilized as the standard side effect vocabulary. The side effect data from other resources were mapped to MedDRA *preferred items*, avoiding the semantic redundancy. For example "*respiratory diseases*" and "*respiration diseases*" were identified as two different side effects in the raw data, and both of them were mapped to the same *preferred item* "*respiratory disease*" in MedDRA.

External test samples

As described in **Table 1**, SIDER is a frequently cited resource for drug side effects. Herein, 98 drugs in SIDER version 2 which were not covered by the drug network were used as external test samples (see the 98 drugs in **Table S1**). Also, the side effects in SIDER were mapped to *preferred items* in MedDRA version 15.1.

Drug indication

FDA-approved indications were obtained from *Citeline Pipeline*, *Thomson Reuters Partnering* and *GeneGo* (see details in **Table 2**). Next, each indication was modified to a MeSH heading. Finally, we obtained 2183 drugs with 6495 clinical side effects and 994 4th level MeSH items.

Drug network construction with side effects (see Figure 1)

Step 1: Build the side effect fingerprint. Herein, each side effect was treated as a feature vector. If a drug displays side effect *i*, then it would be tagged "1" in the element *i*, otherwise, it would be marked "0". After that a 0-1 binary vector was defined as the side effect fingerprint for the drug. For the 2183 drugs with recorded clinical side effect data, each would be assigned a 6495-dimension vector.

Step 2: Calculate the similarity between drugs. The Jaccard index was used to evaluate the similarities of side effect fingerprints. In a given drug pair (labelled A and B), the Jaccard index for the binary vectors could be calculated as the formula I.

$$J(drugA,drugB)=\frac{c}{a+b-c} \quad (I)$$

In this formula, a, b represent the number of side effects for drugs A and B, respectively. c represents the number of side effects shared by drug A and B.

Step 3: Evaluate the side effect similarities between drugs. The difference in the quantity of side effects associated with drugs may lead to similarity bias. It's necessary to evaluate whether the similarities between two drugs are randomly generated. As shown in **Figure 1**, the random side effect fingerprint sets of *drug A* were generated by randomly selecting the same number of side effects from the side effects pool 10000 times. For each random side effect fingerprint of *drug A*, the *J(random A, drug B)* similarity was calculated according to formula I. Then, the random Jaccard index set *S(drug A, drug B)* = {*J(random A 1,drug B)*, *J(random A 2,drug B)*,… *J(random A 10000, drug B)*} between *drug A* and *drug B* was obtained. The *Z score* calculated by formula II was used to test whether the similarities between drug A and drug B were significantly larger than the random distribution. (*Z score*≥2.576 was set as the threshold)

Table 1. Drug side effects resources.

Source	Description
Meyler's Side Effects of Drugs (15th edition)	The International Encyclopaedia of Adverse Drug Reactions, a publication for a history spanning more than 60 years. It has been published every four years since 1980. It is the most comprehensive and authoritative resource of drug side effects, which contains>3,400 drugs and>12,600 side effects.
Side Effects of Drugs Annuals(2007–2012)	The Side Effects of Drugs Annual was first published in 1977. It has been continually published since then as a yearly update to the encyclopaedia *Meyler's Side Effects of Drugs*.
Drugs@FDA Database	Drugs@FDA includes most of the drug products approved by the FDA since 1939. Most patient information, labels, approval letters, reviews, approval packages and other information for drug products approved since 1998 are available.
SIDER	Contains information on 996 marketed drugs and corresponding 4192 recorded adverse drug reactions. The information is extracted from public documents and package inserts.

Table 2. Drug indication resources.

Source	Description
Pipeline	Developed by Citeline. Reputed to have collected information on drugs developed for any disease anywhere in the world since 1980, including their approval dates, companies and related clinical trials.
Thomson Reuters Partnering	The database was formally called IDdb and acquired by Thomson Reuters. The drug pipeline information is integrated from a variety of sources, such as company websites, and over 200 global conferences.
GeneGO	GeneGO is a comprehensive biological database, covering a wide range of data, including pathways, drug information, biomarkers etc. Each drug indication is mapped to a MeSH item.

$$Zscore = \frac{J(drugA,drugB) - mean(S(drugA,drugB))}{std(S(drugA,drugB))} \quad \text{(II)}$$

Step 4: Cutoff optimization. Cutoff optimization is an important process which could directly influence the specificity of the drug network. In this network, drugs sharing similar side effects were expected to be clustered together. Two criteria were considered when optimizing the threshold. First, the selected drug-drug pairs should cover as many drugs as possible. Second, the percentage of drug-drug pairs that share the same indication should be as high as possible. Usually, the two instances are contradictory to each other. When the cutoff is set at Jaccard index = 0, all of the drugs would be covered. A non-sense drug-drug network would be built with lots of totally unrelated drug-drug pairs. On the other hand, if the cutoff is set at Jaccard index = 1, then only a few drug-drug pairs would be selected.

MeSH hierarchy and drug indication prediction

MeSH contains plentiful hierarchically arranged disease information, which makes it convenient to investigate drug indications. In this study, the potential indications of a drug could be predicted according to the MeSH hierarchy distribution of its neighbours (the 4th level of MeSH hierarchy item could well represent an indication).

EASE score [26] is offered as a conservative adjustment to the Fisher exact probability, which was defined in DAVID [27] to evaluate gene-enrichment in pathways. The smaller the *EASE Score*, the higher the enrichment of genes in the pathways (see details in http://david.abcc.ncifcrf.gov/content.jsp?file=functional_annotation.html#fisher).

Herein, we used the *EASE score* to evaluate drug indication enrichment in the network. Taking *drug A* and *indication i* as an example, we built a 2×2 contingency table (See **Table 3**). Sorting the *EASE score in descending order*, we could generate the rank positions of indications for *drug A*.

Herein, the network represents the connected component which contains *drug A*. The connected component is defined as a sub-network in which any two drugs are connected to each other by paths.

Performance evaluation

Normalized discounted cumulative gain (NDCG)[28] was originally used to evaluate web search engine algorithms in the field of information retrieval. It can measure the usefulness of a document based on its position in the result list.

Here we used NDCG to measure the effectiveness of ranking performance for each drug's predicted results (see formula III).

$$NDCG@p = Z\sum_{i=1}^{p} \frac{2^{rel_i} - 1}{\log_2(i+1)} \quad \text{(III)}$$

Z is the normalization constant.

i is the rank position of *indication m*.

rel_i is the relevance value of *indication m*. If *indication m* is the FDA approved indication of *drug A*, rel_i is set to 1, otherwise, rel_i is set to 0.

p is the maximum position.

For example if the FDA approved indications of *drug A* are ranked at *2, 3 & 8*, respectively, while the ideal rank position of *drug A*'s FDA-approved indications should be *1, 2& 3*,then:

$$Z = \frac{1}{\sum_{i=1}^{3} \frac{1}{\log_2(i+1)}} = 0.4693$$

In the top 5 results,

$$NDCG@5 = Z\left(\frac{1}{\log_2(2+1)} + \frac{1}{\log_2(3+1)}\right) = 0.5307$$

Results

Cutoff selection criteria and drug-drug network construction

As mentioned in **Methods**, we investigated variation trends in the percentage of covered drugs and co-indicated drug-drug pairs according to different Jaccard indexes. As shown in **Figure 2**, the percentage of co-indicated drug-drug pairs is positively correlated with the Jaccard index at four MeSH hierarchy levels. This evidence also suits our hypothesis that drugs with similar side effects would display similar functions. From **Figure 2**, it is obvious that the percentage of co-indicated pairs dramatically increases from 26.27% to 62.35% in the inflection area at the Jaccard index [0.2, 0.35] at the fourth level of MeSH hierarchy. Herein, Jaccard index = 0.275 was defined as the cutoff threshold. Then a drug-drug network based on side effect similarities was constructed, which contains 17400 drug-drug pairs, covering 1647 drugs. 1234 drugs with no less than 2 neighbors were used as our test samples. These drugs can be mapped to 81 ATC therapeutic categories including 5337 FDA approved drug-indication pairs, covering 584 indications. On average, 36.87% of the drugs achieved NDCG@5≥0.7, which means the known FDA-approved indications were well predicted. For details, the top 10 categories with NDCG@5≥0.7 were listed in **Table 4** (see full list

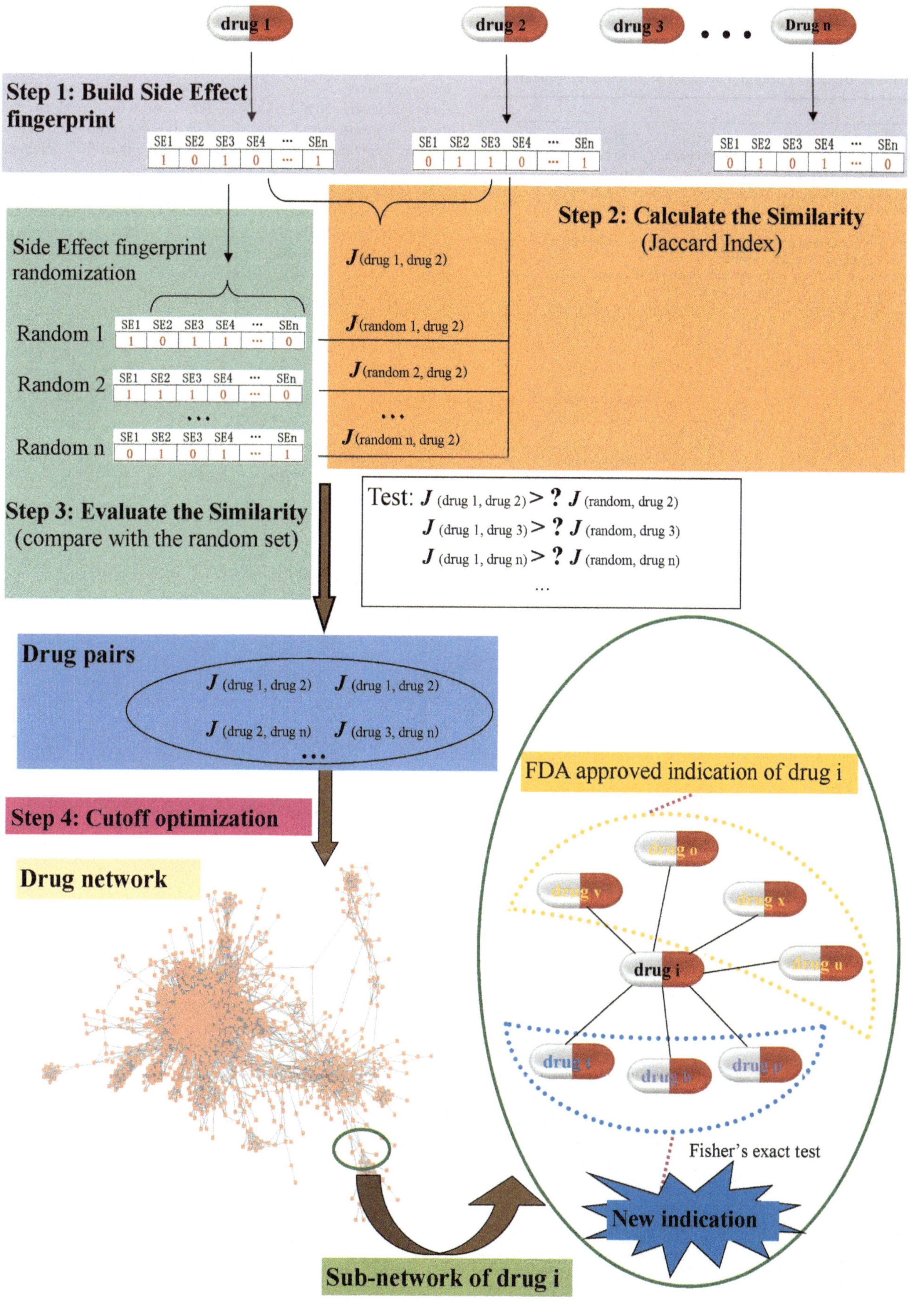

drug 1
drug 2
drug 3
Drug n
Step 1: Build Side Effect fingerprint
SE1 SE2 SE3 SE4 ··· SEn
Step 2: Calculate the Similarity (Jaccard Index)
J (drug 1, drug 2)
J (random 1, drug 2)
J (random 2, drug 2)
J (random n, drug 2)
Side Effect fingerprint randomization
Random 1
Random 2
Random n
Step 3: Evaluate the Similarity (compare with the random set)
Test: J (drug 1, drug 2) > ? J (random, drug 2)
J (drug 1, drug 3) > ? J (random, drug 3)
J (drug 1, drug n) > ? J (random, drug n)
Drug pairs
J (drug 1, drug 2) J (drug 1, drug 2)
J (drug 2, drug n) J (drug 3, drug n)
Step 4: Cutoff optimization
Drug network
FDA approved indication of drug i
drug o
drug v
drug x
drug i
drug u
drug t
drug b
drug p
Fisher's exact test
New indication
Sub-network of drug i

Figure 1. Construction of drug network using side effects.

Table 3. The 2×2 contingency table of *drug A* and indication *i*.

	Drug A's neighbours	The background network
Indication *i*	n -1	r
Other indications	N-n	d-r

n: The number of *drug A*'s neighbors which are approved for indication *i* (n≥2);
N: The number of *drug A*'s neighbors;
r: the number of drugs in the network which are approved for indication *i*;
d: The number of drugs in the network.

in **Table S2**). The drugs for diabetes, obesity, laxatives and antimycobacterials were best predicted with more than 80% of them achieving NDCG@5≥0.7. The drugs for cardiovascular disease (diuretics and agents acting on the renin-angiotensin system) were also well predicted with more than 70% of them achieving NDCG@5≥0.7

Besides that, we also investigated the prediction performance in a different indication range (number of drugs approved for the indication) (see **Table 5**). Totally, 32.77% FDA approved drug-indication pairs could be predicted in the top 5 results, covering 202 (34.59%) indications. It seems that the indications with more drug approvals are likely to be predicted in the top 5 results. Good

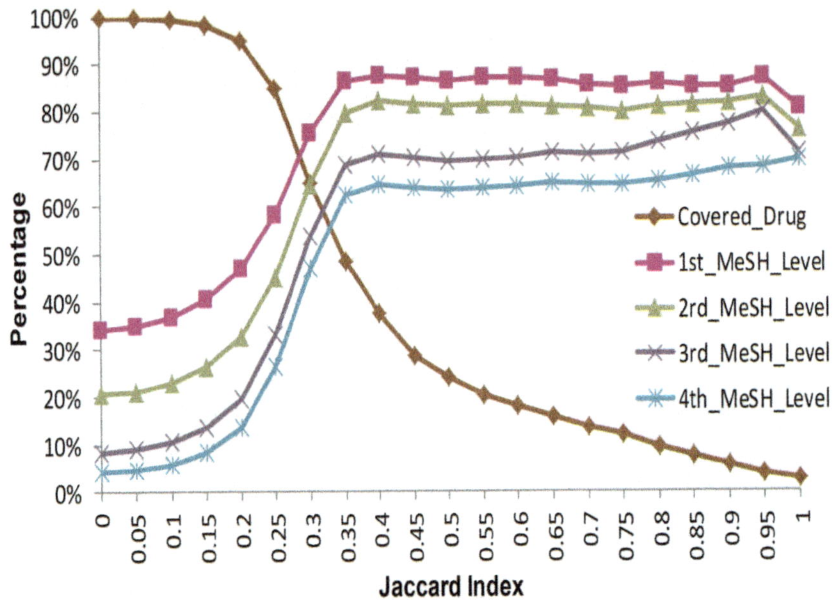

Figure 2. The trends of covered drugs and drug-drug pairs that share the same terms in the MeSH hierarchy.

Table 4. Top 10 ATC therapeutic categories with NDCG@5≥0.7.

ATC code	Therapeutic category	NO. drugs	Percentage of drugs with NDCG@5≥0.7
A10	Drugs used in diabetes	33	84.85%
A08	Antiobesity preparations, excluding diet products	12	83.33%
A06	Laxatives	6	83.33%
J04	Antimycobacterials	6	83.33%
G02	Other gynecologicals	11	72.73%
C09	Agents acting on the renin-angiotensin system	43	72.09%
J05	Antivirals for systemic use	37	70.27%
C03	Diuretics	38	68.42%
B05	Blood substitutes and perfusion solutions	3	66.67%
R07	Other respiratory system products	3	66.67%

Table 5. Prediction performance of the 1234 drugs in different indication range (number of network drugs approved for an indication).

NO. drugs per indication	NO. indications approved by FDA	Top 5 covered indications (percentage)	NO. drug-indication pairs approved by FDA	Top 5 covered drug-indication pairs (percentage)
less than 5	196	11 (5.61%)	430	18 (4.19%)
6~10	130	26 (20.00%)	556	66 (11.87%)
11~15	66	27 (40.91%)	508	92 (18.11%)
16~20	66	32 (62.75%)	560	87 (15.54%)
21~25	38	26 (68.42%)	566	124 (21.91%)
26~30	20	16 (80.00%)	389	99 (25.45%)
31~35	19	17 (89.47%)	412	185 (44.90%)
36~40	14	13 (92.86%)	376	153 (40.69%)
41~45	8	7 (87.50%)	224	58 (25.89%)
46~50	5	5 (100.00%)	163	106 (65.03%)
51~55	8	8 (100.00%)	297	183 (61.62%)
56~60	4	4 (100.00%)	150	92 (61.33%)
more than 60	10	10 (100.00%)	706	486 (68.84%)
Total	584	202 (34.59%)	5337	1749 (32.77%)

performance was generated in the indications with 30~40 and 46~55 approved drugs. The top 5 drug indication pairs in these groups achieved 40.69% and 61.33% of the corresponding FDA approved drug indication pairs respectively. In addition, for indications with 15 or more FDA drug approvals, more than 62.75% of them were ranked with at least one drug-indication pair at the top 5 positions.

Herein, only the FDA approved drug-indication pairs are considered a positive set. The prediction performance may be underestimated due to the fact that drug-indications have not yet been approved though they may well be capable of treating disease. For example, the drug-indications being tested in the clinical studies through phase I, II and III, were also classified as false positive. We manually checked the 1858 drug-indication pairs with an *EASE score*$\leq 10^{-5}$ (see details in **Table S3**). We found that 80.73% of them could be verified by preclinical/clinical studies or scientific literature (see **Table 6**). We further investigated three drugs to understand their predicted results.

Dynastat

Dynastat (also called Parecoxib) is a COX-2 selective inhibitor developed by Pfizer. It was initially approved for pain management by the European Union in 2002. Dynastat relieves pain through modulating prostaglandins levels. It exerts the effect by inhibiting COX-2, which is responsible for converting arachidonic acid to prostaglandin G2 and prostaglandin H2. Prostaglandins also play an important role in the pathogenesis of rheumatoid arthritis (RA) [29]. Prostaglandins were found at elevated levels in rheumatoid synovial fluid, and the bone-resorption activity produced by rheumatoid synovial tissues was shown to be mediated in part by prostaglandin E2 [30], which is one of the downstream products of prostaglandin H2 in the arachidonic acid metabolism pathway. In our predicted results, the neighbours of Dynastat are significantly enriched in pain relief (EASE score $= 1.76\times10^{-14}$) and rheumatoid arthritis (EASE score $= 1.03\times10^{-21}$) management. As shown in **Figure 3**, Dynastat displays a similar side effect profile to 33 RA drugs in addition to the pain drugs. Up to now, a group of COX-2 inhibitors were verified as promising drugs in the treatment of RA. For example, Celecoxib, Rofecoxib and Valdecoxib have already been approved in RA treatment. Considering that Parecoxib is a water-soluble prodrug that can be rapidly hydrolyzed into Valdecoxib [31], it may also be effective in the treatment of RA.

Table 6. Predicted results with evidence supported at an EASE score$\leq 10^{-5}$.

Drug-indication pairs	Number	Percentage
FDA-approved	1336	71.91%
Clinical	132	7.10%
Preclinical	32	1.72%
Unknown	358	19.27%

Tasmar

Tolcapone (brand name Tasmar) developed by Roche, was approved as an effective adjunctive treatment with Levodopa for Parkinson's disease in 1997 [32]. As a catechol-o-methyltransferase (COMT) inhibitor, Tasmar could improve the pharmacokinetic profile of Levodopa in two ways. First, it could directly inhibit the metabolic path from Levodopa to 3-O-methyldopa, which may finally increase the Levodopa half-life. Second, it may facilitate the transport of Levodopa to the brain by reducing 3-O-methyldopa, which may compete with Levodopa in brain barrier penetration [33]. The mechanism of actions also may explain why Tolcapone shares similar side effects with only 4 drugs for Parkinson therapy (*EASE score* $= 0.39$). We found that the indication of Tolcapone's neighbours was significantly enriched in anti-depression functions (15 drugs were approved for depression treatment, EASE score $= 5.09\times10^{-8}$. See **Figure 4**). A group of pharmaco-genetics studies showed that COMT variations are correlated with the effective management of depression [34,35,36,37,38,39]. Besides that, Elin et al's study [40] proved that the Met-variants of COMT Val158Met are risk

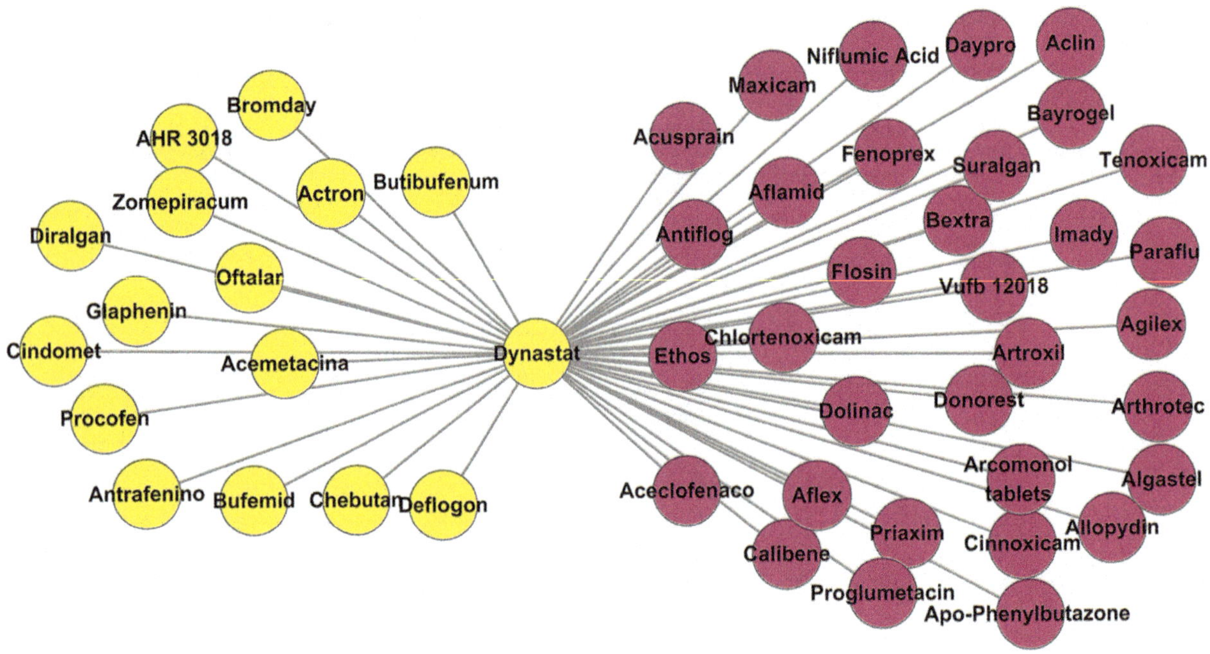

Figure 3. Sub-network of Dynastat. Each node represents a drug. Drugs approved for pain management are marked in yellow. Drugs approved for rheumatoid arthritis therapy are marked in purple.

variants for depression in the Swedish population. All of the available evidence indicates that COMT inhibitors may have an effect on depression. In fact, the application of COMT inhibitors in depression treatment was approved for a US patent in 2005 (US 20050137162 A1). In animal studies, an increase of SAMe in the central nervous system was detected after the administration of Tolcapone [41]. SAMe is a naturally occurring compound with putative antidepressant properties [42]. This effect, coupled with antidepressant properties exhibited in the rat model of chronic mild stress-induced anhedonia [43], suggests that Tolcapone may have significant antidepressant properties. Moreover, in an open study on 21 adults with major depressive disorders, the group treated with Tolcapone showed significant improvement over the placebo group (17-item Hamilton Rating Scale for Depression 19.4+/−2.9 vs 10.7+/−5.5; Clinical Global Impressions Severity 3.9+/−0.6 vs 2.4+/−1.1; Beck Depression Inventory 21.6+/−8.1 vs 12.3+/−8.6) [44]. The preliminary results suggest that Tolcapone may be a promising anti-depressant.

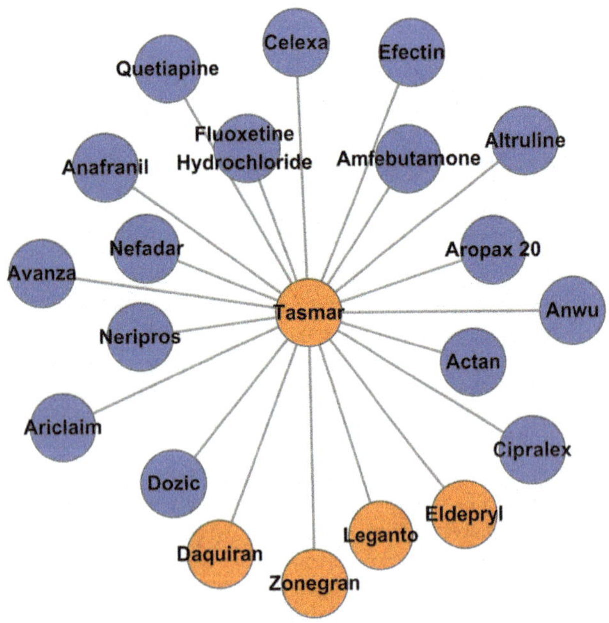

Figure 4. Sub-network of Tasmar. Each node represents a drug. Drugs approved for the treatment of Parkinson's disease are marked in orange. Drugs approved for rheumatoid arthritis therapy are marked in blue.

Adamon

Tramadol hydrochloride (brand name Adamon) is a centrally acting synthetic analgesic used to treat moderately severe pain, which was first approved in 1977 as a product of the German pharmaceutical company Grünenthal GmbH. It is supposed to have an analgesic effect on pain based on two complementary mechanisms of action derived from its affinity for the mu opioid receptor and its blockade of norepinephrine and serotonin reuptake [45,46]. Herein, two systems involved in pain relief are activated by Tramadol; namely, the opioid and the descending monoaminergic pain modulating pathways. In our predicted results, it shares similar side effect profiles with 22 pain management drugs (general pain: EASE score = 0.021; postoperative pain: *EASE score = 0.0063*). As shown in **Figure 5**, Tramadol is also connected to 13 anti-depression drugs (*EASE score* = 9.06×10^{-5}). Desmeules's study [47] suggested that the analgesic action of Tramadol is mainly related to the central monoaminergic mechanism rather than opioid receptor pathways. Antidepressants usually act by inhibiting norepinephrine-serotonin reuptake, which is similar to Tramadol's effect of blocking monoaminergic reuptake [48]. In addition, opioid systems are also influenced in the pathophysiology of depression [49]. All the evidence suggests

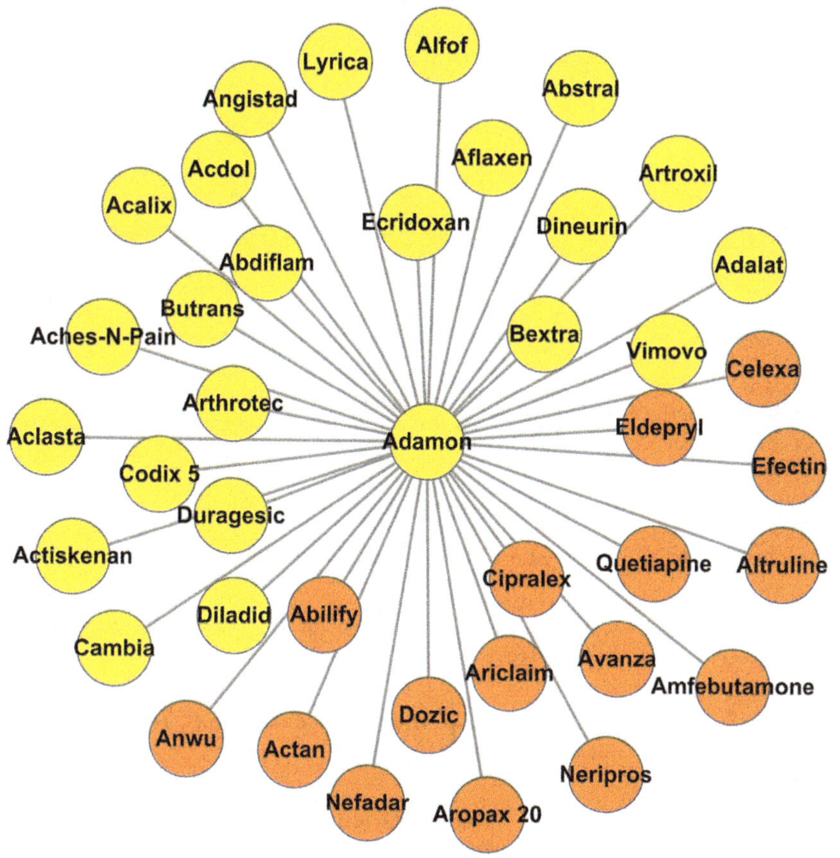

Figure 5. Sub-network of Adamon. Each node represents a drug. Drugs approved for the treatment of Parkinson 's disease are marked in orange. Drugs approved for pain treatment are marked in blue.

that Tramadol may have an effect on depression. In fact, a group of preclinical studies based on several depressive mice models showed the efficacy of Tramadol in depression management, such as the forced swimming test and the tail suspension test [48,50,51]. In 2008, the application of Tramadol in depression treatment was patented by European Union (EP20080011241). More promisingly, according to the pipeline of e-Therapeutics, the indication of Tramadol on depression has already been moved to Phase IIb clinical studies http://www.etherapeutics.co.uk/Information/pipeline.html.

Table 7. The similarity of 98 SIDER drugs in test sample set with the drugs in the network.

Similarity (Jaccard index)	Drugs with more than 2 neighbours (Percentage)
[0,0.15)	5 (5.10%)
[0.15,0.2)	21 (21.43.%)
[0.2,0.225)	11 (11.22%)
[0.225,0.25)	25 (25.51%)
[0.25,0.275)	21 (21.43%)
More than 0.275	15 (15.31%)

External data evaluation

After we tested the predicted results of all drugs in the network, external drugs with side effect data were also tested. 98 drugs exclusively covered in SIDER were used as inputs to our system to calculate similarities with the drugs in the network one by one.

As described in the **Methods**, we calculated similarities between 98 SIDER drugs with the background 2183 drugs. As shown in **Table 7**, 84.69% of SIDER drugs showed similarities to the network drugs with Jaccard index≤0.275. Herein, the Jaccard index = 0.225 in the inflection area [0.2, 0.35] was set as the threshold. Next, 61 drugs with more than 2 neighbours were inputted to evaluate the method. Finally, the indications of 41 drugs could be predicted since they have more than 2 neighbouring drugs approved for the same indication. Among the top 5 predicted results, 36.59% of the drugs reached a performance score NDCG@5≥0.7. In addition, by selecting the

Table 8. Predicted drug-indication pairs of SIDER drugs.

Drug-indication pairs	Number	Percentage
FDA-approved	37	34.91%
Clinical	10	9.43%
Preclinical	7	6.60%
Unknown	52	49.06%

top 5 predicted results of 41 drugs with an EASE score≤0.05, 106 drug- indication pairs were generated (See details in **Table S4**). During the manual check, we found that 50.94% of them were FDA approved or could be verified by clinical trials or scientific literature (See **Table 8**).

Discussion

In this study, we integrated drug side effect data from several different resources. With these data, we built a drug network and screened new indications of drugs based on their network neighbours. Our method performed well at predicting their FDA approved indications in the top 5 positions. In addition to screening new indications of FDA approved drugs, our method could also be extended to candidate drugs with clinical side effect data. Since approved drugs sharing similar side effect profiles with query candidates could be identified, the indications of candidates could be inferred by its neighbours. Especially for drugs which failed in the late clinical stages, the comprehensive side effect data should have been generated in early clinical studies. These side effects can be used as inputs to our repositioning platform so that new indications for these drugs can be predicted.

Our drug repositioning platform has its own limitations. Due to the differences between side effect data resources, during an external data test using 98 drugs exclusively covered by SIDER, we found 58.16% of these SIDER drugs have low side effect similarities with the drugs in the network. Our method is not applicable to these SIDER drugs. Since very few side effect databases are available, many efforts are still needed to build or integrate these resources. For example, clinical case reports or other adverse event reporting systems may supply additional information on drug side effects. Up to now, only the direct neighbours in our network were considered to evaluate the indications in the study. We could quantify the influences of each neighbouring drug in the indication enrichment process according to their side effect similarities. Besides that, considering the fact that side effects vary in severity and frequency of occurrence, the current Jaccard index may not correctly mimic side effect similarities between the drugs. For example, the severity of a given side effect might be tagged as "serious" or "mild", while its frequency of occurrence might be described as "common" or "rare". Actually, these two side effect parameters are also related to the number of clinical patient samples and drug doses in treatment. Further meta-analysis should be carried out to modify the side effect data in order to take account of information regarding the severity and frequency of these side effects. This could certainly improve the accuracy of the predictions.

Drug repositioning is a complicated process. It is impossible that any one computational method alone would be accurate enough to provide promising results. A package of methods from different perspectives could be integrated to make predictions more precise. In our study, we also compared our results to Lun's [21] predicted results. In his study, 14040 drug-indication pairs are proposed. 14.57% of them overlapped with our results (747 drug-indications with EASE score≤0.05, see details in **Table S5**). In particular, five of the drugs (Ziprasidone, Quetiapine, Oxcarbazepine, Clozapine, Sildenafil) mentioned in Lun's paper were able to be used in the treatment of obsessive-compulsive disorder. The associations were also predicted by our method with a low EASE score$\leq 6.35\times10^{-3}$. The overlapping results from different methods, which may integrate comprehensive features in drug repositioning at the chemical levels, the MOA levels, and the phenotypic levels could provide promising predictions as well as cross validations.

Supporting Information

Table S1 The 98 drugs exclusively covered in SIDER.

Table S2 Performance of drugs in 81 ATC therapeutic categories.

Table S3 The predicted 1858 drug-indication pairs with an *EASE score*$\leq 10^{-5}$.

Table S4 The predicted 106 drug-indication pairs in external data evaluation using SIDER.

Table S5 The 747 drug-indication pairs overlapped with Lun's paper.

Acknowledgments

We would like to thank Qi Song and Ming Chen for their help with side effect data extraction. We also appreciate Dr. Weiguo Gao who provided constructive suggestions in this study.

Author Contributions

Conceived and designed the experiments: HY JW. Performed the experiments: HY. Analyzed the data: HY. Contributed reagents/materials/analysis tools: HY QL. Wrote the paper: HY.

References

1. Paul SM, Mytelka DS, Dunwiddie CT, Persinger CC, Munos BH, et al. (2010) How to improve R&D productivity: the pharmaceutical industry's grand challenge. Nat Rev Drug Discov 9: 203–214.
2. David E, Tramontin T, Zemmel R (2009) Pharmaceutical R&D: the road to positive returns. Nat Rev Drug Discov 8: 609–610.
3. Berggren R, Moller M, Moss R, Poda P, Smietana K (2012) Outlook for the next 5 years in drug innovation. Nat Rev Drug Discov 11: 435–436.
4. Kola I, Landis J (2004) Can the pharmaceutical industry reduce attrition rates? Nat Rev Drug Discov 3: 711–715.
5. Ashburn TT, Thor KB (2004) Drug repositioning: identifying and developing new uses for existing drugs. Nat Rev Drug Discov 3: 673–683.
6. Wu Z, Wang Y, Chen L (2013) Network-based drug repositioning. Mol Biosyst 9: 1268–1281.
7. Oprea TI, Mestres J (2012) Drug repurposing: far beyond new targets for old drugs. AAPS J 14: 759–763.
8. Liu X, Zhu F, Ma XH, Shi Z, Yang SY, et al. (2013) Predicting targeted polypharmacology for drug repositioning and multi- target drug discovery. Curr Med Chem 20: 1646–1661.
9. Lamb J, Crawford ED, Peck D, Modell JW, Blat IC, et al. (2006) The Connectivity Map: using gene-expression signatures to connect small molecules, genes, and disease. Science 313: 1929–1935.
10. Luo H, Chen J, Shi L, Mikailov M, Zhu H, et al. (2011) DRAR-CPI: a server for identifying drug repositioning potential and adverse drug reactions via the chemical-protein interactome. Nucleic Acids Res 39: W492–498.
11. Dakshanamurthy S, Issa NT, Assefnia S, Seshasayee A, Peters OJ, et al. (2012) Predicting new indications for approved drugs using a proteochemometric method. J Med Chem 55: 6832–6848.
12. Cheng F, Zhou Y, Li J, Li W, Liu G, et al. (2012) Prediction of chemical-protein interactions: multitarget-QSAR versus computational chemogenomic methods. Mol Biosyst 8: 2373–2384.
13. Sanseau P, Agarwal P, Barnes MR, Pastinen T, Richards JB, et al. (2012) Use of genome-wide association studies for drug repositioning. Nat Biotechnol 30: 317–320.
14. Ye H, Tang K, Yang L, Cao Z, Li Y (2012) Study of drug function based on similarity of pathway fingerprint. Protein Cell 3: 132–139.
15. Ye H, Yang L, Yang L, Cao Z, Tang K, Li Y (2012) A pathway profile-based method for drug repositioning. Chin Sci Bull 57: 2106–2112.

16. Iorio F, Bosotti R, Scacheri E, Belcastro V, Mithbaokar P, et al. (2010) Discovery of drug mode of action and drug repositioning from transcriptional responses. Proc Natl Acad Sci U S A 107: 14621–14626.
17. Gottlieb A, Stein GY, Ruppin E, Sharan R (2011) PREDICT: a method for inferring novel drug indications with application to personalized medicine. Mol Syst Biol 7: 496.
18. Pammolli F, Magazzini L, Riccaboni M (2011) The productivity crisis in pharmaceutical R&D. Nat Rev Drug Discov 10: 428–438.
19. Paolini GV, Shapland RH, van Hoorn WP, Mason JS, Hopkins AL (2006) Global mapping of pharmacological space. Nat Biotechnol 24: 805–815.
20. Kuhn M, Campillos M, Letunic I, Jensen LJ, Bork P (2010) A side effect resource to capture phenotypic effects of drugs. Mol Syst Biol 6: 343.
21. Yang L, Agarwal P (2011) Systematic drug repositioning based on clinical side-effects. PLoS One 6: e28025.
22. Duran-Frigola M, Aloy P (2012) Recycling side-effects into clinical markers for drug repositioning. Genome Med 4: 3.
23. Ye H, Tang K, Li Y (2012) Drug-Drug Network Based on Similarity of Molecular Fingerprint. Journal of East China University of Science and Technology 3: 301–306.
24. Aronson JK (2006) Meyler's Side Effects of Drugs: The International Encyclopedia of Adverse Drug Reactions and Interactions (Fifteenth Edition).
25. Aronson JK (2007~2012) Side Effects of Drugs Annual: A worldwide yearly survey of new data in adverse drug reactions and interactions. Volume 29~34.
26. Hosack DA, Dennis G, Sherman BT, Lane HC, Lempicki RA (2003) Identifying biological themes within lists of genes with EASE. Genome Biol 4: R70.
27. Huang da W, Sherman BT, Lempicki RA (2009) Systematic and integrative analysis of large gene lists using DAVID bioinformatics resources. Nat Protoc 4: 44–57.
28. Jarvelin K, Kekalainen J (2002) Cumulated gain-based evaluation of IR techniques. ACM Transactions on Information Systems 20: 422–446.
29. Sundy JS (2001) COX-2 inhibitors in rheumatoid arthritis. Curr Rheumatol Rep 3: 86–91.
30. Robinson DR, Tashjian AH, Levine L (1975) Prostaglandin-stimulated bone resorption by rheumatoid synovia. A possible mechanism for bone destruction in rheumatoid arthritis. J Clin Invest 56: 1181–1188.
31. Bingham CO (2002) Development and clinical application of COX-2-selective inhibitors for the treatment of osteoarthritis and rheumatoid arthritis. Cleve Clin J Med 69: SI5–12.
32. Truong DD (2009) Tolcapone: review of its pharmacology and use as adjunctive therapy in patients with Parkinson's disease. Clin Interv Aging 4: 109–113.
33. Borges N (2005) Tolcapone in Parkinson's disease: liver toxicity and clinical efficacy. Expert Opin Drug Saf 4: 69–73.
34. Szegedi A, Rujescu D, Tadic A, Muller MJ, Kohnen R, et al. (2005) The catechol-O-methyltransferase Val108/158Met polymorphism affects short-term treatment response to mirtazapine, but not to paroxetine in major depression. Pharmacogenomics J 5: 49–53.
35. Arias B, Serretti A, Lorenzi C, Gasto C, Catalan R, et al. (2006) Analysis of COMT gene (Val 158 Met polymorphism) in the clinical response to SSRIs in depressive patients of European origin. J Affect Disord 90: 251–256.
36. Benedetti F, Colombo C, Pirovano A, Marino E, Smeraldi E (2009) The catechol-O-methyltransferase Val(108/158)Met polymorphism affects antidepressant response to paroxetine in a naturalistic setting. Psychopharmacology (Berl) 203: 155–160.
37. Yoshida K, Higuchi H, Takahashi H, Kamata M, Sato K, et al. (2008) Influence of the tyrosine hydroxylase val81met polymorphism and catechol-O-methyltransferase val158met polymorphism on the antidepressant effect of milnacipran. Hum Psychopharmacol 23: 121–128.
38. Benedetti F, Dallaspezia S, Colombo C, Lorenzi C, Pirovano A, et al. (2010) Effect of catechol-O-methyltransferase Val(108/158)Met polymorphism on antidepressant efficacy of fluvoxamine. Eur Psychiatry 25: 476–478.
39. Spronk D, Arns M, Barnett KJ, Cooper NJ, Gordon E (2011) An investigation of EEG, genetic and cognitive markers of treatment response to antidepressant medication in patients with major depressive disorder: a pilot study. J Affect Disord 128: 41–48.
40. Aberg E, Fandino-Losada A, Sjoholm LK, Forsell Y, Lavebratt C (2011) The functional Val158Met polymorphism in catechol-O-methyltransferase (COMT) is associated with depression and motivation in men from a Swedish population-based study. J Affect Disord 129: 158–166.
41. Prada DM, Borgulya J, Napolitano A, Zurcher G (1994) Improved therapy of Parkinson's disease by tolcapone, a central and peripheral COMT inhibitor with an S-adenosyl-L-methionine sparing effect. Clin Neuropharmacol 17: S26–S37..
42. Bressa GM (1994) S-adenosyl-l-methionine (SAMe) as antidepressant: meta-analysis of clinical studies. Acta Neurol Scand Suppl 154: 7–14.
43. Moreau JL, Borgulya J, Jenck F, Martin JR (1994) Tolcapone: a potential new antidepressant detected in a novel animal model of depression. Behav Pharmacol 5: 344–350.
44. Fava M, Rosenbaum JF, Kolsky AR, Alpert JE, Nierenberg AA, et al. (1999) Open study of the catechol-O-methyltransferase inhibitor tolcapone in major depressive disorder. J Clin Psychopharmacol 19: 329–335.
45. Raffa RB, Friderichs E, Reimann W, Shank RP, Codd EE, et al. (1992) Opioid and nonopioid components independently contribute to the mechanism of action of tramadol, an 'atypical' opioid analgesic. J Pharmacol Exp Ther 260: 275–285.
46. Driessen B, Reimann W (1992) Interaction of the central analgesic, tramadol, with the uptake and release of 5-hydroxytryptamine in the rat brain in vitro. Br J Pharmacol 105: 147–151.
47. Desmeules JA, Piguet V, Collart L, Dayer P (1996) Contribution of monoaminergic modulation to the analgesic effect of tramadol. Br J Clin Pharmacol 41: 7–12.
48. Tayal V, Kalra BS, Chawla S (2008) Evaluation of antidepressant activity of tramadol in mice. Indian J Pharmacol 40: 129–130.
49. Berrocoso E, Sanchez-Blazquez P, Garzon J, Mico JA (2009) Opiates as antidepressants. Curr Pharm Des 15: 1612–1622.
50. Chowta MN, Manjunath M, Gopalakrishna HN, Gokul P (2011) Evaluation of role of noradrenergic system in the antidepressant activity of tramadol using tail suspension test in Albino mice. J Pharmacol Pharmacother 2: 281–282.
51. Rojas-Corrales MO, Gibert-Rahola J, Mico JA (1998) Tramadol induces antidepressant-type effects in mice. Life Sci 63: PL175–180.

14

Human Leukocyte Antigens and Systemic Lupus Erythematosus: A Protective Role for the HLA-DR6 Alleles *DRB1*13:02* and **14:03*

Hiroshi Furukawa[1*], Aya Kawasaki[2], Shomi Oka[1], Ikue Ito[2], Kota Shimada[3,4], Shoji Sugii[3], Atsushi Hashimoto[4], Akiko Komiya[1], Naoshi Fukui[1], Yuya Kondo[5], Satoshi Ito[6], Taichi Hayashi[5], Isao Matsumoto[5], Makio Kusaoi[7], Hirofumi Amano[7], Tatsuo Nagai[8], Shunsei Hirohata[8], Keigo Setoguchi[9], Hajime Kono[10], Akira Okamoto[11], Noriyuki Chiba[12], Eiichi Suematsu[13], Masao Katayama[14], Kiyoshi Migita[15], Akiko Suda[16,17], Shigeru Ohno[16], Hiroshi Hashimoto[18], Yoshinari Takasaki[7], Takayuki Sumida[5], Shouhei Nagaoka[17], Naoyuki Tsuchiya[2☯], Shigeto Tohma[1☯]

1 Clinical Research Center for Allergy and Rheumatology, Sagamihara Hospital, National Hospital Organization, Sagamihara, Japan, **2** Molecular and Genetic Epidemiology Laboratory, Faculty of Medicine, University of Tsukuba, Tsukuba, Japan, **3** Department of Rheumatology, Tokyo Metropolitan Tama Medical Center, Fuchu, Japan, **4** Department of Rheumatology, Sagamihara Hospital, National Hospital Organization, Sagamihara, Japan, **5** Department of Internal Medicine, Faculty of Medicine, University of Tsukuba, Tsukuba, Japan, **6** Department of Rheumatology, Niigata Rheumatic Center, Shibata, Japan, **7** Department of Internal Medicine and Rheumatology, Juntendo University School of Medicine, Tokyo, Japan, **8** Department of Rheumatology and Infectious Disease, Kitasato University School of Medicine, Sagamihara, Japan, **9** Department of Allergy and Immunological Diseases, Tokyo Metropolitan Cancer and Infectious Diseases Center Komagome Hospital, Tokyo, Japan, **10** Department of Internal Medicine, Teikyo University, Tokyo, Japan, **11** Department of Rheumatology, Himeji Medical Center, National Hospital Organization, Himeji, Japan, **12** Department of Rheumatology, Morioka Hospital, National Hospital Organization, Morioka, Japan, **13** Department of Internal Medicine and Rheumatology, Clinical Research Institute, Kyushu Medical Center, National Hospital Organization, Fukuoka, Japan, **14** Department of Internal Medicine, Nagoya Medical Center, National Hospital Organization, Nagoya, Japan, **15** Clinical Research Center, Nagasaki Medical Center, National Hospital Organization, Omura, Japan, **16** Center for Rheumatic Diseases, Yokohama City University Medical Center, Yokohama, Japan, **17** Department of Rheumatology, Yokohama Minami Kyosai Hospital, Yokohama, Japan, **18** Juntendo University School of Medicine, Tokyo, Japan

Abstract

Many studies on associations between human leukocyte antigen (HLA) allele frequencies and susceptibility to systemic lupus erythematosus (SLE) have been performed. However, few protective associations with *HLA-DRB1* alleles have been reported. Here, we sought protective, as well as predispositional, alleles of *HLA-DRB1* in Japanese SLE patients. An association study was conducted for *HLA-DRB1* in Japanese SLE patients. Relative predispositional effects were analyzed by sequential elimination of carriers of each allele with the strongest association. We also explored the association of *DRB1* alleles with SLE phenotypes including the presence of autoantibody and clinical manifestations. Significantly different carrier frequencies of certain *DRB1* alleles were found to be associated with SLE as follows: increased *DRB1*15:01* ($P = 5.48\times10^{-10}$, corrected P (Pc) = 1.59×10^{-8}, odds ratio [OR] 2.17, 95% confidence interval [CI] 1.69–2.79), decreased *DRB1*13:02* ($P = 7.17\times10^{-5}$, $Pc = 0.0020$, OR 0.46, 95% CI 0.34–0.63) and decreased *DRB1*14:03* ($P = 0.0010$, $Pc = 0.0272$, OR 0.34, 95% CI 0.18–0.63). Additionally, the "*15:01/*13:02 or *14:03" genotype tended to be negatively associated with SLE ($P = 0.4209$, OR 0.66), despite there being significant positive associations with **15:01* when present together with alleles other than **13:02* or **14:03* ($P = 1.79\times10^{-11}$, OR 2.39, 95% CI 1.84–3.10). This protective effect of **13:02* and **14:03* was also confirmed in SLE patients with different clinical phenotypes. To the best of our knowledge, this is the first report of a protective association between the carrier frequencies of *HLA-DRB1*13:02* and **14:03* and SLE in the Japanese population.

Editor: Masataka Kuwana, Keio University School of Medicine, Japan

Funding: This work was supported by Grants-in-Aid for Scientific Research (B, C) (22390199, 22591090), for Exploratory Research (25670458) and for Young Scientists (B) (24791018) from the Japan Society for the Promotion of Science, Health and Labour Science Research Grants from the Ministry of Health, Labour and Welfare of Japan, Grants-in-Aid for Clinical Research from National Hospital Organization, Research Grants from Daiwa Securities Health Foundation, Research Grants from Japan Research Foundation for Clinical Pharmacology, Research Grants from The Nakatomi Foundation, Research Grants from Takeda Science Foundation, Research Grants from Mitsui Sumitomo Insurance Welfare Foundation, Research Grants from SENSHIN Medical Research Foundation and research grants from pharmaceutical companies: Abbott Japan Co., Ltd., Astellas Pharma Inc., Chugai Pharmaceutical Co., Ltd., Eisai Co., Ltd., Mitsubishi Tanabe Pharma Corporation, Merck Sharp and Dohme Inc., Pfizer Japan Inc., Takeda Pharmaceutical Company Limited, Teijin Pharma Limited. The funders had no role in study design, data collection and analysis, decision to publish or preparing the manuscript.

Competing Interests: The following funders are supported in whole or in part by the indicated pharmaceutical companies. The Japan Research Foundation for Clinical Pharmacology is run by Daiichi Sankyo, the Takeda Science Foundation is supported by an endowment from Takeda Pharmaceutical Company and the Nakatomi Foundation was established by Hisamitsu Pharmaceutical Co., Inc. The Daiwa Securities Health Foundation was established by Daiwa Securities Group Inc. and Mitsui Sumitomo Insurance Welfare Foundation was established by Mitsui Sumitomo Insurance Co., Ltd. AH was supported by research grants from Mitsubishi Tanabe Pharma Corporation. NT is supported by SENSHIN Medical Research Foundation, which is supported by an endowment from Mitsubishi Tanabe Pharma Corporation. ST was supported by research grants from 9 pharmaceutical companies: Abbott Japan Co., Ltd., Astellas Pharma Inc., Chugai Pharmaceutical Co., Ltd., Eisai Co., Ltd., Mitsubishi Tanabe Pharma Corporation, Merck Sharp and Dohme Inc., Pfizer Japan Inc., Takeda Pharmaceutical Company Limited, Teijin Pharma Limited. The other authors declare no financial or commercial conflict of interest.

* E-mail: h-furukawa@sagamihara-hosp.gr.jp

ᵑ These authors contributed equally to this work.

Introduction

Systemic lupus erythematosus (SLE) is a prototypic autoimmune disease of unknown etiology that affects multiple organs and is associated with the production of several different autoantibodies. It is a systemic inflammatory disease susceptibility to which is associated with genetic and environmental factors [1]. Genetic risk factors for SLE include alleles in *IRF5, STAT4, BLK, TNFAIP3, TNIP1, FCGR2B* and others [2,3,4]; the functional role of the polymorphisms as well as the relationships with other autoimmune diseases such as rheumatoid arthritis were suggested[5,6]. Especially, altered frequencies of human leukocyte antigen (*HLA*) alleles are known to be associated with SLE. Some *HLA-DRB1* alleles are reported to be positively associated with SLE susceptibility in several ethnic groups studied: *DRB1*03:01* and **15:01* in European [7,8], **15:03* in African-American [9], **08:02* in Hispanic [10] and **15:01* and **15:02* in Asian populations [11,12,13,14]. Gene dosage effects were not noted in the associations of *HLA-DRB1* alleles with susceptibility to SLE in that homozygosity for a susceptibility allele does not confer higher disease risk than heterozygosity for that allele. However, only limited information is available concerning protective *DRB1* alleles for SLE, i.e. those with a reduced frequency in patients. Here, we sought protective, as well as predispositional, *HLA-DRB1* alleles in Japanese SLE patients. We also explored associations of *DRB1* alleles with SLE phenotypes including the presence of autoantibody and clinical manifestations of disease.

Materials and Methods

Patients and controls

A first set of 459 SLE patients (with a mean age ± standard deviation (SD) of 48.2±15.4 years) of whom 36 were men was recruited at Sagamihara Hospital, Yokohama Minami Kyosai Hospital, Tama Medical Center, Kitasato University, Komagome Hospital, Teikyo University, Himeji Medical Center, Morioka Hospital, Kyushu Medical Center and Yokohama City University Medical Center and a second set of 389 patients (41.6±13.7 years of age; 31 men) at University of Tsukuba, Juntendo University and the University of Tokyo. A first set of 307 healthy controls (39.5±11.1 years; 2 men) was recruited at Sagamihara Hospital or by the Pharma SNP Consortium (Tokyo, Japan) [15] and a second set of 542 healthy controls (34.0±9.8 years; 245 men) at the University of Tokyo and University of Tsukuba. All patients and healthy individuals were native Japanese living in Japan. All patients with SLE fulfilled the American College of Rheumatology criteria for SLE [16]. This study was reviewed and approved by the research ethics committees of each participating institute, Sagamihara Hospital Research Ethics Committee, Nagasaki Medical Center Research Ethics Committee, Yokohama Minami Kyosai Hospital Research Ethics Committee, Tama Medical Center Research Ethics Committee, University of Tsukuba Research Ethics Committee, Kitasato University Research Ethics Committee, Komagome Hospital Research Ethics Committee, Teikyo University Research Ethics Committee, Himeji Medical Center Research Ethics Committee, Morioka Hospital Research Ethics Committee, Kyushu Medical Center Research Ethics Committee, Nagoya Medical Center Research Ethics Committee, Yokohama City University Medical Center Research Ethics Committee, the University of Tokyo Research Ethics Committee and Juntendo University Research Ethics Committee. Written informed consent was obtained from all study participants. This study was conducted in accordance with the principles expressed in the Declaration of Helsinki.

Genotyping

Genotyping of *HLA-DRB1* and *DQB1* was performed by a polymerase chain reaction technique using sequence-specific oligonucleotide probes (WAKFlow HLA typing kits, Wakunaga, Hiroshima, Japan), using a Bio-Plex 200 system (Bio-Rad, Hercules, CA), or using MPH-2 HLA typing kits (Wakunaga). Results of *HLA-DRB1* genotyping for some of the healthy controls were reported previously [17,18]. Although a small part of second set SLE patients recruited at University of Tsukuba or Juntendo University was overlapped with that in another study which reported susceptible effects of *DRB1*09:01* [14], DNA collection and *HLA-DRB1* genotyping were independently performed for this replication study of protective association with *DRB1*13:02* and **14:03*. *DRB1-DQB1* haplotypes were elucidated by direct counting.

Statistical analysis

Differences of allele carrier frequencies, genotype frequencies, haplotype carrier frequencies or amino acid residue carrier frequencies were analyzed by Fisher's exact test using 2×2 contingency tables. Adjustment for multiple comparisons was performed using the Bonferroni method. Corrected *P* (*P*c) values were calculated by multiplying the *P* value by the number of alleles, haplotypes or amino acid residues tested. Relative predispositional effects (RPE) were analyzed by sequential elimination of carriers of each allele with the strongest association [19]. Correction for multiple testing of SLE with different clinical and phenotypic manifestations was performed by calculating false discovery rate Q-value [20].

Results

Association analysis of the first set of SLE patients and healthy controls

HLA-DRB1 and *DQB1* genotyping was performed in 459 SLE patients and 307 healthy controls in the first set to compare carrier frequencies of each allele or haplotype (Table 1, left column, Table S1). Although the positive association between the carrier frequency of *DRB1*15:01* and SLE failed to reach significance in this set (*P*c = 0.0705, odds ratio [OR] 1.76, 95% confidence interval [CI] 1.22–2.53, Table 1), a significant protective association was found for *DRB1*13:02* and SLE (*P*c = 0.0123, OR 0.42, 95% CI 0.26–0.68). Additionally, the carrier frequency of the *DRB1*14:03* allele was lower in SLE, although this difference was not statistically significant (*P*c = 0.0812, OR 0.30, 95% CI 0.14–0.68). The DR6 (*DRB1*13* and **14*) allele carrier frequency was significantly lower in SLE ($P = 4.34\times10^{-5}$, OR 0.51, 95% CI 0.37–0.70), but DR2 (*DRB1*15* and **16*) was not different (*P* = 0.1743, OR 1.23). A significant negative association was found for *DQB1*06:04* and SLE (*P*c = 0.0499, OR 0.46, 95% CI 0.28–0.77, Table S1). The *DRB1*13:02-DQB1*06:04* haplotype was negatively associated with SLE (*P*c = 0.0414, OR 0.30, 95% CI 0.26–0.72). Thus, we detected certain *DRB1 and DQB1*

Table 1. *HLA-DRB1* allele carrier frequency in the SLE patients and controls.

	1st Set						2nd set						combined						
	Case (n = 459)	Control (n = 307)	*P*	OR	*Pc*	95%CI	Case (n = 389)	Control (n = 542)	*P*	OR	*Pc*	95%CI	Case (n = 848)	Control (n = 849)	*P*	OR	*Pc*	95%CI	*P* (RPE)
*DRB1*01:01*	41 (8.9)	27 (8.8)	1.0000	1.02	NS		34 (8.7)	65 (12.0)	0.1312	0.70	NS		75 (8.8)	92 (10.8)	0.1921	0.80	NS		
*DRB1*04:01*	19 (4.1)	4 (1.3)	0.0292	3.27	0.8189	(1.10–9.71)	15 (3.9)	15 (2.8)	0.3546	1.41	NS		34 (4.0)	19 (2.2)	0.0371	1.82	NS	(1.03–3.23)	
*DRB1*04:03*	15 (3.3)	15 (4.9)	0.2612	0.66	NS		16 (4.1)	29 (5.4)	0.4403	0.76	NS		31 (3.7)	44 (5.2)	0.1560	0.69	NS		0.0117
*DRB1*04:05*	94 (20.5)	68 (22.1)	0.5890	0.91	NS		79 (20.3)	125 (23.1)	0.3357	0.85	NS		173 (20.4)	193 (22.7)	0.2621	0.87	NS		
*DRB1*04:06*	17 (3.7)	26 (8.5)	0.0062	0.42	0.1738	(0.22–0.78)	10 (2.6)	36 (6.6)	0.0053	0.37	0.1533	(0.18–0.76)	27 (3.2)	62 (7.3)	0.0002	0.42	0.0052	(0.26–0.66)	0.0020
*DRB1*04:10*	15 (3.3)	10 (3.3)	1.0000	1.00	NS		10 (2.6)	15 (2.8)	1.0000	0.93	NS		25 (2.9)	25 (2.9)	1.0000	1.00	NS		
*DRB1*08:02*	59 (12.9)	31 (10.1)	0.2549	1.31	NS		40 (10.3)	32 (5.9)	0.0176	1.83	0.5114	(1.13–2.96)	99 (11.7)	63 (7.4)	0.0029	1.65	0.0848	(1.18–2.30)	0.0082
*DRB1*08:03*	93 (20.3)	50 (16.3)	0.1855	1.31	NS		61 (15.7)	76 (14.0)	0.5119	1.14	NS		154 (18.2)	126 (14.8)	0.0673	1.27	NS		0.0151
*DRB1*09:01*	139 (30.3)	72 (23.5)	0.0394	1.42	NS	(1.02–1.97)	118 (30.3)	151 (27.9)	0.4208	1.13	NS		257 (30.3)	223 (26.3)	0.0670	1.22	NS		
*DRB1*11:01*	11 (2.4)	18 (5.9)	0.0192	0.39	0.5378	(0.18–0.85)	15 (3.9)	16 (3.0)	0.4639	1.32	NS		26 (3.1)	34 (4.0)	0.3576	0.76	NS		
*DRB1*12:01*	37 (8.1)	20 (6.5)	0.4836	1.26	NS		36 (9.3)	43 (7.9)	0.4771	1.18	NS		73 (8.6)	63 (7.4)	0.3730	1.18	NS		
*DRB1*12:02*	12 (2.6)	6 (2.0)	0.6330	1.35	NS		14 (3.6)	24 (4.4)	0.6156	0.81	NS		26 (3.1)	30 (3.5)	0.6839	0.86	NS		
*DRB1*13:02*	30 (6.5)	44 (14.3)	0.0004	0.42	0.0123	(0.26–0.68)	39 (10.0)	93 (17.2)	0.0022	0.54	0.0646	(0.36–0.80)	69 (8.1)	137 (16.1)	5.21×10^{-7}	0.46	1.51×10^{-5}	(0.34–0.63)	7.17×10^{-5}
*DRB1*14:03*	9 (2.0)	19 (6.2)	0.0029	0.30	0.0812	(0.14–0.68)	5 (1.3)	21 (3.9)	0.0247	0.32	0.7156	(0.12–0.86)	14 (1.7)	40 (4.7)	0.0004	0.34	0.0127	(0.18–0.63)	0.0010
*DRB1*14:05*	14 (3.1)	11 (3.6)	0.6836	0.85	NS		10 (2.6)	28 (5.2)	0.0635	0.48	NS		24 (2.8)	39 (4.6)	0.0715	0.60	NS		
*DRB1*14:06*	9 (2.0)	12 (3.9)	0.1176	0.49	NS		4 (1.0)	11 (2.0)	0.2962	0.50	NS		13 (1.5)	23 (2.7)	0.1284	0.56	NS		
*DRB1*14:54*	33 (7.2)	20 (6.5)	0.7727	1.11	NS		18 (4.6)	29 (5.4)	0.6521	0.86	NS		51 (6.0)	49 (5.8)	0.8375	1.04	NS		
*DRB1*15:01*	119 (25.9)	51 (16.6)	0.0025	1.76	0.0705	(1.22–2.53)	98 (25.2)	65 (12.0)	3.07×10^{-7}	2.47	8.90×10^{-6}	(1.75–3.49)	217 (25.6)	116 (13.7)	5.48×10^{-10}	2.17	1.59×10^{-8}	(1.69–2.79)	5.48×10^{-10}
*DRB1*15:02*	69 (15.0)	63 (20.5)	0.0514	0.69	NS		76 (19.5)	116 (21.4)	0.5118	0.89	NS		145 (17.1)	179 (21.1)	0.0414	0.77	NS	(0.61–0.98)	
DR2 (*DRB1*15, *16*)	187 (40.7)	110 (35.8)	0.1743	1.23			170 (43.7)	183 (33.8)	0.0026	1.52		(1.16–1.99)	357 (42.1)	293 (34.5)	0.0014	1.38		(1.13–1.68)	
DR6 (*DRB1*13, *14*)	98 (21.4)	107 (34.9)	4.34×10^{-5}	0.51		(0.37–0.70)	83 (21.3)	180 (33.2)	6.68×10^{-5}	0.55		(0.40–0.74)	181 (21.3)	287 (33.8)	1.06×10^{-8}	0.53		(0.43–0.66)	

SLE: systemic lupus erythematosus, OR: odds ratio, CI: confidence interval, *Pc*: corrected *P* value, NS: not significant, RPE: relative predispositional effects. Allele carrier frequencies are shown in parenthesis (%). Alleles with more than 1% of the frequency in controls are shown. Association was tested by Fisher's exact test using 2×2 contingency tables. RPE were tested by sequential elimination of carriers of each of the alleles *DRB1*15:01, *13:02, *14:03, *04:06, *08:02, *08:03* and **04:03*.

alleles which either conferred protection against or susceptibility to SLE.

Replication in the second set and combined analysis

We then sought to confirm these findings in an independent set of SLE patients and healthy controls by *DRB1* genotyping the second set of 389 SLE patients and 542 healthy controls (Table 1, central column). In this case, a significant positive association was found for *DRB1*15:01* and SLE ($Pc = 8.90 \times 10^{-6}$, OR 2.47, 95% CI 1.75–3.49) and it was the protective association with *DRB1*13:02* which just failed to achieve significance ($Pc = 0.0646$, OR 0.54, 95% CI 0.36–0.80). As in the first set, the protective association with *DRB1*14:03* also failed to reach significance ($Pc = 0.7156$, OR 0.32, 95% CI 0.12–0.86). Carrier frequencies of DR6 ($P = 6.68 \times 10^{-5}$, OR 0.55, 95% CI 0.40–0.74) and DR2 ($P = 0.0026$, OR 1.52, 95% CI 1.16–1.99) alleles were significantly lower and higher, respectively, in SLE.

We further explored associations between these *DRB1* alleles and SLE in a combined analysis, using RPE testing [19]. RPE were analyzed by sequential elimination of carriers of each allele with the strongest association (Table 1, right column). The strongest association was between *DRB1*15:01* and SLE, confirmed in this combined analysis ($P = 5.48 \times 10^{-10}$, $Pc = 1.59 \times 10^{-8}$, OR 2.17, 95% CI 1.69–2.79). The second round of comparisons was conducted after the elimination of *DRB1*15:01* carriers, revealing the next strongest association to be between *DRB1*13:02* and SLE ($P = 7.17 \times 10^{-5}$, $Pc = 0.0020$). The third round was after the elimination of both *DRB1*15:01* or **13:02* carriers, now showing the strongest association to be between *DRB1*14:03* and SLE ($P = 0.0010$, $Pc = 0.0272$). Further rounds after elimination of *DRB1*15:01*, **13:02* or **14:03* carriers revealed only tendential associations between the remaining *DRB1* alleles and SLE, particularly for *DRB1*04:06* ($P = 0.0020$, $Pc = 0.0509$), **08:02* ($P = 0.0082$, $Pc = 0.2040$), **08:03* ($P = 0.0151$, $Pc = 0.3615$) and **04:03* ($P = 0.0117$, $Pc = 0.2683$). We therefore focused on the *DRB1* alleles with the strongest SLE associations, namely *DRB1*15:01*, **13:02* and **14:03*.

Genotype analysis of HLA-DRB1*15:01, *13:02 and *14:03

We next compared genotype frequencies of *HLA-DRB1*15:01*, **13:02* and **14:03* to seek associations with SLE (Table 2). A significant positive association was found for "*DRB1*15:01/allele other than *15:01*" ($P = 4.83 \times 10^{-9}$, OR 2.14, 95% CI 1.65–2.76). On the other hand, "*DRB1*13:02/allele other than *13:02*" and the "**13:02/*13:02*" genotypes were both negatively associated with SLE ($P = 6.47 \times 10^{-6}$, OR 0.49, 95% CI 0.36–0.67 and $P = 0.0211$, OR 0.11, 95% CI 0.01–0.87, respectively). A negative association of the "**13:02 or *14:03*/alleles other than **13:02* or **14:03*" genotype with SLE was also observed ($P = 5.53 \times 10^{-9}$, OR 0.43, 95% CI 0.33–0.58), again although a significant positive association for the genotype "alleles other than **13:02* or **14:03*/ alleles other than **13:02* or **14:03*" was present ($P = 3.69 \times 10^{-10}$, OR 2.41, 95% CI 1.82–3.19). A significant positive association was found with "**15:01*/alleles other than **13:02* or **14:03*" ($P = 1.79 \times 10^{-11}$, OR 2.39, 95% CI 1.84–3.10). Thus, protective effects of **13:02* and **14:03* are dominant over the predisposing effects of **15:01* in SLE.

Associations of DRB1 with SLE of different clinical and phenotypic manifestations

We analyzed the associations of genotype frequencies of **15:01*, **13:02* and **14:03* separately in SLE patients with different clinical and autoantibody phenotypes to confirm the protective effects of **13:02* and **14:03* in SLE patients with different manifestations. The significant positive association of the genotype "**15:01*/alleles other than **13:02* or **14:03*" with SLE of a certain phenotype was confirmed for almost all factors assessed (Table 3, left column). The same was true for the negative association of the "**15:01/*13:02* or **14:03*" genotype with SLE regardless of phenotype (Table 3, right column). Thus, the protective effects of **13:02* and **14:03* were confirmed in all the different phenotypic manifestations of SLE.

Amino acid residues in the DRβ chain are associated with SLE

Amino acid residues in the HLA-DRβ chain were also analyzed for associations with SLE. The amino acid residue 13S in the DRβ chain showed strong protective associations with SLE ($P = 2.24 \times 10^{-8}$, $Pc = 7.63 \times 10^{-7}$, OR 0.55, 95%CI 0.45–0.68, Figure 1) and is shared by **13:02* and **14:03*, whereas the amino acid residues 32H ($P = 9.76 \times 10^{-5}$, $Pc = 0.0033$, OR 0.67, 95%CI 0.55–0.82), 67L ($P = 0.0003$, $Pc = 0.0118$, OR 0.70, 95%CI 0.58–0.85), and 71E ($P = 1.84 \times 10^{-5}$, $Pc = 0.0006$, OR 0.53, 95%CI 0.40–0.71) showed only moderate protective associations and are possessed by **13:02* and **14:03*, **14:03*, and **13:02*, respectively. Thus, association analysis suggested roles for certain defined amino acid residues in the DRβ chain in SLE susceptibility.

Discussion

Several studies have shown that certain *HLA-DR* alleles are positively associated with SLE. However, few studies have focused on negative associations of *HLA* alleles with SLE. To the best of our knowledge, this is the first report of a negative association of the HLA-DR6 alleles *DRB1*13:02 and *14:03* with Japanese SLE, although a lower frequency of DR5 [21] or DR6 [22] alleles in Asian patients with SLE has been reported before. Several studies have noted positive associations of *DRB1*15:01* [11,21,23], **15:02* [12,13] or **09:01* [3,14,24,25] alleles with SLE in Asians. However, here we only confirmed the association with **15:01*, but not **15:02* or **09:01* in Japanese SLE patients in general (Table 1). The association of **15:02* with SLE has never been reported in a Japanese population, suggesting that this allele may not be the primary genetic factor in itself, but a marker for a nearby gene. Since the allele frequencies between Thai and Japanese are comparable [13,18], the differences in allele frequencies could not explain the reason of the lack of association of **15:02* in Japanese SLE. Because HLA is the strongest genetic factor for SLE, it is quite difficult to explain the reason by other genetic backgrounds than *HLA* region. Since the amino acid sequences of **15:01* and **15:02* are almost same, presented peptide will be same. Environmental background could not explain the reason. HLA region is in strong linkage disequilibrium. Therefore, we cannot rule out the possibility that another causative genes, namely *DRB5* or *DQA1* genes, might exist in the *HLA* region in linkage disequilibrium with the culprit gene in the *DRB1* locus.

In the genotype analysis of *HLA-DRB1*15:01*, **13:02* and **14:03*, a nominally lower frequency of the "**15:01/*13:02* or **14:03*" genotype in SLE was observed, although a positive association was revealed for the genotype of "**15:01*/alleles other than **13:02* or **14:03*" (Table 2). The protective effects of **13:02* or **14:03* thus seem to overcome the predispositional effects of **15:01* in SLE. *DRB1*13:02* commonly belongs to the haplotype *DRB1*13:02-DQB1*06:04-DPB1*04:01* positively selected in Japanese in recent history [26]. The *DRB1*13:02* allele is also a protective allele for cervical cancer caused by human papilloma

Table 2. *HLA-DRB1* genotype frequency in the SLE patients and controls.

	Case (n = 848)	Control (n = 849)	*P*	OR	95%CI
*15:01/alleles other than *15:01	198 (23.3)	106 (12.5)	4.83×10^{-9}	2.14	(1.65–2.76)
*15:01/*15:01	19 (2.2)	10 (1.2)	0.0958	1.92	
*13:02/alleles other than *13:02	68 (8.0)	128 (15.1)	6.47×10^{-6}	0.49	(0.36–0.67)
*13:02/*13:02	1 (0.1)	9 (1.1)	0.0211	0.11	(0.01–0.87)
*15:01/*13:02	8 (0.9)	12 (1.4)	0.5009	0.66	
*15:01/alleles other than *15:01 or *13:02	190 (22.4)	94 (11.1)	3.30×10^{-10}	2.32	(1.77–3.03)
*14:03/alleles other than *14:03	13 (1.5)	40 (4.7)	0.0002	0.31	(0.17–0.59)
*14:03/*14:03	1 (0.1)	0 (0.0)	0.4997	3.01	
*15:01/*14:03	2 (0.2)	3 (0.4)	1.0000	0.67	
*13:02/*14:03	0 (0.0)	1 (0.1)	1.0000	0.33	
*15:01/alleles other than *15:01, *13:02 or *14:03	188 (22.2)	91 (10.7)	1.58×10^{-10}	2.37	(1.81–3.11)
*13:02 or *14:03/any alleles	83 (9.8)	176 (20.7)	3.69×10^{-10}	0.41	(0.31–0.55)
*13:02 or *14:03/alleles other than *13:02 or *14:03	81 (9.6)	166 (19.6)	5.53×10^{-9}	0.43	(0.33–0.58)
*13:02 or *14:03/*13:02 or *14:03	2 (0.2)	10 (1.2)	0.0379	0.20	(0.04–0.91)
alleles other than *13:02 or *14:03/alleles other than *13:02 or *14:03	765 (90.2)	673 (79.3)	3.69×10^{-10}	2.41	(1.82–3.19)
*15:01/*13:02 or *14:03	10 (1.2)	15 (1.8)	0.4209	0.66	
*15:01/alleles other than *13:02 or *14:03	207 (24.4)	101 (11.9)	1.79×10^{-11}	2.39	(1.84–3.10)

SLE: systemic lupus erythematosus, OR: odds ratio, CI: confidence interval. Genotype frequencies are shown in parenthesis (%). Association was tested by Fisher's exact test using 2×2 contingency tables.

virus infection [27] and *DPB1*04:01* is protective for hepatitis B infection [28].

The *DRB1* and *DQB1* alleles which showed significant associations are in strong linkage disequilibrium. In order to elucidate which of the *DRB1* and *DQB1* genes was responsible for

Table 3. *HLA-DRB1* genotype frequency in the SLE patients and controls relative to SLE phenotype.

	n	*15:01/alleles other than *13:02, or *14:03	*P*	OR	*Q*	95%CI	*15:01/*13:02, or *14:03	*P*	OR	*Q*	95%CI
age of onset < 20	144	36 (25.0)	7.58×10^{-5}	2.47	0.0001	(1.60–3.80)	1 (0.7)	0.4920	0.39	0.8806	
anti-Ro/SS-A antibodies (+)	326	80 (24.5)	2.13×10^{-7}	2.41	6.04×10^{-7}	(1.74–3.34)	4 (1.2)	0.6138	0.69	0.8806	
anti-La/SS-B antibodies (+)	70	14 (20.0)	0.0591	1.85	0.0628		1 (1.4)	1.0000	0.81	1.0000	
anti-RNP antibodies (+)	240	60 (25.0)	1.62×10^{-6}	2.47	3.07×10^{-6}	(1.72–3.53)	1 (0.4)	0.2192	0.23	0.8806	
anti-Sm antibodies (+)	220	51 (23.2)	5.14×10^{-5}	2.23	7.49×10^{-5}	(1.53–3.25)	2 (0.9)	0.5478	0.51	0.8806	
anti-dsDNA antibodies (+)	603	148 (24.5)	5.53×10^{-10}	2.41	3.13×10^{-9}	(1.82–3.18)	7 (1.2)	0.3916	0.65	0.8806	
antiphospholipid syndrome (+)	165	37 (22.4)	0.0007	2.14	0.0009	(1.41–3.26)	1 (0.6)	0.4925	0.34	0.8806	
malar rash (+)	301	90 (25.4)	2.08×10^{-8}	2.52	8.85×10^{-8}	(1.83–3.45)	2 (0.7)	0.2655	0.37	0.8806	
discoid rash (+)	116	84 (27.9)	5.28×10^{-10}	2.87	3.13×10^{-9}	(2.07–3.97)	2 (1.7)	1.0000	0.98	1.0000	
photosensitivity (+)	238	28 (24.1)	0.0007	2.36	0.0009	(1.47–3.78)	3 (1.3)	0.7770	0.71	0.8806	
arthritis (+)	410	60 (25.2)	1.44×10^{-6}	2.50	3.06×10^{-6}	(1.74–3.57)	4 (1.0)	0.3336	0.55	0.8806	
serositis (+)	161	96 (23.4)	3.46×10^{-7}	2.26	8.41×10^{-7}	(1.66–3.08)	0 (0.0)	0.1477	0.17	0.8806	
renal disorder (+)	380	35 (21.7)	0.0015	2.06	0.0017	(1.34–3.16)	5 (1.3)	0.6354	0.74	0.8806	
neurologic disorder (+)	130	93 (24.5)	7.01×10^{-8}	2.40	2.38×10^{-7}	(1.76–3.28)	3 (2.3)	0.7219	1.31	0.8806	
hemolytic anemia (+)	95	35 (26.9)	1.84×10^{-5}	2.73	3.14×10^{-5}	(1.76–4.24)	2 (2.1)	0.6857	1.20	0.8806	
lymphopenia (+)	459	18 (18.9)	0.0708	1.73	0.0708		4 (0.9)	0.2335	0.49	0.8806	
thrombocytopenia (+)	180	122 (26.6)	5.58×10^{-11}	2.68	9.49×10^{-10}	(2.00–3.60)	2 (1.1)	0.7513	0.62	0.8806	
Control	849	101 (11.9)					15 (1.8)				

SLE: systemic lupus erythematosus, OR: odds ratio, CI: confidence interval. Genotype frequencies are shown in parenthesis (%). Associations were tested by Fisher's exact test using 2×2 contingency tables. To correct for multiple testing, the false discovery rate Q-value was calculated.

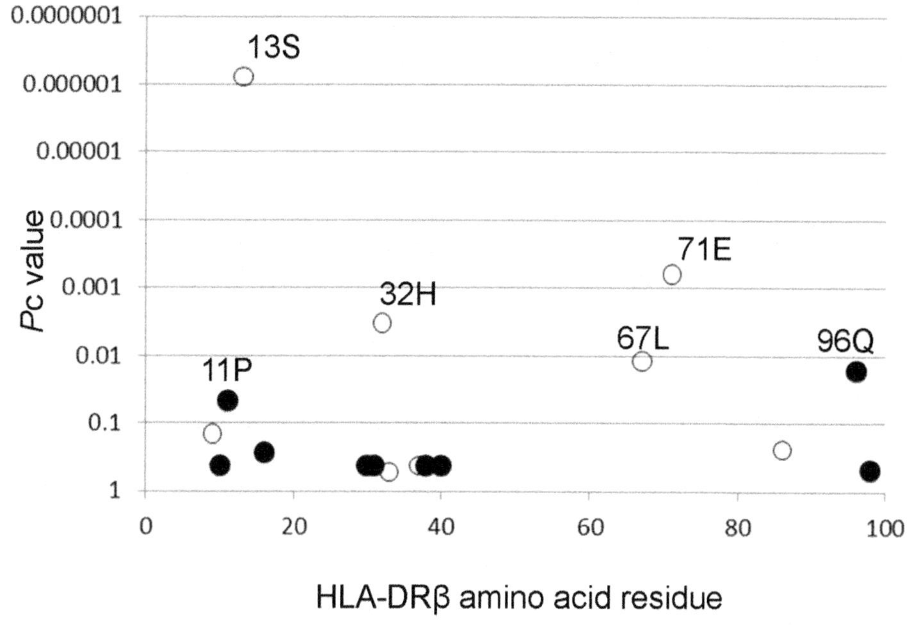

Figure 1. Associations of amino acid residues in the DRβ chain with SLE. Corrected *P* (*Pc*) values were calculated by multiplying the *P* value by the number of amino acid residues tested. Associations were established by Fisher's exact test using 2×2 contingency tables. Positive associations were indicated in filled circles and negative in open circles.

primary association, haplotype analysis of *DRB1-DQB1* was performed. A significant negative association was found for the *DQB1*06:04* allele and the *DRB1*13:02-DQB1*06:04* haplotype with SLE in the first set comparison (Table S1). The primary role of *DRB1* or *DQB1* was not elucidated, because the strong linkage disequilibrium between *DRB1*13:02* and *DQB1*06:04* results in a low frequency of *DRB1*13:02* in patients without *DQB1*06:04* and similarly a low frequency of *DQB1*06:04* in patients without *DRB1*13:02*.

It was reported that anti-Ro/SS-A-positive rheumatoid arthritis patients were more frequently *DRB1*08:03*-positive and an association of *DRB1*15:01* and anti-La/SS-B antibodies has been reported in Japanese rheumatoid arthritis patients [29]. In the present study, a significant positive association of *DRB1*04:05* with the presence of anti-Ro/SS-A antibodies in SLE patients was found; in contrast, the *DRB1*12:02* allele was associated with the presence of anti-La/SS-B antibodies. These four *DRB1* alleles are in linkage disequilibrium with *DPB1*05:01* in the Japanese population [30], suggesting a role for *DPB1*in the production of autoantibodies to ribonucleoprotein. Susceptibility alleles for background diseases, *DRB1*15:01* in SLE or *DRB1*04:05* in rheumatoid arthritis, might not be easily detected as autoantibody-associated alleles in a comparison of antibody-positive and -negative patients. Alternatively, these findings could be explained by differences in the pathogenesis of rheumatoid arthritis and SLE.

Amino acid residues 13, 32, 67 and 71 of the HLA-DRβ chain were found to be associated with SLE (Figure 1). Residues 13, 32, 67 and 71 form the HLA-DR peptide-binding groove [31]. These data suggest the involvement of peptide antigens bound to specific HLA molecules in controlling the development of SLE.

The negative association with *HLA-DR6* alleles needs to be confirmed in future independent studies. Because the allelic distribution of *HLA* in other ethnic populations is different from the Japanese, the protective role of some *DRB1* alleles in SLE in other populations should be determined.

This is the first identification of a negative association of *HLA-DRB1*13:02 and *14:03* with SLE. Our findings support the dominantly protective role of *HLA-DR6* alleles in the pathogenesis of SLE.

Acknowledgments

We thank Ms. Mayumi Yokoyama (Sagamihara Hospital) for secretarial assistance.

Author Contributions

Conceived and designed the experiments: HF NT ST. Performed the experiments: HF A. Kawasaki S. Oka II. Analyzed the data: HF. Contributed reagents/materials/analysis tools: HF K. Shimada SS AH A. Komiya NF YK SI TH IM M. Kusaoi HA TN SH K. Setoguchi HK AO NC ES M. Katayama KM AS S. Ohno HH YT TS SN NT ST. Wrote the paper: HF NT ST. Collected clinical information: HF K. Shimada SS AH A. Komiya NF YK SI TH IM M. Kusaoi HA TN SH K. Setoguchi HK AO NC ES M. Katayama KM AS S. Ohno HH YT TS SN NT ST.

References

1. Rahman A, Isenberg DA (2008) Systemic lupus erythematosus. N Engl J Med 358: 929–939.
2. Koga M, Kawasaki A, Ito I, Furuya T, Ohashi J, et al. (2011) Cumulative association of eight susceptibility genes with systemic lupus erythematosus in a Japanese female population. J Hum Genet 2011: 12.

3. Kim I, Kim YJ, Kim K, Kang C, Choi CB, et al. (2009) Genetic studies of systemic lupus erythematosus in Asia: where are we now? Genes Immun 10: 421–432.
4. Furukawa H, Kawasaki A, Oka S, Shimada K, Matsui T, et al. (2013) Association of a single nucleotide polymorphism in the SH2D1A intronic region with systemic lupus erythematosus. Lupus 22: 497–503.
5. Deng FY, Lei SF, Zhang YH, Zhang ZL, Guo YF (2013) Functional relevance for associations between genetic variants and systemic lupus erythematosus. PLoS One 8: e53037.
6. Perricone C, Ceccarelli F, Valesini G (2011) An overview on the genetic of rheumatoid arthritis: a never-ending story. Autoimmun Rev 10: 599–608.
7. Black CM, Welsh KI, Fielder A, Hughes GR, Batchelor JR (1982) HLA antigens and Bf allotypes in SLE: evidence for the association being with specific haplotypes. Tissue Antigens 19: 115–120.
8. Tsuchiya N, Kawasaki A, Tsao BP, Komata T, Grossman JM, et al. (2001) Analysis of the association of HLA-DRB1, TNFalpha promoter and TNFR2 (TNFRSF1B) polymorphisms with SLE using transmission disequilibrium test. Genes Immun 2: 317–322.
9. Suggs MJ, Majithia V, Lewis RE, Cruse JM (2011) HLA DRB1*1503 allelic haplotype predominance and associated immunodysregulation in systemic lupus erythematosus. Exp Mol Pathol 91: 548–562.
10. Reveille JD, Moulds JM, Ahn C, Friedman AW, Baethge B, et al. (1998) Systemic lupus erythematosus in three ethnic groups: I. The effects of HLA class II, C4, and CR1 alleles, socioeconomic factors, and ethnicity at disease onset. LUMINA Study Group. Lupus in minority populations, nature versus nurture. Arthritis Rheum 41: 1161–1172.
11. Hashimoto H, Nishimura Y, Dong RP, Kimura A, Sasazuki T, et al. (1994) HLA antigens in Japanese patients with systemic lupus erythematosus. Scand J Rheumatol 23: 191–196.
12. Lu LY, Ding WZ, Fici D, Deulofeut R, Cheng HH, et al. (1997) Molecular analysis of major histocompatibility complex allelic associations with systemic lupus erythematosus in Taiwan. Arthritis Rheum 40: 1138–1145.
13. Sirikong M, Tsuchiya N, Chandanayingyong D, Bejrachandra S, Suthipinittharm P, et al. (2002) Association of HLA-DRB1*1502-DQB1*0501 haplotype with susceptibility to systemic lupus erythematosus in Thais. Tissue Antigens 59: 113–117.
14. Shimane K, Kochi Y, Suzuki A, Okada Y, Ishii T, et al. (2013) An association analysis of HLA-DRB1 with systemic lupus erythematosus and rheumatoid arthritis in a Japanese population: effects of *09:01 allele on disease phenotypes. Rheumatology (Oxford) 52: 1172–1182.
15. Kamatani N, Kawamoto M, Kitamura Y, Harigai M, Okumoto T, et al. (2004) Establishment of B-cell lines derived from 996 Japanese individuals. Tissue Culture Res Commun 23: 71–80.
16. Hochberg M (1997) Updating the American College of Rheumatology revised criteria for the classification of systemic lupus erythematosus. Arthritis Rheum 40: 1725.
17. Shibue T, Tsuchiya N, Komata T, Matsushita M, Shiota M, et al. (2000) Tumor necrosis factor alpha 5'-flanking region, tumor necrosis factor receptor II, and HLA-DRB1 polymorphisms in Japanese patients with rheumatoid arthritis. Arthritis Rheum 43: 753–757.
18. Furukawa H, Oka S, Shimada K, Sugii S, Ohashi J, et al. (2012) Association of human leukocyte antigen with interstitial lung disease in rheumatoid arthritis: A protective role for shared epitope. PLoS ONE 7: e33133.
19. Payami H, Joe S, Farid NR, Stenszky V, Chan SH, et al. (1989) Relative predispositional effects (RPEs) of marker alleles with disease: HLA-DR alleles and Graves disease. Am J Hum Genet 45: 541–546.
20. Benjamini Y, Hochberg Y (1995) Controlling the false discovery rate: a practical and powerful aproach to multiple testing. J R Statist Soc B 57: 289–300.
21. Zhang J, Ai R, Chow F (1997) The polymorphisms of HLA-DR and TNF B loci in northern Chinese Han nationality and susceptibility to systemic lupus erythematosus. Chin Med Sci J 12: 107–110.
22. Doherty DG, Ireland R, Demaine AG, Wang F, Veerapan K, et al. (1992) Major histocompatibility complex genes and susceptibility to systemic lupus erythematosus in southern Chinese. Arthritis Rheum 35: 641–646.
23. Lee HS, Chung YH, Kim TG, Kim TH, Jun JB, et al. (2003) Independent association of HLA-DR and FCgamma receptor polymorphisms in Korean patients with systemic lupus erythematosus. Rheumatology (Oxford) 42: 1501–1507.
24. Hong GH, Kim HY, Takeuchi F, Nakano K, Yamada H, et al. (1994) Association of complement C4 and HLA-DR alleles with systemic lupus erythematosus in Koreans. J Rheumatol 21: 442–447.
25. Li CF, He XH, Teng Q, Jiang ZF (2003) Association of HLA-A, B, and DR haplotypes with genotype in Chinese children with systemic lupus erythematosus. Zhonghua Er Ke Za Zhi 41: 422–425.
26. Kawashima M, Ohashi J, Nishida N, Tokunaga K (2012) Evolutionary analysis of classical HLA class I and II genes suggests that recent positive selection acted on DPB1*04:01 in Japanese population. PLoS One 7: e46806.
27. Madeleine MM, Johnson LG, Smith AG, Hansen JA, Nisperos BB, et al. (2008) Comprehensive analysis of HLA-A, HLA-B, HLA-C, HLA-DRB1, and HLA-DQB1 loci and squamous cell cervical cancer risk. Cancer Res 68: 3532–3539.
28. Kamatani Y, Wattanapokayakit S, Ochi H, Kawaguchi T, Takahashi A, et al. (2009) A genome-wide association study identifies variants in the HLA-DP locus associated with chronic hepatitis B in Asians. Nat Genet 41: 591–595.
29. Furukawa H, Oka S, Shimada K, Sugii S, Hashimoto A, et al. (2013) Association of increased frequencies of HLA-DPB1*05:01 with the presence of anti-Ro/SS-A and anti-La/SS-B antibodies in Japanese rheumatoid arthritis and systemic lupus erythematosus patients. PLoS ONE 8: e53910.
30. Nakajima F, Nakamura J, Yokota T (2001) Analysis of HLA haplotypes in Japanese, using high resolution allele typing. MHC 8: 1–32.
31. Jardetzky TS, Brown JH, Gorga JC, Stern LJ, Urban RG, et al. (1994) Three-dimensional structure of a human class II histocompatibility molecule complexed with superantigen. Nature 368: 711–718.

Confounding by Indication Probably Distorts the Relationship between Steroid Use and Cardiovascular Disease in Rheumatoid Arthritis: Results from a Prospective Cohort Study

Alper M. van Sijl*, Maarten Boers, Alexandre E. Voskuyl, Michael T. Nurmohamed

Department of Rheumatology, VU University Medical Center, Amsterdam, the Netherlands

Abstract

Objective: To evaluate the risk of cardiovascular disease in patients with rheumatoid arthritis exposed to glucocorticoids.

Methods: Retrospective analysis of exposure to glucocorticoids in a prospective cohort of 353 patients with rheumatoid arthritis followed from June 2001 up to November 2011 for incident cardiovascular disease in a hospital-based outpatient cohort in the Netherlands. Hazard ratios with 95%-confidence intervals were calculated for the association between different types of exposure to glucocorticoids and incident cardiovascular disease. Associations were adjusted for demographics, cardiovascular risk factors and disease related parameters.

Results: Recent and current exposure to glucocorticoids were associated with incident cardiovascular disease, as was a longer duration of exposure and cumulative exposure to glucocorticoids. Adjustment for disease activity and severity negated the association.

Conclusion: In observational studies the finding of incident cardiovascular disease in patients with rheumatoid arthritis exposed to glucocorticoids is strongly confounded by indication due to high disease activity. The adverse cardiovascular effects of glucocorticoids might be balanced by positive effects working through inflammation control.

Editor: Masataka Kuwana, Keio University School of Medicine, Japan

Funding: The authors have no support or funding to report.

Competing Interests: The authors have declared that no competing interests exist.

* E-mail: Alper.vanSijl@vumc.nl

Introduction

Glucocorticoids (GC) are one of the most effective anti-rheumatic drugs, but concerns over long-term side effects have not been resolved. [1] In rheumatoid arthritis (RA), GC are disease-modifying agents as they rapidly provide symptomatic relief, suppress disease activity and, slow progression of radiological damage. [2,3] However, recent studies suggest that cumulative exposure to GCs is associated with an increased risk of cardiovascular (CV) disease, perhaps in part through worsening of the CV risk profile. [4,5].

Considering the systemic inflammatory process in RA, also responsible for the increased CV risk in this group, GC use might enhance or mitigate the pre-existing CV risk. The net effect of GC use on the risk of developing CV disease therefore remains elusive.

Materials and Methods

A total of 353 individuals were followed in the prospective hospital-based outpatient cohort of the CArdiovascular Risk in patients with RhEumatoid arthritis (CARRÉ) study. The purpose of the CARRÉ study is to investigate CV disease and its risk factors in RA patients. [6] In 2000, a random sample of RA patients registered at the Jan van Breemen Research Institute - Reade in Amsterdam, the Netherlands, was drawn. Patients fulfilled the 1987 American College of Rheumatology classification criteria for RA, and were aged between 50 and 75 years. The local ethics committees and institutional review board of the VU University Medical Center in Amsterdam, the Netherlands, approved the study protocol and all participants gave their written informed consent for the study in accordance to the declaration of Helsinki.

At inclusion, prior medication use, baseline disease activity and CV risk factors were assessed. From clinical notes we collected data on GC exposure at baseline by ascertaining the duration of exposure, last exposure by date, mean dose of GC and cumulative exposure in grams. GC exposure was calculated as prednisone equivalents. Individuals, aged 50–75 years with a diagnosis of RA, were followed for approximately 10 years for the development of CV disease. Follow-up duration was calculated as time from enrolment in the study until follow-up measurement or occurrence of a (non-) fatal CV event. During the follow-up period, all CV events were recorded and adjudication of CV events was performed on the basis of standardized criteria by an independent trained person according to the ICD-9 codes for myocardial infarction (MI) (410.0–9), stroke (436) or transient ischemic attack (TIA) (435.9), a history of peripheral arterial reconstruction, carotid endarterectomy, percutaneous coronary intervention (PCI) (8036), coronary artery by-pass surgery (CABG) (8038) and sudden death, cause unknown (798). Data on the participants' vital status on December 1, 2011 were collected from the local municipalities and general practitioners. For each subject, we determined whether or not an incident CV disease had occurred. If a patient had moved out of town, information on vital status was obtained from the new local municipalities. Information on health status could not be obtained for 31 (8.8%) participants.

The association between GC exposure at baseline and incident CV disease was analyzed using Cox proportional hazard analyses. Multivariate Cox proportional hazard analyses assessed whether this association was independent of: 1. age, gender, and 10-year estimated CV risk according to SCORE, and 2. age, gender, SCORE, Disease activity score in 28 joints (DAS-28), and the Health Assessment Questionnaire – Disability Index (HAQ-DI). Possible confounders were considered according to available literature and by selecting variables on the basis of the effect on the original estimate of the exposure effect. Results are described as hazard ratios (HR) with 95%-confidence intervals (95%-CI) expressing the risk of a CV event. Analyses were performed again with steroid exposure during follow-up period as independent variables, adjusting for demographic factors, CV risk, cumulative DAS28, cumulative HAQ and steroid use at baseline. Two sided p-values less than 0.05 were considered statistically significant. All analyses were performed by SPSS 17.0 (Chicago, IL, USA).

Results

The study comprised of 353 individuals of whom 59 (17%) were on GC treatment at the time of inclusion. During the study period 95 (27%) individuals used GC at any given moment during follow-up. The median (interquartile range) duration of exposure of patients on GC before inclusion was 2.2 (0.6–4.8) years and the cumulative exposure before inclusion was 8.7 grams (2.5–25.4). After a total follow-up experience of 2.361 years, 58 (16.5%) participants developed an incident CV disease, yielding an incidence rate of 24.6/1.000 patient years.

Compared to patients without, cases with incident CV disease included significantly more GC users at baseline, were treated with GC for a longer period and at higher cumulative doses. The associations remained similar after adjustment for age, gender and SCORE-estimated CV risk at baseline (Table 1: crude estimate and model 1, respectively). However, additional adjustment for disease activity (28-joint disease activity score, DAS28) and disability (Health Assessment Questionnaire – Disability Index (HAQ-DI), which is a measure that reflects both current inflammatory activity and the effects of cumulative joint damage) completely erased the associations of GC with incident CV disease (Figure 1). The standard error estimates of the regression coefficients did not increase substantially after correction for covariates, suggesting robustness of our observations. We can therefore assume the effect of GC remained present in most individuals at risk during follow-up. In addition, statistical analyses performed with prospective data on steroid use during follow-up period, with adjustment for cumulative DAS28 and HAQ, yielded essentially similar results, albeit in this analysis the results were not statistically significant.(data not shown) Furthermore, subgroup-analysis for patients who were not on concomittant NSAIDs did not reveal essentially different results.(data not shown).

Discussion

We hypothesize that GC use in uncontrolled populations represents a marker of high RA disease activity; high disease activity itself represents an increased risk of CV disease. Thus the observed relationship of GC with CV disease in RA patients is strongly confounded by indication. Intensive treatment of systemic inflammation and disease activity remains an essential part of treatment of RA. In this setting, it is possible that the adverse CV effects of GC are balanced by positive effects working through inflammation control.

Prior studies found an increased risk of CV disease in patients who used steroids. A nested-case control study from a general practice database showed that individuals who currently use steroids were at increased risk of developing cardiovascular disease, cerebrovascular disease or heart failure. These results remained similar for patients with a diagnosis of RA and chronic obstructive pulmonary disease (COPD). A dose-response association with higher cumulative doses was not found. [7] In addition, two retrospective population cohort studies investigated the incidence of CV disease in patients with RA who used steroids. [4,5] Both studies found an up to threefold increased risk of CV events in patients with RA who used steroids, especially in patients with rheumatoid factor positivity, higher cumulative exposure to steroids and exposure to steroids for more than 5 years. One of these studies even found that the use of low-dose glucocorticoids was associated with the development of a CV event. [5].

The present study confirms these findings, as we also found an increased risk of CV events in RA patients treated currently with steroids, patients treated for more than 5 years and patients treated with high cumulative doses. With additional adjustment for demographic parameters and cardiovascular risk, the association remained similar. However, when adjusted for disease activity and disability, the association is negated, thus reflecting an effect confounded by indication.

Previously, the relationship between steroid use and CV disease was always thought to be an unfavourable one. This study shows that this association is strongly mitigated by the disease activity and disability of the disease itself. The current guidelines on CV risk in rheumatoid arthritis state that "an adequate disease activity control is necessary to lower the CV risk", while "glucocorticoids should be used in the lowest dose possible". [8] If we extrapolate the findings from this study to the clinical situation that physicians and patients face on a daily basis, we would recommend that glucocorticoid use should be limited to small dosages and short periods of exposure. However, in patients with active RA, our data support the use of glucocorticoids to gain rapid disease control.

Strengths and weaknesses of this study merit careful consideration. Strengths of the present study include the recording of CV- and RA-related factors as well as medication use, which were all performed by three physicians using the same protocol. In addition, this study provides a well-defined study population with a long-term follow-up period that can investigate the effects of medication use on incident CV disease. However, our study has several limitations that should be acknowledged. First, we did not use a control population of healthy subjects and therefore were not able to compare the present findings in RA-patients with matched non-RA patients. Second, small number of incident cases and soft events (elective PCI or CABG) might have caused a relatively low power. Therefore, we restricted confounding analyses to a minimum of variables. Third, relatively diminished use of steroids in the follow-up period limited our power for analyses of prospective steroid use and the risk of incident CV disease.

Table 1. Cox-proportional hazard analyses of exposure to glucocorticoids at baseline and incident CV disease in patients with rheumatoid arthritis.

	Crude	Adjusted model 1[¶]	Adjusted model 2[§]
Steroid use			
- Ever vs. never	1.68 (0.92–3.07)	1.77 (0.68–4.63)	0.89 (0.26–3.09)
- Recent (<1 year) vs. never	1.93 (1.00–3.72)*	2.03 (0.72–5.74)	1.11 (0.27–4.53)
- Current vs. never	2.18 (1.12–4.27)*	2.91 (1.06–8.00)*	1.34 (0.31–5.88)
Duration of steroids, years	1.15 (1.01–1.31)*	1.18 (0.90–1.41)	1.14 (0.83–1.58)
- No steroids	1.00 (ref)	1.00 (ref)	1.00 (ref)
- =<5 years	1.00 (0.46–2.19)	1.02 (0.28–3.67)	0.71 (0.15–3.27)
- >5 years	4.64 (2.12–10.14)*	4.33 (1.31–14.29)*	1.48 (0.21–10.45)
Cumulative steroid use, grams	1.02 (1.01–1.04)*	1.04 (1.01–1.07)*	1.05 (0.99–1.11)
- No steroids	1.00 (ref)	1.00 (ref)	1.00 (ref)
- =<10 gram	0.92 (0.36–2.37)	0.43 (0.06–3.33)	0.42 (0.05–3.30)
- >10 gram	2.34 (1.15–4.77)*	3.88 (1.39–3.33)*	1.80 (0.37–8.74)
- No steroids	1.00 (ref)	1.00 (ref)	1.00 (ref)
- 1st tertile	1.53 (0.60–3.92)	0.59 (0.08–4.67)	0.54 (0.07–4.36)
- 3rd tertile	3.52 (1.72–7.18)*	5.21 (1.79–15.17)*	2.420.45–13.00)

*p<0.05. Results presented as hazard ratios (95%-confidence interval).
¶Correction for age, gender, and 10-year estimated CV risk according to SCORE.
§Correction for age, gender, SCORE, Disease activity score in 28 joints (DAS-28), and the Health Assessment Questionnaire – Disability Index (HAQ-DI).

In conclusion, this study suggests that glucocortioid use is a risk factor for CV events in RA, but that this association is strongly confounded by disease activity and disability.

Author Contributions

Conceived and designed the experiments: AMS MB AEV MTN. Performed the experiments: AMS MB AEV MTN. Analyzed the data: AMS MB AEV MTN. Contributed reagents/materials/analysis tools: AMS MB AEV MTN. Wrote the paper: AMS MB AEV MTN.

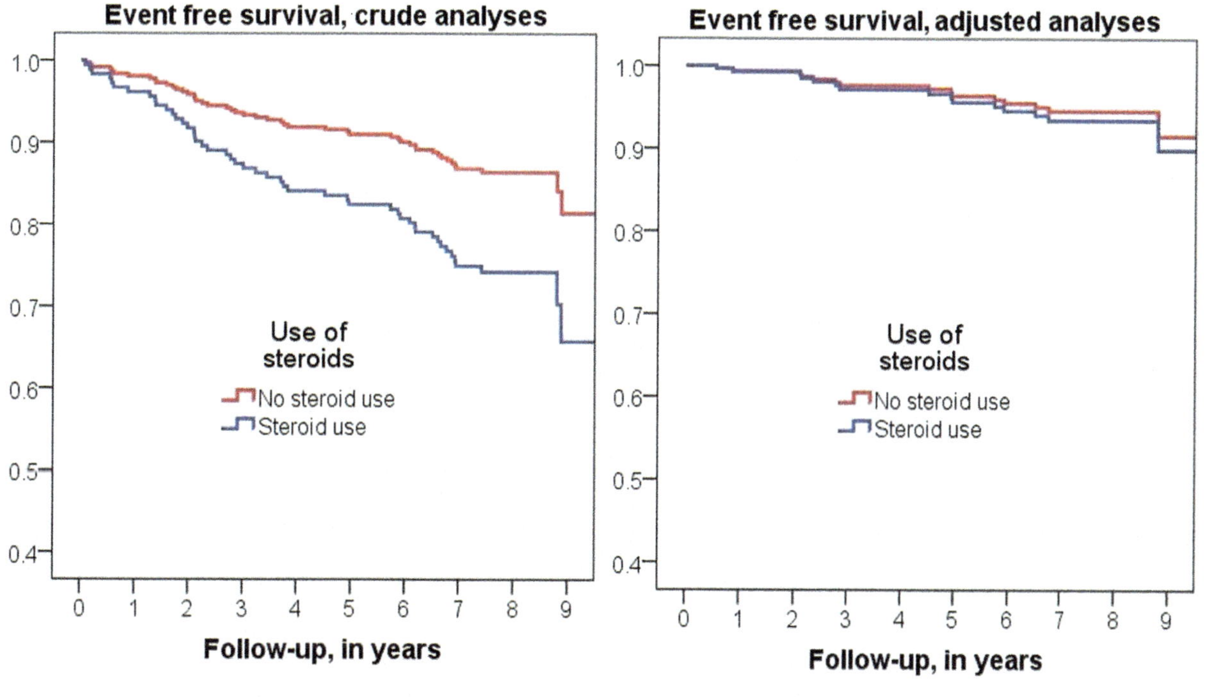

Figure 1. Kaplan-Meier survival curve of individuals who were using steroids at baseline vs. individuals who were not using steroids at baseline, both crude as well as fully adjusted for disease activity–/severity.

References

1. Da Silva JA, Jacobs JW, Kirwan JR, Boers M, Saag KG, et al. (2006) Safety of low dose glucocorticoid treatment in rheumatoid arthritis: published evidence and prospective trial data. Ann Rheum Dis 65: 285–293.
2. Gorter SL, Bijlsma JW, Cutolo M, Gomez-Reino J, Kouloumas M, et al. (2010) Current evidence for the management of rheumatoid arthritis with glucocorticoids: a systematic literature review informing the EULAR recommendations for the management of rheumatoid arthritis. Ann Rheum Dis 69: 1010–1014.
3. Boers M, Verhoeven AC, Markusse HM, van de Laar MA, Westhovens R, et al. (1997) Randomised comparison of combined step-down prednisolone, methotrexate and sulphasalazine with sulphasalazine alone in early rheumatoid arthritis. Lancet 350: 309–318.
4. Davis JM, Maradit Kremers H, Crowson CS, Nicola PJ, Ballman KV, et al. (2007) Glucocorticoids and cardiovascular events in rheumatoid arthritis: a population-based cohort study. Arthritis Rheum 56: 820–830.
5. Mazzantini M, Talarico R, Doveri M, Consensi A, Cazzato M, et al. (2010) Incident Comorbidity Among Patients with Rheumatoid Arthritis Treated or Not with Low-dose Glucocorticoids: A Retrospective Study. J Rheumatol 37(11): 2232–6.
6. Peters MJL, van Halm VP, Voskuyl AE, Smulders YM, Boers M, et al. (2009) Does rheumatoid arthritis equal diabetes mellitus as an independent risk factor for cardiovascular disease? A prospective study. Arthritis Rheum 61(11);1571–9.
7. Souverein PC, Berard A, van Staa TP, Cooper C, Egberts ACG, et al. (2004) Use of oral glucocorticoids and risk of cardiovascular and cerebrovascular disease in a population based case-control study. Heart 90;859–65.
8. Duru N, van der Goes MC, Jacobs JW, Andrews T, Boers M, et al. (2013) EULAR evidence-based and consensus-based recommendations on the management of medium to high-dose glucocorticoid therapy in rheumatic diseases. Ann Rheum Dis 72(12);1905–13.

16

Performance of the 2010 Classification Criteria for Rheumatoid Arthritis: A Systematic Literature Review and a Meta-Analysis

Garifallia Sakellariou[1]*, Carlo Alberto Scirè[1], Antonella Zambon[2], Roberto Caporali[1], Carlomaurizio Montecucco[1]

1 Chair and Division of Rheumatology, IRCCS Policlinico San Matteo Foundation, Pavia, Italy, **2** Department of Biostatistics Statistics and Quantitative Methods, University of Milano-Bicocca, Milano, Italy

Abstract

Objectives: To evaluate the performance of the American College of Rheumatology (ACR)/European League Against Rheumatism (EULAR) 2010 classification criteria for rheumatoid arthritis (RA) with a systematic literature review and a meta-analysis.

Methods: PubMed, Embase, Cochrane Library and the abstracts of the ACR and EULAR meetings (2010–2012) were searched for original articles or abstracts with the following inclusion criteria: 1) recent onset arthritis, with at least one swollen joint and no alternative diagnosis; 2) the ACR/EULAR 2010 criteria as index test; 3) the prescription of methotrexate (MTX) or disease modifying antirheumatic drugs (DMARDs) at any time during follow-up as reference standard. Data were pooled using the bivariate model. Three meta-analyses were performed with MTX (primary analysis), DMARDs or their combination (secondary analyses) as reference standard. Heterogeneity was formally tested and explored performing an influence analysis.

Results: The search identified 1,277 references. Six full papers and 4 abstracts met the inclusion criteria. With MTX as reference standard, sensitivity (95% confidence interval, CI) was 0.80 (0.74,0.85), specificity 0.61 (0.56,0.67), positive likelihood ratio (LR) 2.11 (1.92,2.32), negative LR 0.31 (0.25,0.38) and the diagnostic odds ratio (DOR) was 6.74 (5.49,8.28). Using DMARDs as reference standard, sensitivity was 0.73 (0.64,0.80), specificity was 0.74 (0.68,0.79), LR+2.85 (2.53,3.22), LR− 0.35 (0.27,0.45) and DOR 8.03 (6.4,10.09). Using the combination of MTX and DMARDs as reference standard, intermediate results were obtained. The influence analysis detected one potentially influential study. However, its exclusion from the meta-analysis did not have a clinically relevant impact on the results.

Conclusions: The new classification criteria have good sensitivity, lower specificity and an overall moderate diagnostic accuracy. These results confirm that the criteria have classificative and not diagnostic function.

Editor: Adrian V. Hernandez, Universidad Peruana de Ciencias Aplicadas (UPC), Peru

Funding: The authors have no support or funding to report.

Competing Interests: The authors have declared that no competing interests exist.

* E-mail: filiciasak@gmail.com

Introduction

In the last few decades, the recognition of the central role of an early diagnosis and the early administration of disease modifying antirheumatic drugs (DMARDs), particularly methotrexate (MTX), greatly improved the management of rheumatoid arthritis (RA) [1]. The more effective diagnostic and treatment strategies led to a better control of the disease with a deeper suppression of synovitis [2] and the prevention of radiological progression of bone erosions in the joints [3]. All these improvements have led to a great reduction of the risk of permanent disability [4,5] which is the most significant long-term detrimental consequence of the disease.

For these reasons, the early recognition of RA has become a central issue in clinical practice, although the absence of a single and reliable test to identify the disease does not always allow an immediate diagnosis. The American College of Rheumatology (ACR) proposed in 1987 a set of classification criteria, developed in patients with longstanding disease with the aim to be specific rather than sensitive [6]. These criteria, that were initially meant for the enrolment of patients in clinical trials, but in some cases are used for diagnosis, have shown an unsatisfactory performance in the setting of early arthritis, especially due to a low sensitivity [7]. The inadequate performance of the 1987 criteria led in recent years to the development of prognostic algorithms, meant to discriminate, at the time of symptom onset, patients with higher probability of persistent disease amenable to treatment with DMARDs from those with self-limiting arthritis [8,9].

In 2010 the ACR and the European League Against Rheumatism (EULAR) jointly developed new classification criteria, aiming to allow earlier patient classification, treatment and inclusion in clinical trials [10]. The new criteria were developed from inceptional cohorts of inflammatory arthritis data [11] which subsequently integrated with expert opinion [12] and finally validated in external early arthritis cohorts. For their development, the reference standard for diagnosis was the prescription of MTX or other DMARDs within the first year of observation. This was considered the best available reference standard, reflecting the risk of chronicity and erosive damage [10]. Since the criteria were developed using a reference standard that can be fulfilled after a follow-up, their value is not only classificative, but also prognostic. The opinion of an expert rheumatologist was not considered an acceptable reference standard because the widespread knowledge of the 1987 classification criteria would have likely lead to a circularity bias.

The 2010 criteria include tender and swollen joint count, acute phase reactants, anti-cyclic citrullinated peptide antibodies (ACPA) or rheumatoid factor (RF), and symptom duration (Table 1). These clinical and laboratory data are combined into a score ranging from 0 to 10. In the validation cohorts, the areas under the Receiving Operator Characteristics (ROC) curve (AUC) for the new criteria ranged from 0.66 to 0.82, and the score that determined an optimal discrimination was between 6 and 7. The cut-off of 6 was afterwards chosen in order to improve sensitivity. However, detailed information on the sensitivity and specificity of the new criteria, along with the corresponding likelihood ratios (LR), has not been reported in the original paper. Moreover, there was a certain variability in accuracy measures across different cohorts [13].

After their first presentation at the ACR congress in 2009, the new criteria have been tested in a number of external early arthritis cohorts with a wide variability in the overall performance [14–17]. These studies are slightly different in terms of population,

Table 1. 2010 ACR/EULAR classification criteria for rheumatoid arthritis.

A Joint involvement	
1 large joint	0
2–10 large joints	1
1–3 small joints	2
4–10 small joints	3
>10 joints	5
B Serology	
Negative RF and negative ACPA	0
Low-positive RF or low-positive ACPA	2
High-positive RF or high-positive ACPA	3
C Acute-phase reactants	
Normal CRP and normal ESR	0
Abnormal CRP or Abnormal ESR	1
D Duration of symptoms	
<6 weeks	0
≥6 weeks	1

The criteria are meant to be applied in patients with at least one swollen joint, after the exclusion of other causes of synovitis. Patients with a score ≥6 are classified as having RA. Also subjects with typical bone erosions can be classified as RA regardless of the score. Modified from Aletaha D, et al. RF: rheumatoid factor; ACPA: anti-cyclic citrullinated peptide antibodies; CRP: C-reactive protein; ESR: erythrocyte sedimentation rate.

but the main differences are in the assessment of the reference standard. In fact, many studies considered expert opinion as reference standard [15], as well as disease persistency, appearance of bone erosions or the 1987 classification criteria [17]. Only some of the studies considered the prescription of MTX or other DMARDs as reference standard for diagnosis as indicated in the newly developed criteria.

Because of the increasing knowledge on the 2010 RA classification criteria it seemed timely to summarise the results of the available literature. The present study aims to evaluate the performance of the 2010 ACR/EULAR classification criteria in populations of individuals with early arthritis. For this purpose, we performed a systematic literature review and subsequent meta-analyses in which we considered the 2010 classification criteria a s index test, the prescription of MTX or other DMARDs as reference standard for the classification of RA as done during the development of the criteria.

Methods

The Preferred Reporting Items for Systematic Reviews and Meta-analyses (PRISMA) guidelines for the reporting of systematic reviews and meta-analysis were followed to conduct this review [18]. A pre-specified protocol, including research question, search strategy, inclusion criteria for the articles and methods for the analysis, was developed before the beginning of the study.

Data Sources and Search

The search was performed by one of the authors (GS) and a control search by a second author (CAS). We searched Medline (PubMed), Embase and Cochrane databases from November 2009 (when the criteria were presented for the first time) to May 2012. The search strategies are shown in table 2. The search strategy was based on terms related to RA, classification and diagnosis. The references of the included studies were manually screened to search for further papers. The abstracts of the ACR (2010 and 2011) and EULAR congresses (2010, 2011, 2012) were examined to look for additional studies. No language or publication restrictions were applied and studies were not selected based on quality. Filters developed for the identification of diagnostic studies were not utilised since such filters may result in omission of relevant studies [19].

Study Selection

Studies should include subjects presenting with recent onset arthritis, with at least one swollen joint and no definite diagnosis that could explain symptoms (that is, the same population in which classification criteria should be applied) [10]. Finally, only data on patients with RA or undifferentiated polyarthritis (UPA) at baseline were included. The 2010 classification criteria were the index test, in the score format; the presence of bone erosions was not included since it was not tested in the data-driven phase of the development. Moreover, a definition of typical erosions had not yet been presented during the timespan that we examined. The prescription of MTX or DMARDs was considered as reference standard. In particular, we included studies that considered MTX (alone) as reference standard or overall DMARDs (including also MTX). Corticosteroids were not included.

Diagnostic cohort studies (prospective and retrospective) and case control studies were eligible for inclusion in the review. The presence of sufficient data to build a 2×2 table of diagnostic performance was required. Two reviewers independently screened titles and abstracts. The full-text of the potentially eligible articles was obtained; inclusion assessment was performed by one reviewer

Table 2. Search strategy.

PubMed	1 "rheumatoid arthritis"
	2 Arthritis, rheumatoid[Mesh]
	3 #1 OR #2
	4 "classification"
	5 "diagnostic criteria"
	6 "ACR EULAR"
	7 #4 OR #5 OR #6
	8 #3 AND #7
Embase	1 'rheumatoid arthritis'/exp AND [embase]/lim
	2 'classification criteria' AND [embase]/lim
	3 acr AND eular
	4 #2 OR #3
	5 #1 AND #4 AND [embase]/lim AND [1-6-2009]/sd AND [2009-2012]/py
Cochrane	#1 MeSH descriptor Arthritis, Rheumatoid, this term only
	#2 rheumatoid arthritis
	#3 (#1 OR #2)
	#4 classification
	#5 diagnostic criteria
	#6 ACR EULAR
	#7 (#4 OR #5 OR #6)
	#8 (#3 AND #7)

Limits: humans, adults, from November 2009.

and checked by a second. Disagreements were resolved by consensus. Only the most recent and complete report was included in the case of studies reported in multiple publications or abstracts.

Data Extraction and Quality Assessment

We extracted data using a standardised form. Results were extracted as 2×2 tables. Studies were assessed for methodological quality by using the modified version of the Quality Assessment of Diagnostic Accuracy Studies (QUADAS) tool proposed by the Cochrane Collaboration [20]. Data extraction and quality assessment were done by one reviewer and checked by a second reviewer.

Data Synthesis and Analysis

Sensitivity and specificity were calculated for each 2×2 set of data. Heterogeneity among n included studies was visually evaluated plotting sensitivity and specificity on a ROC graph, and separately tested by the Chi-square test using $n-1$ degree of freedom [21].

In the presence of heterogeneity and negative correlation between sensitivity and specificity, as commonly seen in diagnostic studies, the bivariate model was used to estimate summary sensitivity and specificity with 95% confidence intervals (CI) and to derive a hierarchical summary receiving operator characteristic (HSROC) curve [22–24].Summary positive and negative likelihood ratios (LR+, LR−) and the diagnostic odds ratio (DOR) were derived for each analysis.

Three different analyses were performed. Primary analysis used MTX as reference standard for diagnosis. Secondary analysis used DMARDs as reference standard for diagnosis. Since MTX is a particular type of DMARDs, and in order to increase the number of available studies and hence the precision of the meta-analysis, a third analysis used MTX or DMARDs as reference standard was performed. For this analysis, if data on both MTX and DMARDs were reported separately, data on DMARDs were used.

To evaluate the robustness of our findings, we performed an influence analysis calculating Cook's distance for each study. This index is a measure of the influence of a study on the model parameters and can be used to check for particularly influential study. Studies with Cook's distance ≥1 were considered potentially influent. A further meta-analysis was then performed after excluding these potentially influential studies.

Publication bias was indirectly evaluating the symmetry on the funnel plot of logDOR. Forest plots were used to represent sensitivity and specificity of the primary studies.

Finally to verify the presence of publication bias, a funnel plot was implemented.

Review Manager (RevMan) version 5 (The Nordic Cochrane Centre, The Cochrane Collaboration, Copenhagen) was used to build the forest plot showing sensitivity and specificity of single studies and the risk of bias tables. Stata, version 11, (StataCorp, College Station, Texas) was used to perform all analyses. In particular the generalized linear mixed model approach to bivariate meta-analysis of sensitivity and specificity was obtained using the 'metandi' command of Stata.

Results

The search strategy identified 1277 studies. Figure 1 reports the flow-chart of the process of study selection. 6 articles were included after the evaluation of all titles and abstracts [14,16,25–28]. Moreover, 4 abstracts from the ACR and EULAR congresses were eligible for inclusion [29–32]. In total, 4 papers used MTX as unique reference standard, 3 used DMARDs as unique reference standard, while 3 studies reported separate data on both MTX and DMARDs. Two studies [15,33] were excluded since they used a composite reference standard based on concomitant expert opinion and DMARDs and expert opinion was not considered an acceptable reference standard for this review. Table 3 and Figure 2 summarise the main features of the included studies. Figure 2 shows the point estimates with 95% CIs of sensitivity and specificity for the included studies. Sensitivity ranged from 0.68 to 0.88 when MTX was considered as reference standard, and from 0.59 to 0.87 when DMARDs were used. The specificity ranged from 0.50 to 0.72 with MTX as reference standard, and from 0.64 to 0.88 with DMARDs.

The evaluation of the methodological quality of the included studies is shown in Figure 3. All studies had a low risk of bias for most of the items except for blinding that was not explicitly mentioned in any of the studies. For this reason, the blinding of the results of the reference standard and the index test was considered unclear. All the included studies had an overall low risk of bias; for this reason, additional analyses, excluding those for low-quality studies, were not performed, since the results of the meta-analysis would not be affected by a low methodological quality.

Both sensitivity and specificity showed significant heterogeneity, with a Chi-square for differences across studies of 29.01 ($p<0.0001$) and 17.09 ($p=0.009$) respectively.

Table 4 summarises the results of all the meta-analyses. Using MTX as reference standard, pooled sensitivity (95% CI) was 0.80 (0.74, 0.85) and pooled specificity (95% CI) was 0.61 (0.56, 0.67), a LR+ of 2.11 (1.92, 2.32) and a LR− of 0.31 (0.25, 0.38).

Using DMARDs as reference standard, sensitivity was 0.73 (0.64,0.80), specificity was 0.74 (0.68,0.79), LR+ was 2.85 (2.53,3.22) and LR− was 0.35 (0.27,0.45).

The third analysis, combining MTX and DMARDs, led to intermediate results (Figure 4).

The influence analysis using the Cook's distance identified Van Der Linden's study as a potentially influential [27]. After removing this study the pooled sensitivity changed from 0.80 (0.74, 0.85) to 0.79 (0.72, 0.84), and specificity from 0.61 (0.56, 0.67) to 0.60 (0.53, 0.68). The influence of each single study is reported in Figure 5.

Funnel plot did not show any systematic asymmetry suggesting the absence of publication bias (Figure 6).

Discussion

Since the new classification criteria for RA were first presented, several studies have provided a wide range of results by evaluating their performance in the setting of early arthritis. These studies were different in terms of population (mainly due to the recruitment criteria and calendar year into the existing cohorts) and reference standard. Moreover, treatment patterns differed significantly among them. This variability did not allow the drawing of consistent conclusions from a single study. Therefore it seemed appropriate to review the available literature on this topic.

We adopted a search strategy meant to be sensitive rather than specific; the limited time period under exam allowed this approach. We did not use pre-specified filters for diagnostic accuracy studies [19]. Since the search was designed to be as broad as possible, it is unlikely that relevant studies were missed. Even in this way, the number of studies that were eligible for the inclusion was limited. This is the main limitation of this review, since it did not allow to investigate the causes of heterogeneity in detail and, for the same reason, subgroup analyses were not feasible.

The majority of the validation studies did not use the same reference standard highlighted in the development of the criteria and many of them used expert opinion or the 1987 ACR criteria. In particular, 13 studies that were selected for detailed review have afterwards been excluded because of a wrong reference standard. These studies were excluded because of the possibility of the introduction of considerable circularity bias. Same reference standard used to develop the new criteria were adopted, that is the prescription of MTX or other DMARDs [10]. The results obtained showed an overall moderate performance of the criteria with acceptable values of sensitivity through all reference standards. One the other hand, specificity was lower in the analyses based on MTX, and MTX with DMARDs. The analysis based on overall DMARDs as reference standard showed a better specificity of the 2010 classification criteria. In fact, MTX might not have been given to all patients that would require it due to contraindications or national differences in prescriptions. On the other hand sensitivity does not increase accordingly because a twofold higher increase of subjects treated with DMARDs not fulfilling the 2010 criteria is observed.

The values of LR+ were around 2.5, far from the values of LR+ >10 that ideally identify a test having the power to detect the disease. However, LR− were around 0.3, which is closer to the optimal values of LR− <0.1 [34]. This indicates the patients not fulfilling the 2010 classification criteria have high probability of not having RA (and will not develop it later, if we consider that the criteria identify patients that might fulfil an outcome after a follow-up), while patients fulfilling them will not certainly develop RA. In contrast with this consideration, the DORs suggest a good

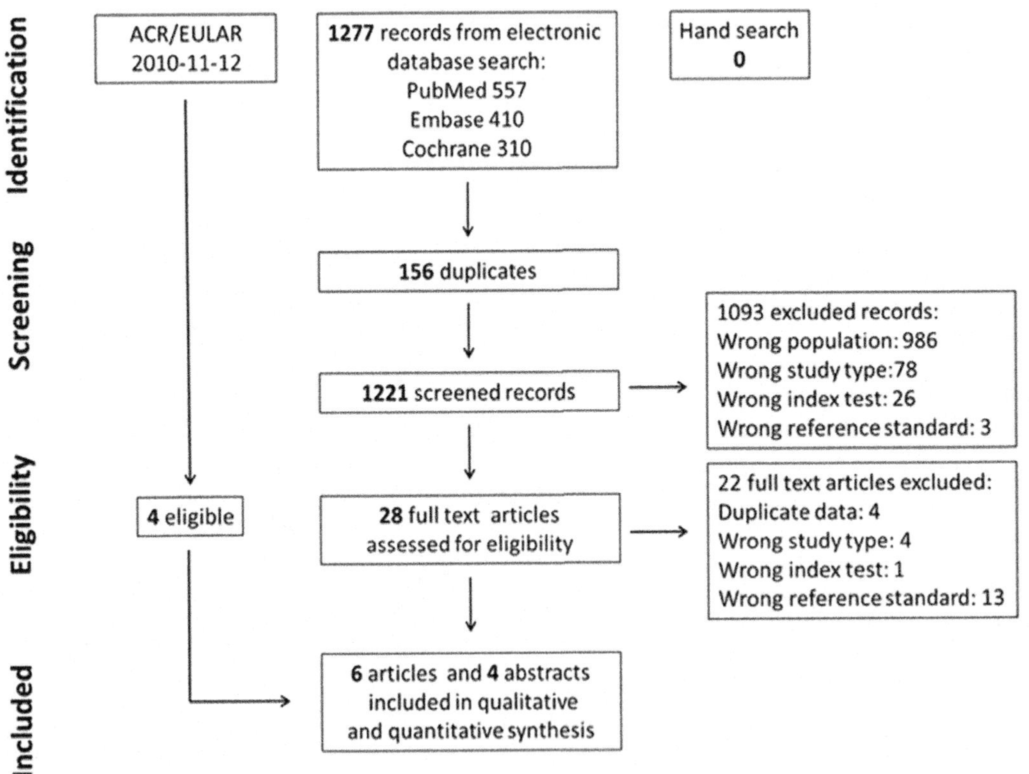

Figure 1. PRISMA flow-chart describing the selection process in the systematic literature review.

A

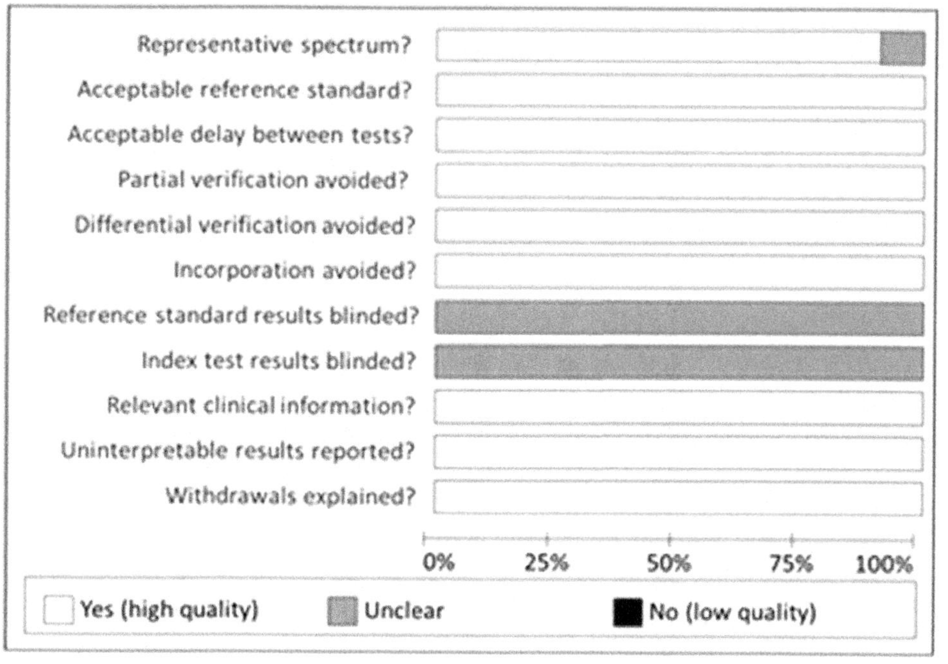

B

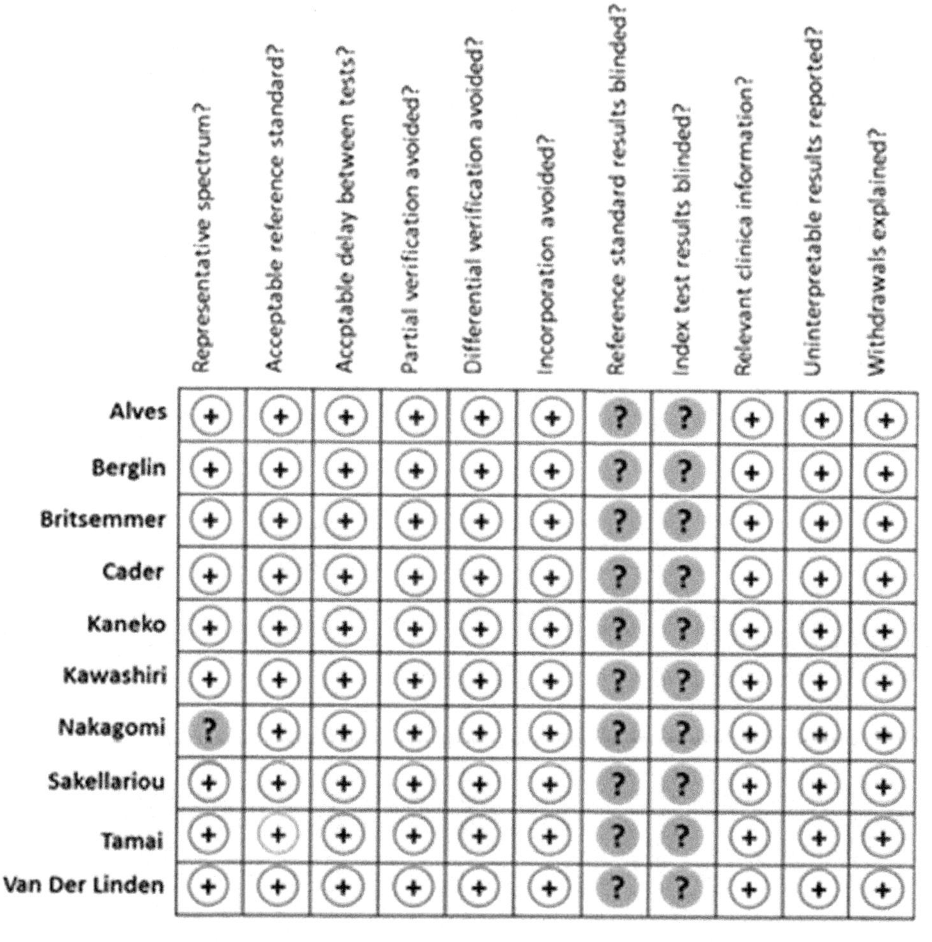

Figure 2. Sensitivity and specificity of the included studies. A) methotrexate as reference standard **B)** disease modifying antirheumatic drugs as reference standard **C)** methotrexate+ disease modifying antirheumatic drugs as reference standard.

Table 3. Characteristics of the included studies.

Study	Clinical setting	Population	Calendar year	Index test	Reference standard	Study design	N	Follow-up duration	RF/ACPA (%)	Symptoms duration	Joint count
Alves	Early arthritis	≥1 swollen joint for less than 1 year; ≥16 years old, no history of trauma or exertion. MTX: 64/231	2004–2008	ACR/EULAR 2010 classification criteria	MTX	Retrospective cohort	231	12 months	26/19	3.47 months	44
Berglin	Early arthritis	≥1 swollen joint; no alternative diagnosis; ≤1 year symptom duration; ≥1 year of follow-up. MTX: 230/313	n.a.	ACR/EULAR 2010 classification criteria	MTX	Retrospective cohort	313	12 months	60/64	4 months	n.a.
Britsemmer	Early arthritis	>18 years old; ≥2 swollen joints; symptom duration of <2 years; no prior DMARDs. MTX: 354/455	2000–n.a.	ACR/EULAR 2010 classification criteria	MTX	Retrospective cohort	455	12 months	42.6/52	5.6 months	n.a.
Cader	Early arthritis	≥1 swollen joint;; ≤3 months of symptom duration; ≥18 months follow-up. MTX: 74/205; DMARDs: 102/205	n.a.	ACR/EULAR 2010 classification criteria	MTX DMARDs	Retrospective cohort	205	18 months	56/59	1.37 months	66
Kanenko	Early arthritis	joint symptoms (arthralgia, joint swelling and morning stiffness); no previous treatment; no diagnosis DMARDs: 54/82	2009–2010	ACR/EULAR 2010 classification criteria	DMARDs	Retrospective cohort	82	0–3 months	66/61	4 months	n.a.
Kawashiri	Early arthritis	suspicion of RA; symptom duration <1 year; no alternative diagnosis; no previous DMARDs. DMARDs: 37/69	2010–2011	ACR/EULAR 2010 classification criteria	DMARDs	Prospective cohort	69	3 months	49/36	4 months	n.a.
Nakagomi	Early arthritis	musculoskeletal symptoms <3 years; no alternative diagnosis. MTX:83/117	n.a.	ACR/EULAR 2010 classification criteria	MTX	Prospective cohort	117	12 months	n.a./n.a.	n.a.	28
Sakellariou	Early arthritis	patients with RA or UPA. MTX: 202/26; DMARDs: 211/266	2005–2010	ACR/EULAR 2010 classification criteria	MTX DMARDs	Retrospective cohort	266	12 months	33/n.a.	3.07 months	44
Tamai	Early arthritis	early arthritis; no alternative diagnosis. DMARDs: 97/138	n.a.	ACR/EULAR 2010 classification criteria	DMARDs	Prospective cohort	138	12 months	n.a.	3 months	n.a.
Van der Linden	Early arthritis	arthritis confirmed by physical examination; <2 years symptom duration. MTX: 445/2258; DMARDs: 1066/2258	1993–2009	ACR/EULAR 2010 classification criteria	MTX DMARDs	Retrospective cohort	2258	12 months	30/29	5.7 months	66

N: number of patients included; n.a.: not available; RF: rheumatoid factor; ACPA: anti-ciclic citrullinated peptide antibodies; MTX: methotrexate; DMARDS: disease modifying antirheumatic drugs; RA: rheumatoid arthritis; UPA: undifferentiated polyarthritis.

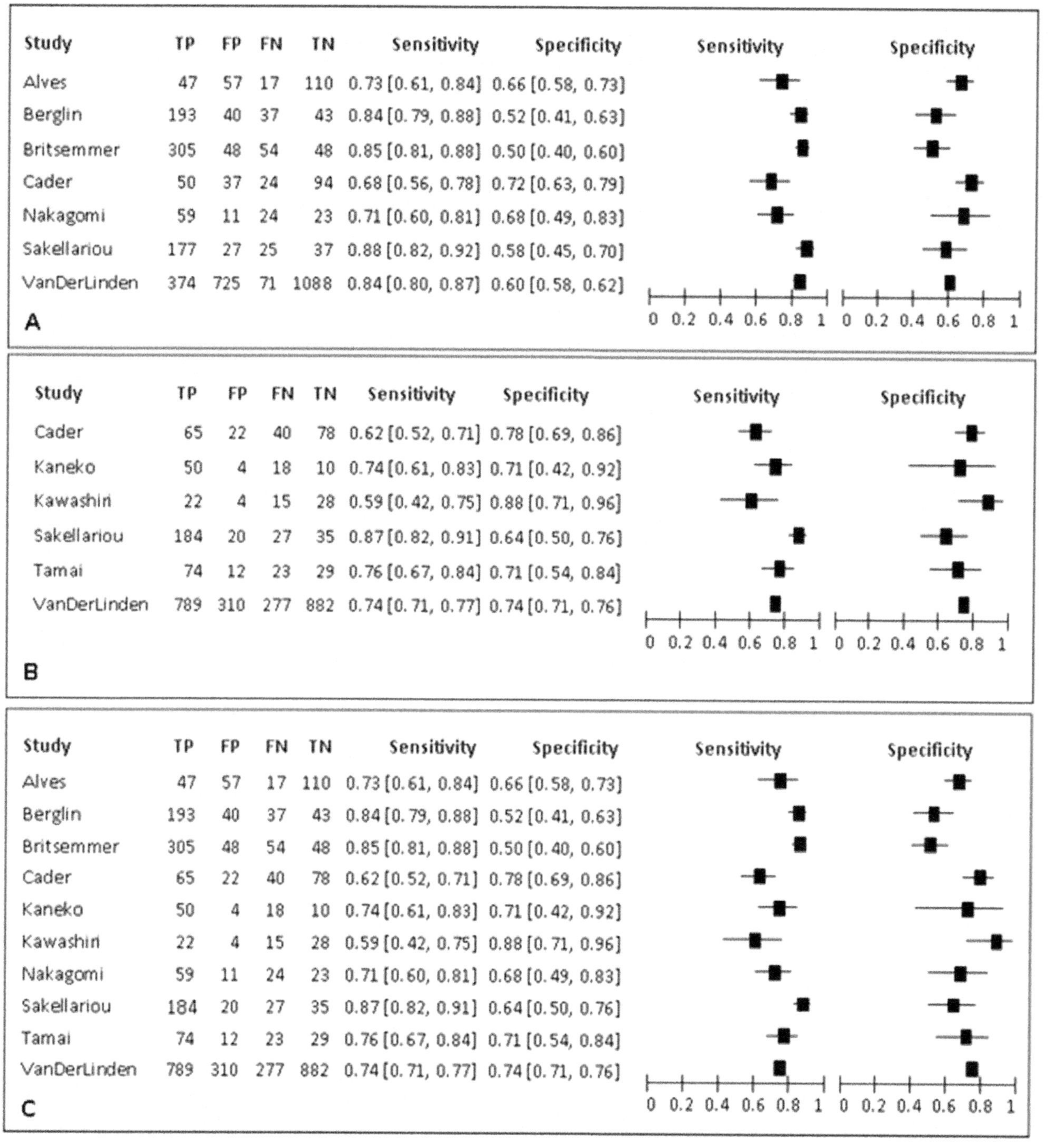

Figure 3. Assessment of the risk of bias in the included studies. 3A) Methodological quality graph: authors' judgment about each methodological quality item presented as percentages across all included studies. 3B) Methodological quality summary: authors' judgment about each methodological quality item for each included study. +: low risk of bias; ?: unclear risk of bias; -: high risk of bias.

performance, though this is probably driven by low values of LR−.

The need to perform differential diagnosis before the application of the criteria might have determined the underestimation of their accuracy even if the majority of studies excluded patients that were afterwards diagnosed with disease other than RA or UPA. Differential diagnosis is not always feasible in the early stages; this might have increased the number of false positives resulting in the reduction of specificity.

In the original presentation paper, detailed data on sensitivity, specificity and performance were not reported. The values of the areas under the ROC curve (AUC) reported in the validation cohorts ranged from 0.66 to 0.82. The best performance was achieved in the Norwegian cohort of early arthritis, while in the remaining two the AUCs were <0.7; this indicates a test with

Table 4. Results of meta-analyses.

Reference standard	Studies (n)	Sensitivity (95% CI)	Specificity (95% CI)	LR+(95% CI)	LR– (95% CI)	DOR (95% CI)
MTX	7	0.80 (0.74,0.85)	0.61 (0.56,0.67)	2.11 (1.92,2.32)	0.31 (0.25,0.38)	6.74 (5.49,8.28)
DMARDs	6	0.73 (0.64,0.80)	0.74 (0.68,0.79)	2.82 (2.53,3.22)	0.35 (0.27,0.45)	8.03 (6.40,10.09)
MTX+DMARDs	10	0.76 (0.71,0.81)	0.69 (0.61,0.75)	2.48 (2.08,2.95)	0.33 (0.29,0.38)	7.38 (6.33,8.62)

95% CI: 95% confidence interval; LR+: positive likelihood ratio; LR−: negative likelihood ratio; DOR: diagnostic odds ratio; MTX: methotrexate; DMARDs: disease modifying antirheumatic drugs.

moderate performance [10]. The differences between the populations could be due to differences in recruitment and treatment. In the external validation cohorts, only the proportion of patients correctly classified was reported, while overall estimates of accuracy were not presented. Since not all information on the performance of the 2010 criteria is provided in the original paper, results could not be directly compared our with data from the inception of the criteria.

As expected, significant heterogeneity was found among diagnostic studies. This finding did not permit the separate combination of sensitivity and specificity. For this reason we adopted a bivariate model that allows for the negative correlation between sensitivity and specificity. Given the low number of studies, investigating heterogeneity by stratified meta-analysis or meta-regression was not feasible. For this reason we evaluated the robustness of our results by performing an influence analysis [21]. However, though one study was demonstrated to be potentially influential, a subsequent meta-analysis after the exclusion of the influential study led to comparable results.

All the included studies had an overall good methodological quality. The items dealing with blinding were not explicitly addressed by the papers, therefore the risk of bias related to these points was considered unclear for all studies. Despite this, given to the retrospective design and the unavailability of the criteria at the time of the clinical assessment and therapeutic decision, this did not clearly biased the results. The last two items (on the report of uninterpretable results and withdrawals), even though not directly reported, were considered satisfactory, since, as suggested by the Cochrane collaboration, they probably had no influence on the results [20]. Since the methodological quality of all the included studies was good, the results of the meta-analysis have likely not been affected by the methodological quality of the primary studies.

A meta-analysis on the diagnostic performance of the 1987 ACR classification criteria demonstrated an overall sensitivity and specificity of 0.77 in the subgroup of patients with early arthritis and a better performance among cases of established arthritis [7]. These results are not substantially different from those of our meta-analyses: the new criteria, specifically designed for early arthritis, do not perform better than the old ones in the same setting. However, it has to be kept in mind that the 1987 criteria were developed based on expert opinion while the 2010 criteria

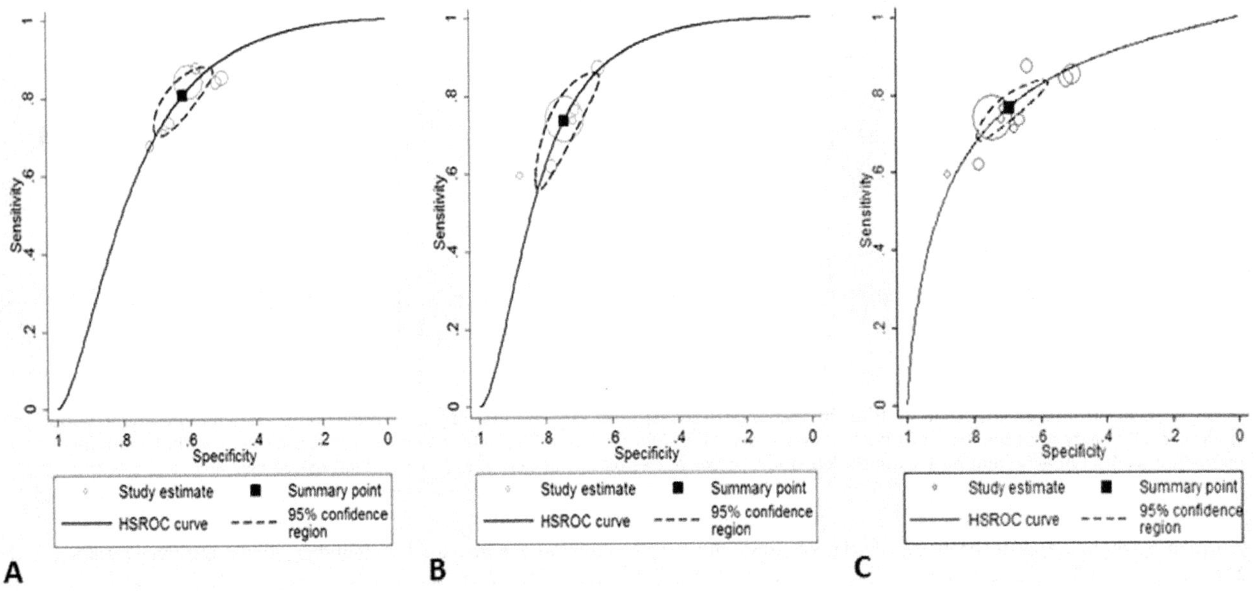

Figure 4. Results of the meta-analyses. A) methotrexate as reference standard; 7 studies included, 3845 participants. **B)** disease modifying antirheumatic drugs s as reference standard; 6 studies included, 3018 participants. **C)** methotrexate+disease modifying antirheumatic drugs as reference standard; 10 studies included, 4134 participants. The black square indicates the point estimate of sensitivity and specificity for the meta-analysis, the dotted line indicates the 95% confidence interval. The continuous line is the hierarchical summary receiving operator characteristics curve. The dots represent the primary studies.

	Sensitivity (95% CI)	Specificity (95% CI)
Overall	0.805 (0.749,0.0851)	0.619 (0.566,0.670)
Alves	0.814 (0.755,0.861)	0.612 (0.550,0.671)
Berglin	0.797 (0.729,0.851)	0.629 (0.575,0.681)
Britsemmer	0.794 (0.727,0.849)	0.631 (0.580,0.679)
Cader	0.823 (0.777,0.861)	0.601 (0.555,0.646)
Nakagomi	0.817 (0.763,0.861)	0.609 (0.554,0.663)
Sakellariou	0.792 (0.731,0.842)	0.629 (0.571,0.684)
VanDerLinden	0.794 (0.726,0.849)	0.609 (0.533,0.680)

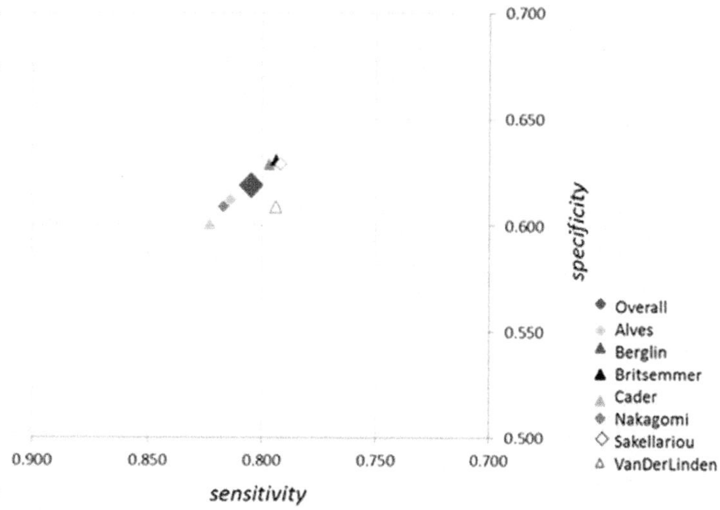

Figure 5. Results of meta-analyses excluding single studies. Overall meta-analysis, based on the primary analysis using methotrexate as reference standard, and meta-analysis excluding a single study are reported. The table and the legend refer to the study that has been excluded.

used a more practical reference standard, such as the use of specific treatment regimes. Therefore, the 2010 criteria could be more useful in a clinical setting because they classify patients based on a relevant prognostic aspect of the disease with an impact on clinical management. Nevertheless, the function of the criteria is classification, and not diagnosis; based on current knowledge the 2010 criteria should not be used as a guide to start specific treatments for RA.

The external validation studies in the meta-analysis on 1987 criteria had a cross-sectional case-control design that overestimates the accuracy while the cohort study design (such as in the development of the criteria) tends to underestimate accuracy [35], and this might have influenced our results as well.

One of the merits of the 2010 classification criteria is the fact that it is not necessary to reach six weeks of symptom duration to classify a patient as having RA. Only one study [14] applied the new criteria in a population of very early arthritis, but their performance did not seem substantially different that in the remaining early arthritis population.

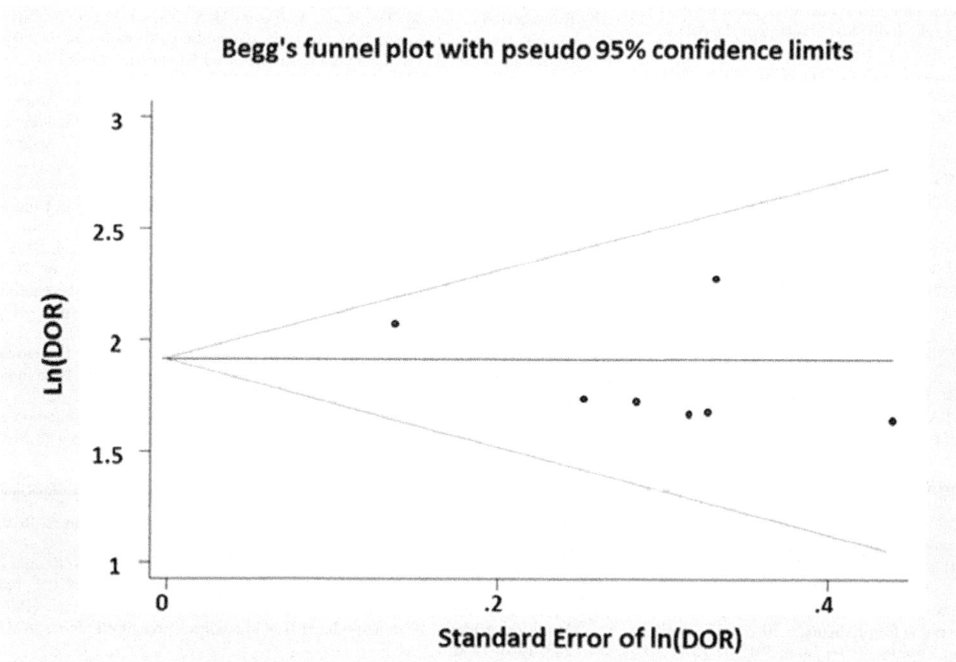

Figure 6. Funnel plot. The distribution of the studies in the funnel plot does not suggest the presence of publication bias. In fact, studies are distributed by each side of the plot, with moreover a lower number of studies with positive results. In the case of publication bias, the opposite situation would have been expected.

The creation of an optimal tool for the classification of rheumatic disease, with RA in particular, has always been challenging. This is mainly due to the absence of gold standards for diagnosis. The decision to prescribe either DMARDs or MTX is dependent from expert opinion and reflects a judgement on the severity of arthritis, for this reason their performance does not seem to be superior to the old ones. However developing the criteria avoiding to use expert opinion as reference standard gives an opportunity to innovate clinical practice, and we could expect that the presentation of the new classification criteria might significantly modify the approach to RA. In fact, the results of the present meta-analysis evaluate the 2010 criteria in the setting of the current management of RA by rheumatologists, but the final judgement on the criteria will probably be drawn after prospective studies, evaluating their long-term impact on disease outcomes.

Author Contributions

Conceived and designed the experiments: CAS CM RC GS. Performed the experiments: GS CAS. Analyzed the data: CAS AZ. Contributed reagents/materials/analysis tools: CAS AZ RC CM. Wrote the paper: GS CAS AZ RC CM.

References

1. McInnes IB, O'Dell JR (2010) State-of-the-art: rheumatoid arthritis. Ann Rheum Dis 69: 1898–1906.
2. Sakellariou G, Scirè CA, Montecucco C, Caporali R (2013) In patients with early rheumatoid arthritis, the new ACR/EULAR definition of in clinical remission identifies patients with persistent absence of functional disability and suppression of ultrasonographic synovitis. Ann Rheum Dis 72: 245–249.
3. Breedveld FC, Combe B (2011) Understanding emerging treatment paradigms in rheumatoid arthritis. Arthritis Res Ther 13: S3.
4. Scirè CA, Verstappen SM, Mirjafari H, Bunn DK, Lunt M, et al. (2011) Reduction of functional disability in inflammatory polyarthritis by early and persistent suppression of joint inflammation: results from the Norfolk Arthritis register. Arthritis Care Res (Hoboken) 63: 945–952.
5. Knevel R, Schoels M, Huizinga TW, Aletaha D, Burmester GR, et al. (2010) Current evidence for a strategic approach to the management of rheumatoid arthritis with disease-modifying antirheumatic drugs: a systematic literature review informing the EULAR recommendations for the management of rheumatoid arthritis. Ann Rheum Dis 69: 987–994.
6. Arnett FC, Edworthy SM, Bloch DA, McShane DJ, Fries JF, et al. (1988) The America Rheumatism Association 1987 revised criteria for the classification of rheumatoid arthritis. Arthritis Rheum 31: 315–324.
7. Banal F, Dougados M, Combescure C, Gossec L (2009) Sensitivity and specificity of the American College of Rheumatology 1987 criteria for the diagnosis of rheumatoid arthritis according to disease duration: a systematic literature review and meta-analysis. Ann Rheum Dis 68: 1184–1191.
8. Visser H, le Cessie S, Vos K, Breeedveld FC, Hazes JM (2004) How to diagnose rheumatoid arthritis early: a prediction model for persistent (erosive) arthritis. Arthritis Rheum 46: 357–365.
9. van der Helm-van Mil AH, le Cessie S, van Dongen H, Breedveld FC, Toes RE (2007) A Prediction Rule for Disease Outcome in Patients With Recent-Onset Undifferentiated Arthritis. How to Guide Individual Treatment Decisions. Arthritis Rheum 56: 433–440.
10. Aletaha D, Neogi T, SIlman A, Funovits J, Felson DT, et al. (2010) 2010 rheumatoid arthritis classification criteria: an America College of Rhuematology/European League Against Rheumatism collaborative initiative. Ann Rheum Dis 69: 1580–1588.
11. Funovits J, Aletaha D, Bykerk V, Combe B, Dougados M, et al. (2010) The 2010 American College of Rheumatology/European league Against Rheumatism classification criteria for rheumatoid arthritis: methodological report phase I. Ann Rheum Dis 69: 1589–1595.
12. Neogi T, Aletaha D, Silman AJ, Naden RL, Felson DT, et al. (2010) The 2010 American College of Rheumatology/European League Against Rheumatism classification criteria for rheumatoid arthritis: Phase 2 methodological report. Arthritis Rheum 62: 2582–2591.
13. Corrao S, Calvo L, Licata G (2011) The new criteria for classification of rheumatoid arthritis: what we need to know for clinical practice. Eur J Intern Med 22: 217–219.
14. Cader MZ, Filer A, Hazlehurst J, de Pablo P, Buckley CD, et al. (2011) Performance of the 2010 ACR/EULAR criteria for rheumatoid arthritis: comparison with the 1987 ACR criteria in a very early synovitis cohort. Ann Rheum Dis 70: 949–955.
15. Varache S, Cornec D, Morvan J, Devauchelle-Pensec V, Berthelot J,et al. (2011) Diagnostic accuracy of ACR/EULAR 2010 criteria for rheumatoid arthritis in a 2-year cohort. J Rheumatol 2011;38: 1250–1257.
16. Kaneko y, Kuwana M, Kamed H, Takeuchi T (2011) Sensitivity and specificity of 2010 rheumatoid arthritis classification criteria. Rheumatology (Oxford) 50: 1268–1274.
17. Cornec D, Varache S, Morvan J, Devauchelle-Pensec V, Berthelot JM, et al. (2012) Comparison of the 1987 ACR criteria for predicting a 10-year diagnosis of rheumatoid arthritis. Joint Bone Spine doi:10.1016/j.jbspin.2012.01.015.
18. Moher D, Liberati A, Tetzlaff J, Altman DG, the PRISMA group (2009) Preferred reporting items for systematic reviews and meta-analyses: the PRISMA statement. J Clin Epidemiol 62: 1006–1012.
19. Leeflang MM, Scholten RJ, Rutjes AW, Reitsma JB, Bossuyt PM (2006) Use of methodological search filters to identify diagnostic accuracy studies can lead to the omission of relevant studies. J Clin Epidemiol 59: 234–240.
20. Reitsma JB, Rutjes AWS, Whiting P, Vlassov VV, Leeflang MMG, et al. (2009) Chapter 9: Assessing methodological quality. In: Deeks JJ, Bossuyt PM, Gatsonis C (editors), *Cochrane Handbook for Systematic Reviews of Diagnostic Test Accuracy* Version 1.0.0. The Cochrane Collaboration. Available from: http://srdta.cochrane.org/.
21. Dinnes J, Deeks J, Kirby J, Roderick P (2005) A methodological review of how heterogeneity has been examined in systematic reviews of diagnostic test accuracy. Health Technology Assess 9: 1–113.
22. Harbord RM, Deeks JJ, Egger M, Whiting P, Sterne JA (2007) A unification of models for meta-analysis of diagnostic accuracy studies. Biostatistics 8: 239–251.
23. Harbord RM, Whiting P (2009) metandi: Meta-analysis of diagnostic accuracy using hierarchical logistic regression. Stata J 9: 211–229.
24. Reitsma H (2011) Meta-analysis of diagnostic accuracy data. Diagnostic test accuracy author training, Amsterdam, 2011. http://srdta.cochrane.org/sites/srdta.cochrane.org/files/uploads/10_Stat_Methods_2011.pdf.
25. Alves C, Luime JJ, van Zeben D, Huisman A, Weel AEAM, et al. (2011) Diagnostic performance of the ACR/EULAR 2010 criteria for rheumatoid arthritis and two diagnostic algorithms in an early arthritis clinic (REACH). Ann Rheum Dis 70: 1645–1647.
26. Britsemmer K, Ursum J, Gerritsen M, van Tuyl L, van Schaardenburg D (2011) Validation of the 2010 ACR/EULAR classification criteria for rheumatoid arthritis: slight improvement over the 1987 ACR criteria. Ann Rheum Dis 70: 1468–1470.
27. Kawashiri SY, Suzuki T, Okada A, Yamasaki S, Tamai M, et al. (2013) Musculoskeletal ultrasonography assists the diagnostic performance of the 2010 classification criteria for rheumatoid arthritis. Mod Rheumatol 23: 36–43.
28. van der Linden MM, Knevel R, Huizinga TWJ, van der Helm-van Mil AHM (2011) Classification of rheumatoid arthritis. Comparison of the 1987 America College of Rheumatology criteria and the 2010 American College of Rheumatology/American League Against Rheumatism Criteria. Arthritis Rheum 63: 37–42.
29. Berglin EH, Rantapaa-Dahlqvist SM (2011) Comparison of the 1987 ACR and 2010 ACR/EULAR Classification Criteria for Rheumatoid Arthritis in Clinical Practice. Arthritis Rheum 63 (S10): S117.
30. Nakagomi D, Ikeda K, Okubo A, Iwamoto T, Suzuki Y, et al. (2012) Ultrasonographic assessment of synovitis improves the accuracy of 2010 America College of Rheumatology/American League against rheumatism classification criteria for rheumatoid arthritis to predict development of a methotrexate-requiring disease. Ann Rheum Dis 71 (S3): 98.
31. Sakellariou G, Scirè CA, Montecucco C, Caporali R (2012) Diagnostic performance of the 2010 ACR/EULAR classification criteria for rheumatoid arthritis in a cohort of early arthritis. Ann Rheum Dis 71 (S3): 334.
32. Tamai M, Arima K, Uetani M, Iwamoto N, Kita J, et al. (2011) Evaluation of the Patients with Early Arthritis by 2010 RA Criteria in Conjunction with MRI of Wrists and Finger Joints. Arthritis Rheum 63 (S10): 318.
33. Chitale S, Goodson NJ, Sharpley DW, Thompson RL, Moots RJ, et al. (2010) New 2010 ACR-EULAR rheumatoid arthritis classification criteria are highly sensitive in patients with early rheumatoid arthritis. Arthritis Rheum 62 (S10): S733.
34. Jaeschke R, Guyatt G, Lijmer J (2002) Diagnostic tests. In: Guyatt G, Rennie D editors. User's guides to the medical literature. Chicago: AMA press, 121–140.
35. Lijmer JG, Mol BW, Heisterkamp S, Bonsel GJ, Prins MH, et al. (1999) Empirical evidence of design-related bias in studies of diagnostic tests. JAMA 282: 1061–1066.

17

Accelerated Development of Cervical Spine Instabilities in Rheumatoid Arthritis: A Prospective Minimum 5-Year Cohort Study

Takashi Yurube[1], Masatoshi Sumi[2]*, Kotaro Nishida[1], Hiroshi Miyamoto[3], Kozo Kohyama[4], Tsukasa Matsubara[5], Yasushi Miura[1], Hiroaki Hirata[1], Daisuke Sugiyama[6], Minoru Doita[1]

1 Department of Orthopaedic Surgery, Kobe University Graduate School of Medicine, Chuo-ku, Kobe, Japan, **2** Department of Orthopaedic Surgery, Kobe Rosai Hospital, Chuo-ku, Kobe, Japan, **3** Department of Orthopaedic Surgery, Kobe Medical Center, Suma-ku, Kobe, Japan, **4** Department of Orthopaedic Surgery, Kohnan Kakogawa Hospital, Kanno-cho, Kakogawa, Japan, **5** Department of Orthopaedic Surgery, Matsubara Mayflower Hospital, Fujita, Kato, Japan, **6** Department of Evidence-Based Laboratory Medicine, Kobe University Graduate School of Medicine, Chuo-ku, Kobe, Japan

Abstract

Objective: To clarify the incidence and predictive risk factors of cervical spine instabilities which may induce compression myelopathy in patients with rheumatoid arthritis (RA).

Methods: Three types of cervical spine instability were radiographically categorized into "moderate" and "severe" based on atlantoaxial subluxation (AAS: atlantodental interval >3 mm versus ≥10 mm), vertical subluxation (VS: Ranawat value < 13 mm versus ≤10 mm), and subaxial subluxation (SAS: irreducible translation ≥2 mm versus ≥4 mm or at multiple). 228 "definite" or "classical" RA patients (140 without instability and 88 with "moderate" instability) were prospectively followed for >5 years. The endpoint incidence of "severe" instabilities and predictors for "severe" instability were determined.

Results: Patients with baseline "moderate" instability, including all sub-groups (AAS^+ [VS^- SAS^-], VS^+ [SAS^- $AAS^\pm$], and SAS^+ [$AAS^\pm$ $VS^\pm$]), developed "severe" instabilities more frequently (33.3% with AAS^+, 75.0% with VS^+, and 42.9% with SAS^+) than those initially without instability (12.9%; $p<0.003$, $p<0.003$, and $p=0.061$, respectively). The incidence of cervical canal stenosis and/or basilar invagination was also higher in patients with initial instability (17.5% with AAS^+, 37.5% with VS^+, and 14.3% with SAS^+) than in those without instability (7.1%; $p=0.028$, $p<0.003$, and $p=0.427$, respectively). Multivariable logistic regression analysis identified corticosteroid administration, Steinbrocker stage III or IV at baseline, mutilating changes at baseline, and the development of mutilans during the follow-up period correlated with the progression to "severe" instability ($p<0.05$).

Conclusions: This prospective cohort study demonstrates accelerated development of cervical spine involvement in RA patients with pre-existing instability—especially VS. Advanced peripheral erosiveness and concomitant corticosteroid treatment are indicators for poor prognosis of the cervical spine in RA.

Editor: Chi Zhang, University of Texas Southwestern Medical Center, United States of America

Funding: The authors have no support or funding to report.

Competing Interests: The authors have declared that no competing interests exist.

* E-mail: sumim@kobeh.rofuku.go.jp

Introduction

Rheumatoid arthritis (RA) is a chronic inflammatory disease, which affects 0.5–1% of the adult population [1]. The cervical spine is a popular focus of RA synovitis and enthesitis [2]. Rheumatoid arthritis often causes three characteristic instabilities in the cervical spine: atlantoaxial subluxation (AAS) [3–11], vertical subluxation (VS) of the axis [12–14], and subaxial subluxation (SAS) [15]. These subluxations should be noted as one of the most serious pathologies in patients with RA since they can introduce irreversible neural impairment, non-ambulation, respiratory dysfunction, or sudden death [16]. However, the prevalence of cervical spine instabilities which may lead to complications has not been fully profiled. Predictive risk factors for severe aggravation have not been comprehensively evaluated. While many studies have investigated the progression of instabilities retrospectively, limited prospective studies have been published [7,8,10,17–22].

We previously presented a prospective multicenter cohort study for the cervical spine in established RA patients [23,24]. The first study described the progression of instabilities, but not of lesions with impending neurological deficit [23]. The second study aimed to identify predictors for the aggravation of instabilities; however, this had limited inclusion criteria, small sample size, and did not provide conclusive evidence [24]. Thus, the hypothesis-generating data from these two studies revealed the necessity of larger-scale, more comprehensive studies for the development of instabilities which may induce compression myelopathy and their predictive factors. Therefore, in the current study, we examined the >5-year incidence of myelopathy-inducing cervical spine subluxations in 228 known RA patients. Various predictors were analyzed using multivariable logistic regression. The objective of this study was to elucidate the prognosis of the cervical spine in patients with RA.

Materials And Methods

Ethics Statement

This prospective cohort study was conducted at 21 investigation sites (Himeji St. Mary's Hospital, Himeji; Hyogo Prefectural Awaji Hospital, Awaji; Hyogo Prefectural Kakogawa Hospital, Kakogawa; Hyogo Prefectural Nishinomiya Hospital, Nishinomiya; Hyogo Rehabilitation Center, Kobe; Kakogawa City Hospital, Kakogawa; Kanzaki General Hospital, Kanzaki; Kasai City Hospital, Kasai; Kobe Century Memorial Hospital, Kobe; Kobe Medical Center, Kobe; Kobe Rosai Hospital, Kobe; Kobe University Hospital, Kobe; Kohnan Hospital, Kobe; Kohnan Kakogawa Hospital, Kakogawa; Matsubara Mayflower Hospital, Kato; Miki City Hospital, Miki; Miki Sanyo Hospital, Miki; Rokko Island Hospital, Kobe; Saiseikai Hyogoken Hospital, Kobe; Sanda City Hospital, Sanda; and Takasago City Hospital, Takasago, all located in Japan). The study protocol was approved by the institutional review board at each facility. Written informed consent was obtained from each patient. The study was conducted in concordance with the principles of the Declaration of Helsinki and with the laws and regulations of Japan.

Patients

Between 2001 and 2002, in 21 facilities, 634 outpatients who fulfilled the American Rheumatism Association 1958 criteria for "definite" or "classical" RA [25] and the American College of Rheumatology 1987 revised criteria for RA [26] were enrolled in our study [23,24]. Cervical radiographs were taken at baseline, and three types of cervical spine instability were categorized into two levels of severity; "moderate" and "severe" criteria were applied as described below. Five hundred and three of 634 cases were identified as patients initially without instability or with "moderate" instability. Between 2006 and 2008, 223 of 503 cases were prospectively followed as outpatients every three months and radiographically reassessed at >5-year follow-up. Additionally, five patients underwent cervical spine surgery for myelopathy during the follow-up period; the last pre-operative radiographs and clinical data were used for evaluation. Therefore, the current study population consisted of the total 228 of 503 patients without any "severe" category of pre-existing cervical spine instability (45.3%) with a mean follow-up period of 6.0±0.8 years. The profile of the cohort and its surgical incidence is shown in **Figure 1**. All data from this study is included in the article.

Radiographic evaluation

Lateral cervical radiographs, obtained in full-flexion, neutral, and full-extension positions with the standardized protocol (exposure time 80 msec; distance 150 cm; current 250 mA; voltage 72 kV), were used for evaluating cervical spine instability. Cervical radiographs were measured twice at one-week intervals by each of four rheumatologists who were not associated with clinical follow-up of the patients, and the presence of instabilities was determined using the average length of measured values.

Instability was defined as AAS in patients with the anterior atlantodental interval (ADI) >3 mm [3,4], VS in patients with the Ranawat value <13 mm [12], and SAS in patients with irreducible vertebral translation ≥2 mm without osteophyte formation [15].

"Severe" instability, which indicates impending neurological deficit, was defined as AAS in patients with ADI ≥10 mm [10], VS in patients with Ranawat value ≤10 mm [16,27,28], and SAS in patients with irreducible translation ≥4 mm or ≥2 mm at multiple levels [15,29].

"Moderate" instability was defined in patients with instability who did not meet the "severe" criteria.

Cervical canal stenosis, which is severe enough to induce compression myelopathy, was identified in patients with space available for the spinal cord (SAC) (also called the posterior ADI) ≤13 mm due to "severe" AAS or "severe" VS at C1–C2 level [30] or SAC ≤12 mm due to "severe" SAS at C2–C7 levels [31].

Basilar invagination, which may compress the brainstem and result in life-threatening symptoms, was recognized in patients with the tip of the odontoid process above the McRae line due to "severe" VS [32].

Bilateral hand radiographs were used for classifying the severity of peripheral joint destruction into five categories: Steinbrocker classification stages I–IV [33] and mutilating changes [34,35]. Mutilating changes were defined in patients with three or more "mutilans fingers [34]" as previously established [35]. Patients with the development of stages I–IV into mutilating changes during the follow-up period were separately categorized. Steinbrocker stages and mutilating changes were decided by accepting the majority decision of three rheumatologists blinded to the research purpose.

Clinical evaluation

Patient age (<55 [11,15] and ≥65 [36] years), sex (male [6,9]), the duration of RA (≥15 years [11]), and previous joint surgery for RA [14,22,37,38] were recorded at baseline. In addition, each patient's follow-up period was compared with the mean duration of 6.0 years.

C-reactive protein (CRP) level was quantified at baseline and assessed whether ≥3.8 mg/dl, a reported average value in RA patients with myelopathic deterioration [39].

Rheumatoid factor (RF) was measured at baseline and positivity was assessed [6,8,11,40].

At baseline, patients received intensive use of disease modifying anti-rheumatic drugs (DMARDs): methotrexate (MTX) (≤8 mg/week), salazosulfapyridine (≤1,000 mg/day), D-penicillamine (≤100 mg/day), or intramuscular gold (≤25 mg/2 weeks). Afterward, MTX, approved for RA since 1999 in Japan, rapidly replaced other DMARDs. Oral corticosteroids were allowed to relieve RA symptoms (≤10 mg/day prednisolone). In more aggressive cases, biologic therapies—infliximab (3 mg/kg/8 weeks), etanercept (10–25 mg/twice a week), adalimumab (40 mg/2 weeks), or tocillizumab (8 mg/kg/4 weeks)—were applied. Patients were categorized based on drug administration at baseline and through more than half of the follow-up period. Since no biologic agent was approved for RA until 2003, patients who had biologic administration for more than half of the follow-up period were similarly identified.

Statistical analysis

Patients were divided into four groups based on pre-existing cervical spine involvement: no instability, "moderate" AAS alone (shown as AAS^{+}), "moderate" VS without SAS but with or without AAS (shown as VS^{+}), and "moderate" SAS with and/or without either AAS and/or VS (shown as SAS^{+}). To elucidate the influence of baseline instability on the development of cervical spine involvement in RA, the >5-year incidence of the progression of prior instabilities and/or the development of additional instabilities including "severe" instabilities, canal stenosis, and

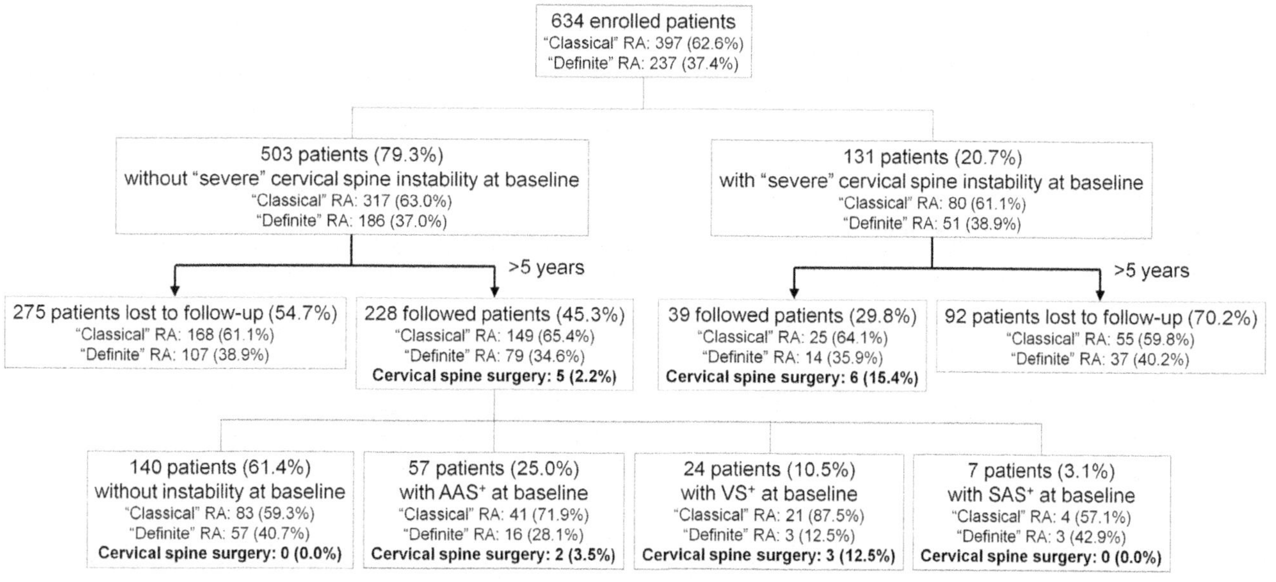

Figure 1. Numbers of patients enrolled, followed, and lost to follow-up with the baseline proportion of "classical" and "definite" rheumatoid arthritis (RA) in the American Rheumatism Association 1958 criteria and the >5-year incidence of cervical spine surgery for myelopathy. Patients were grouped by the type of pre-existing cervical spine involvement: no instability, atlantoaxial subluxation (AAS) alone (shown as AAS$^+$), vertical subluxation (VS) without subaxial subluxation (SAS) but with or without AAS (shown as VS$^+$), and SAS with and/or without either AAS and/or VS (shown as SAS$^+$) and by the level of severity—"moderate" and "severe".

basilar invagination for each group was compared. Distributions of parameters for cervical spine involvement and of RA stages and mutilating changes were compared between baseline and >5-year follow-up. The χ^2 test, Fisher exact test, paired t-test, or Wilcoxon signed-rank test was used. In addition, intra-class correlation coefficient or κ coefficient was calculated to determine intra- and inter-observer reliabilities for the measurement of radiographic parameters.

Multivariable logistic regression analysis was performed to identify independent predictive risk factors for "severe" instability. Baseline and >5-year differences associated with an increased risk of cervical spine involvement in RA were compared between patients who developed "severe" instabilities versus those who did not; the χ^2 test, Fisher exact test, Student t-test, or Welch t-test was used. Variables eligible for inclusion in the multivariable models had p values of <0.20 in the univariable analyses and were clinically and/or biologically plausible as described previously [41]. In the multivariable models, the goodness of fit was assessed by the Hosmer-Lemeshow test and the discriminatory ability was assessed by the c-statistic [42]. A random classifier has the c-statistic of 0.5. The c-statistic for a perfect classifier is equal to 1, representing 100% sensitivity (0% false negative rate) and 100% specificity (0% false positive rate). In the present analysis, the false positive rate indicates the percentage of patients with identified predictive factors but without the development of "severe" instabilities. The false negative rate indicates the percentage of patients without the predictors but with "severe" instabilities at > 5-year follow-up.

Data analyses were performed with PASW Statistics 18 (SPSS, Chicago, IL). All statistical tests were two-sided. Statistical significance was assessed with $p<0.05$ and $p<0.01$. When the incidence of cervical spine lesions was compared between patients with AAS$^+$, VS$^+$, or SAS$^+$ and those without instability at baseline, the Bonferroni adjustment to the threshold for significance was performed; therefore, statistical significance was evaluated with $p<0.05/3=0.017$ and $p<0.01/3=0.003$.

Results

Baseline radiographic analysis of the cervical spine identified that 228 patients consisted of 140 without any instability, 57 with AAS$^+$, 24 with VS$^+$, and 7 with SAS$^+$. Baseline demographics and disease characteristics of the patients are shown in **Table S1**. There were no significant differences in these variables between 21 investigation sites.

In radiographic measurements, intra-observer reliabilities for parametric ADI, Ranawat value, SAC, and subaxial translation were 0.90–0.94, 0.80–0.85, 0.89–0.95, and 0.81–0.84 by intra-class correlation coefficient. Inter-observer reliabilities were 0.95, 0.90, 0.94, and 0.91. Intra-observer reliabilities for non-parametric basilar invagination and RA stages with mutilating changes were 0.79–0.83 and 0.74–0.79 by κ coefficient. Inter-observer reliabilities were 0.87 and 0.86. All the values indicated an acceptable reproducibility.

Incidence of cervical spine instabilities and "severe" cervical spine instabilities

To understand the total incidence of cervical spine subluxations, we investigated the incidence of instabilities which consisted of "moderate" and "severe" categories. Then, to clarify the incidence of compression myelopathy-inducing subluxations, we examined the incidence of "severe" instabilities. Forty-three point six percent of 140 patients without cervical spine instability at baseline developed instabilities at >5-year follow-up: AAS in 32.1%, VS in 11.4%, and SAS in 16.4% with some combinations. Furthermore, 12.9% of patients initially without instability presented with "severe" instabilities—"severe" AAS in 3.6%, "severe" VS in 6.4%, and "severe" SAS in 5.0% (**Table 1**).

Fifty-seven patients with AAS$^+$ at baseline developed VS in 22.8% at >5-year follow-up, which was higher than those without instability at baseline (11.4%) with a trend toward significance ($p=0.041$). Moreover, 33.3% of patients initially with AAS$^+$ exhibited "severe" instabilities at a significantly higher rate than

Table 1. Incidence of cervical spine instabilities and "severe" cervical spine instabilities at >5-year follow-up in 228 patients without "severe" cervical spine instability at baseline.

	Cervical spine involvement at baseline				
Cervical spine involvement at >5-year follow-up	No instability (n = 140)	AAS⁺ (n = 57)	VS⁺ (n = 24)	SAS⁺ (n = 7)	Total (n = 228)
Total instability, no. (%)*	61 (43.6)	57 (100.0)††	24 (100.0)††	7 (100.0)†	149 (65.4)
"Moderate" or "severe" AAS, no. (%)	45 (32.1)	56 (98.2)††	18 (75.0)††	4 (57.1)	123 (53.9)
"Moderate" or "severe" VS, no. (%)	16 (11.4)	13 (22.8)$^{p=0.041}$	24 (100.0)††	2 (28.6)	55 (24.1)
"Moderate" or "severe" SAS, no. (%)	23 (16.4)	12 (21.1)	10 (41.7)†	7 (100.0)††	52 (22.8)
"Severe" instability, no. (%)*	18 (12.9)	19 (33.3)††	18 (75.0)††	3 (42.9)	58 (25.4)
"Severe" AAS, no. (%)	5 (3.6)	11 (19.3)††	3 (12.5)	0 (0.0)	19 (8.3)
"Severe" VS, no. (%)	9 (6.4)	4 (7.0)	17 (70.8)††	2 (28.6)	32 (14.0)
"Severe" SAS, no. (%)	7 (5.0)	6 (10.5)	5 (20.8)$^{p=0.017}$	2 (28.6)	20 (8.8)

Patients were grouped by pre-existing cervical spine involvement: no instability, "moderate" atlantoaxial subluxation (AAS) alone (shown as AAS⁺), "moderate" vertical subluxation (VS) without subaxial subluxation (SAS) but with or without AAS (shown as VS⁺), and "moderate" SAS with and/or without either AAS and/or VS (shown as SAS⁺).
*Including patients fulfilling multiple criteria.
†$p<0.05/3=0.017$, ††$p<0.01/3=0.003$ when compared to the incidence in patients initially without instability by the χ^2 test or Fisher exact test with the Bonferroni adjustment to the threshold for significance.

that of patients initially without instability (12.9%; p<0.003)—especially "severe" AAS in 19.3% (versus 3.6%; p<0.003) (**Table 1**)

In 24 patients with VS⁺ at baseline, the >5-year incidence of SAS was 41.7%, which was significantly higher than in those without instability at baseline (16.4%; p = 0.010). "Severe" instabilities were developed in 75.0% of patients initially with VS⁺, also more frequently than those initially without instability (12.9%; p<0.003)—notably "severe" VS in 70.8% (versus 6.4%; p<0.003). In addition, the incidence of "severe" SAS in 20.8% of patients with baseline VS⁺ was higher than in those without baseline instability (5.0%), and trended toward significance (p = 0.017) (**Table 1**).

Of seven patients with SAS⁺ at baseline, 42.9% developed "severe" instabilities at >5-year follow-up, which was higher than that of patients without instability at baseline (12.9%) although the comparison did not reach significance (p = 0.061). "Severe" VS occurred in 28.6% of patients initially with SAS⁺ (versus 6.4% of those initially without instability; p = 0.087). "Severe" SAS appeared in 28.6% of patients with baseline SAS⁺ (versus 5.0% of those without baseline instability; p = 0.060) (**Table 1**).

In distributions of radiographic parameters, the ADI significantly increased during >5 years only in patients initially without instability and those with AAS⁺ (p<0.01 for both groups). The Ranawat value decreased in all patient groups (p<0.01 for patients without instability, with AAS⁺, and with VS⁺ and p = 0.04 for those with SAS⁺) (**Figure 2**).

Incidence of cervical canal stenosis and basilar invagination

While 4.3% of patients without baseline instability developed cervical canal stenosis with decreased SAC (SAC ≤13 mm at C1–C2 in 2.9% and SAC ≤12 mm at C2–C7 in 2.1%), 15.8% of those with baseline AAS⁺ exhibited stenosis (p = 0.014)—particularly SAC ≤13 mm at C1–C2 in 10.5% (p = 0.036). Patients with baseline VS⁺ presented with cervical stenosis in 16.7% (p = 0.041) who all showed SAC ≤13 mm at C1–C2 (p = 0.017). Patients with baseline SAS⁺ developed stenosis in 14.3% (p = 0.295) who demonstrated SAC ≤12 mm at C2–C7 (p = 0.179) (**Table 2**).

Basilar invagination with cranial migration of the odontoid tip was detected in 2.9% of patients initially without instability whereas it was found in 33.3% of those initially with VS⁺ (p< 0.003) and 5.3% of those with AAS⁺ (p = 0.415) (**Table 2**).

Therefore, the >5-year incidence of cervical canal stenosis and/or basilar invagination, which may fully progress to myelopathy and/or brainstem symptoms, was higher in patients with baseline instability (17.5% in those with AAS⁺, 37.5% in those with VS⁺, and 14.3% in those with SAS⁺) than in patients without instability (7.1%; p = 0.028, p<0.003, and p = 0.427, respectively) (**Table 2**).

In distributions of radiographic parameters, the SAC at C1–C2 significantly decreased during >5 years in every patient group (p< 0.01 for patients without instability, with AAS⁺, and with VS⁺ and p = 0.04 for those with SAS⁺) (**Figure 2**).

Predictive risk factors for the development of "severe" cervical spine instabilities

Radiographic cervical spine analysis at baseline and at >5-year follow-up identified the development of "severe" instabilities in 58 of 228 patients (25.4%), as summarized in **Table 1**. Radiographic peripheral assessment disclosed a significant shift in the distribution of RA stages and mutilating changes (p<0.01). Patients with stage I or II decreased from 49 (21.5%) to 18 (7.9%; p<0.01) while those with stage III or IV increased from 162 (71.1%) to 182 (79.8%; p = 0.03) and those with mutilating changes increased from 17 (7.5%) to 28 (12.3%; p = 0.08). Eleven patients (4.8%) initially with stages I–IV developed mutilating changes during the follow-up period. Baseline and >5-year demographics and disease characteristics in patients who developed "severe" instabilities and those who did not develop are shown in **Table 3**.

In the univariable analysis, previous joint surgery, CRP ≥ 3.8 mg/dl, corticosteroid administration, Steinbrocker stage III or IV at baseline (without the development of mutilating changes during the follow-up period), mutilating changes at baseline, and the development of stages I–IV into mutilating changes during the

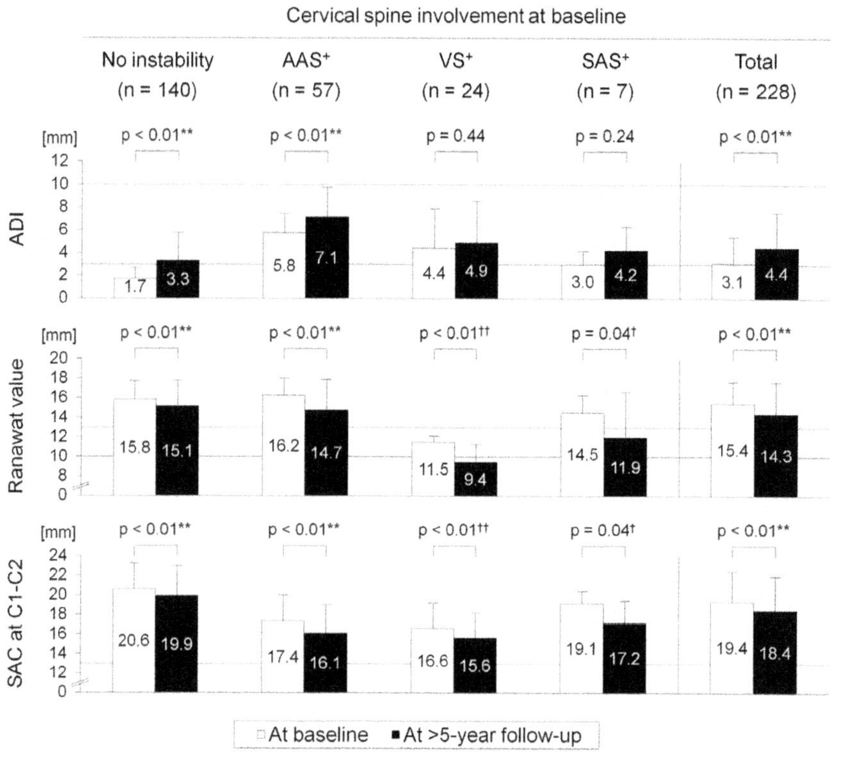

Figure 2. Baseline and >5-year distributions of radiographic parameters for upper cervical spine involvement, the atlantodental interval (ADI), Ranawat value, and space available for the spinal cord (SAC) at C1–C2, in 228 patients without "severe" cervical spine instability at baseline. Patients were grouped by pre-existing cervical spine involvement: no instability, "moderate" atlantoaxial subluxation (AAS) alone (shown as AAS$^+$), "moderate" vertical subluxation (VS) without subaxial subluxation (SAS) but with or without AAS (shown as VS$^+$), and "moderate" SAS with and/or without either AAS and/or VS (shown as SAS$^+$). Data are expressed as mean ± standard deviation. **$p<0.01$ by the paired t-test. $^\dagger p<0.05$, $^{\dagger\dagger}p<0.01$ by the Wilcoxon signed-rank test because of the small number of cases.

follow-up period were statistically significant for the development of "severe" cervical spine instabilities at >5-year follow-up ($p<0.05$) (**Table 4**). Rheumatoid factor positive was not significant for "severe" instability with p of <0.20. Methotrexate, other DMARDs, and biologic agent administration was not statistically significant with p of ≥0.20 but was thought to be clinically and biologically relevant in the progression of rheumatoid involvement.

Table 2. Incidence of cervical canal stenosis and basilar invagination at >5-year follow-up in 228 patients without "severe" cervical spine instability at baseline.

	Cervical spine involvement at baseline				
	No instability (n = 140)	AAS$^+$ (n = 57)	VS$^+$ (n = 24)	SAS$^+$ (n = 7)	Total (n = 228)
Cervical spine involvement at >5-year follow-up					
Cervical canal stenosis, no. (%)*	6 (4.3)	9 (15.8)†	4 (16.7)$^{P=0.041}$	1 (14.3)	20 (8.8)
SAC ≤13 mm at C1–C2, no. (%)	4 (2.9)	6 (10.5)$^{P=0.036}$	4 (16.7)$^{P=0.017}$	0 (0.0)	14 (6.1)
SAC ≤12 mm at C2–C7, no. (%)	3 (2.1)	4 (7.0)	2 (8.3)	1 (14.3)	10 (4.4)
Basilar invagination, no. (%)	4 (2.9)	3 (5.3)	8 (33.3)††	0 (0.0)	26 (11.4)
Cervical canal stenosis and/or basilar invagination, no. (%)*	10 (7.1)	10 (17.5)$^{P=0.028}$	9 (37.5)††	1 (14.3)	30 (13.2)

Patients were grouped by pre-existing cervical spine involvement: no instability, "moderate" atlantoaxial subluxation (AAS) alone (shown as AAS$^+$), "moderate" vertical subluxation (VS) without subaxial subluxation (SAS) but with or without AAS (shown as VS$^+$), and "moderate" SAS with and/or without either AAS and/or VS (shown as SAS$^+$).

*Including patients fulfilling multiple criteria.

$^\dagger p<0.05/3=0.017$, $^{\dagger\dagger}p<0.01/3=0.003$ when compared to the incidence in patients initially without instability by the χ^2 test or Fisher exact test with the Bonferroni adjustment to the threshold for significance.

SAC, space available for the spinal cord.

Table 3. Baseline and >5-year demographics and disease characteristics in 228 patients with and without "severe" cervical spine instability at >5-year follow-up.

	Patients with "severe" cervical spine instability (n = 58)	Patients without "severe" cervical spine instability (n = 170)	p Value*
At baseline			
Demographics and clinical characteristics			
Age, mean ± SD years	61.4±9.3	60.6±10.8	0.62
<55, no. (%)	17 (29.3)	50 (29.4)	0.80
55–64, no. (%)	15 (25.9.)	51 (30.0)	
≥65, no. (%)	26 (44.8)	69 (40.6)	
Male sex, no. (%)	11 (19.0)	34 (20.0)	0.86
RA duration, mean ± SD years	14.0±9.5	12.9±11.0	0.52
≥15, no. (%)	21 (36.2)	47 (27.6)	0.22
Previous joint surgery, no. (%)	36 (62.1)	60 (35.3)	<0.01[††]
CRP, mean ± SD mg/dl	2.5±1.9	1.5±1.8	<0.01[††]
≥3.8, no. (%)	14 (24.1)	20 (11.8)	0.02[†]
RF positive, no. (%)	50 (86.2)	131 (77.1)	0.14
Medications			
Corticosteroids, no. (%)	49 (84.5)	89 (52.4)	<0.01[††]
MTX, no. (%)	30 (51.7)	78 (45.9)	0.44
Other DMARDs, no. (%)	28 (48.3)	90 (52.9)	0.54
RA stages and mutilating changes			
Stage I or II, no. (%)	4 (6.9)	45 (26.5)	<0.01[††]
Stage III or IV, no. (%)	43 (74.1)	119 (70.0)	
Mutilating changes, no. (%)	11 (19.0)	6 (3.5)	
At >5-year follow-up			
Demographics and clinical characteristics			
Follow-up period, mean ± SD years	5.9±1.2	6.1±0.6	0.371
≥6.0, no. (%)	30 (51.7%)	96 (56.5%)	0.53
Medications			
Biologic agents, no. (%)	4 (6.9)	6 (3.5)	0.28
RA stages and mutilating changes			
Development of stages I–IV into mutilating changes, no. (%)	7 (12.1)	4 (2.4)	<0.01[††]

*Tested by the χ^2 test, Fisher exact test, Student t-test, or Welch t-test.
[†]p<0.05. [††]p<0.01.
CRP, C-reactive protein; DMARD, disease modifying anti-rheumatic drug; MTX, methotrexate; RA, rheumatoid arthritis; RF, rheumatoid factor; SD, standard deviation.

In the multivariable analysis, we established a multivariable logistic regression model including the variables described above (**Table 4**). This multivariable model identified four variables as significant predictive risk factors for the progression to "severe" instability: corticosteroid administration (odds ratio [OR] 4.65, 95% confidence interval [95% CI] 1.98–10.91, p<0.01), Steinbrocker stage III or IV at baseline (OR 3.65, 95% CI 1.02–13.13, p = 0.047), mutilating changes at baseline (OR 21.23, 95% CI 3.97–113.57, p<0.01), and the development of stages I–IV into mutilating changes during the follow-up period (OR 13.44, 95% CI 2.24–80.55, p<0.01). The high ORs of pre-existing mutilating changes, new development of mutilating changes, and then established Steinbrocker stage III or IV suggest a direct association of the severity of peripheral erosions with the development of cervical spine instabilities in RA patients. Accordingly, the high OR of the administration of corticosteroids could be explained by concomitant severe disease activity. Previous joint surgery was not significant but showed a weak correlation (OR 1.93, 95% CI 0.95–3.90, p = 0.07). As the ORs of the presence of surgically treated joints, high CRP, and positive RF were modest, these factors would be supportive, but not strong enough to estimate RA severity in the cervical spine. The administration of MTX, other DMARDs, and biologic agents did not show a strong association with the development of "severe" instabilities in this study. This model had a good predictive ability, with the c-statistic of 0.80.

To reduce the risk for overfitting variables [43], we designed an additional multivariable model based on backward stepwise variable selection (**Table 4**). This multivariable model also detected the same four significant variables: corticosteroid administration (OR 4.57, 95% CI 1.98–10.53, p<0.01), stage III or IV at baseline (OR 3.92, 95% CI 1.11–13.81, p = 0.03), mutilating changes at baseline (OR 23.29, 95% CI 4.51–120.34, p<0.01), and the development of stages I–IV into mutilating changes during the follow-up period (OR 14.65, 95% CI 2.56–83.88, p<0.01). Previous joint surgery was marginally significant

Table 4. Odds ratios (ORs), 95% confidence intervals (95% CIs), and p values for "severe" cervical spine instability by univariable and multivariable logistic regression analyses.

	Univariable analysis		Multivariable analysis*		Stepwise multivariable analysis**	
	OR (95% CI)	p Value	Adjusted OR (95% CI)	p Value	Adjusted OR (95% CI)	p Value
Demographics and clinical characteristics						
<55 years old	1.16 (0.52–2.56)	0.72	Not included		Not included	
≥65 years old	1.28 (0.62–2.66)	0.51	Not included		Not included	
Male sex	0.94 (0.44–1.99)	0.86	Not included		Not included	
RA duration ≥15 years	1.49 (0.79–2.80)	0.22	Not included		Not included	
Previous joint surgery	3.00 (1.62–5.56)	<0.01††	1.93 (0.95–3.90)	0.07	1.89 (0.96–3.75)	0.07
CRP ≥3.8 mg/dl	2.39 (1.11–5.11)	0.03†	1.37 (0.57–3.27)	0.48	Not included	
RF positive	1.86 (0.81–4.26)	0.14	1.26 (0.50–3.14)	0.62	Not included	
Follow-up period ≥6.0 years	0.83 (0.45–1.50)	0.53	Not included		Not included	
Medications						
Corticosteroids	4.96 (2.29–10.72)	<0.01††	4.65 (1.98–10.91)	<0.01††	4.57 (1.98–10.53)	<0.01††
MTX	1.26 (0.70–2.30)	0.44	0.70 (0.30–1.63)	0.41	Not included	
Other DMARDs	0.83 (0.46–1.51)	0.54	0.81 (0.36–1.82)	0.62	Not included	
Biologic agents	2.02 (0.55–7.44)	0.29	1.04 (0.23–4.60)	0.96	Not included	
RA stages and mutilating changes						
Stage III or IV at baseline (without the development of mutilating changes)	4.83 (1.42–16.45)	0.012†	3.65 (1.02–13.13)	0.047†	3.92 (1.11–13.81)	0.03†
Mutilating changes at baseline	27.50 (5.93–127.60)	<0.01††	21.23 (3.97–113.57)	<0.01††	23.29 (4.51–120.34)	<0.01††
Development of stages I–IV into mutilating changes	26.25 (4.82–143.06)	<0.01††	13.44 (2.24–80.55)	<0.01††	14.65 (2.56–83.88)	<0.01††

*The Hosmer-Lemeshow goodness-of-fit χ^2 p = 0.85 (8 degrees of freedom) and the c-statistic for the model = 0.80.
**The Hosmer-Lemeshow goodness-of-fit χ^2 p = 0.93 (7 degrees of freedom) and the c-statistic for the model = 0.79.
†p<0.05. ††p<0.01.
CRP, C-reactive protein; DMARD, disease modifying anti-rheumatic drug; MTX, methotrexate; RA, rheumatoid arthritis; RF, rheumatoid factor.

(OR 1.89, 95% CI 0.96–3.75, p = 0.07). This model also had an acceptable predictive ability, with the c-statistic of 0.79.

Discussion

In the current study, we assessed and compared the >5-year incidence of cervical spine instabilities with impending neurological deficit in 228 established RA patients with and without baseline instability, which demonstrated that the development of these serious lesions was accelerated in response to the type of baseline cervical spine instability—especially VS. Multivariable logistic regression analysis identified advanced peripheral erosiveness, concomitant corticosteroid treatment, and marginally previous joint surgery as independent risk factors for the development of severe cervical spine instabilities in RA. This study clarifies these clinically important findings with statistically robust, more conclusive evidence, which provides a comprehensive understanding of the progression of cervical spine involvement in patients with RA.

The incidence of cervical spine instabilities depends on the diagnostic criteria for subluxation and the severity of RA. In this study, we used previously validated criteria [24] and enrolled patients with "definite" or "classical" RA only. During 6.0±0.8 years, 43.6% of patients without pre-existing cervical spine instability developed instabilities. Patients initially without instability further developed "severe" instabilities in 12.9% and canal stenosis and/or basilar invagination in 7.1%. The detailed occurrence rate and pattern of each lesion were described in our previous report [24]. The observed percentage of patients who developed instabilities at endpoint is comparable to the previously reported incidence of instabilities in patients with long-standing RA (46.7%) in a mean 6.1-year follow-up study [17]. This supports that our diagnostic criteria and radiographic measurement are acceptable for the assessment of patients with known RA. In the current study, in order to elucidate the progression of cervical spine involvement, we designed a comparative cohort study for the incidence of instabilities in established RA patients with and without pre-existing instability.

"Severe" cervical spine instabilities occurred in 33.3–75.0% of patients with baseline "moderate" instability, while these lesions only appeared in 12.9% of patients initially without instability. In patients initially with AAS$^+$, 19.3% progressed to "severe" AAS and 22.8% developed VS. Notably, in patients initially with VS$^+$, 70.8% progressed to "severe" VS, 41.7% newly developed SAS, and 20.8% further developed "severe" SAS. Patients initially with SAS$^+$ also frequently had the progression of instabilities, although no statistical significance was obtained due to the small number of cases. Additionally, distributions of radiographic parameters support this higher progression tendency of instabilities in patients with initial instability. These results indicate accelerated development of cervical spine involvement in RA patients with pre-existing instability—especially VS.

Cervical canal stenosis and/or basilar invagination occurred in 14.3–37.5% of patients with baseline "moderate" instability, while these complications only appeared in 7.1% of patients initially without instability. The highest incidence of both these lesions was detected in patients initially with VS$^+$. In our previous study, we found that patients with pre-existing VS and/or SAS had substantially worse cervical spine instabilities [23]. The current analysis further demonstrates that patients with pre-existing VS are highly likely to develop myelopathy and/or brainstem symptoms, which is similar to other studies [8–10,17,22,27–30]. This study lacks data relating RA and neurological symptoms due to the difficulties in standardizing assessment between multiple centers. However, the observed incidence of cervical spine surgery may suggest neurological deterioration. Surgery was most frequently seen in patients initially with VS$^+$. The development of cervical canal stenosis and/or basilar invagination, severe enough to induce spinal cord and/or brainstem compression, are accelerated in patients with pre-existing instability—especially VS.

Recently, advances in RA therapies have drastically changed the clinical course even in patients with active disease [44], and may require careful interpretation of our results in treated populations for its effect on incidence. The impact of biologic therapies on cervical spine instability in RA is still poorly understood. A mean 4.4-year follow-up study of patients with the compliant >2-year administration of MTX and biologic agents demonstrated that only 8.3% without baseline instability developed instabilities while 80.8% with baseline instability had the progression of prior instabilities and/or development of additional instabilities [45]. A similar finding was observed in hip, knee, and ankle joints [46]; under biologic therapies, the development of radiographic damage was suppressed in joints with baseline Larsen grades 0 to II [47] but damaged joints with baseline Larsen grades III and IV showed further progression. These lines of evidence suggest potential effectiveness of intensive biologic therapies on preventing the development of cervical spine involvement in the early course of RA rather than on reducing the progression of pre-existing instabilities with the structural damage of the joints, bones, and ligaments. Also, this supports the early initiation of biologic therapies for the management of RA, corresponding with the European League Against Rheumatism recommendations [48]. Further studies need to be conducted.

Reported evidence indicates that patients with "severe" cervical spine instabilities, narrowed spinal canals, and/or cranial migration of the odontoid process are at risk for irreversible neurological damage [9,10,15,17,27–31]. The soft-tissue pannus as well as bone can induce symptomatic compression of the spinal cord in patients with RA [30]. In the present study, intra-observer reliabilities for the Ranawat value and subaxial translation were relatively low. Variations in radiographic technique and evaluation can easily affect the accuracy and precision of these radiographic measurements, which are more challenging to measure in RA patients because of generalized osteopenia, multiple subluxations, and erosions [12,14,17]. Therefore, RA patients with these advanced cervical spine lesions should receive not only radiographic but also magnetic resonance imaging examinations in the cervical spine.

Our multivariable analysis identified independent predictive risk factors for the development of "severe" instabilities: corticosteroid administration, Steinbrocker stage III or IV at baseline, mutilating changes at baseline, and the development of stages I–IV into mutilating changes during the follow-up period. These four variables, with significance in all the univariable, multivariable, and stepwise multivariable analyses, are relatively robust predictors for the progression of cervical spine involvement in RA. In addition, the consistent results from these analyses support further validation of the clinically-led multivariable model before applying stepwise approach.

Prolonged and high dose administration of corticosteroids is shown to aggravate cervical subluxations in RA patients [5,6,8,15,49,50]. Increased incidence of SAS, directly related to the duration of corticosteroid therapy, is reported even in non-RA patients [51]. Our results also indicate a negative effect of corticosteroids on the cervical spine in RA; however, we cannot conclude whether it is explained by concomitant severe disease activity or by corticosteroid-mediated structural damage. Biologically, corticosteroids induce the loss of bone mineral density [52] and articular chondrocyte death [53]. Further investigations for possible pathomechanisms are needed.

This study, which began in 2001, detected no obvious therapeutic effect of MTX and biologic therapies. However, their ineffectiveness cannot be concluded because their approval occurred in 1999 and 2003, respectively, and our patients had long RA histories predating these treatments. In addition, the dosages of medications used were lower than those used in Western countries. Reduced effectiveness of RA therapies indicates our results should be carefully interpreted.

Mutilating changes are reported to highly correlate with aggressive cervical instabilities in RA [22,35,39,40,50]. A prior multivariable analysis further demonstrated that patients with ≥ 10% peripheral joint damage at 5 years were 15.9 times more likely to develop AAS at 8–13 years than those with <10% [36]. In the context of this evidence, our multivariable models indicate that, in addition to patients with established mutilans, those without mutilans have the potential to develop severe cervical spine involvement with simultaneous development of their peripheral erosiveness into mutilans.

Steinbrocker stage III or IV was also statistically significant for the progression to "severe" instability. Previous joint surgery was a marginally significant predictor; a high prevalence of cervical spine instabilities in RA patients undergoing joint surgery is often reported [14,22,37,38]. Based on the ORs and 95% CIs of these variables, we propose that RA patients not only with mutilating changes but also with stage III or IV and severe disease activity—long-term corticosteroid administration and/or previous joint surgery—should receive radiological follow-up in the cervical spine.

This study is limited in that the duration of RA ranged widely. The currently used classification system for the severity of RA might be a somewhat obsolete and insensitive method of assessment. The biggest limitation is a low follow-up rate of 45.3%. As shown in **Table S1**, followed patients were younger than patients lost to follow-up. In addition, patients with baseline "severe" instability, speculated to have worse conditions, showed a lower follow-up rate. This indicates that many older, advanced RA outpatients potentially drop out due to polyarthralgia, worsening general condition, and/or cervical problems. Furthermore, patients who developed "severe" instabilities during the follow-up period might be lost more frequently, implying that the endpoint incidence of "severe" instabilities is higher than the observed data suggests. Taken together, patients' loss to follow-up is likely not completely random in this study.

Survival analyses such as the Cox proportional hazards analysis should provide more useful information for identifying predictive factors for "severe" instability when cervical radiographs obtained at multiple time points are available. The mixed-effects model may also be more suitable in the case of data missing at random between patients with and without the development of "severe" instabilities. The application of these statistical analysis methods is an issue to be considered in future studies.

Conclusions

This prospective cohort study demonstrates accelerated development of cervical spine involvement in RA patients with pre-existing instability—especially VS. Established mutilating changes and progressive development of non-mutilating into mutilating changes strongly indicate poor prognosis of the cervical spine in patients with RA. Steinbrocker stage III or IV, corticosteroid treatment, and possibly previous joint surgery also correlate with the progression of cervical spine instabilities in RA.

Acknowledgments

The authors would like to thank all the patients for their permission to use the data as well as all the members of Kobe Spine Conference (Kobe, Japan) for their help in acquiring the data. We especially thank Drs. Koichiro Maeno, Kenichiro Kakutani, and Zhongying Zhang (Department of Orthopaedic Surgery, Kobe University Graduate School of Medicine, Kobe, Japan) for their help in analyzing the data. We also thank Dr. Tiffany R. Dugan and Messrs. David C.L. Phillibert and Kevin Ngo (Department of Orthopaedic Surgery, University of Pittsburgh, Pittsburgh, PA) for their help in preparing the manuscript.

Author Contributions

Conceived and designed the experiments: TY MS. Performed the experiments: TY MS HH. Analyzed the data: TY MS DS. Contributed reagents/materials/analysis tools: TY MS KN HM KK TM YM MD. Wrote the paper: TY MS.

References

1. Alamanos Y, Drosos AA (2005) Epidemiology of adult rheumatoid arthritis. Autoimmun Rev 4: 130–136.
2. Ball J (1971) Enthesopathy of rheumatoid and ankylosing spondylitis. Ann Rheum Dis 30: 213–223.
3. Sharp J, Purser DW (1961) Spontaneous atlanto-axial dislocation in ankylosing spondylitis and rheumatoid arthritis. Ann Rheum Dis 20: 47–77.
4. Martel W (1961) The occipito-atlanto-axial joints in rheumatoid arthritis and ankylosing spondylitis. Am J Roentgenol Radium Ther Nucl Med 86: 223–240.
5. Lourie H, Stewart WA (1961) Spontaneous atlantoaxial dislocation. A complication of rheumatoid disease. N Engl J Med 265: 677–681.
6. Mathews JA (1969) Atlanto-axial subluxation in rheumatoid arthritis. Ann Rheum Dis 28: 260–266.
7. Isdale IC, Conlon PW (1971) Atlanto-axial subluxation. A six-year follow-up report. Ann Rheum Dis 30: 387–389.
8. Mathews JA (1974) Atlanto-axial subluxation in rheumatoid arthritis. A 5-year follow-up study. Ann Rheum Dis 33: 526–531.
9. Weissman BN, Aliabadi P, Weinfeld MS, Thomas WH, Sosman JL (1982) Prognostic features of atlantoaxial subluxation in rheumatoid arthritis patients. Radiology 144: 745–751.
10. Rana NA (1989) Natural history of atlanto-axial subluxation in rheumatoid arthritis. Spine (Phila Pa 1976) 14: 1054–1056.
11. Halla JT, Hardin JG Jr (1990) The spectrum of atlantoaxial facet joint involvement in rheumatoid arthritis. Arthritis Rheum 33: 325–329.
12. Ranawat CS, O'Leary P, Pellicci P, Tsairis P, Marchisello P, et al. (1979) Cervical spine fusion in rheumatoid arthritis. J Bone Joint Surg Am 61: 1003–1010.
13. Redlund-Johnell I, Pettersson H (1984) Radiographic measurements of the cranio-vertebral region. Designed for evaluation of abnormalities in rheumatoid arthritis. Acta Radiol Diagn (Stockh) 25: 23–28.
14. Kauppi M, Sakaguchi M, Konttinen YT, Hamalainen M (1990) A new method of screening for vertical atlantoaxial dislocation. J Rheumatol 17: 167–172.
15. Yonezawa T, Tsuji H, Matsui H, Hirano N (1995) Subaxial lesions in rheumatoid arthritis. Radiographic factors suggestive of lower cervical myelopathy. Spine (Phila Pa 1976) 20: 208–215.
16. Casey AT, Crockard HA, Bland JM, Stevens J, Moskovich R, et al. (1996) Surgery on the rheumatoid cervical spine for the non-ambulant myelopathic patient-too much, too late? Lancet 347: 1004–1007.
17. Pellicci PM, Ranawat CS, Tsairis P, Bryan WJ (1981) A prospective study of the progression of rheumatoid arthritis of the cervical spine. J Bone Joint Surg Am 63: 342–350.
18. Winfield J, Cooke D, Brook AS, Corbett M (1981) A prospective study of the radiological changes in the cervical spine in early rheumatoid disease. Ann Rheum Dis 40: 109–114.
19. Winfield J, Young A, Williams P, Corbett M (1983) Prospective study of the radiological changes in hands, feet, and cervical spine in adult rheumatoid disease. Ann Rheum Dis 42: 613–618.
20. Paimela L, Laasonen L, Kankaanpaa E, Leirisalo-Repo M (1997) Progression of cervical spine changes in patients with early rheumatoid arthritis. J Rheumatol 24: 1280–1284.
21. Neva MH, Kaarela K, Kauppi M (2000) Prevalence of radiological changes in the cervical spine—a cross sectional study after 20 years from presentation of rheumatoid arthritis. J Rheumatol 27: 90–93.
22. Fujiwara K, Owaki H, Fujimoto M, Yonenobu K, Ochi T (2000) A long-term follow-up study of cervical lesions in rheumatoid arthritis. J Spinal Disord 13: 519–526.
23. Yurube T, Sumi M, Nishida K, Takabatake M, Kohyama K, et al. (2011) Progression of cervical spine instabilities in rheumatoid arthritis: a prospective cohort study of outpatients over 5 years. Spine (Phila Pa 1976) 36: 647–653.
24. Yurube T, Sumi M, Nishida K, Miyamoto H, Kohyama K, et al. (2012) Incidence and aggravation of cervical spine instabilities in rheumatoid arthritis: a prospective minimum 5-year follow-up study of patients initially without cervical involvement. Spine (Phila Pa 1976) 37: 2136–2144.
25. Ropes MW, Bennett GA, Cobb S, Jacox R, Jessar RA (1958) 1958 Revision of diagnostic criteria for rheumatoid arthritis. Bull Rheum Dis 9: 175–176.
26. Arnett FC, Edworthy SM, Bloch DA, McShane DJ, Fries JF, et al. (1988) The American Rheumatism Association 1987 revised criteria for the classification of rheumatoid arthritis. Arthritis Rheum 31: 315–324.
27. Casey AT, Crockard HA, Geddes JF, Stevens J (1997) Vertical translocation: the enigma of the disappearing atlantodens interval in patients with myelopathy and rheumatoid arthritis. Part I. Clinical, radiological, and neuropathological features. J Neurosurg 87: 856–862.
28. Casey AT, Crockard HA, Stevens J (1997) Vertical translocation. Part II. Outcomes after surgical treatment of rheumatoid cervical myelopathy. J Neurosurg 87: 863–869.
29. Clark CR, Goetz DD, Menezes AH (1989) Arthrodesis of the cervical spine in rheumatoid arthritis. J Bone Joint Surg Am 71: 381–392.
30. Boden SD, Dodge LD, Bohlman HH, Rechtine GR (1993) Rheumatoid arthritis of the cervical spine. A long-term analysis with predictors of paralysis and recovery. J Bone Joint Surg Am 75: 1282–1297.
31. Kataoka O, Kurihara A (1977) The role of dynamic canal stenosis in cervical spondylotic myelopathy. J West Pacific Orthop Assoc 14: 1–22.
32. McRae DL, Barnum AS (1953) Occipitalization of the atlas. Am J Roentgenol Radium Ther Nucl Med 70: 23–46.
33. Steinbrocker O, Traeger CH, Batterman RC (1949) Therapeutic criteria in rheumatoid arthritis. J Am Med Assoc 140: 659–662.
34. Belt EA, Kaarela K, Kauppi MJ, Savolainen HA, Kautiainen HJ, et al. (1999) Assessment of mutilans-like hand deformities in chronic inflammatory joint diseases. A radiographic study of 52 patients. Ann Rheum Dis 58: 250–252.
35. Laiho K, Belt E, Kauppi M (2001) The cervical spine in mutilant rheumatoid arthritis. Rheumatol Int 20: 225–228.
36. Neva MH, Isomaki P, Hannonen P, Kauppi M, Krishnan E, et al. (2003) Early and extensive erosiveness in peripheral joints predicts atlantoaxial subluxations in patients with rheumatoid arthritis. Arthritis Rheum 48: 1808–1813.
37. Collins DN, Barnes CL, FitzRandolph RL (1991) Cervical spine instability in rheumatoid patients having total hip or knee arthroplasty. Clin Orthop Relat Res 272: 127–135.
38. Grauer JN, Tingstad EM, Rand N, Christie MJ, Hilibrand AS (2004) Predictors of paralysis in the rheumatoid cervical spine in patients undergoing total joint arthroplasty. J Bone Joint Surg Am 86: 1420–1424.
39. Fujiwara K, Fujimoto M, Owaki H, Kono J, Nakase T, et al. (1998) Cervical lesions related to the systemic progression in rheumatoid arthritis. Spine (Phila Pa 1976) 23: 2052–2056.
40. Conlon PW, Isdale IC, Rose BS (1966) Rheumatoid arthritis of the cervical spine. An analysis of 333 cases. Ann Rheum Dis 25: 120–126.
41. Olsen MA, Nepple JJ, Riew KD, Lenke LG, Bridwell KH, et al. (2008) Risk factors for surgical site infection following orthopaedic spinal operations. J Bone Joint Surg Am 90: 62–69.
42. Hosmer DW, Lemeshow S (2000) Applied logistic regression (2nd edition). New York, NY: John Wiley & Sons.
43. Peduzzi P, Concato J, Kemper E, Holford TR, Feinstein AR (1996) A simulation study of the number of events per variable in logistic regression analysis. J Clin Epidemiol 49: 1373–1379.
44. Lipsky PE, van der Heijde DM, St Clair EW, Furst DE, Breedveld FC, et al. (2000) Infliximab and methotrexate in the treatment of rheumatoid arthritis. Anti-Tumor Necrosis Factor Trial in Rheumatoid Arthritis with Concomitant Therapy Study Group. N Engl J Med 343: 1594–1602.
45. Kaito T, Hosono N, Ohshima S, Ohwaki H, Takenaka S, et al. (2012) Effect of biological agents on cervical spine lesions in rheumatoid arthritis. Spine (Phila Pa 1976) 37: 1742–1746.

46. Seki E, Matsushita I, Sugiyama E, Taki H, Shinoda K, et al. (2009) Radiographic progression in weight-bearing joints of patients with rheumatoid arthritis after TNF-blocking therapies. Clin Rheumatol 28: 453–460.
47. Larsen A, Dale K, Eek M (1977) Radiographic evaluation of rheumatoid arthritis and related conditions by standard reference films. Acta Radiol Diagn (Stockh) 18: 481–491.
48. Smolen JS, Landewe R, Breedveld FC, Dougados M, Emery P, et al. (2010) EULAR recommendations for the management of rheumatoid arthritis with synthetic and biological disease-modifying antirheumatic drugs. Ann Rheum Dis 69: 964–975.
49. Smith PH, Benn RT, Sharp J (1972) Natural history of rheumatoid cervical luxations. Ann Rheum Dis 31: 431–439.
50. Rasker JJ, Cosh JA (1978) Radiological study of cervical spine and hand in patients with rheumatoid arthritis of 15 years' duration: an assessment of the effects of corticosteroid treatment. Ann Rheum Dis 37: 529–535.
51. Rudge SR, Drury PL, Lloyd-Jones JK (1981) Long-term corticosteroids and cervical subluxation in non-rheumatoid patients. Rheumatol Rehabil 20: 102–105.
52. Grossman JM, Gordon R, Ranganath VK, Deal C, Caplan L, et al. (2010) American College of Rheumatology 2010 recommendations for the prevention and treatment of glucocorticoid-induced osteoporosis. Arthritis Care Res (Hoboken) 62: 1515–1526.
53. Farkas B, Kvell K, Czompoly T, Illes T, Bardos T (2010) Increased chondrocyte death after steroid and local anesthetic combination. Clin Orthop Relat Res 468: 3112–3120.

18

The Status of Rheumatoid Factor and Anti-Cyclic Citrullinated Peptide Antibody Are Not Associated with the Effect of Anti-TNFα Agent Treatment in Patients with Rheumatoid Arthritis: A Meta-Analysis

Qianwen Lv[1]☯, Yufeng Yin[1]☯, Xin Li[1]☯, Guangliang Shan[2], Xiangni Wu[1], Di Liang[1], Yongzhe Li[1], Xuan Zhang[1]*

1 Department of Rheumatology & Clinical Immunology, Peking Union Medical College Hospital, Chinese Academy of Medical Sciences and Peking Union Medical College, Beijing, China, **2** Department of Epidemiology and Statistics, Institute of Basic Medical Sciences, Chinese Academy of Medical Sciences and School of Basic Medicine, Peking Union Medical College, Beijing, China

Abstract

Objectives: This meta-analysis was conducted to investigate whether the status of rheumatoid factor (RF) and anti-cyclic citrullinated peptide (anti-CCP) antibody are associated with the clinical response to anti-tumor necrosis factor (TNF) alpha treatment in rheumatoid arthritis (RA).

Methods: A systemic literature review was performed using the MEDLINE, SCOPUS, Cochrane Library, ISI Web of Knowledge, and Clinical Trials Register databases, and Hayden's criteria of quality assessment for prognostic studies were used to evaluate all of the studies. The correlation between the RF and anti-CCP antibody status with the treatment effect of anti-TNFα agents was analyzed separately using the Mantel Haenszel method. A fixed-effects model was used when there was no significant heterogeneity; otherwise, a random-effects model was applied. Publication bias was assessed using Egger's linear regression and a funnel plot.

Results: A total of 14 studies involving 5561 RA patients meeting the inclusion criteria were included. The overall analysis showed that the pooled relative risk for the predictive effects of the RF and anti-CCP antibody status on patient response to anti-TNFα agents was 0.98 (95% CI: 0.91–1.05, $p = 0.54$) and 0.88 (95% CI: 0.76–1.03, $p = 0.11$), respectively, with I^2 values of 43% ($p = 0.05$) and 67% ($p < 0.01$), respectively. Subgroup analyses of different anti-TNFα treatments (infliximab vs. etanercept vs. adalimumab vs. golimumab), response criteria (DAS28 vs. ACR20 vs. EULAR response), follow-up period (≥6 vs. <6 months), and ethnic group did not reveal a significant association for the status of RF and anti-CCP.

Conclusions: Neither the RF nor anti-CCP antibody status in RA patients is associated with a clinical response to anti-TNFα treatment.

Editor: Oreste Gualillo, SERGAS, Santiago University Clinical Hospital, IDIS Research Laboratory 9, NEIRID Lab, Spain

Funding: This work was supported by the grants from the National Natural Science Foundation of China (81325019, 81172859, and 81273312), Beijing Municipal Natural Science Foundation (7141008), the Research Special Fund for Public Welfare Industry of Health (20120217), the Capital Health Research and Development of Special (2011-4001-02), and the National laboratory Special Fund (2060204). The funders had no role in study design, data collection and analysis, decision to publish, or preparation of the manuscript.

Competing Interests: The authors have declared that no competing interests exist.

* E-mail: zxpumch2003@sina.com

☯ These authors contributed equally to this work.

Introduction

Rheumatoid arthritis (RA) is a chronic inflammatory autoimmune disease that affects approximately 1% of the population worldwide [1]. OLE_LINK10Although the introduction of anti-TNFα agents has dramatically improved the outcome of RA, there unfortunately remains a proportion of RA patients who do not exhibit an adequate response to this treatment. Considering the high cost and potential side effects of anti-TNFα treatment, it is important to identify those RA patients who will be more likely to respond to these agents. Indeed, numerous studies have been conducted to investigate potential predictors for patient response to anti-TNFα therapy [2–4].

Both rheumatoid factor (RF) and antibodies against cyclic citrullinated peptide (anti-CCP) are regarded as serological markers of RA [5,6]. Some studies have suggested that the status of RF or anti-CCP antibody in RA patients is associated with a clinical response to anti-TNFα treatment [7–14], whereas such a correlation was not found in other studies [15–19]. Thus, no definite conclusion has been reached to date.

Flowchart of the selection process of included studies for meta-analysis

Bolded risk ratio highlight statistically significant results.

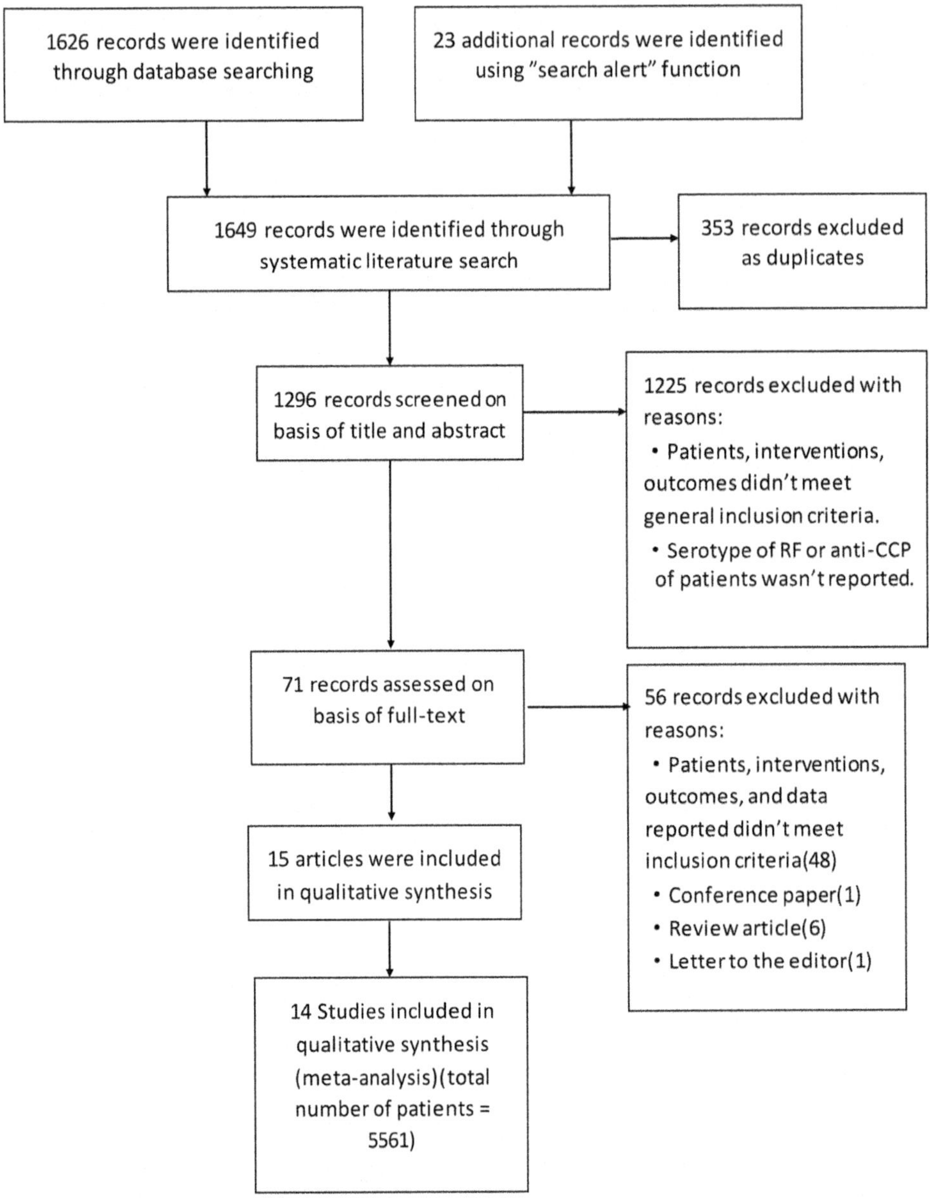

Figure 1. Flowchart of the study selection.

We performed a meta-analysis to investigate whether RF and anti CCP have predictive value for a clinical response to anti-TNFα treatment. Suitable studies investigating an association of the status of RF or anti-CCP and response to anti-TNFα treatment were searched and included. We also performed subgroup analyses on different variables to explore potential sources of independent predictive factors for an effect of anti-TNFα treatment.

Methods

Search strategy

A literature search was performed for all studies evaluating an association between the status of RF or anti-CCP antibody and a response to anti-TNFα therapy in RA patients using the Medline, Cochrane Library, SCOPUS (including EMbase), ISI Web of Knowledge, and Clinical Trials Register (clinical trials.gov) databases. The following keywords were searched: rheumatoid arthritis, anti-TNFα, rheumatoid factor, anti-cyclic citrullinated peptide antibody, clinical trials, and systematic review. Synonyms and spelling variations were taken into account (Search strategy for Scopus was listed in Table S1 in File S1). There was a limitation with regard to language, i.e., we only considered English publications, but not the year of publication. We also contacted authors to request a full-text review or specific data from studies when there was no electronic version of the full text or sufficient data for the meta-analysis. Citations were reviewed to search

Table 1. Data extracted from the included studies.

Study	Study design	No. of patients	Disease duration (yrs)	Age (yrs)	Gender (female%)	No. of swollen joints	No of tender joints	DAS28	Prior biologic used#	Intervention	Country	Primary clinical outcome (response criteria)	Study duration	Antibody measurement	Cut-off value of antibody
Braun2006	Pro*	30	12 (8.9)	50.6 (13.9)	73%	N/A	N/A	7.4 (0.95)	N/A	INF+86.7%MTX	Israel	EULAR	3.5 m	Anti-CCP: ELISA	5 IU/ml
Hyrich2006	Pro	2879	14 (9)	55 (12)	78%	12 (6)	16 (7)	6.7 (1.0)	N/A	ETA+28%MTX: 1267 pts; INF+86%MTX: 1612 pts	Britain	EULAR	6 m	N/A	N/A
Bobbio 2007	Pro	126	8.3 (6.9)	57.3 (12.5)	76.5%	9.6 (5.7)	16.0 (9.9)	5.87 (0.99)	N/A	INF/ADA/ETA+CSs/ NSAIDs allowed	Italy	EULAR	12 m	RF: immunone-phelometry; Anti-CCP: ELISA	15 IU/ml; 5 IU/ml
Lequerre 2007	Pro	76	10.5(8.6)	53.8 (12.4)	81.6%	13.8(6)	10.7 (7.3)	5.8(1)	N/A	INF+MTX/LEF	France	EULAR	3.5 m	RF: latex agglutination test;; Anti-CCP: ELISA	N/A
Mancarella 2007	Retro	591	11.6 (7.6)	53.3 (12.7)	67%	10.4 (7.1)	17.1 (9.4)	5.9 (1.2)	N/A	INF/ETA/ADA	Italy	EULAR	6 m	N/A	20 IU/ml
Wijbrandts 2007	Pro	103	10.4 (9.2)	55 (13)	69%	N/A	N/A	5.9 (1.1)	None	INF+CSs/NSAIDs allowed	The Netherlands	DAS28	4 m	N/A	N/A
Cuchacovich 2008	Pro	59	11.7	48.9	87%	16.2	20	N/A	N/A	ADA+DMARDs/ NSAIDs allowed	Chile	ACR20	6 m	Anti-CCP: ELISA	25 IU/ml
Wouter2008	Pro	172	8.5	53.7	79.3%	N/A	N/A	5.1	N/A	ADA+74%MTX+ 34%CSs	The Netherlands	EULAR	7 m	RF: ELISA; Anti-CCP: ELISA	30 IU/ml; 5 AU/ml
Alexandra 2009	Pro	36	10.2 (5.8)	50.5 (10.2)	75%	7.4 (5.3)	9.5 (5)	5.2 (0.9)	None	INF+91.6%MTX	France	EULAR	12 m	RF: quantitative nephelometric test; Anti-CCP: ELISA	1000 IU/ml; 200 IU/ml
Keystone 2009	Pro	179	5.3	52	80.9%	12.5	24.5	6.008	N/A	GOL+MTX	From 12 countries	ACR20	3.5 m	N/A	N/A
Potter2009	Pro	642	14 (10)	57 (11)	78%	N/A	N/A	6.7 (1)	N/A	ADA: 62 pts; ETA: 241 pts; INF: 218 pts	Britain	EULAR	6 m	RF; immunotur-bidimetry; Anti-CCP: ELISA	40 U/ml; 5 U/ml
Soto2010	Pro	52	11.9	50	88.5%	16.9	21.4	5.8	N/A	ADA+stable DMARDs/ NSAIDs/CSs allowed	Chile	DAS28; ACR20/ 50/70	6 m	RF: ELISA; Anti-CCP: ELISA	N/A; 25 IU/ml
Vasilopoulos 2011	Pro	100	13.6 (6.5)	57.4 (10.8)	92%	N/A	N/A	5.6 (0.2)	N/A	INF+MTX: 24 pts; ETA±MTX: 26 pts; ADA±MTX/LEF:50 pts	Greece	DAS28	6 m	RF: immunone-phelometry; Anti-CCP: ELISA	15 IU/ml; 5 U/ml
Canhao2012	Pro	516	10.4 (8.6)	50.9–54.1	88%	8 (5.4)	11.5 (7.3)	5.8 (1.2)	None	INF/ADA/ETA± DMARDs/CSs	Portugal	EULAR	6 m	RF: ELISA	IgM:5 IU/ml; IgA:20 IU/ml

*Pro, prospective clinical trial; Retro, retrospective study; N/A, not available; INF, infliximab; ADA, adalimumab; ETA, etanercept; MTX, methotrexate; LEF, leflunomide; NSAIDs, non-steroidal anti-inflammatory drugs; DMARDs, disease-modifying anti-rheumatic drugs; CSs, corticosteroids.

#Different prior biologic agents used may introduce potential heterogeneity, though the available data were insufficient for a sub-analysis.

Disease of duration, age, No. of swollen joints, No. of tender joints, DAS28 are presented as the mean (SD).

Table 2. The results of an assessment for bias in accordance with Hayden's criteria.

Study	Assessment domain						
	study participation	study attrition	prognostic factor measurement	outcome measurement	confounding measurement and account	analysis	total score
Braun, 2006	moderate	low	moderate	low	low	low	10
Hyrich, 2006	low	low	unsure	low	moderate	low	9*
Bobbio, 2007	low	low	low	low	high	low	10
Lequerre, 2007	low	low	moderate	low	moderate	low	10
Mancarella, 2007	low	high	moderate	low	high	low	7
Wijbrandts, 2007	low	moderate	low	low	moderate	low	10
Cuchacovich, 2008	moderate	moderate	low	low	moderate	low	10
Wouter, 2008	low	low	low	low	moderate	low	11
Alexandra, 2009	moderate	low	moderate	low	moderate	low	9
Keystone, 2009	high	low	moderate	low	low	low	9
Potter, 2009	low	moderate	low	low	moderate	low	10
Soto, 2010	moderate	low	moderate	low	moderate	low	9
Vasilopoulos, 2011	low	low	low	low	moderate	low	11
Canhao, 2012	low	moderate	moderate	low	moderate	low	9

Unsure: not enough information to evaluate.
Low, low risk of bias; moderate, moderate risk of bias; high, high risk of bias.
*One of the domains was assessed as "unsure" due to unavailable information even after the authors were contacted.

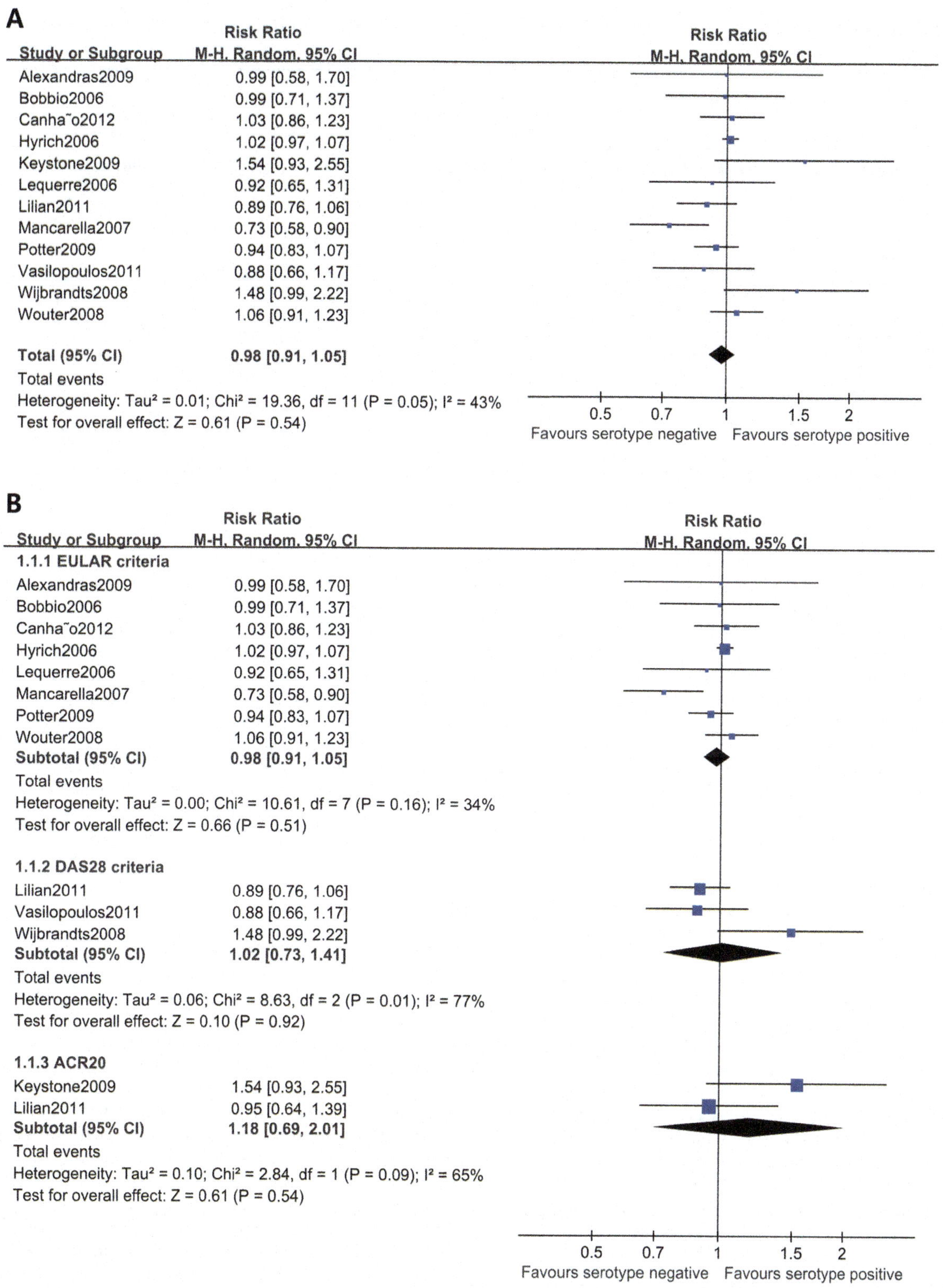

Figure 2. Forest graphs of the meta-analysis of RF status and response to anti-TNFα agents. The overall analysis of RF status showed a pooled RR of 0.98 (95% CI: 0.91–1.05, p = 0.54) and an I^2 of 43%. Subgroup analyses on different response criteria revealed no significant differences.

relevant original studies, and an electronic search alert was set to cover recent studies.

Study selection

There were 1649 references identified by the literature search. Three individual investigators (QL, YY, & XL) evaluated the

Table 3. Subgroup meta-analysis of RF and RA patient response according to different anti-TNFα agents, follow-up periods, response criteria, and ethnic groups.

				Test of association			Test of heterogeneity		
Subgroup	**Population**	**No. of studies**	**No. of patients**	**RR**	**95%CI**	**P value**	**Model**	**P value**	**I^2**
	overall	12	5374	0.98	0.91–1.05	0.54	R	0.05	43%
Anti-TNFα agent*	infliximab	4	1827	1.03	0.89–1.19	0.71	R	0.28	23%
	adalimumab	2	248	0.98	0.81–1.18	0.8	R	0.09	65%
	etanercept	1	1267	1.05	0.97–1.12	0.21	NA	NA	NA
	golimumab	1	178	1.54	0.93–2.55	0.09	NA	NA	NA
Follow up period	≥6 months	9	5017	0.96	0.90–1.03	0.27	R	0.13	37%
	<6 months	3	357	1.25	0.87–1.78	0.22	R	0.11	54%
Ethnic group	European	10	5146	0.98	0.91–1.06	0.59	R	0.10	39%
	South American	1	50	0.89	0.76–1.06	0.19	NA	NA	NA

R, random-effects model; NA, not applicable.
*The number of studies and number of patients receiving individual anti-TNFα agent in this table are those that we could identified after literature review and contacting the authors.

references, and the decision of inclusion was made by consensus. A study was included based on the following criteria: 1) the patients were older than 16 years old, diagnosed with RA using ACR criteria, and treated with at least one anti-TNFα agent (adalimumab, infliximab, etanercept, certolizumab, or golimumab); 2) efficacy was measured using EULAR or ACR or DAS28 criteria after a minimum duration of 12 weeks; and 3) the status of RF or anti-CCP antibody at baseline and sufficient data to calculate the risk ratio (RR) were reported in the study. The following information was extracted from each study: the study design, patients' characteristics, baseline status of RF or anti-CCP antibody, interventions, outcomes, and study duration.

Study assessment

All of the studies included were evaluated for potential bias using Hayden's criteria of the quality assessment of prognostic studies [20] (The details of the modified criteria were provided in Table S2 in File S2). Six domains were considered in the bias assessment method: "study participation", "study attrition", "prognostic factor measurement", "outcome measurement", "confounding measurement and account", and "analysis". Scores of "0", "1", or "2" represented "high bias", "partial bias", and "low bias", respectively. If the available information was insufficient to obtain a decision after contacting the authors, "unsure" was used, and no score was calculated. The total scores were calculated to show the level of study quality; studies with a score of "11–12" were rated as having relatively high quality, with "9–10" as moderate, and "less than 8" as low quality. The evaluation was performed independently by three investigators (QL, YY, & XL) to improve the validity of the results.

Statistical analysis

We estimated the risk ratio of the RF or anti-CCP antibody status for a response to anti-TNFα treatment. The point estimate of the risk ratio (RR) and 95% confidence intervals (CI) were calculated for each study, and a Mantel Haenszel analysis was used to calculate the pooled RR and 95% CI. The heterogeneity of the effects across studies was assessed using the Chi square test and qualified by I^2 values, which represent the proportion of between-study variability that is attributable to heterogeneity rather than to chance; I^2 values of 25%, 50%, and 75% are referred to as low, moderate, and high heterogeneity effects, respectively. A fixed-effects model was used when there was no significant heterogeneity, whereas a random-effects model was used in other cases. Subgroup analyses were performed to investigate potential sources of heterogeneity by stratifying the different anti-TNFα agents, response criteria, duration of follow-up, and ethnic group. In addition, a sensitivity analysis was performed by the sequential omission of individual studies. Publication bias was estimated by funnel plots and an Egger's test, with $p<0.05$ considered as representing significant bias. All of the statistical analyses were performed using Review Manager 5.0 software, and the results of the publication bias were estimated using STATA 12.0 software.

Results

Characteristics of the included studies

Figure 1 describes the flowchart of our literature search. According to pre-determined criteria, fifteen articles, published between 2006 and 2012, were included [7,9–19,21–23] (A list of articles excluded and the reasons for exclusion were presented in Table S3 in File S1). As two described the same cohort [11,21], fourteen studies were ultimately included in this meta-analysis [7,9,10,12–19,21–23]. These studies comprised a total of 5561 RA patients: 5374 patients had their status of RF detected, and 1283 patients had their status of anti-CCP antibody detected. All but one were prospective cohort studies. All of the participants in the 14 studies had active RA, as evaluated by the number of swollen and tender joints, or DAS28 value, and the patients in all but one_ENREF_7 study had exhibited failure for at least one type of Disease-modifying Anti-Rheumatic Drug (DMARD) treatment [13]. Almost all of the patients had established RA, with a mean disease duration from 5 to 14 years. The data extracted from the 14 studies are summarized in Table 1. With regard to the anti-TNFα agents utilized, 10 studies involved infliximab, 8 involved adalimumab, 6 involved etanercept, and 1 involved golimumab.

There was no study that involved patients receiving certolizumab. Only four studies investigated the status of RF, with only two investigating anti-CCP; the other eight studies measured both RF

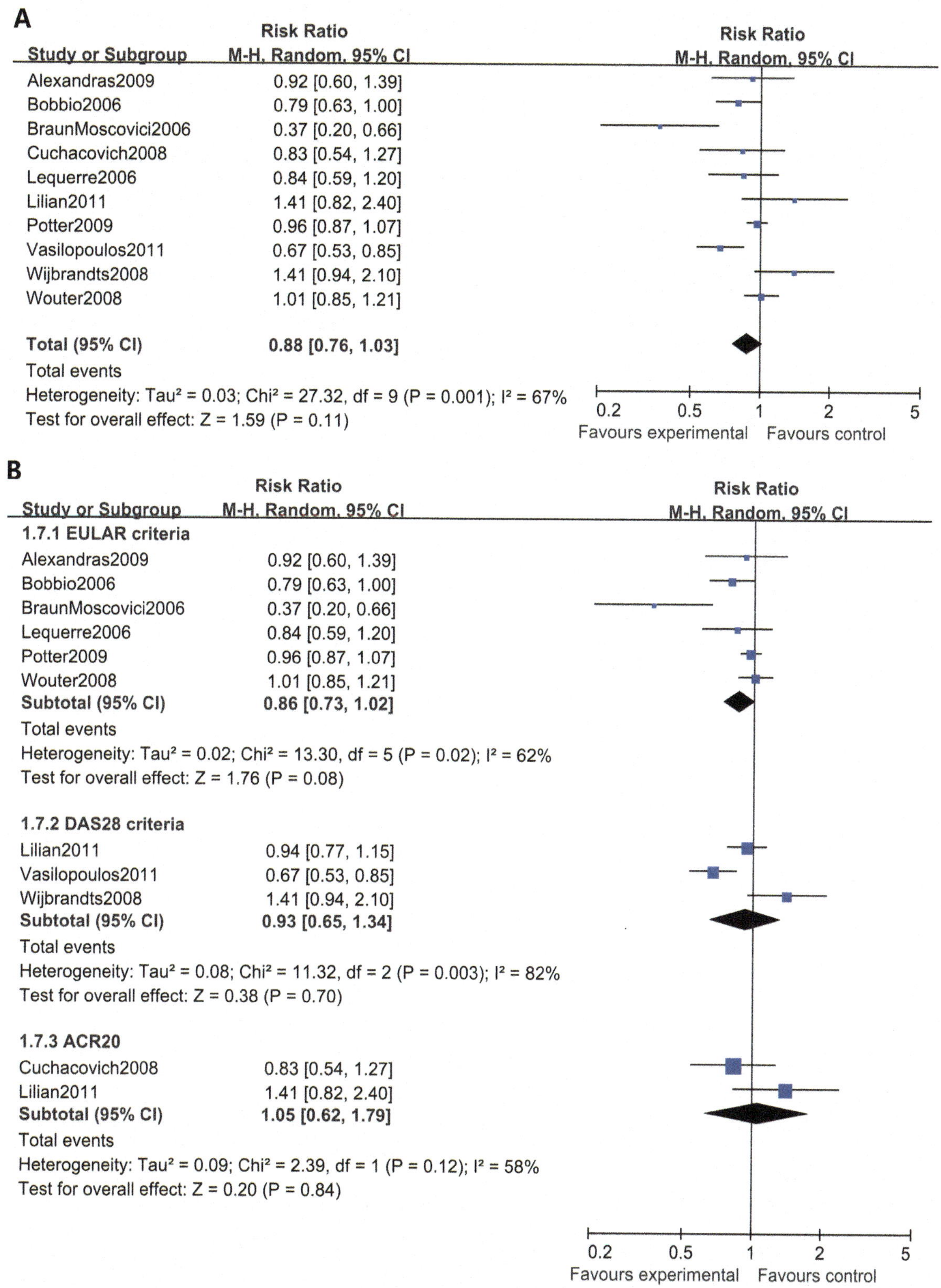

Figure 3. Forest graphs of the meta-analysis of anti-CCP antibody status and response to anti-TNFα agents. The overall analysis of anti-CCP antibody status showed a pooled RR of 0.88 (95% CI: 0.76–1.03, p = 0.11) and an I^2 of 67%. Subgroup analyses on different response criteria revealed no significant differences.

Table 4. Subgroup meta-analysis of anti-CCP and RA patient response according to different anti-TNFα agents, follow-up periods, response criteria, and ethnic groups.

				Test of association			Test of heterogeneity		
Subgroup	**Population**	**No. of studies**	**No. of patients**	**RR**	**95%CI**	**P value**	**Model**	**P value**	**I^2**
	overall	10	1283	0.88	0.76–1.03	0.11	R	<0.01	67%
Anti-TNFα agent*	infliximab	5	345	0.79	0.55–1.13	0.19	R	<0.01	78%
	adalimumab	3	297	1.01	0.88–1.17	0.86	F	0.69	0%
Follow up period	≥6 months	7	1074	0.90	0.80–1.01	0.06	R	0.09	46%
	<6 months	3	209	0.78	0.40–1.53	0.47	R	<0.01	86%
Ethnic group	European	7	1144	0.90	0.79–1.04	0.17	R	0.02	60%
	South American	2	109	1.01	0.79–1.30	0.91	F	0.38	0
	Asian	1	30	0.37	0.20–0.66	<0.05	NA	NA	NA

F, fixed-effects model; R, random-effects model; NA, not applicable.
*The number of studies and number of patients receiving individual anti-TNFα agent in this table are those that we could identified after literature review and contacting the authors.

and anti-CCP. The follow-up duration of these 14 studies ranged from 14 weeks to 48 weeks.

Study quality

Our assessment was performed on the basis of Hayden's criteria for prognostic studies [20]. The results revealed that only one of the included studies was considered to be of low quality, with a score of 7; the other thirteen studies were considered as having moderate or high quality (11 moderate and 2 high) (Table 2).

Association evaluation of RF/anti-CCP antibody status and patient response to anti-TNFα agents

Twelve of the included studies, with a total of 5374 patients, examined the predictive effect of the RF status for patient response

Egger's test

Std_Eff	Coef.	Std. Err.	t	P>|t|	[95% Conf.	Interval]
slope	.0065257	.0396738	0.16	0.873	-.0818731	.0949245
bias	-.1727359	.594678	-0.29	0.777	-1.497761	1.152289

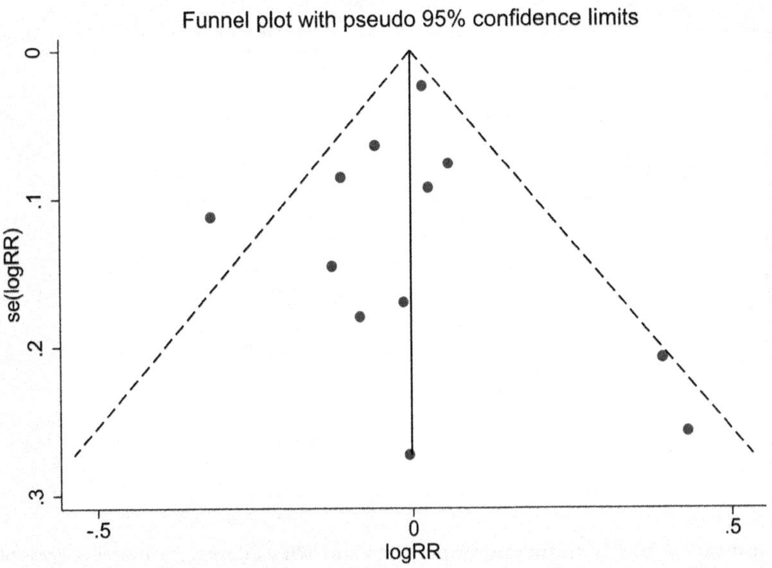

Figure 4. Overall analysis of publication bias on the effect of RF status on the response to anti-TNFα treatment. Egger's linear regression test was performed to quantify publication bias. The p values of the RF status analysis were 0.777. The funnel plot showed no significant evidence of asymmetry.

Egger's test

Std_Eff	Coef.	Std. Err.	t	P>|t|	[95% Conf. Interval]	
slope	.005925	.1270781	0.05	0.964	-.2871176	.2989677
bias	-.955509	1.129908	-0.85	0.422	-3.561082	1.650064

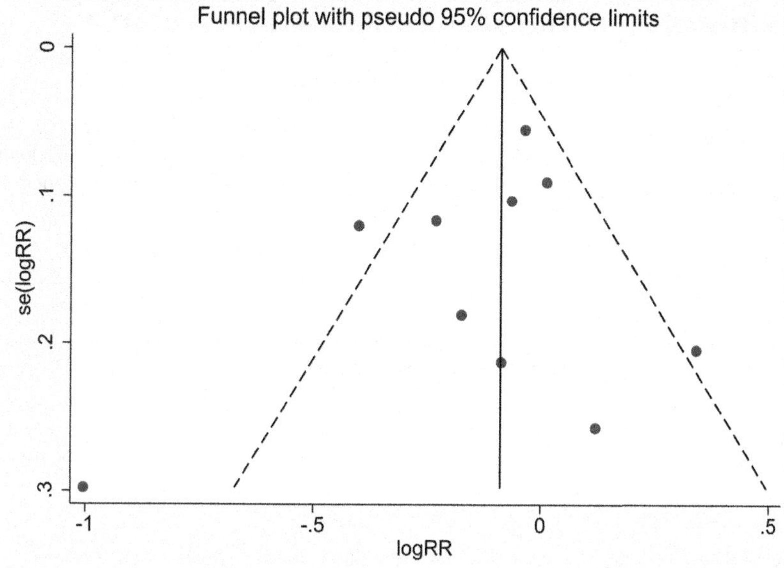

Figure 5. Overall analysis of publication bias on the effect of anti-CCP antibody status on the response to anti-TNFα treatment. Egger's linear regression test was performed to quantify publication bias. The p values of the anti-CCP antibody status analysis were 0.422. The funnel plot showed no significant evidence of asymmetry.

to anti-TNFα agents. The overall analysis revealed that the pooled RR was 0.98 (95% CI: 0.91–1.05, p = 0.54) and that I^2 was 43% (Figure 2a), suggesting that the RF status was not associated with a patient's response to anti-TNFα treatment, with a moderate heterogeneity observed. Subgroup analyses on the different anti-TNFα agents, follow-up periods, response criteria, and ethnic groups were performed to investigate sources of this heterogeneity, though the results revealed no significant differences (Figure 2b, Table 3).

Ten studies, with a total of 1283 RA patients, were analyzed for an association of anti-CCP antibody status and patient response to anti-TNFα treatment. The overall meta-analysis showed no association between the status of anti-CCP antibody and a patient's response to anti-TNFα treatment, with a pooled RR of 0.88 (95% CI: 0.76–1.03, p = 0.11) and an I^2 of 67% (Figure 3a). When we performed a subgroup analysis to explore potential heterogeneity, we did not identify any association by stratifying the studies using either different anti-TNFα agents, follow-up periods, response criteria, or ethnic groups (Figure 3b, Table 4).

Sensitivity and publication bias

Sensitivity analyses were performed based on the results of the bias assessments, Hayden's criteria of quality assessment for prognostic studies, by the sequential omission of individual studies, and the result revealed that the significance estimate of the overall pooled RR was not influenced by omitting any single study. The publication bias was evaluated by a funnel plot, which showed no significant evidence of asymmetry (Figures 4–5). We also performed an Egger's linear regression test to quantify the publication bias. The p values of the RF and anti-CCP antibody status analyses were 0.777 and 0.422 (Figures 4–5), and all other Egger's test p values in this meta-analysis were >0.05, suggesting no significant bias in the analysis.

Discussion

Previous single studies have suggested that the presence of RF and anti-CCP antibody is associated with a reduced response to anti-TNFα treatment [7–14];_ENREF_9 however, a number of studies have reported a contrasting conclusion [15–19]. Thus, to investigate whether the status of RF or anti-CCP antibody in RA patients has predictive value for a clinical response to anti-TNFα treatment, we performed a meta-analysis by a comprehensive literature search and inclusion of all of the available qualifying studies. The results of our meta-analysis demonstrated that there was no association between the status of RF and patient response to anti-TNFα treatment. Furthermore, the status of anti-CCP antibody was also not associated with patient response, with a pooled RR of 0.88 and 95% CI of 0.76–1.03 (p = 0.11), indicating a tendency of association between the absence of anti-CCP antibodies and a patient's response to anti-TNFα therapy. Therefore the cumulative results did not support or completely reject the association between the presence of RF and/or anti-CCP and the effect of treatment with TNFα inhibitors. Anti-CCP is an independent predictor of radiological damage and progression in RA patients [24,25], and anti-CCP-positive patients have a relatively worse prognosis. As a result, patients with a different anti-CCP antibody status may have a different baseline of the disease, which could influence their response to anti-TNFα agents. To explore this influence, analyses should be performed to investigate potential differences in the baseline characteristics between groups stratified by the status of anti-CCP antibody. Alternatively, only analyses based on studies with placebo groups are powered to definitively identify such an association. Unfortunately, such information was not available for the included studies.

This meta-analysis does have some limitations. First, only 14 studies were included in this meta-analysis, with 12 studies reporting the status of RF and 10 studies reporting the status of anti-CCP antibody. Nonetheless, after a comprehensive literature search covering five databases and the selection of eligible studies by three different investigator strictly according to the inclusion criteria, most of the included studies were assessed with moderate-to-high quality. Therefore, it is reasonable to obtain a conclusion based on the studies included in this meta-analysis. However, as potential heterogeneity exists between studies after subgroup analyses were performed, the result of our analyses should be interpreted with caution, and our conclusions should be updated using new, larger studies in the future. Secondly, all of the patients in the studies included in our meta-analysis had long-standing disease, with a mean value of disease duration ranging from 5 to 14 years, and had previously shown failure with at least one type of DMARD. Indeed, patients with more severe chronic disease as a result of irreversible joint damage may be less likely to respond to anti-TNFα treatment [17]. Thirdly, most of the included studies reported a combined treatment of DMARDs in a proportion of the patients enrolled. Because studies have demonstrated improved outcomes among patients receiving combination therapy with MTX plus anti-TNFα [17], the heterogeneity of combined therapy among the studies may have introduced potential bias.

In summary, our meta-analysis indicated that the status of RF and anti-CCP are not associated with the clinical response to anti-TNFα treatment in RA patients.

Supporting Information

File S1 File includes Tables S1–S3. Table S1: Search strategy for Scopus. Table S2: Guidelines for assessing quality in prognostic studies. Table S3: A list of the article not included in the study (and the reasons).

Author Contributions

Conceived and designed the experiments: YY XL XZ. Performed the experiments: QL YY XL. Analyzed the data: QL YY XL. Contributed reagents/materials/analysis tools: XW DL GS YL. Wrote the paper: QL.

References

1. Harris ED (1990) Rheumatoid Arthritis. New England Journal of Medicine 322: 1277–1289.
2. Radovits BJ, Kievit W, Fransen J, van de Laar MA, Jansen TL, et al. (2009) Influence of age on the outcome of antitumour necrosis factor alpha therapy in rheumatoid arthritis. Ann Rheum Dis 68: 1470–1473.
3. Kristensen LE, Kapetanovic MC, Gulfe A, Soderlin M, Saxne T, et al. (2008) Predictors of response to anti-TNF therapy according to ACR and EULAR criteria in patients with established RA: results from the South Swedish Arthritis Treatment Group Register. Rheumatology (Oxford) 47: 495–499.
4. Gibbons LJ, Hyrich KL (2009) Biologic therapy for rheumatoid arthritis: clinical efficacy and predictors of response. BioDrugs 23: 111–124.
5. Pruijn GJ, Wiik A, van Venrooij WJ (2010) The use of citrullinated peptides and proteins for the diagnosis of rheumatoid arthritis. Arthritis Research & Therapy 12: 203.
6. Avouac J, Gossec L, Dougados M (2006) Diagnostic and predictive value of anti-cyclic citrullinated protein antibodies in rheumatoid arthritis: a systematic literature review. Ann Rheum Dis 65: 845–851.
7. Vasilopoulos Y, Bagiatis V, Stamatopoulou D, Zisopoulos D, Alexiou I, et al. (2011) Association of anti-CCP positivity and carriage of TNFRII susceptibility variant with anti-TNF-alpha response in rheumatoid arthritis. Clinical & Experimental Rheumatology 29: 701–704.
8. Tanaka Y, Takeuchi T, Inoue E, Saito K, Sekiguchi N, et al. (2008) Retrospective clinical study on the notable efficacy and related factors of infliximab therapy in a rheumatoid arthritis management group in Japan: one-year clinical outcomes (RECONFIRM-2). Modern Rheumatology 18: 146–152.
9. Potter C, Hyrich KL, Tracey A, Lunt M, Plant D, et al. (2009) Association of rheumatoid factor and anti-cyclic citrullinated peptide positivity, but not carriage of shared epitope or PTPN22 susceptibility variants, with anti-tumour necrosis factor response in rheumatoid arthritis. Ann Rheum Dis 68: 69–74.
10. Mancarella L, Bobbio-Pallavicini F, Ceccarelli F, Falappone PC, Ferrante A, et al. (2007) Good clinical response, remission, and predictors of remission in rheumatoid arthritis patients treated with tumor necrosis factor-alpha blockers: the GISEA study.[Erratum appears in J Rheumatol. 2007 Sep;34(9):1947]. Journal of Rheumatology 34: 1670–1673.
11. Klaasen R, Cantaert T, Wijbrandts CA, Teitsma C, Gerlag DM, et al. (2011) The value of rheumatoid factor and anti-citrullinated protein antibodies as predictors of response to infliximab in rheumatoid arthritis: an exploratory study. Rheumatology 50: 1487–1493.
12. Cuchacovich M, Catalan D, Wainstein E, Gatica H, Soto L, et al. (2008) Basal anti-cyclic citrullinated peptide (anti-CCP) antibody levels and a decrease in anti-CCP titres are associated with clinical response to adalimumab in rheumatoid arthritis. Clinical & Experimental Rheumatology 26: 1067–1073.
13. Canhao H, Rodrigues AM, Mourao AF, Martins F, Santos MJ, et al. (2012) Comparative effectiveness and predictors of response to tumour necrosis factor inhibitor therapies in rheumatoid arthritis. Rheumatology (Oxford) 51: 2020–2026.
14. Braun-Moscovici Y, Markovits D, Zinder O, Schapira D, Rozin A, et al. (2006) Anti-cyclic citrullinated protein antibodies as a predictor of response to anti-tumor necrosis factor-alpha therapy in patients with rheumatoid arthritis. Journal of Rheumatology 33: 497–500.
15. Soto L, Sabugo F, Catalan D, Wurmann P, Cermenatti T, et al. (2011) The presence of anti-citrullinated protein antibodies (ACPA) does not affect the clinical response to adalimumab in a group of RA patients with the tumor necrosis factor (TNF) alpha-308[NON-BREAKING SPACE]G/G promoter polymorphism. Clinical Rheumatology 30: 391–395.
16. Lequerre T, Jouen F, Brazier M, Clayssens S, Klemmer N, et al. (2007) Autoantibodies, metalloproteinases and bone markers in rheumatoid arthritis patients are unable to predict their responses to infliximab. Rheumatology 46: 446–453.
17. Hyrich KL, Watson KD, Silman AJ, Symmons DPM, British Society for Rheumatology Biologics R (2006) Predictors of response to anti-TNF-alpha therapy among patients with rheumatoid arthritis: results from the British Society for Rheumatology Biologics Register. Rheumatology 45: 1558–1565.
18. Bobbio-Pallavicini F, Caporali R, Alpini C, Avalle S, Epis OM, et al. (2007) High IgA rheumatoid factor levels are associated with poor clinical response to tumour necrosis factor alpha inhibitors in rheumatoid arthritis. Annals of the Rheumatic Diseases 66: 302–307.
19. Alexandra, Nicaise-Roland P, Hayem G, Palazzo E, Dieude P, et al. (2009) Prospective cohort study of effects of infliximab on rheumatoid factor, anti-cyclic citrullinated peptide antibodies and antinuclear antibodies in patients with long-standing rheumatoid arthritis. Joint, Bone, Spine: Revue du Rhumatisme 76: 248–253.
20. Hayden JA,-te' PC, Bombardier C (2006) Evaluation of the Quality of Prognosis Studies in Systematic Reviews. Ann Intern Med 144: 427–437.
21. Wijbrandts CA, Dijkgraaf MG, Kraan MC, Vinkenoog M, Smeets TJ, et al. (2008) The clinical response to infliximab in rheumatoid arthritis is in part dependent on pretreatment tumour necrosis factor alpha expression in the synovium. Ann Rheum Dis 67: 1139–1144.
22. Bos WH, Bartelds GM, Wolbink GJ, de Koning MHMT, van de Stadt RJ, et al. (2008) Differential response of the rheumatoid factor and anticitrullinated protein antibodies during adalimumab treatment in patients with rheumatoid arthritis. Journal of Rheumatology 35: 1972–1977.
23. Keystone EC, Genovese MC, Klareskog L, Hsia EC, Hall ST, et al. (2009) Golimumab, a human antibody to tumour necrosis factor {alpha} given by monthly subcutaneous injections, in active rheumatoid arthritis despite methotrexate therapy: the GO-FORWARD Study. Annals of the Rheumatic Diseases. pp. 789–796.
24. Forslind K, Ahlmen M, Eberhardt K, Hafstrom I, Svensson B (2004) Prediction of radiological outcome in early rheumatoid arthritis in clinical practice: role of antibodies to citrullinated peptides (anti-CCP). Ann Rheum Dis 63: 1090–1095.
25. Bongi SM, Manetti R, Melchiorre D, Turchini S, Boccaccini P, et al. (2004) Anti-cyclic citrullinated peptide antibodies are highly associated with severe bone lesions in rheumatoid arthritis anti-CCP and bone damage in RA. Autoimmunity 37: 495–501.

19

Association of MASP-2 Levels and *MASP2* Gene Polymorphisms with Rheumatoid Arthritis in Patients and Their Relatives

Isabela Goeldner[1]*, Thelma Skare[2], Angelica B. W. Boldt[1], Flavia R. Nass[1], Iara J. Messias-Reason[1], Shirley R. Utiyama[3]

1 Department of Medical Pathology, Federal University of Paraná, Curitiba, Brazil, **2** Rheumatology Unit, Evangelical University Hospital, Curitiba, Brazil, **3** Department of Clinical Analysis, Federal University of Paraná, Curitiba, Brazil

Abstract

Background: Mannan-binding lectin-associated serine protease 2 (MASP-2) is a key protein of the lectin pathway of complement. MASP-2 levels have been associated with different polymorphisms within *MASP2* gene as well as with the risk for inflammatory disorders and infections. Despite its clinical importance, MASP-2 remains poorly investigated in rheumatoid arthritis (RA).

Methods: In this case-control study, we measured MASP-2 serum levels in 156 RA patients, 44 patient relatives, and 100 controls from Southern Brazil, associating the results with nine *MASP2* polymorphisms in all patients, 111 relatives, and 230 controls genotyped with multiplex SSP-PCR.

Results: MASP-2 levels were lower in patients than in controls and relatives (medians 181 vs. 340 or 285 ng/ml, respectively, P<0.0001). Conversely, high MASP-2 levels were associated with lower susceptibility to RA and to articular symptoms independently of age, gender, ethnicity, smoking habit, anti-CCP and rheumatoid factor positivity (OR = 0.05 [95%CI = 0.019–0.13], P<0.0001 between patients and controls; OR = 0.12, [95%CI = 0.03–0.45], P = 0.002 between patients and relatives; OR = 0.06, [95%CI = 0.004–0.73], P = 0.03 between relatives with and without articular symptoms). *MASP2* haplotypes **2A1* and **2B1-i* were associated with increased susceptibility to RA (OR = 3.32 [95%CI = 1.48–7.45], P = 0.004). Deficiency-causing *p.120G* and *p.439H* substitutions were associated with five times increased susceptibility to articular symptoms in relatives (OR = 5.13 [95%CI = 1.36–20.84], P = 0.02). There was no association of MASP-2 levels or *MASP2* polymorphisms with autoantibodies, Sjögren's syndrome, nodules and functional class.

Conclusions: In this study, we found the first evidence that MASP-2 deficiency might play an important role in the development of RA and articular symptoms among relatives of RA patients.

Editor: Deyu Fang, Northwestern University Feinberg School of Medicine, United States of America

Funding: This work was partially supported by grants from the Araucária Foundation (no. 412/2009, protocol 5103, http://www.fundacaoaraucaria.org.br/), as well as by fellowships from the National Counsel of Technological and Scientific Development (CNPq) and Coordination for the Improvement of Higher Level Personnel (CAPES). The funders had no role in study design, data collection and analysis, decision to publish, or preparation of the manuscript.

Competing Interests: The authors have declared that no competing interests exist.

* E-mail: igoeldner@gmail.com.br

Introduction

Rheumatoid arthritis (RA) is an autoimmune disorder with complex etiology which affects approximately 0.5–1.1% of the world population and has an annual incidence of 3 per 10 000 adults [1]. RA represents a substantial economic burden due to frequent hospitalizations, disability and productivity loss faced by the patients, culminating with 2–3 times increased mortality rates [2]. Despite the increasing number of studies aiming at the development of new RA therapy strategies, up to 50% RA patients do not achieve disease remission [3]. The failure to recognize the disease in early stages, as well as treatment side effects, are still the main obstacles to be overcome.

The disease is characterized by intense destructive inflammation promoted by immune deregulation. Similarly to other autoimmune diseases, multiple factors are known to contribute to its development. Recent genome-wide association studies have confirmed that genetic factors play an important role in the etiology of RA, but many of these factors need to be validated in the Brazilian population [4–6]. The important genetic contribution in the development of RA turns relatives of RA patients to be more susceptible to the disease [7–9]. Furthermore, familial RA aggregation is associated to autoantibody positivity and poorer disease prognosis [10,11].

The complement system is an important arm of the innate immunity and plays a crucial role in the first line defense of the host. Complement activation has been shown to be an important mediator of inflammation in RA, being associated with severity of joint destruction [12]. The lectin pathway leads to complement activation through the pattern recognition molecules mannan-binding lectin (MBL) and ficolins, which in association with mannan-binding lectin-associated serine protease 1 and 2 (MASP-1 and -2), recognize a wide variety of microorganisms and cell debris, leading to complement activation and their clearance. Thus, MASPs play a relevant role in complement activation by the lectin pathway [13,14]. So far investigations have been made aiming to clarify the role of MBL in the pathogenesis of RA [15]. Despite the importance of MASP-2 in the activation of complement, studies regarding its role in this context are still scarce [16–19].

MASP-2 is a protein analogous to the C1s and C1r serine proteases of the classical complement pathway [20]. It is composed of well-defined domains, including the CUB1 (C1r/C1s, Uegf and bone morphogenetic protein-1 domains), EGF (epidermal growth factor), CUB2, CCP1 (complement control protein 1), CCP2 and SP (serine protease) domains [21]. The *MASP2* gene is located on chromosome 1p36.3–36.2, in a region that has been found associated with RA and other inflammatory autoimmune conditions in recent studies [22–24]. Its single nucleotide polymorphisms (SNPs) are associated with different MASP-2 levels which are stable in adult healthy individuals but not in the pediatric population [25–27]. The *p.D120G* SNP is located in exon 3 of *MASP2* gene and affects the CUB1 domain and the binding of MASP-2 to ficolins or MBL. In the homozygous state, it determines MASP-2 deficiency in approximately 0.3% of European individuals [25,28]. In addition, amino acid substitutions caused by *p.P126L* (first CUB domain), *p.V377A* (second CCP domain) and *p.R439H* (SP domain) are also known to reduce MASP-2 concentration and, in the case of *p.R439H*, impair complement activation [25]. We recently described ten *MASP2* haplotypes combined with five other SNPs distributed from the promoter to the last exon (5′untranslated region) [26].

Only few disease association studies on *MASP2* polymorphisms and MASP-2 levels have been reported so far, none in RA [29–32]. In the present study, we aimed to investigate whether MASP-2 serum levels and *MASP2* polymorphisms could influence the susceptibility to RA and its clinical presentation in a population from Southern Brazil. We found an association between low MASP-2 levels and deficiency-causing substitutions and RA, as well as an association between high MASP-2 levels and lower susceptibility to RA in relatives from patients.

Materials and Methods

Ethics statement

The Ethics Research Committee from Evangelical Beneficent Society, Curitiba, Brazil, approved this study and the experiments were performed in accordance with the Declaration of Helsinki. All subjects provided written informed consent, which was approved by the Ethics Committee.

Subjects and samples

One-hundred and fifty-six adult RA patients from the urban population of Paraná's capital (Curitiba) were diagnosed according to the American College of Rheumatology criteria in the Rheumatological Unit of the Evangelical Hospital of Curitiba (Brazil) [33], and consecutively included in the study from August 2007 to April 2009 (84.6% female, 15.4% male, mean age 51.5 years, range 24 to 77 years, with 1–60 years of documented disease).

Clinical and demographic data were obtained from medical records and interviews using a standard questionnaire (Table 1). To access the extent of physical disability in RA patients, the Steinbrocker functional classification was applied. This index of disease activity rates on a four-level scale, ranging from class I, complete functional capacity, to class IV, largely or wholly incapacitated. Functional classes III and IV were grouped due to its low sample number. Detailed description of anti-CCP and rheumatoid factor determinations has been given elsewhere [9]. Two hundred thirty healthy unrelated individuals matched for age and gender with RA patients were used as a control group (82.6% female, 17.4% male, mean age 45.8 years, range 24 to 89 years). To reduce the potential for selection bias, we selected controls from different sources: 202 blood donors from three different blood banks in Curitiba (58 from the Hospital de Clínicas – UFPR, 144 from the Biobanco of the Hospital Evangélico) and 28 volunteers without RA from the Curitiba's surrounding (Witmarsum).

Patients, relatives and controls were defined as being from major European, African or Amerindian ancestry based on physical characteristics and informed ethnic background. Based on HLA allelic frequencies of South Brazilian population samples identified in the same way, Euro-Brazilians have an average sub-Saharan African component of 9% and an average Amerindian component of 5%, whereas Afro-Brazilians have at least 40% of African and 6% of Amerindian ancestry [34,35]. Patients and control subjects had the same socioeconomic status and were from the same geographical area.

During the routine medical appointment of RA patients, their relatives were invited to participate on the study. From about 150 relatives invited, 111 (74%) relatives accepted to participate and had their blood samples collected (57.6%, 64/111 female, 42.4%, 47/11 male, mean age 38.5 years, range 7 to 73 years). Using a questionnaire and clinical examination, relatives were investigated for articular symptoms suggestive of RA (swollen or tender joints).

Venous blood was collected using anticoagulant and genomic DNA was extracted from mononuclear peripheral cells through Genomic Blood DNA Purification kit, GE Healthcare (São Paulo,

Table 1. Clinical and demographic data of RA patients.

Characteristic	Patients % (n = 156)
Anti-CCP positivity	72.3 (119)
Rheumatoid factor positivity	69.2 (108)
Females	84.6 (132)
Age at disease onset	
<40 years	39.1 (61)
≥40 years	60.9 (95)
Disease duration	
6 to 24 months	17.3 (27)
>2 to 10 years	51.9 (81)
>10 years	30.8 (48)
Steinbrocker functional class	
Class I	48.1 (75)
Class II	40.4 (63)
Class III	9.6 (15)
Class IV	1.9 (3)
Extra-articular manifestations	
Rheumatoid nodules (139)[a]	7.9 (11)
Sjögren syndrome (114)[a]	32.4 (37)

[a]: Total number of samples with available data for the extra-articular manifestation.

Brazil). In addition, venous blood was collected without anticoagulant, centrifuged at 800 g^{-1} for 15 minutes, aliquoted and stored at −80°C until the assays for MASP-2 levels could be performed.

MASP-2 levels measurement

We measured MASP-2 concentrations in sera of 156 RA patients, 44 patient relatives and 100 healthy individuals by ELISA according to the manufacturer's protocol (HK326 kit, Hycult Biotechnology, Uden, The Netherlands). For economic reasons, MASP-2 concentrations were determinate in randomly chosen subgroups of relatives and controls. The minimum measurable MASP-2 concentration of the ELISA kit used was 1.6 ng/ml. The color intensity was evaluated at 450 nm in an ELISA reader. Samples with a mean absorbance above the absorbance for the highest standard concentration were repeated using a higher dilution. MASP-2 levels lower than 200 ng/ml were considered low MASP-2 levels (cut-off adopted by others [26,36]).

MASP2 haplotyping

We genotyped the following single nucleotide polymorphisms (SNPs) NG007289.1: *g.4847A>C* (SNP database: rs7548659), *p.R99Q* (rs61735600), *p.D120G* (rs72550870) and *p.P126L* (rs56392418) in exon 3, *g.21081C>T* (rs17409276) in intron 9, *p.D371Y* (rs12711521) and *p.V377A* (rs2273346) in exon 10, *p.R439H* (rs12085877) and *g.24762C>T* (rs1782455) in exon 12. These polymorphisms were previously associated with variation of MASP-2 levels [37]. The phase between the SNPs was determinate using sequence-specific primer polymerase chain reactions (PCR-SSP). A simple PCR-SSP was designed to identify the *p.D120G* mutation and the remaining SNPs were identified using two multiplex PCRs (I and II), as described [26]. Interpretation was based on the presence or absence of bands corresponding to the amplified fragments in agarose gel electrophoresis.

Statistical analyses

Tests of independence between RA patients and the comparison groups were performed with binary logistic regression, using the Intercooled STATA 9.2 program (STATACorp). Using the same program, the number of included variables was gradually minimized, first eliminating those with a Wald's test p value higher than 0.20 and finally those with p values higher than 0.05 (whose contribution to final adjustment is almost insignificant), to end up with a reduced model of binary logistic regression. The comparison of MASP-2 levels between the groups was done through nonparametric Kruskal-Wallis or Mann-Whitney tests. Correlation analysis was done using Spearman correlation coefficient for nonparametric data. This statistical analysis was undertaken using the GraphPad Prism 3.0 software package (GraphPad Software Inc.). Two-tailed P-values less than 5% were considered significant. Direct counting was used to estimate genotype, allele and haplotype frequencies. SNPs distributed in the promoter and exon 3, intron 9, exon 10 and exon 12 could be phased with the SSP primers. The phase between distantly situated SNPs could be deduced due to strong linkage disequilibrium between the variants. Deviations from Hardy–Weinberg equilibrium and from the hypothesis of homogeneity between haplotype distributions (exact test of population differentiation of Raymond and Rousset) were tested using the ARLEQUIN software package version 3.1 (http://anthro.unige.ch/arlequin/). Linkage disequilibrium analysis (D′ and r2) between the *MASP2* SNPs was performed with the Haploview v.3.2 program (Broad Institute of MIT and Harvard).

Results

MASP-2 levels

MASP-2 levels were significantly lower in RA patients than in controls and relatives (median 181 [21–1200 ng/ml, IQR = 199 ng/ml] vs. 340 ng/ml [42–1200 ng/ml, IQR = 398 ng/ml] and median 181 vs. 285 ng/ml [30–1646 ng/ml, IQR = 329 ng/ml], respectively, Mann-Whitney P<0.0001, Figure 1), but did not differ between patient groups with different clinical characteristics. On the other hand, high MASP-2 levels were associated with lower susceptibility to RA independently of age, gender and ethnicity (P<0.0001).

Whereas anti-CCP positivity increases almost seven times the susceptibility to RA between relatives, high MASP-2 levels decreases this susceptibility independently of age, gender, ethnicity, smoking habit and anti-CCP and rheumatoid factor positivity (Table 2).

In addition, relatives with articular symptoms had lower MASP-2 levels than controls, being similar to patients (median 196 ng/ml vs. 340 ng/ml, Mann-Whitney P = 0.0339, Figure 1), whereas relatives without those complaints presented similar values to the controls, i.e., with higher MASP-2 levels than patients (median 315.5 vs. 181 ng/ml, Mann-Whitney P<0.0001, Figure 1). There was also a difference in MASP-2 levels between relatives with and without articular symptoms (median 196 ng/ml vs. 315.5 ng/ml, Mann-Whitney P = 0.0143, Figure 1). High MASP-2 levels decreases the susceptibility to articular symptoms in otherwise healthy relatives, independently of age, gender, ethnic group, smoking habit and anti-CCP and rheumatoid factor positivity (Table 2). In contrast, anti-CCP and rheumatoid factor levels had no effect in the development of symptoms (P = 0.17 and 0.28, respectively, binary logistic regression) and did not correlate with MASP-2 levels (P = 0.9618, r = −0.0039 for anti-CCP and P = 0.3909, r = −0.0796 for rheumatoid factor, Spearman correlation coefficient test).

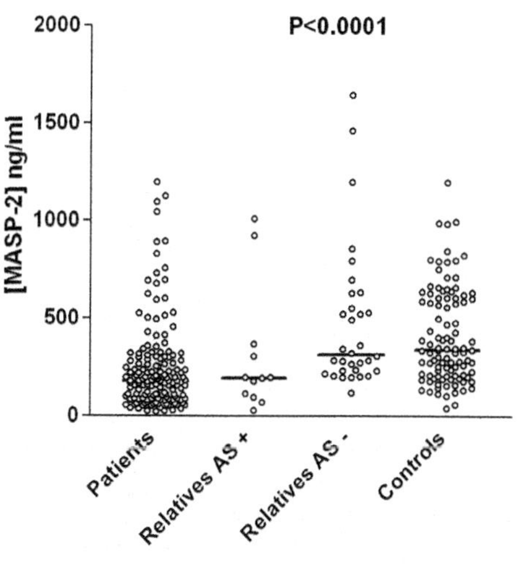

Figure 1. Differences between MASP-2 levels of patients, relatives with and without articular symptoms, and controls. Data is shown in medians and interquartile ranges, differences were calculated with Mann-Whitney tests (P<0.0001 between patients and controls, and patients and asymptomatic relatives; P = 0.0339 between symptomatic relatives and controls and P = 0.0143 between symptomatic and asymptomatic relatives). AS: articular symptom.

Table 2. Reduced binary logistic regression models for rheumatoid arthritis.

Patients vs. Controls (P<0.00001)	n = 256	OR	95%CI	P
MASP-2		0.05	0.019–0.13	<0.0001
*2A1 and/or *2B1-i[a]		3.32	1.48–7.45	0.004
Patients vs. relatives (P<0.00001)	**n = 200**			
MASP-2		0.12	0.03–0.45	0.002
Anti-CCP positivity		6.45	2.38–17.45	<0.0001
Rheumatoid factor positivity		5.19	1.55–17.40	0.008
Age		1.04	1.004–1.074	0.026
Relatives with vs. without articular symptoms		**&**		
MASP-2 (P = 0.011)	n = 44	0.06	0.004–0.73	0.03
*1C2-l and/or *2B2B-l[b] (P = 0.024)	n = 111	5.13	1.26–20.84	0.02

The original model included age, gender and ethnicity for all observations; smoking habit, anti-CCP and RF positivity for patients and relatives. Significance of the model is given in parentheses. MASP-2 levels were normalized as logarithms on base 10 (Log_{10}). anti-CCP: anti-cyclic citrullinated peptide antibodies; n: number of included observations; &: not independent; OR: odds ratio;
[a]: with intermediary levels,
[b]: with low MASP-2 levels.

MASP2 haplotypes

Genotype frequencies were in Hardy-Weinberg equilibrium. We found most of the pairs of evaluated SNPs to be in absolute linkage disequilibrium (data not shown) and identified eleven *MASP2* haplotypes in patients, relatives and healthy controls. One of them (**2B2A-i.1B1-h*) is a recombinant haplotype identified for the first time in this study (Table 3).

There was, as expected, a significant association between MASP-2 levels and high, intermediary and low MASP-2-producing genotypes in all investigated groups, but patient MASP-2 levels were always lower compared to all other groups (Figure 2). Two haplotypes were associated with three times increased susceptibility to RA: **2A1* and **2B1-i*, of which the last one is associated with intermediary MASP-2 levels (44/312 or

Table 3. *MASP2* haplotypes nomenclature and frequencies (% ± SD).

Haplotype[a]	Human Genome Variation Society[b]	Controls n = 460	Relatives n = 222	Patients n = 312
*1A	[g.4847C; p.99R; p.120D; p.126P; g.21081C; p.371D; p.377V; p.439R; g.24762C]	5.2±1.0	6.3±1.6	4.8±1.2
*1B1-h	[g.4847C; p.99R; p.120D; p.126P; g.21081T; p.371D; p.377V; p.439R; g.24762C]	13.9±1.6	14.4±2.4	16.0±2.1
*1B2-h	[g.4847C; p.99Q; p.120D; p.126P; g.21081T; p.371D; p.377V; p.439R; g.24762C]	1.1±0.5	0	0.6±0.4
*1C1-l	[g.4847C; p.99R; p.120D; p.126L; g.21081C; p.371D; p.377V; p.439R; g.24762C]	1.3±0.5	0	0
*1C2-l	[g.4847C; p.99R; p.120D; p.126L; g.21081C; p.371D; p.377V; p.439H; g.24762C]	0.6±0.4	1.8±0.9	1.9±0.8
*2A1	[g.4847C; p.99R; p.120D; p.126P; g.21081C; p.371D; p.377V; p.439R; g.24762T]	0.4±0.3	1.4±0.8	2.6±0.9
*2A2-l	[g.4847C; p.99R; p.120D; p.126P; g.21081C; p.371D; p.377A; p.439R; g.24762T]	4.6±1.0	2.7±1.0	2.2±0.8
*2B1-i	[g.4847C; p.99R; p.120D; p.126P; g.21081C; p.371Y; p.377V; p.439R; g.24762T]	5.6±1.0	10.8±2.1	11.5±1.8
*2B2A-i	[g.4847A; p.99R; p.120D; p.126P; g.21081C; p.371Y; p.377V; p.439R; g.24762T]	65.4±2.2	59.9±3.3	59±2.8
*2B2B-l	[g.4847A; p.99R; p.120G; p.126P; g.21081C; p.371Y; p.377V; p.439R; g.24762T]	1.5±0.6	2.7±1.1	1.3±0.6
***2B2A-i. 1B1-h**	**[g.4847A; p.99R; p.120D; p.126P; g.21081T; p.371D; p.377V; p.439R; g.24762C]**	**0.2±0.2**	**0**	**0**

[a]: phylogenetic nomenclature according to [26] and [38], where "h", "i" and "l" refer to *MASP2* haplotypes associated with low (<200 ng/ml), intermediary (200–600 ng/ml) and high (≥600 ng/ml) MASP-2 levels (cut off adopted by [26] and [35]),
[b]: reference sequence NT_021937 (GenBank sequence); anti-CCP: anti-cyclic citrullinated peptide antibodies; n: number of chromosomes; SD: standard deviation. In bold: recombinant haplotype.

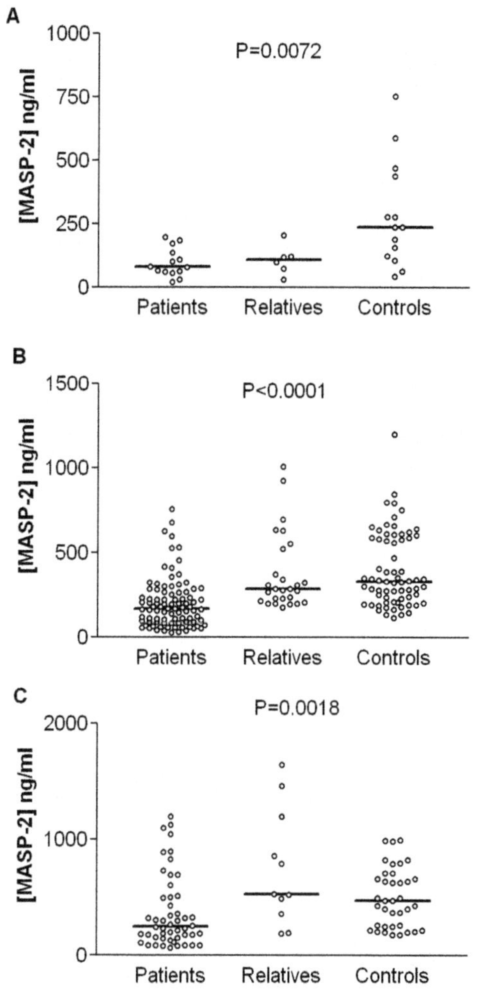

Figure 2. MASP-2 levels in RA patients, relatives and controls according to haplotype producing profiles. Data is shown with medians, differences were calculated with Kruskal-Wallis test A: Low MASP-2 producing haplotypes (**2B2B-l/*1A, *2B2A-i/*2B2B-l, 2B2B-l/2A1, *2B2A-i/*2A2-l, 2B1-i/2A2-l, *2B1-i/*1C2-l, *1C2-l/*1C2-l, *2B2A-i/*1C2-l, *2B2B-l/*1C2-l, *2A2-l/*1C2-l*); B: Intermediary MASP-2 producing haplotypes (**2B2A-i/*2B2A-i, *2B2A-i/*1A, *2B2A-i/*2B1-i, *2B1-i/*1A, *2B1-i/2A1, *2B1-i/*2B1-i*); C: High MASP-2 producing haplotypes (**2B2A-i/*1B1-h, *2B2A-i/*1B2-h, *2B1-i/*1B1-h, *1B1-h/*1B1-h, *1A/*1B1-h, *2A1/1B1-h, *2A1/*2A1, *2B2A-i/*2A1, *2A1/*1A, *2B2A-i.1B1-h/1B1-h*).

14.1% in the patients vs. 28/460 or 6.1% in the controls, binary logistic regression P = 0.004, Tables 2 and 3). There was no association between *MASP2* haplotypes and clinical characteristics such as time of disease duration, functional class and extra-articular manifestations (data not shown).

The deficiency-causing *p.120G* and/or *p.439H* amino acid substitutions (embedded in the **2B2B-l* and **1C2-l* haplotypes, respectively), were associated with five times increased susceptibility to articular symptoms among relatives, independently of age, gender, ethnic group, smoking habit and anti-CCP and rheumatoid factor positivity (in relatives with and without articular symptoms, 5/50 or 10% vs. 5/172 or 2.9%, respectively, binary logistic regression P = 0.02, Table 3).

Discussion

RA is a complex and still not entirely understood disease. Environmental, genetic and immunological factors are known to contribute for its development, however the identification of components that determine disease establishment remains a great challenge [39,40]. Although the complement system has already been related to RA development and clinical presentation [41,42], this is, to our knowledge, the first study to examine the association between the central serine protease of the lectin pathway of complement, MASP-2, and human RA.

In this study, high MASP-2 levels decreased the susceptibility to RA and to the onset of articular symptoms among patient relatives. Protection against RA was independent of classical markers of disease establishment and progression such as rheumatoid factor and anti-CCP antibodies. More surprising, these well-established markers did not show any significant association with articular symptoms. Since relatives from RA patients are characterized as a risk group for the development of RA [9], this leads us to suggest that MASP-2 levels might be used as an independent biomarker to follow-up individuals with familiar RA predisposition.

In the present study, MASP-2 levels in patients were almost always lower than in controls and relatives, independently from genotypes. A possible explanation for lower MASP-2 levels in RA patients could be related to protein consumption and/or lower gene expression, also described by Ip et al (2000), which found similar results for MBL in the southern Chinese [41]. Reduced MASP-2 levels due to protein consumption were also recently associated with ischemia-related necrotic myocardial injury in a human cohort [31]. On the other hand, *MASP2* expression may be impaired in detriment to the expression of other proteins such as MBL-associated protein of 19 kDa, an alternative splice product of the *MASP2* gene [26]. Concomitantly, the synovial permeability of joints is slightly augmented in RA, which enhances protein diffusion from plasma into synovial fluid. In addition, the synovial fluid/plasma ratio of complement proteins have been already described to be higher in RA in comparison to other arthropathies, suggesting a sequestration and consumption of complement proteins in the synovial fluid in RA patients [18].

Studies have shown that cytokines such as interleukin 6 and the binding protein STAT3 can modify the expression of *MASP2* genes [43,44]. Interleukin 6 is highly expressed by synoviocytes in RA patients and has been shown to down regulate the expression of complement system proteins, including MASP-2 [43,45]. Thus, the consequences of the interaction between pro-inflammatory cytokines, such as interleukin 6, and MASP-2 might play an important role on the development of RA.

The reduction of MASP-2 serum levels in RA patients could also be due to hormonal alterations, such as from thyroid and growth hormones, and acute phase response, since the expression of some complement proteins can be influenced by these conditions [46,47].

In the present study, the **2A1* and **2B1-i MASP2* haplotypes increased susceptibility to RA, which might be rather the result of a variant linked to these haplotypes. On the other hand, the deficiency-associated variants *p.120G* and *p.439H* (**2B2B-l* and **1C2-l*, respectively), which turn mature MASP-2 proteins unable to activate complement, increase the susceptibility to articular symptoms in individuals with familiar RA predisposition. This leads us to suggest that the ability to activate the lectin pathway of complement might play a critical role on disease onset, which is in accordance with other studies pointing to the importance of complement deficiency in the immunopathology of RA [41,42]. In

Norwegian patients with juvenile rheumatoid arthritis, MBL deficiency was found associated with early disease onset and was also shown to favor disease remission, pointing a dual role of this protein in this rheumatic disease [48]. Further studies should clarify if MASP-2 follows this trend as well.

Conclusion

In this study, we found the first evidence that MASP-2 deficiency might play an important role in the development of RA and articular symptoms among relatives of RA patients.

Acknowledgments

We are grateful to the subjects of this investigation. We thank also the medical staff of the Rheumatology Unit at the Evangelical Hospital from Curitiba for patient recruitment, and Dr. Renato M. Nisihara for the excellent technical assistance.

Author Contributions

Conceived and designed the experiments: IG TS IJMR SRU. Performed the experiments: IG TS ABWB FRN. Analyzed the data: IG ABWB. Contributed reagents/materials/analysis tools: TS IJMR SRU. Wrote the paper: IG ABWB IJMR SRU.

References

1. Silman AJ, Pearson JE (2002) Epidemiology and genetics of rheumatoid arthritis. Arthritis Res 4:265–72.
2. Gabriel SE, Crowson CS, O'Fallon WM (1999) Mortality in rheumatoid arthritis: have we made an impact in 4 decades? J Rheumatol 26:2529–33.
3. Van Vollenhoven RF (2009) Treatment of rheumatoid arthritis: state of the art 2009. Nat Rev Rheumatol 5;531–41.
4. Eleftherohorinou H, Hoggart CJ, Wright VJ, Levin M, Coin LJ (2011) Pathway-driven gene stability selection of two rheumatoid arthritis GWAS identifies and validates new susceptibility genes in receptor mediated signalling pathways. Hum Mol Genet 20:3494–506.
5. Myouzen K, Kochi Y, Okada Y, Terao C, Suzuki A, et al. (2012) Functional variants in NFKBIE and RTKN2 involved in activation of the NF-κB pathway are associated with rheumatoid arthritis in Japanese. PLoS Genet 8:e1002949.
6. Okada Y, Terao C, Ikari K, Kochi Y, Ohmura K, et al. (2012) Meta-analysis identifies nine new loci associated with rheumatoid arthritis in the Japanese population. Nat Genet 44:511–6.
7. Michou L, Rat AC, Lasbleiz S, Bardin T, Cornélis F (2008) Prevalence and distribution of autoimmune diseases in 368 rheumatoid arthritis families. J Rheumatol 35:790–6.
8. Guthrie KA, Tishkevich NR, Nelson JL. (2009) Non-inherited maternal human leukocyte antigen alleles in susceptibility to familial rheumatoid arthritis. Ann Rheum Dis 68:107–9.
9. Goeldner I, Skare TL, de Messias Reason IT, Nisihara RM, Silva MB, et al. (2010) Anti-cyclic citrullinated peptide antibodies and rheumatoid factor in rheumatoid arthritis patients and relatives from Brazil. Rheumatology (Oxford) 49:1590–3.
10. Rojas-Villarraga A, Diaz FJ, Calvo-Páramo E, Salazar JC, Iglesias-Gamarra A, et al. (2009) Familial disease, the HLA-DRB1 shared epitope and anti-CCP antibodies influence time at appearance of substantial joint damage in rheumatoid arthritis. J Autoimmun 32:64–9.
11. Ärlestig L, Mullazehi M, Kokkonen H, Rocklöv J, Rönnelid J, et al. (2012) Antibodies against cyclic citrullinated peptides of IgG, IgA and IgM isotype and rheumatoid factor of IgM and IgA isotype are increased in unaffected members of multicase rheumatoid arthritis families from northern Sweden. Ann Rheum Dis 71:825–9.
12. Jacobsen S, Garred P, Madsen HO, Heegaard NH, Hetland ML, et al. (2009) Mannose-binding lectin gene polymorphisms are associated with disease activity and physical disability in untreated, anti-cyclic citrullinated peptide-positive patients with early rheumatoid arthritis. J Rheumatol 36:731–5.
13. Thiel S (2007) Complement activating soluble pattern recognition molecules with collagen-like regions, mannan-binding lectin, ficolins and associated proteins. Mol Immunol 44:3875–88.
14. Degn SE, Jensen L, Hansen AG, Duman D, Tekin M, et al. (2012) Mannan-binding lectin-associated serine protease (MASP)-1 is crucial for lectin pathway activation in human serum, whereas neither MASP-1 nor MASP-3 is required for alternative pathway function. J Immunol 189:3957–69.
15. Martiny FL, Veit TD, Brenol CV, Brenol JC, Xavier RM, et al. (2012) Mannose-binding Lectin Gene Polymorphisms in Brazilian Patients with Rheumatoid Arthritis. J Rheumatol 39:6–9.
16. Messias-Reason IT, Bosco DG, Nisihara RM, Jakobsen LH, Petzl-Erler ML, et al. (2008) Circulating levels of mannan-binding lectin (MBL) and MBL-associated serine protease 2 in endemic pemphigus foliaceus. Clin Exp Dermatol 33:495–7.
17. Banda NK, Takahashi M, Levitt B, Glogowska M, Nicholas J, et al. (2010) Essential role of complement mannose-binding lectin-associated serine proteases-1/3 in the murine collagen antibody-induced model of inflammatory arthritis. J Immunol 185:5598–606.
18. Ammitzboll CG, Thiel S, Ellingsen T, Deleuran B, Jorgensen A, et al. (2012) Levels of lectin pathway proteins in plasma and synovial fluid of rheumatoid arthritis and osteoarthritis. Rheumatol Int 32:1457–63.
19. Boldt AB, Goeldner I, de Messias-Reason IJ (2012) Relevance of the lectin pathway of complement in rheumatic diseases. Adv Clin Chem 56:105–53.
20. Hajela K, Kojima M, Ambrus G, Wong KH, Moffatt BE, et al. (2002) The Biological Functions of MBL-Associated Serine Proteases (MASPs). Immunobiology 205:467–75.
21. Stover C, Endo Y, Takahashi M, Lynch NJ, Constantinescu C, et al. (2001) The human gene for mannan-binding lectin-associated serine protease-2 (MASP-2), the effector component of the lectin route of complement activation, is part of a tightly linked gene cluster on chromosome 1p36.2-3. Genes Immun 2:119–27.
22. Herráez DL, Martínez-Bueno M, Riba L, de la Torre IG, Sacnún M, et al. (2013) Rheumatoid Arthritis in Latin Americans Enriched for Amerindian Ancestry is Associated With Loci in Chromosomes 1, 12, and 13, and the HLA Class II Region. Arthritis Rheum 65:1457–67.
23. The International Multiple Sclerosis Genetics Consortium (IMSGC) (2011) Genetic risk and a primary role for cell-mediated immune mechanisms in multiple sclerosis. Nature 10:214–9.
24. Jostins L, Ripke S, Weersma RK, Duerr RH, McGovern DP, et al. (2012) Host-microbe interactions have shaped the genetic architecture of inflammatory bowel disease. Nature 491:119–24.
25. Thiel S, Steffensen R, Christensen IJ, Ip WK, Lau YL, et al. (2007) Deficiency of mannan-binding lectin associated serine protease-2 due to missense polymorphisms. Genes Immun 8:154–63.
26. Boldt AB, Grisbach C, Steffensen R, Thiel S, Kun JF, et al. (2011) Multiplex sequence specific polymerase chain reaction reveals new MASP2 haplotypes associated with MASP-2 and MAp19 serum levels. Hum Immunol 72:753–60.
27. Sallenbach S, Thiel S, Aebi C, Otth M, Bigler S, et al. (2011) Serum concentrations of lectin-pathway components in healthy neonates, children and adults: mannan-binding lectin (MBL), M-, L-, and H-ficolin, and MBL-associated serine protease-2 (MASP-2). Pediatr Allergy Immunol 22:424–30.
28. Stengaard-Pedersen K, Thiel S, Gadjeva M, Møller-Kristensen M, Sørensen R, et al. (2003) Inherited deficiency of mannan-binding lectin-associated serine protease 2. N Engl J Med 349:554–60.
29. Schafranski MD, Ferraria LP, Scherner D, Torres R, de Messias-Reason IJ (2008) Functional MASP2 gene polymorphism in patients with history of rheumatic fever. Hum Immunol 69:41–4.
30. Boldt AB, Luz PR, Messias-Reason IJ (2011) MASP2 haplotypes are associated with high risk of cardiomyopathy in chronic Chagas disease. Clin Immunol 140:63–70.
31. Zhang M, Hou YJ, Cavusoglu E, Lee DC, Steffensen R, et al. (2013) MASP-2 activation is involved in ischemia-related necrotic myocardial injury in humans. Int J Cardiol 166:499–504.
32. Boldt ABW, Goeldner I, Stahlke ERS, Thiel S, Jensenius JC, et al. (2013) Leprosy association with low MASP-2 levels generated by MASP2 haplotypes and polymorphisms flanking MAp19 exon 5. PLoS One In press.
33. Arnett FC, Edworthy SM, Bloch DA, McShane DJ, Fries JF, et al. (1988) The American Rheumatism Association 1987 revised criteria for the classification of rheumatoid arthritis. Arthritis Rheum 31:315–24.
34. Braun-Prado K, Vieira Mion AL, Farah PN, Culpi L, Petzl-Erler ML (2000) HLA class I polymorphism, as characterised by PCR-SSOP, in a Brazilian exogamic population. Tissue Antigens 56:417–27.
35. Probst CM, Bompeixe EP, Pereira NF, de O Dalalio MM, Visentainer JE, et al. (2000) HLA polymorphism and evaluation of European, African, and Amerindian contribution to the white and mulatto populations from Parana, Brazil. Hum Biol 72:597–617.
36. Schlapbach LJ, Aebi C, Otth M, Leibundgut K, Hirt A, et al. (2009) Deficiency of mannose-binding lectin-associated serine protease-2 associated with increased risk of fever and neutropenia in pediatric cancer patients. Pediatr Infect Dis J 26:989–94.
37. Vallès X, Sarrias MR, Casals F, Farnós M, Piñer R, et al. (2009) Genetic and structural analysis of MBL2 and MASP2 polymorphisms in south-eastern African children. Tissue Antigens 74:298–307.
38. Nebert DW (2000) Proposal for an allele nomenclature system based on the evolutionary divergence of haplotypes. Hum Mutat 20:463–72.
39. Bergstrom U, Jacobsson LT, Nilsson JA, Berglund G, Turesson C (2011) Pulmonary dysfunction, smoking, socioeconomic status and the risk of developing rheumatoid arthritis. Rheumatology (Oxford) 50:2005–13.
40. van de Stadt LA, de Koning MH, van de Stadt RJ, Wolbink G, Dijkmans BA, et al. (2011) Development of the anti-citrullinated protein antibody repertoire prior to the onset of rheumatoid arthritis. Arthritis Rheum 63:3226–33.

41. Ip WK, Lau YL, Chan SY, Mok CC, Chan D, et al. (2000) Mannose-binding lectin and rheumatoid arthritis in southern Chinese. Arthritis Rheum 43:1679–87.
42. Troelsen LN, Garred P, Christiansen B, Torp-Pedersen C, Christensen IJ, et al. (2010) Double role of mannose-binding lectin in relation to carotid intima-media thickness in patients with rheumatoid arthritis. Mol Immunol 47:713–8.
43. Endo Y, Takahashi M, Kuraya M, Matsushita M, Stover CM, et al. (2002) Functional characterization of human mannose-binding lectin-associated serine protease (MASP)-1/3 and MASP-2 promoters, and comparison with the C1s promoter. Int Immunol 14:1193–201.
44. Unterberger C, Hanson S, Klingenhoff A, Oesterle D, Frankenberger M, et al. (2007) Stat3 is involved in control of MASP2 gene expression. Biochem Biophys Res Commun 364:1022–5.
45. Srirangan S, Choy EH (2010) The role of interleukin 6 in the pathophysiology of rheumatoid arthritis. Ther Adv Musculoskelet Dis 2:247–56.
46. Sorensen CM, Hansen TK, Steffensen R, Jensenius JC, Thiel S (2006) Hormonal regulation of mannan-binding lectin synthesis in hepatocytes. Clin Exp Immunol 145:173–82.
47. Thiel S, Jensen L, Degn SE, Nielsen HJ, Gál P, et al. (2012) Mannan-binding lectin (MBL)-associated serine protease-1 (MASP-1), a serine protease associated with humoral pattern-recognition molecules: normal and acute-phase levels in serum and stoichiometry of lectin pathway components. Clin Exp Immunol 169:38–48.
48. Dolman KM, Brouwer N, Frakking FN, Flatø B, Tak PP, et al. (2008) Mannose-binding lectin deficiency is associated with early onset of polyarticular juvenile rheumatoid arthritis: a cohort study. Arthritis Res Ther 10:R32.

20

Association of Autoimmune Addison's Disease with Alleles of STAT4 and GATA3 in European Cohorts

Anna L. Mitchell[1]*, Katie D. R. Macarthur[1], Earn H. Gan[1], Lucy E. Baggott[1], Anette S. B. Wolff[2], Beate Skinningsrud[3,4], Hazel Platt[5], Andrea Short[5], Anna Lobell[6], Olle Kämpe[6], Sophie Bensing[6,7], Corrado Betterle[8], Anna Kasperlik-Zaluska[9], Magdalena Zurawek[10], Marta Fichna[10], Ingrid Kockum[11], Gabriel Nordling Eriksson[12], Olov Ekwall[13], Jeanette Wahlberg[14], Per Dahlqvist[15], Anna-Lena Hulting[7], Marissa Penna-Martinez[16], Gesine Meyer[16], Heinrich Kahles[16], Klaus Badenhoop[16], Stephanie Hahner[17], Marcus Quinkler[18], Alberto Falorni[19], Amanda Phipps-Green[20], Tony R. Merriman[20], William Ollier[5], Heather J. Cordell[1], Dag Undlien[3,4], Barbara Czarnocka[21], Eystein Husebye[2,22], Simon H. S. Pearce[1]

1 Institute of Genetic Medicine, Newcastle University, Newcastle, United Kingdom, **2** Department of Clinical Science, University of Bergen, Bergen, Norway, **3** Department of Medical Genetics, Oslo University Hospital, Oslo, Norway, **4** University of Oslo, Oslo, Norway, **5** CIGMR, Institute of Population Health, University of Manchester, Manchester, United Kingdom, **6** Uppsala University, Uppsala, Sweden, **7** Karolinska Institutet, Stockholm, Sweden, **8** Department of Medicine, University of Padua School of Medicine, Padua, Italy, **9** Department of Endocrinology, Center for Postgraduate Medical Education, Warsaw, Poland, **10** Institute of Human Genetics, Polish Academy of Sciences, Poznan, Poland, **11** Neuroimmunology Unit, Department of Clinical Neuroscience and Centrum for Molecular Medicine, Karolinska Institutet, Stockholm, Sweden, **12** Department of Molecular Medicine and Surgery, Karolinska Institutet, Stockholm, Sweden, **13** The Sahlgrenska Academy, University of Gothenburg, Gothenburg, Sweden, **14** Department of Medical and Health Sciences, Division of Endocrinology, Faculty of Health Sciences, Linköping University, Linköping, Sweden, **15** Department of Public Health and Clinical Medicine, Umeå University, Umeå, Sweden, **16** Department Medicine (Division Endocrinology), University Hospital Frankfurt, Goethe-University, Frankfurt, Germany, **17** University Hospital Wuerzburg (Department of Medicine, Endocrinology and Diabetology), Wuerzburg, Germany, **18** Clinical Endocrinology, Charité Campus Mitte, Charité University Medicine Berlin, Berlin, Germany, **19** Department of Internal Medicine, University of Perugia, Perugia, Italy, **20** Department of Biochemistry, University of Otago, Otago, New Zealand, **21** Department of Biochemistry and Molecular Biology, Center for Postgraduate Medical Education, Warsaw, Poland, **22** Department of Medicine, Haukeland University Hospital, Bergen, Norway

Abstract

Background: Gene variants known to contribute to Autoimmune Addison's disease (AAD) susceptibility include those at the MHC, MICA, CIITA, CTLA4, PTPN22, CYP27B1, NLRP-1 and CD274 loci. The majority of the genetic component to disease susceptibility has yet to be accounted for.

Aim: To investigate the role of 19 candidate genes in AAD susceptibility in six European case-control cohorts.

Methods: A sequential association study design was employed with genotyping using Sequenom iPlex technology. In phase one, 85 SNPs in 19 genes were genotyped in UK and Norwegian AAD cohorts (691 AAD, 715 controls). In phase two, 21 SNPs in 11 genes were genotyped in German, Swedish, Italian and Polish cohorts (1264 AAD, 1221 controls). In phase three, to explore association of GATA3 polymorphisms with AAD and to determine if this association extended to other autoimmune conditions, 15 SNPs in GATA3 were studied in UK and Norwegian AAD cohorts, 1195 type 1 diabetes patients from Norway, 650 rheumatoid arthritis patients from New Zealand and in 283 UK Graves' disease patients. Meta-analysis was used to compare genotype frequencies between the participating centres, allowing for heterogeneity.

Results: We report significant association with alleles of two STAT4 markers in AAD cohorts (rs4274624: $P = 0.00016$; rs10931481: $P = 0.0007$). In addition, nominal association of AAD with alleles at GATA3 was found in 3 patient cohorts and supported by meta-analysis. Association of AAD with CYP27B1 alleles was also confirmed, which replicates previous published data. Finally, nominal association was found at SNPs in both the NF-κB1 and IL23A genes in the UK and Italian cohorts respectively.

Conclusions: Variants in the STAT4 gene, previously associated with other autoimmune conditions, confer susceptibility to AAD. Additionally, we report association of GATA3 variants with AAD: this adds to the recent report of association of GATA3 variants with rheumatoid arthritis.

Editor: Francesco Dotta, University of Siena, Italy

Funding: This study was funded by a European Union Framework 7 grant 201167 to the Euradrenal Consortium. Financial support for the Swedish contribution was also provided through the regional agreement on medical training and clinical research (ALF) between Stockholm County Council and Karolinska Institutet, The Swedish Society for Medical Research, the Swedish Society of Medicine, the NovoNordisk Foundation, Karolinska Institutet, and the Åke Wiberg Foundation. The funders had no role in study design, data collection and analysis, decision to publish, or preparation of the manuscript.

Competing Interests: The authors have declared that no competing interests exist.

* E-mail: annamitchell@doctors.org.uk

Introduction

Autoimmune Addison's disease (AAD) is a rare autoimmune endocrinopathy with a prevalence of 110–140 cases per million in Caucasian European populations [1,2]. Like many autoimmune endocrine conditions, AAD has a strong and oligo-genetic basis. The first case report of monozygotic twins concordant for AAD, suggesting a genetic aetiology, was published more than 40 years ago [3] and a number of similar cases have since been reported [4–6]. The observation that AAD, in common with many other autoimmune conditions, sometimes clusters within families also supports a genetic basis for the condition [7,8]. Furthermore, individuals with AAD are predisposed to develop other organ-specific autoimmune diseases which suggests shared susceptibility loci for these conditions. Most cases of AAD are not attributable to Mendelian abnormalities, but are a complex genetic trait, whereby currently unknown environmental factors interact with a number of genetic variants to cause disease.

The hypothesis-driven candidate gene approach has been used to investigate numerous complex diseases to date. In this method, plausible candidates are selected for investigation based on what is known of the biology and pathophysiology of a disease, on known allelic associations with mechanistically-related diseases and from information gained from the investigation of monogenic forms of a condition. In AAD such a monogenic form exists, as the autoimmune polyendocrinopathy syndrome type 1 (APS1), caused by loss of function mutations to both alleles of the *AIRE* gene [9]. In the investigation of complex AAD, the candidate gene approach has seen a number of successes, most notably the finding, and replication, of association of *MHC* alleles [10–13] and polymorphisms in *PTPN22* [14,15] and *CTLA4* [16,17] with AAD, all of which were investigated after having been associated with related autoimmune conditions. In AAD, previous candidate gene studies have been relatively small and some findings have proved difficult to replicate [18,19]. Therefore, in order to attain adequate power in candidate gene studies, large case-control cohorts are needed. The EURADRENAL consortium has recently provided a platform for collaboration between researchers in Europe and has, for the first time, allowed a large number of AAD DNA samples to be aggregated for genetic analysis.

This study aimed to investigate the role of 19 candidate genes in the pathogenesis of AAD in six European case-control cohorts using the Sequenom iPlex genotyping platform.

Subjects and Methods

Ethical approval for this work was obtained in each participating country as follows: Padua, Italy - Regione del Veneto Azienda Ospedaliera di Padova (ref 1583P); Perugia, Italy - CEAS Umbria (1247/08); Poznan, Poland - Ethics Committee at the Poznan University of Medical Sciences (18.06.2009; decision # 540/09); Warsaw, Poland - Ethical committee at the Center of Postgraduate Medical Education (April 18, 2007); Sweden - Regionala etikprövningsnämnden i Stockholm Dnr 2008/296-31/2; Oslo, Norway – Oslo Regional Ethics committee; Bergen, Norway - Regional Ethics Committee West; Newcastle, UK - Leeds (East) Research Ethics Committee, 2005 (REC reference number 05/Q1206/144); Frankfurt, Germany - Ethical committee of the University Hospital, Goethe-University, Frankfurt am Main (Reference-No 49/09); New Zealand - The New Zealand Multi-Region Ethics Committee (reference OTA/99/02/007).

Informed, written consent was sought from each study participant at all centres with the exception of the Norwegian controls. These samples were gathered through the national blood donor scheme. All blood donors are informed of ongoing research through written information and are given the opportunity to opt out should they wish to do so. All samples collected in this way are anonymised at source.

In each subject with AAD, the clinical diagnosis was confirmed by either a low basal cortisol with a high ACTH level or a subnormal response to the short synacthen test (250 μg parenteral synthetic $ACTH_{1-24}$). Patients with primary adrenal failure due to adrenal gland infiltration or infection, with secondary adrenal failure, or with APS1 (on the grounds of mucocutaneous candidiasis, hypoparathyroidism, and/or ectodermal dystrophy) were excluded. In total, DNA samples from 1,955 individuals with AAD and 1,936 healthy controls from 6 European countries were available for analysis. Available cohort characteristics are shown in table 1. 21-hydroxylase (21OH) autoantibody status was not available for all AAD cases included in this study, as it is not routinely tested in all participating countries. In total, 1,204 cases (61.6% of the total cohort) were known to be 21OH autoantibody positive (21OH+): 53 from UK, 290 from Norway, 73 from Poland, 154 from Germany, 266 from Italy and 368 from Sweden. All control samples included were Caucasian and had no personal or family history of autoimmune disease. Clinically silent autoimmune disease was not excluded in these controls by checking autoantibody levels, adrenal or thyroid function, however 21OH positivity in controls is known to be very rare.

Members of the EURADRENAL consortium selected 19 candidate genes for investigation, based on current knowledge of immunological pathways and the aetiology of autoimmune conditions. These included genes influencing $CD4^+$ lymphocyte fate (*GATA3, GATA binding protein 3; IL17A, interleukin 17A; IL17RA, interleukin 17 receptor A; IL21, interleukin 21; IL23A, interleukin 23 alpha subunit p19; RORA, RAR-related orphan receptor A; RORC, RAR-related orphan receptor C; STAT2, signal transducer and activator of transcription 2; STAT4, signal transducer and activator of transcription 4* and *TBX21, T-box 21*), transcription factors which alter the immune response (*NFATC2, nuclear factor of activated T-cells, cytoplasmic, calcineurin-dependent 2, NFKB1, nuclear factor of kappa light polypeptide gene enhancer in B-cells 1* and *REL, v-rel reticuloendotheliosis viral oncogene homolog*) and those genes important for innate immune mechanisms (*CYP2R1, vitamin D 25-hydroxylase; CYP24A1, 1,25-dihydroxyvitamin D3 24-hydroxylase; CYP27B1, 25-hydroxyvitamin D-1 alpha hydroxylase; GC, vitamin D binding protein; IFIH1, interferon induced with helicase C domain 1* and *VDR, vitamin D receptor*).

SNPs in these candidate genes were selected for genotyping using the HapMap database tag-SNP picker (www.Hapmap.org) [20]. SNPs were chosen with consideration of linkage disequilibrium (LD) patterns in CEU subjects which were studied in Haploview [21], to ensure that the major haplotypes across each gene were represented in the data collected, as far as possible. Independent SNPs (those with an r^2 of less than 0.4) with a minor allele frequency (MAF) of greater than 0.1 were preferentially selected for genotyping.

In this study, all SNP genotyping was carried out using Sequenom MassARRAY technology (Sequenom, San Diego) at either CIGMR, Manchester University, UK or NewGene, Newcastle University, UK. PCR reactions were set up in a 10 μl volume and contained 30 ng of template DNA, 1.25× PCR buffer, 1 mM $MgCl_2$, 500 μM dNTPs and 0.5 U/reaction of Fast Start Taq polymerase (Roche). A pool of primers (Metabion) was made to give a final concentration of each primer of 100 nM. Primer sequences are available from the authors on request. The thermal cycling conditions for the reaction included an initial

Table 1. Cohort information.

AAD cohort	Cohort size (cases/controls)	Mean age of onset (range)	Male:Female	Additional autoimmune comorbidities*		
				All (% of cohort)	Autoimmune thyroid disease (%)	Type 1 diabetes (%)
UK	309/335	39 (10–83 years)	1:3.3	57	43	6
Norway	382/380	53 (18–95 years)	1:1.7	66	47	12
Germany	341/235	51 (22–88 years)	1:1.3	55	47	7
Italy	280/322	38 (6–84 years)	1:2.0	72	61	12
Poland	275/296	38 (9–76 years)	1:3.0	77	38	10
Sweden	368/368	34 (0–71 years)	1:1.6	62	49	11

Information for each of the six included AAD cohorts.
*Additional autoimmune comorbidities include type 1 diabetes, autoimmune thyroid disease (Graves' and autoimmune hypothyroidism), pernicious anaemia, vitiligo, autoimmune hepatitis, rheumatoid arthritis, SLE, Sjogren's disease, Coeliac disease, premature ovarian failure, alopecia.

denaturation step at 94°C for 15 minutes, followed by 35 cycles of 94°C for 20 seconds, 56°C for 30 seconds and 72°C for 1 minute, followed by a final extension step of 72°C for 3 minutes. The iPlex^{TM} assay was then followed according to manufacturer's instructions (http://www.sequenom.com).

Genotyping was undertaken in three phases, with a statistical analysis performed after each phase. In the first phase, 85 tag SNPs in and around the 19 chosen candidate genes were genotyped in the UK (309 AAD, 335 controls) and Norwegian (382 cases, 380 controls) cohorts. Genes associated with one or both cohorts in this analysis were then selected for replication in phase 2 of this study, where 21 SNPs in 11 genes were genotyped in AAD case and control cohorts from Germany (341 AAD, 235 controls), Poland (275 AAD, 296 controls), Italy (280 AAD, 322 controls) and Sweden (368 AAD, 368 controls). Finally, in phase 3 of the study, 15 SNPs in the *GATA3* gene were genotyped in AAD cases and controls from the UK (335 AAD, 302 controls) and from Norway (352 AAD, 1,353 controls). In addition, to determine whether the association with *GATA3* polymorphisms extended to other autoimmune conditions, these SNPs were also genotyped in a cohort of 1,195 type 1 diabetes patients and matched controls from Norway, in 650 rheumatoid arthritis patients from New Zealand and 452 ancestrally-matched controls and in a cohort of 283 UK Graves' disease patients.

Data management, Quality Control and Statistical analysis

Genotyping call rates were first calculated (AA+Aa+aa/sample number ×100) and any SNP with a call rate of less than 95% was excluded from further analysis. Control genotype data were used to check for Hardy-Weinberg equilibrium (HWE). SNPs out of HWE ($P<0.01$) in the control population were excluded from further analysis. The prevalence of genotypes (AA vs Aa vs aa) and alleles (A = 2xAA+Aa, a = 2xaa+Aa) was calculated for all SNPs. χ^2 testing on 2×2 and 3×2 contingency tables was used to analyse the data for association. To account for multiple testing, a Bonferroni correction was applied (0.05/number of independent loci tested). Independent loci were defined as those with an r^2 value, derived from Hapmap CEU data, of less than 0.4.

A meta-analysis, using the Review Manager (RevMan) Version 5.0 program (The Nordic Cochrane Centre, Copenhagen, Denmark [22]), was then undertaken, using a random effects model to calculate odds ratios, confidence intervals and two-sided p-values. The impact of heterogeneity between the cohorts was estimated using an I^2 index. Results are stated as P-values.

Results

Phase 1

Phase 1 UK cohort results. In total, alleles of 13 SNPs in 9 genes showed nominal association ($P<0.05$) with AAD in the UK cohort (table 2). Maximal association was seen with the *NF-κB1* gene. Six SNPs were genotyped in, and close to, this gene. Alleles at 3 SNPs in moderate LD (r^2 0.39–0.68), *rs10026278*, *rs230532* and *rs4698861*, were associated with AAD in the UK cases compared to controls. Strongest evidence for association was at *rs4698861*, where the frequency of the minor (G) allele was 27.4% in AAD cases vs 37.4% in controls [odds ratio (OR) 0.63, 95% confidence interval (CI) 0.50–0.80; $P=0.00017$)]. Haplotype analysis in UNPHASED [23] revealed that the marker *rs4698861* accounts for all of the association with disease: if conditioned upon, no association with other markers in close proximity is seen. Nominal allelic association was also found at markers in *CYP24A1, CYP27B1, GATA3, IL17A, IL21, IL23A, REL* and *STAT2* (table 2). Allowing for 54 independent loci tested (P $0.05/54 = \leq 0.00096$), two of the above associations, both in the *NF-κB1* gene (*rs230532* $P_{allele}=0.00041$; *rs4698861* $P_{allele}=0.00017$) meet the threshold for significance. Full genotype results for all cohorts can be found in File S1.

Phase 1 Norwegian cohort results. In total, 6 SNPs in 6 genes were associated with AAD in the Norwegian cohort (table 2). Maximal association was seen at *rs4274624* in the *STAT4* gene. In total, 9 SNPs were genotyped at this locus, but in this cohort, 2 were excluded (*rs10931481* and *rs4853543*) due to low genotyping call rates. Of the remaining 7 SNPs, only alleles at *rs4274624* were associated with AAD, with the minor (C) allele frequency being 26.9% in cases and 19.5% in controls ($P=0.00045$, OR 1.52, [95% CI 1.20–1.94]). SNPs in an additional 5 genes, *IL17A, CYP24A1, GATA3, NFKB1* and *RORA* showed nominal significance. However, accounting for multiple comparisons, only *rs4274624* in *STAT4* remained significantly associated ($P=0.00045$) in the Norwegian cohort.

Phase 2

Phase 2 European cohort results. Analysis of genotype data for each of the six different European control cohorts using χ^2 testing indicated significant genetic heterogeneity between the

Table 2. Associations with AAD in the UK and Norwegian cohorts in phase 1 of genotyping.

	Gene	SNPs typed	SNPs excluded	rs ID	Minor allele	MAF cases/ controls	$P_{genotype}/P_{allele}$	OR [95% CI]	LD between associated markers*
UK	**NFKB1**	6	0	rs10026278	T	0.27/0.35	**0.012/0.0034**	0.69 [0.54–0.88]	Moderate
				rs230532	T	0.30/0.40	**0.0016/0.00041**	0.65 [0.52–0.82]	
				rs4698861	G	0.27/0.37	**0.00084/0.00017**	0.63 [0.50–0.80]	
	CYP27B1	3	1	rs4646536	G	0.26/0.33	**0.012/0.0091**	0.72 [0.56–0.92]	Significant
				rs703842	G	0.27/0.33	**0.027/0.014**	0.74 [0.58–0.94]	
	IL23A	1	0	rs11170816	A	0.05/0.09	N/A/**0.0047**	0.53 [0.34–0.84]	
	REL	2	1	rs13017599	A	0.41/0.33	**0.0099/0.0028**	1.40 [1.12–1.76]	
	GATA3	4	0	rs569421	C	0.26/0.19	**0.0092/0.003**	1.50 [1.15–1.96]	Low
				rs444929	C	0.21/0.28	**0.012/0.0053**	0.69 [0.54–0.90]	
	IL21	2	1	rs907715	T	0.32/0.39	**0.015/0.012**	0.74 [0.59–0.93]	
	STAT2	2	1	rs2066808	G	0.05/0.09	**0.039/0.012**	0.57 [0.36–0.90]	
	CYP24A1	9	3	rs4809959	G	0.48/0.53	**0.012/0.046**	0.80 [0.64–0.99]	
	IL17A	3	0	rs16882180	T	0.32/0.38	0.13/**0.043**	0.79 [0.63–1.00]	
Norway	***STAT4***	*11*	*2*	*rs4274624*	*C*	*0.27/0.19*	***0.0013/0.00045***	*1.52 [1.20–1.94]*	
	RORA	*4*	*1*	*rs1234805*	*T*	*0.37/0.30*	***0.0068/0.0018***	*1.41 [1.13–1.75]*	
	GATA3	*4*	*0*	*rs3802604*	*G*	*0.32/0.37*	***0.04/0.038***	*0.79 [0.64–0.98]*	
	NFKB1	*6*	*2*	*rs228611*	*A*	*0.43/0.49*	*0.063/**0.024***	*0.79 [0.65–0.97]*	
	CYP24A1	*9*	*1*	*rs2209314*	*C*	*0.25/0.25*	***0.031**/0.91*	*0.99 [0.78–1.25]*	
	IL17A	*3*	*1*	*rs4711998*	*A*	*0.22/0.27*	*0.060/**0.039***	*0.77 [0.61–0.98]*	

Nominally significant associations with AAD in the UK and Norwegian (italic text) cohorts in phase 1 of genotyping - no association was observed with alleles at *NFATC2, RORC, TBX21, CYP2R1, GC, IFIH1, IL17RA* and *VDR* (data not shown). $P_{genotype}$ and P_{allele} denote the P values derived from 2×3 and 2×2 chi squared testing respectively.
*Low LD = $r^2<0.40$, moderate LD = r^2 0.40–0.79, significant LD = $r^2>0.79$.
If the minor genotype was not represented in the dataset, the $P_{genotype}$ result is recorded as N/A.

populations studied (table 3), with the highest levels of heterogeneity between control cohorts from Italy and the UK and the least heterogeneity between the German and Swedish cohorts.

The phase 2 results for each population are summarised in table 4. Allowing for correction in the testing of 15 independent loci in the individual cohorts (P 0.05/15 = ≤0.0033), alleles at 1 marker only were significantly associated with AAD in the Italian cohort (*rs11171806* in *IL23A*; P = 0.0028).

Meta-analysis. Meta-analysis was performed using genotype data from each of the 6 different patient cohorts. In total, 4 SNPs in 3 genes remained associated with AAD. Maximal association was seen with alleles of two SNPs in moderate LD ($r^2 = 0.59$) in the *STAT4* gene (*rs4274624* P = 0.00016; *rs10931481* P = 0.0007) (figure 1). The intronic SNP, *rs4646536*, in *CYP27B1* was also nominally associated in the whole cohort (P = 0.03). This marker is in moderate LD with another genotyped SNP, *rs10876993* ($r^2 = 0.45$), however no association was seen with this SNP and AAD (figure 1). Finally, *rs3802604*, an independent SNP in *GATA3*, was also nominally associated with AAD (P = 0.03) (figure 1).

When the meta-analysis was repeated including only 21OH+ AAD individuals (1,204 21OH+ compared to 1,955 individuals in the whole AAD cohort), maximal association was again observed at *rs4274624* in *STAT4* (P = 0.0003). *rs3802604* in *GATA3* also remained nominally associated (P = 0.04). In addition, *rs13017599* in *REL* was associated (P = 0.03) although the result for this SNP in the whole AAD cohort was only marginally significant at P = 0.05.

Table 3. Genetic heterogeneity between the six different European control cohorts.

	UK	Norway	Germany	Italy	Poland	Sweden
UK		16.7%	21.4%	73.3%	53.3%	46.7%
Norway			7.7%	64.3%	30.8%	14.3%
Germany				50.0%	5.3%	0.0%
Italy					60.0%	57.1%
Poland						20.0%
Sweden						

Genetic heterogeneity between the six different European control cohorts. Allele frequencies were compared between all control populations using a chi squared test. The percentage of comparisons where a statistically significant result was seen ($P<0.05$) is shown in the table. A low percentage indicates that there were few markers at which allele frequencies differed between 2 populations of interest suggesting that there is little genetic heterogeneity between those two populations. A high percentage indicates that allele frequencies between two populations differed significantly at multiple markers, suggesting significant genetic heterogeneity between those two populations. Between the German and Swedish control cohorts, allele frequencies did not differ significantly at a single marker, suggesting that these populations are relatively genetically similar. By contrast, the UK and Italian control cohorts differed significantly at 73% of markers tested, suggesting significant genetic heterogeneity between these two cohorts.

No association was observed with *rs10931481* in *STAT4* (P = 0.07) or with *rs4646536* in *CYP27B1* (P = 0.16).

Extension of GATA3 analysis

The nominal association of *GATA3* alleles with AAD in UK, Norwegian and Polish cohorts, that remained associated following meta-analysis, was a novel finding (tables 2 and 4), as at the time of this study, polymorphisms in the *GATA3* gene have not previously been associated with autoimmune conditions. This locus was therefore selected for more detailed genotyping in the AAD cohorts and in additional disease cohorts: 1,195 Norwegian subjects with type 1 diabetes, 650 New Zealand subjects with rheumatoid arthritis and 283 UK subjects with Graves' disease.

GATA3 results

Allowing for 5 independent comparisons at the *GATA3* locus (P 0.05/5 = ≤0.01), 2 SNPs in the UK AAD cohort (*rs569421* P = 0.0096; *rs422628* = P 0.01) remained significantly associated. A further SNP in the New Zealand rheumatoid arthritis cohort (*rs3802604* P = 0.0096) would also meet the significance threshold. *rs3802604* was associated with AAD in the meta-analysis, however in AAD the minor G allele appears to confer protection from disease in contrast to rheumatoid arthritis, where the G allele confers disease susceptibility.

Table 4. Associations with AAD in the German, Swedish, Italian and Polish cohorts in phase 2 of genotyping.

Gene	SNPs typed	SNPs excluded	rs ID	Minor allele	MAF cases/controls	$P_{genotype}/P_{allele}$	OR [95% CI]	LD between associated markers*
Germany								
IL21	2	0	rs907715	T	0.24/0.31	**0.0078/0.018**	0.73 [0.56–0.95]	
Sweden								
STAT4	3	0	rs4274624	C	0.29/0.24	0.056/**0.017**	1.33 [1.10–1.68]	
Italy								
STAT4	3	0	rs10931481	G	0.36/0.29	**0.016/0.0056**	1.41 [1.11–1.80]	Moderate
			rs4274624	C	0.28/0.22	0.059/**0.02**	1.37 [1.10–1.78]	
IL23A	1	0	rs11171806	A	0.06/0.03	**0.012/0.0028**	2.37 [1.32–4.23]	
NFKB1	3	0	rs10026278	T	0.27/0.23	**0.049**/0.078	1.27 [0.97–1.65]	
STAT2	2	0	rs2066808	G	0.07/0.04	**0.037/0.014**	1.93 [1.13–3.28]	Significant
			rs2066807	G	0.06/0.03	**0.023/0.0063**	2.18 [1.23–3.85]	
Poland								
IL21	2	0	rs2221903	C	0.31/0.38	**0.04/0.02**	0.75 [0.58–0.96]	
CYP24A1	1	0	rs4809959	G	0.56/0.49	0.11/**0.03**	1.29 [1.02–1.64]	
GATA3	3	0	rs444929	C	0.18/0.21	**0.03**/0.12	0.79 [0.59–1.06]	

Nominally significant associations with AAD in the German, Swedish, Italian and Polish cohorts in phase 2 of genotyping. No association was observed with alleles at *RORA, IL17A, CYP27B1* and *REL* (data not shown).
*Low LD = $r^2<0.40$, moderate LD = r^2 0.40–0.79, significant LD = $r^2>0.7$.

A

Cohort	Cases Events	Cases Total	Controls Events	Controls Total	Weight (%)	Odds ratio M-H, Random, 95% CI
Germany	152	664	99	462	14.1	1.09 [0.82, 1.45]
Italy	152	552	140	644	16.1	1.37 [1.05, 1.78]
Norway	202	750	146	750	18.5	1.52 [1.20, 1.94]
Poland	140	540	129	590	15.2	1.25 [0.95, 1.65]
Sweden	214	736	172	730	19.6	1.33 [1.05, 1.68]
UK	147	618	151	650	16.6	1.03 [0.80, 1.34]
Total (95% CI)		**3860**		**3826**	**100**	**1.27 [1.12, 1.42]**
Heterogeneity I^2	20%					
Test for overall effect: Z	3.91 (P <0.0001)*					

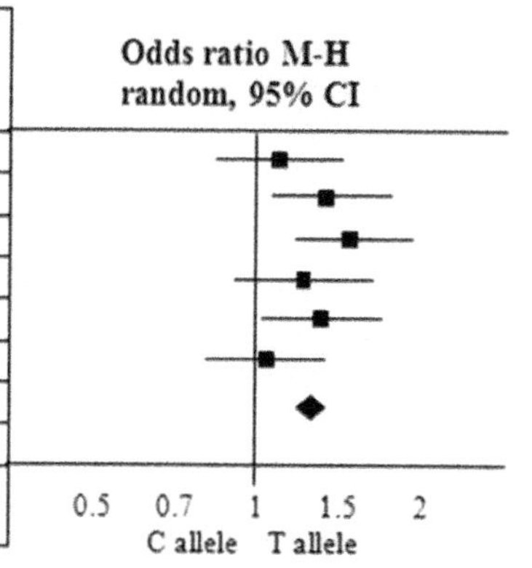

B

Cohort	Cases Events	Cases Total	Controls Events	Controls Total	Weight (%)	Odds ratio M-H, Random, 95% CI
Germany	211	666	136	454	21.7	1.08 [0.84, 1.40]
Italy	199	550	184	642	24.5	1.41 [1.11, 1.80]
Norway	0	0	0	0		Not estimable
Poland	177	540	168	588	22.7	1.22 [0.95, 1.57]
Sweden	268	736	233	728	31.1	1.22 [0.98, 1.51]
UK	0	0	0	0		Not estimable
Total (95% CI)		**2492**		**2412**	**100**	**1.23 [1.09, 1.39]**
Heterogeneity I^2	0%					
Test for overall effect: Z	3.37 (P = 0.0007)					

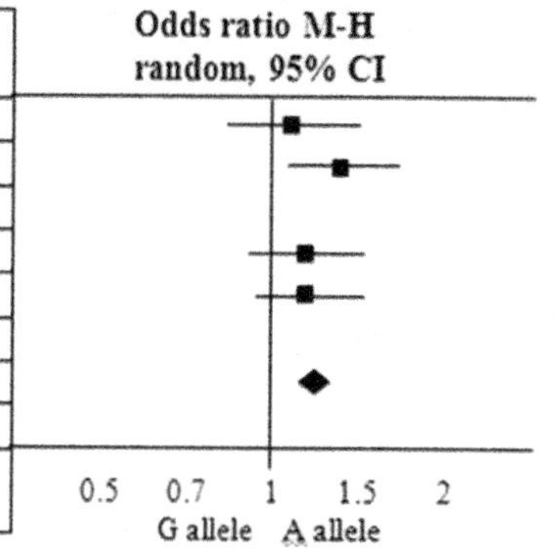

C

Cohort	Cases Events	Cases Total	Controls Events	Controls Total	Weight (%)	Odds ratio M-H, Random, 95% CI
Germany	206	666	149	460	14.4	0.93 [0.72, 1.21]
Italy	137	550	163	644	13.6	0.98 [0.75, 1.27]
Norway	256	742	267	736	20.6	0.93 [0.75, 1.15]
Poland	175	540	210	590	15.4	0.87 [0.68, 1.11]
Sweden	255	736	257	722	20.3	0.96 [0.77, 1.19]
UK	158	600	211	636	15.6	0.72 [0.56, 0.92
Total (95% CI)		**3834**		**3788**	**100**	**0.90 [0.81, 0.99]**
Heterogeneity I^2	0%					
Test for overall effect: Z	2.23 (P = 0.03)					

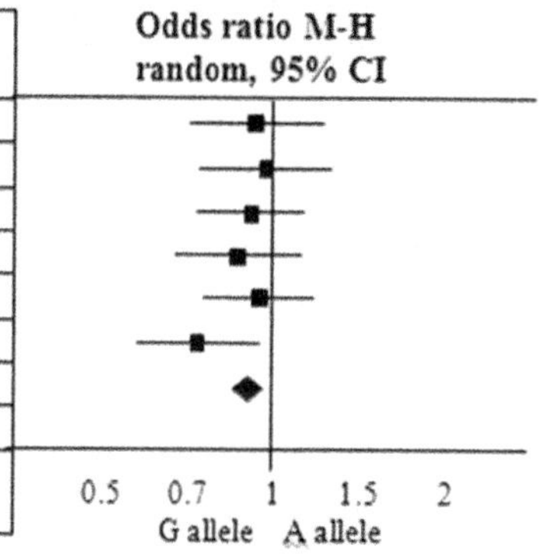

D

Cohort	Cases Events	Cases Total	Controls Events	Controls Total	Weight (%)	Odds ratio M-H, Random, 95% CI
Germany	247	664	180	462	14.6	0.93 [0.73, 1.18]
Italy	214	550	245	642	16.0	1.03 [0.82, 1.30]
Norway	236	738	278	746	19.0	0.79 [0.64, 0.98]
Poland	167	536	215	590	14.2	0.79 [0.62, 1.01]
Sweden	266	736	276	730	19.4	0.93 [0.75, 1.15]
UK	220	614	241	654	16.7	0.96 [0.76, 1.20]
Total (95% CI)		**3838**		**3824**	**100**	**0.90 [0.82, 0.99]**
Heterogeneity I^2	0%					
Test for overall effect: Z	2.21 (P = 0.03)					

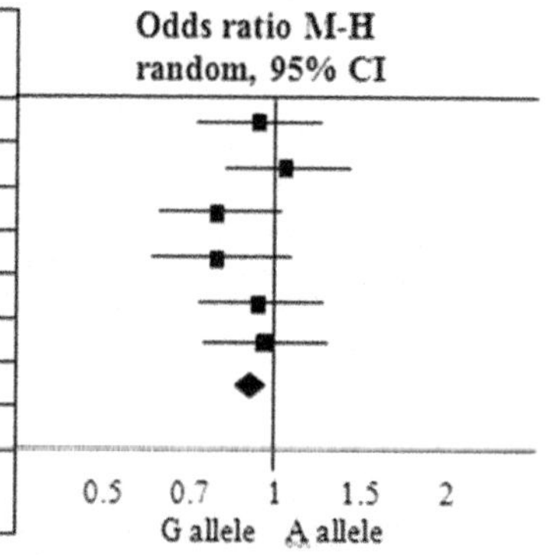

Figure 1. Forest plots of significant meta-analysis results in AAD. Meta-analysis of *rs4274624* and *rs10931481* in the *STAT4* gene (panel A, B), *rs4646536* SNP in the *CYP27B1* gene (panel C) and *rs3802604* SNP in the *GATA3* gene (panel D) in 6 European AAD cohorts. To be included in the analysis, the genotyping call rate per SNP had to be 95% or more for each cohort, in both cases and controls, and the control data set had to not deviate significantly from Hardy Weinberg Equilibrium (P>0.01). Pooled analysis showed little heterogeneity amongst the cohorts ($I^2 \leq 20\%$). Using a random effects model, the meta-analysis confirms association between alleles at these four SNPs and AAD. Maximum association was noted at *rs4274624* (panel A), with an odds ratio (OR) of 1.27 [95% CI 1.12–1.42], P<0.0001. (*P value = 0.00016 when data analysed under a random effects model in Stata). In panel B, data for the UK and Norwegian cohorts is not presented as the quality control inclusion criteria were not met in these cohorts.

Discussion

This is the largest study of AAD genetics to date, including almost 2,000 AAD subjects from six European countries. It implicates a number of biomolecular pathways in the pathogenesis of this rare autoimmune condition.

The most robust finding of this study is association of AAD with alleles at two *STAT4* markers. The STAT4 transcription factor is known to have a role in $CD4^+$ cell fate, being necessary for generation of T_H1 responses, and also plays a role in T_H17 cell differentiation. Variation at the *STAT4* locus is well established as having a role in several different autoimmune conditions including rheumatoid arthritis [24,25], SLE [23] and primary Sjögren's disease [26]. In the study by Remmers *et al.* [24] the minor allele at *STAT4* marker *rs7574865* was significantly associated with both rheumatoid arthritis ($P = 4.64 \times 10^{-8}$, OR 1.27 [95% CI 1.16–1.36]) and SLE ($P = 1.87 \times 10^{-9}$, OR 1.55 [95% CI 1.34–1.79] in a meta-analysis. The minor allele of this SNP, in addition to three others in intron 3 of *STAT4*, was also associated with rheumatoid arthritis in the Korean population ($P = 0.0065$, OR 1.27 [95% CI 1.11–1.45]) [25] and with primary Sjögren's syndrome in a small study ($P = 0.01$, OR 1.47 [95% CI 1.09–1.97]) [26]. The marker most associated with AAD in the meta-analysis performed in this study, *rs4274624*, is in significant LD ($r^2 = 0.90$) with SNP *rs7574865*. The other associated marker, *rs10931481*, in the meta-analysis, is in moderate LD with both *rs4274624* ($r^2 = 0.59$) and *rs7574865* ($r^2 = 0.53$) and was further associated with rheumatoid arthritis and SLE directly in the study by Remmers ($P = 0.005$, 0.025 respectively) [24], but to a lesser degree than *rs7574865*. These SNPs are all within a large intron in the *STAT4* gene which raises the possibility that they are tagging a variant which, rather than disrupting protein structure and/or function directly as deleterious mutations in the coding regions might, may result in splice variation or disrupt non-coding regulatory components to result in disease susceptibility.

Furthermore, we demonstrated nominally significant association of *GATA3* polymorphisms in UK, Norwegian and Polish AAD populations, and meta-analysis of the whole European AAD cohort further supported this association. GATA3 has been implicated in the homeostasis and regulation of CD8+ T-lymphocytes [27] and could therefore contribute to primary T-lymphocyte dysregulation in autoimmune Addison's disease. Extension of *GATA3* analysis to other autoimmune disease cohorts showed only association with alleles at a single SNP, *rs3802604*, in the New Zealand rheumatoid arthritis population, replicating a recent finding in a large multinational RA patient cohort [28]. This is the SNP that was associated in the AAD cohort meta-analysis, however for AAD, the minor G allele is protective (OR 0.90), whereas in rheumatoid arthritis, the minor G allele confers susceptibility (OR 1.27). Although this may represent a novel but different association in rheumatoid arthritis, reflecting the different immunopathogenesis of this disease compared to AAD, the overall degree of association in AAD is weak and this finding needs further replication in larger datasets.

We have also replicated the association of *CYP27B1* polymorphisms with AAD. Association of a promoter polymorphism in this gene with German autoimmune cohorts, including AAD, Hashimoto's thyroiditis, Graves' disease and type 1 diabetes was first reported in 2004 [29]. This finding was later replicated in small AAD cohorts from the UK and Poland [30,31]. In this study, we have used meta-analysis to establish an association with an intronic variant in this gene and AAD in European cohorts. There is strong linkage disequilibrium in this region which encompasses the entire *CYP27B1* gene and therefore these associated SNPs may be tagging a more distant causative variant yet to be defined. Alternatively, polymorphisms in *CYP27B1*, also associated with type 1 diabetes [32] may have a role in regulating vitamin D 1-alpha hydroxylation in a tissue-specific manner [33].

Finally, we report significant association with alleles at *NF-κB1* polymorphisms and AAD in the UK cohort and between alleles of an *IL23A* polymorphism and AAD in the Italian cohort. The NF-κB pathway is a highly conserved innate immune mechanism which allows a vigorous and rapid inflammatory response to a myriad of potentially harmful stimuli, and IL23A has a role in $CD4^+$ cell fate and the T_H1 response, therefore these are both plausible candidates for AAD. However, the significance of these isolated findings is currently unclear and these results will need to be confirmed by replication.

We observed significant genetic heterogeneity between the 6 European control cohorts, particularly between geographically distant countries such as the UK and Italy and this may explain the different patterns of associations between the 6 European AAD cohorts. Genetic heterogeneity may also be contributing to the differences observed in the clinical characteristics of the participating European cohorts, for example the age at onset of AAD and the proportion of each cohort with additional autoimmune conditions. However, variation between countries in diagnostic criteria and how these data are recorded and collected is also likely to be a contributing factor to these observed differences. Previous studies have also demonstrated significant genetic heterogeneity between European countries, even when non-Caucasian individuals are excluded. For example, a study by Cross *et al.* published in 2010 [34] compared allele frequencies of 51 SNPs in 19,027 self-reported white Caucasians. Between individuals from Scandinavia, the UK, Germany and Eastern Europe, minor allele frequencies differed significantly (i.e. $P<0.05$) at 19 (37.3%) SNPs. The difference was particularly marked (i.e. $P<0.0001$) at 5 (9.8%) of the 51 SNPs analysed. The significant heterogeneity observed between the 6 countries included in this study may account for the different patterns of association in each population and clearly highlights the importance of carefully matching cases with controls in genetic studies.

Conclusion

This is the largest genetic study of AAD to date and includes almost 2,000 carefully phenotyped individuals from 6 European countries. We have demonstrated significant heterogeneity between control cohorts of the participating European countries. We report that variants in the *STAT4* gene, previously associated with other autoimmune conditions including rheumatoid arthritis and SLE, appear to confer susceptibility to AAD, as demonstrated by data derived from the Italian, Norwegian and Swedish populations studied. We are also able to confirm a nominal association of *GATA3* variants with another autoimmune condition, namely AAD, in UK, Norwegian and Polish Europeans. On further investigation, a single SNP was also associated with rheumatoid arthritis in a cohort from New Zealand, however, the findings could not be replicated in type 1 diabetes or Graves' disease. In addition, we have replicated a previous association with *CYP27B1* polymorphisms with AAD in the UK cohort, with the result supported by meta-analysis in the six European cohorts together. We have found that variants in two genes, *NF-κB1* and *IL23A*, not previously associated with AAD, contribute to susceptibility in the UK and Italian populations respectively, however these findings require replication. Further research, perhaps by genome-wide association studies in large, collaborative cohorts, or whole exome/genome sequencing in selected individuals, is now warranted to determine the genetic factors which make up the remaining hidden heritability of AAD.

Author Contributions

Conceived and designed the experiments: ALM BS OK SB CB AKZ MF AL ALH KB AF WO DU EH SHSP. Performed the experiments: ALM KDRM HP. Analyzed the data: ALM KDRM EHG LEB HP APG HJC SHSP. Contributed reagents/materials/analysis tools: ASBW BS AS OK SB CB AKZ BC MZ MF IK GNE OE JW PD ALH MPM GM HK MQ AF TRM WO DU EH SHSP SH. Wrote the paper: ALM SHSP. All coauthors provided assistance with manuscript revisions and approved the final version of the manuscript prior to submission.

References

1. Lovas K, Husebye ES (2002) High prevalence and increasing incidence of Addison's disease in western Norway. Clin Endocrinol (Oxf). 56: 787–91.
2. Laureti S, Vecchi L, Santeusanio F, Falorni A (1999) Is the prevalence of Addison's disease underestimated? J Clin Endocrinol Metab 84: 1762.
3. Smith ME, Gough J, Galpin OP (1963) ADDISON'S DISEASE IN IDENTICAL TWINS. Br Med J 2: 1316.
4. Heggarty H (1968) Addison's disease in identical twins. Br Med J 1: 559.
5. Russell GA, Coulter JB, Isherwood DM, Diver MJ, Smith DS (1991) Autoimmune Addison's disease and thyrotoxic thyroiditis presenting as encephalopathy in twins. Arch Dis Child 66: 350–2.
6. Simmonds JP, Lister J (1978) Auto-immune Addison's disease in identical twins. Postgrad Med J 54: 552–4.
7. Fairchild RS, Schimke RN, Abdou NI (1980) Immunoregulation abnormalities in familial Addison's disease. J Clin Endocrinol Metab 51: 1074–7.
8. Hewitt PH (1957) Addison's disease occurring in sisters. Br Med J 2: 1530–1.
9. Lander ES, Schork NJ (1994) Genetic dissection of complex traits. Science 265: 2037–48.
10. Maclaren NK, Riley WJ (1986) Inherited susceptibility to autoimmune Addison's disease is linked to human leukocyte antigens-DR3 and/or DR4, except when associated with type I autoimmune polyglandular syndrome. J Clin Endocrinol Metab 62: 455–9.
11. Myhre AG, Undlien DE, Løvås K, Uhlving S, Nedrebø BG, et al. (2002) Autoimmune adrenocortical failure in Norway autoantibodies and human leukocyte antigen class II associations related to clinical features. J Clin Endocrinol Metab 87: 618–23.
12. Gombos Z, Hermann R, Kiviniemi M, Nejentsev S, Reimand K, et al. (2007) Analysis of extended human leukocyte antigen haplotype association with Addison's disease in three populations. Eur J Endocrinol 157: 757–61.
13. Skinningsrud B, Lie BA, Lavant E, Carlson JA, Erlich H, et al. (2011) Multiple loci in the HLA complex are associated with Addison's disease. J Clin Endocrinol Metab 96: 1703–8.
14. Kahles H, Ramos-Lopez E, Lange B, Zwermann O, Reincke M, et al. (2005) Sex-specific association of PTPN22 1858T with type 1 diabetes but not with Hashimoto's thyroiditis or Addison's disease in the German population. Eur J Endocrinol 153: 895–9.
15. Velaga MR, Wilson V, Jennings CE, Owen CJ, Herington S, et al. (2004) The codon 620 tryptophan allele of the lymphoid tyrosine phosphatase (LYP) gene is a major determinant of Graves' disease. J Clin Endocrinol Metab 89: 5862–5.
16. Blomhoff A, Lie BA, Myrhe AG, Kemp EH, Weetman AP, et al. (2004) Polymorphisms in the cytotoxic T lymphocyte antigen-4 gene region confer susceptibility to Addison's disease. J Clin Endocrinol Metab 89: 3474–6.
17. Vaidya B, Imrie H, Geatch DR, Perros P, Ball SG, et al. (2000) Association analysis of the cytotoxic T lymphocyte antigen-4 (CTLA-4) and autoimmune regulator-1 (AIRE-1) genes in sporadic autoimmune Addison's disease. J Clin Endocrinol Metab 85: 688–91.
18. Pani MA, Regulla K, Segni M, Hofmann S, Hüfner M, et al. (2002) A polymorphism within the vitamin D-binding protein gene is associated with Graves' disease but not with Hashimoto's thyroiditis. J Clin Endocrinol Metab 87: 2564–7.
19. Skinningsrud B, Lie BA, Husebye ES, Kvien TK, Førre Ø, et al. (2010) A CLEC16A variant confers risk for juvenile idiopathic arthritis and anti-cyclic citrullinated peptide antibody negative rheumatoid arthritis. Ann Rheum Dis 69: 1471–4.
20. The International HapMap Consortium (2003) The International HapMap Project. Nature 426: 789–96.
21. Barrett JC, Fry B, Maller J, Daly MJ (2005) Haploview: analysis and visualization of LD and haplotype maps. Bioinformatics 21: 263–5.
22. The Cochrane Collaboration (2011) Review Manager (RevMan) [Computer program]. Version 5.0. Copenhagen: The Nordic Cochrane Centre.
23. Dudbridge F (2008) Likelihood-based association analysis for nuclear families and unrelated subjects with missing genotype data. Hum Hered 66: 87–98.
24. Remmers EF, Plenge RM, Lee AT, Graham RR, Hom G, et al. (2007) STAT4 and the risk of rheumatoid arthritis and systemic lupus erythematosus. N Engl J Med 357: 977–86.
25. Lee HS, Remmers EF, Le JM, Kastner DL, Bae SC, et al. (2007) Association of STAT4 with rheumatoid arthritis in the Korean population. Mol Med 13: 455–60.
26. Korman BD, Alba MI, Le JM, Alevizos I, Smith JA, et al. (2008) Variant form of STAT4 is associated with primary Sjögren's syndrome. Genes Immun 9: 267–70.
27. Tai TS, Pai SY, Ho IC (2013) GATA-3 regulates the homeostasis and activation of CD8+ T cells. J Immunol 190: 428–37.
28. Eyre S, Bowes J, Diogo D, Lee A, Barton A, et al. (2012) High density genetic mapping identifies new susceptibility loci for rheumatoid arthritis. Nature Genetics 44: 1336–1340.
29. Lopez ER, Zwermann O, Segni M, Meyer G, Reincke M, et al. (2004) A promoter polymorphism of the CYP27B1 gene is associated with Addison's disease, Hashimoto's thyroiditis, Graves' disease and type 1 diabetes mellitus in Germans. Eur J Endocrinol 151: 193–7.
30. Jennings CE, Owen CJ, Wilson V, Pearce SH (2005) A haplotype of the CYP27B1 promoter is associated with autoimmune Addison's disease but not with Graves' disease in a UK population. J Mol Endocrinol 34: 859–63.
31. Fichna M, Zurawek M, Januszkiewicz-Lewandowska D, Gryczyñska M, Fichna P, et al. (2010) Association of the CYP27B1 C(-1260)A polymorphism with autoimmune Addison's disease. Exp Clin Endocrinol Diabetes 118: 544–9.
32. Cooper JD, Smyth DJ, Walker NM, Stevens H, Burren OS, et al. (2011) Inherited variation in vitamin D genes is associated with predisposition to autoimmune disease type 1 diabetes. Diabetes 60: 1624–31.
33. Badenhoop K, Kahles H, Penna-Martinez M (2012) Vitamin D, immune tolerance, and prevention of type 1 diabetes. Curr Diab Rep 12: 635–42.
34. Cross DS, Ivacic LC, Stefanski EL, McCarty CA (2010) Population based allele frequencies of disease associated polymorphisms in the Personalized Medicine Research Project. BMC Genet 11: 51.

21

Peripheral CD4CD8 Double Positive T Cells with a Distinct Helper Cytokine Profile Are Increased in Rheumatoid Arthritis

Dagmar Quandt, Kathrin Rothe, Roger Scholz, Christoph W. Baerwald, Ulf Wagner*

Clinics for Gastroenterology and Rheumatology, Division of Rheumatology, University of Leipzig, Leipzig, Saxony, Germany

Abstract

Peripheral CD4CD8 double positive (DP) T cells have been reported to play a role in several autoimmune diseases, virus infections and cancer. In rheumatoid arthritis (RA), both CD4 and CD8 single positive (SP) T cells are known to be involved in the pathogenesis, but the role of peripheral CD4CD8 DP T cells has not been investigated in detail. Anti cyclic citrullinated antibodies (ACPA) positive and ACPA negative RA patients, patients with systemic lupus erythematodes (SLE) and age matched healthy donors (HD) were enrolled in the analysis. The frequencies and phenotype of DP T cells in PBMC were investigated. In addition, DP T cells were quantified in biopsies from rheumatoid synovium. After in vitro restimulation, the cytokine production of DP T cells was investigated in cultures of PBMC. CMV specific cytokine secretion as well as proliferation was analyzed following antigen specific restimulation after an appropriate culture duration. DP T cells were found more frequently in RA patients than in healthy controls or patients with SLE. These DP T cells express αβ TCRs, are of a memory phenotype and share features of both CD4 as well as CD8 SP T cells. Importantly, DP T cells were found to also be present in the rheumatoid synovium. Further characterization of DP T cells from RA patients revealed increased production of IL-21 and IL-4, implying a possible role as T helper cells. In addition, DP T cells in RA seem to contribute to the inflammatory process, because they produce significantly more IFNγ than counterparts from HD and are increased in CMV+ RA patients. Given their capacity to produce a variety of cytokines (IL4, IL21 and IFNγ), their association with ACPA positive RA and their presence in the synovium, we suggest an important role of double positive T cells in the pathogenesis of rheumatoid arthritis.

Editor: Oliver Frey, University Hospital Jena, Germany

Funding: This study was supported by the German Research Foundation (WA 2765/3-1). The author(s) acknowledge support from the German Research Foundation (DFG) and Leipzig University within the program of Open Access Publishing. The funders had no role in study design, data collection and analysis, decision to publish, or preparation of the manuscript.

Competing Interests: The authors declare that they have no competing interest.

* E-mail: ulf.wagner@medizin.uni-leipzig.de

Materials and Methods

Patients and Healthy Individuals

A total of 59 RA patients according to the 2010 EULAR/ACR criteria (female: 46, male: 13, mean age 59.4 years, range 34–79 years) were recruited, among them 39 $ACPA^+$ and 20 $ACPA^-$ patients. 39% of the RA patients were treated with biologicals in combination with conventional standard therapy. Sex and age distribution in $ACPA^+$ versus $ACPA^-$ patients was similar. In addition, 8 SLE patients (all female, mean age 44.3 years, range 21–54 years) were included. Blood of 36 HD (female: 21, male: 15, mean age of 57.1 years, range 25–71 years) who never had evidence of a chronic inflammatory disorder were recruited as controls. The 4 RA patients undergoing knee surgery (2 male, 2 female) were all $ACPA^+$.

Ethics Statement

Written consents were obtained from all patients and healthy donors. The local ethics committee of the University of Leipzig approved the study.

Antibodies and Reagents

RPMI 1640 was from Lifetechnologies. X-Vivo15 media was supplied by Lonza. aCD3, aCD4, aCD8 (recognizing the α chain), aCD28, aCD45RO, aCD56, aCCR7, a-IL17, aTCRα24-Jα18 (clone: 6B11), cytokine secretion assays for IFNγ and IL-4, a-fibroblast microbeads and Cytostim were purchased from Miltenyi. Collagenase, Hyaluronidase and DNAse were all from Sigma-Aldrich. aCD45 and aCD38 were from Immunotools. CFDA-SE was purchased from Molecular Probes/Invitrogen. Intra staining Kit, aCD16, aCD8β and aCD3 were from Beckton Dickinson. aCXCR5 was supplied by R&D Systems and aIL21 was from ebioscience. The Beta Mark TCRVβ Repertoire Kit was supplied by Beckman Coulter. The antibodies were used in different conjugates of FITC, PE, PerCp, APC, APC-Vio770 and PE-Cy7.

PBMC Generation and FACS Analysis *ex vivo*

PBMCs were isolated from EDTA whole blood or buffy coats. Plasma was always discarded from whole blood samples prior to Ficoll-gradient for PBMCs isolation. Subsequently a erythrocyte lysis step with lysis-buffer was applied. Cells were stained with different antibodies and kept on ice throughout the assay. Live Cell analysis (use of PI) with doublet exclusion (LSR II) were performed on a FACS Calibur ™ or a LSR II (both Beckton Dickinson) using Cellquest, FACS DIVA and FlowJo software.

CMV Specific Cytokine Production and Proliferation

These assays were performed as described recently. [1] In brief, 1×10^6 PBMC were CFDA-SE labeled and cultured for 7 days (proliferation) or left unlabeled and cultured for 4 hrs (2×10^6, IFNγ secretion) in the presence of CMV lysate/control lysate (Microbrix Biosystems Inc) of 3 μg/ml in 24-well plates in X-VIVO 15 medium.

Short Term Culture and Staining for Cytokine Analysis

PBMCs were cultured in X-Vivo 15 supplemented with 1% of each glutamin and penicillin/streptomycin in a density of 5×10^6 for cytostim (1:50) or 3×10^6 for PMA (20 ng/ml and Ionomycin (0.5 μg/ml). Culture time was 4 hrs for both and Monensin (2 μM) was added to the last 3 hrs of PMA/Ionomycin cultures. Cytokines were either detected with cytokine secretion assays (IFN-γ and IL-4) following the manufactures protocol by Miltenyi or by intracellular staining (IL-21 and IL-17) using an intra staining Kit.

Tissue Digestions and Leucocyte Extraction

Synovial biopsies from RA patients undergoing surgery were obtained and leucocyte isolation was performed as follows. Tissue was cut into pieces and incubated with an enzyme solution (collagenase, hyaluronidase, DNAse in RPMI) for 90 min and 37° under constant rotation. Single cell suspension was obtained using gauze and smooth mechanical disruption of digested tissue. Subsequently cells were sorted for non-fibroblasts using anti-fibroblast microbeads from Miltenyi. Non-fibroblast were used for FACS analysis and CD45 staining was used additionally to other antibodies in order to discriminate non-leucocytes.

Statistics

Statistical evaluation was performed using Prism version 3.0cx software. Mann-Whitney test, unpaired student's t-test and correlation analysis with spearmen were applied.

Introduction

Peripheral CD4CD8 double positive (DP) T cells have first been identified more than 20 years ago. Like their progenitors in the thymus, they express the coreceptors CD4 and CD8 simultaneously, but in contrast to immature double positive thymocytes, they show varying degrees of coreceptor expression, and display a memory phenotype but no markers of recent thymic emigrants [2–4]. DP T cells can be found in the blood of healthy individuals where they account for about 1% of all T cells within PBMCs, but are also present in the skin of melanoma patients and in systemic sclerosis [5,6]. During the cause of severe virus infections such as HIV and Hepatitis, increased frequency of DP T cells have been described, which are Ag-specific and of high effector potential. [2,7]. DP T cells can provide B cell help both by production of appropriate cytokines and by cell contact due to their T helper like phenotype [5,6], but they can also acquire killer like capacity [7,8].

In rheumatoid arthritis, CD4+ Th cells play a pivotal role in the pathogenesis, as indicated by numerous genetic associations of the disease with polymorphisms in T cell related genes as well as by the clinical efficacy of CD28 co-stimulation [10] and CD4 co-receptor blockade [9] [11]. The peripheral CD4+ T cell pool in RA is characterized by several alterations including a paucity of naïve T cells and recent thymic emigrants, an increased memory pool and a global loss of T cell receptor diversity accompanied by large clonal expansions [12,13].

B cell autoreactivity is also essential in RA pathogenesis, as indicated by autoantibody production and by the clinical efficacy of B cell depletion [14]. The T cell help required for this has been suggested to involve CD40-CD40L interactions [15], but additionally other receptors such as BAFF-R [16] have been identified more recently. The result is the production of disease relevant autoantibodies like anti-citrullinated peptide antibodies (ACPA), anti-RA33, RF and others. ACPA positive RA in particular has been associated with more severe joint destruction [1], frequent extraarticular manifestations and enhanced subclinical artheriosclerosis [17].

A possible role of CD4CD8 DP T cells in the pathogenesis of RA has not been investigated.

Here we report, that CD4CD8 double positive T cells are expanded in the peripheral blood in ACPA$^+$ RA and can also be found in the rheumatoid synovium. DP T cells in RA show features of T helper cells by the production of IL-4 and IL-21. Interestingly, CMV$^+$ RA patients show increased frequencies of these cells and their number correlates positively with CMV specific IFNγ producers. In line with this, a high number of these cells have lost the CD28 costimulator and DP T cells of RA patients show higher amounts of IFNγ producers than HD counterparts. Our data are the first demonstrating a role for CD4CD8 double positive T cells in RA.

Results

ACPA$^+$ RA Patients have Increased Frequencies of Peripheral DP T cells

Total CD4CD8 DP T cells were quantified as percentage of total CD3$^+$ T cells in PBMC, and three subpopulations (CD4^{hi}CD8^{lo}, CD4^{hi}CD8^{hi} and CD4^{lo}CD8^{hi}) according to the level of coreceptor expression could be distinguished as shown in figure 1A. CD4^{hi}CD8^{lo} DP T cells are the most prominent of the DP cell populations and were found to be significantly more frequent in PBMC from ACPA positive RA patients when compared to healthy controls, SLE patients or ACPA negative RA patients (mean%: RA ACPA$^+$1.93, RA ACPA$^-$ 1.07, HD 1.24 and SLE 0.58, figure 1B). Total frequencies of CD4CD8 DP T cells were also higher in ACPA positive than in ACPA negative patients (figure 1C). The total CD4CD8 DP population will be used in all subsequent displays throughout the manuscript, unless otherwise stated. In the RA patient population no influence of age on the frequency of DP T cells was discernible (figure 1 D). Such a correlation was demonstrated for healthy individuals by others [18] and was also found in our own data for HD. (data not shown) A trend towards a further decrease of DP T cells in SLE patients compared to age matched controls did not reach statistical significance.

DP T cells in RA Belong to the Memory Pool of TCRαβ T cells and Display No Marker of iNKT cells

The previously described expansion of the memory pool in RA patients [12] was apparent in the analysis of CD4 SP T cells, 70% of which had a central memory phenotype characterized by expression of CD45RO and CCR7 (figure 2A). In agreement with previous reports [2,7], the majority of CD4CD8 DP T cells was also found to belong to the memory pool (87.9%). Analysis of CD45RO and CCR7 expression identified 58.4% as central memory cells (see figure 2A) and 29.5% as effector memory cells.

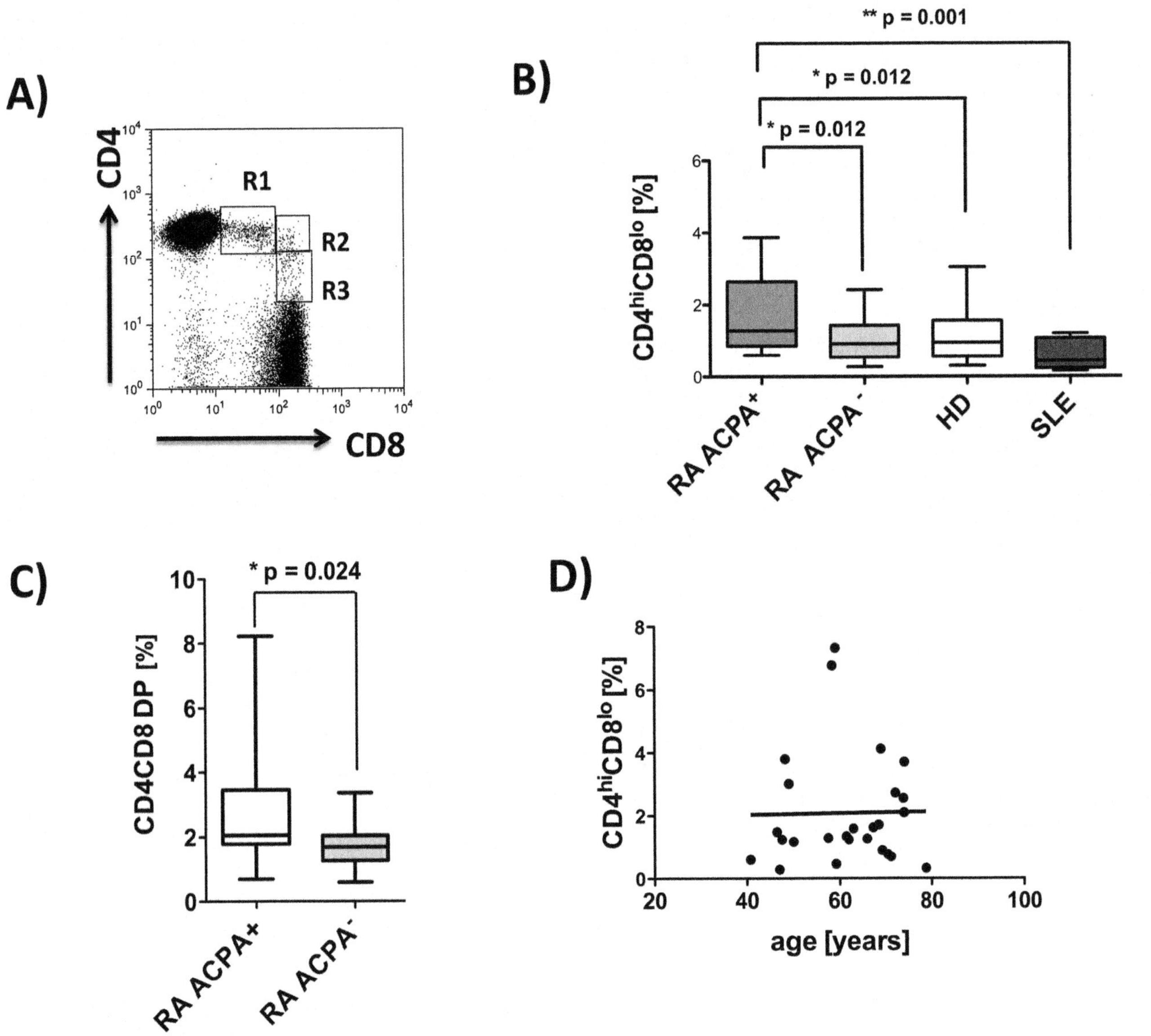

Figure 1. Increased frequencies of peripheral CD4CD8 DP T cells in ACPA$^+$ rheumatoid arthritis patients. PBMC were isolated from RA patients (ACPA$^+$, n = 37, ACPA$^-$, n = 20), healthy donors (n = 36), and patients with SLE (n = 8), and FACS analyses from live cells (PI staining used for exclusion of dead cells) were performed. Analyses for CD4CD8 double positive T cells are always pregated on CD3 positive T cells. **A)** Representative FACS plot from one RA patient, showing CD4CD8 double positive T cells, R1 = CD4^{hi}CD8^{lo}, R2 = CD4^{hi}CD8^{hi} and R3 = CD4^{lo}CD8^{hi} **B)** Comparison of frequencies of CD4^{hi}CD8^{lo}T cells in PBMCs of ACPA$^+$/− RA, HD and SLE patients. **C)** Total CD4CD8 DP T cells in ACPA$^+$ (n = 19) and ACPA$^-$ (n = 20) RA patients. **D)** Correlation analysis for frequencies of CD4^{hi}CD8^{lo} T cells with age in ACPA$^+$ RA patients. Box plots depict median, interquartile range and 10–90 percentile. Significance as given, *$p<0.05$, **$p<0.01$.

The described spectrum of memory markers on DP T cells from RA patients did not differ from healthy controls (data not shown).

With regards to activation markers, DP T cells did not differ from CD4 and CD8 SP cells in their expression of CD38. Expression of the T cell activation marker HLA-DR [19], however, was found on DP T cells more frequently than on CD4 SP cells, but less frequently than on CD8$^+$ SP lymphocytes (figure 2B). In healthy donors, in contrast, HLA-DR expression on DP T cells did not differ from that of CD4 SP T cells (data not shown. CD56, which can also serve as activation marker for T cells [34], was also found significantly more frequently on DP T cells than on CD4 SP T cells (figure 2D). Other markers associated with activation/regulation like CD69 and CTLA-4 were not expressed on DP T cells (data not shown).

In peripheral blood from RA patients, CD4CD8 DP T cells expressed almost exclusively (99,3%) $\alpha\beta$ T cell receptors, which was comparable to CD4 SP T cells (99,3%, figure 2 C). DP T cells were not $\gamma\delta$ T cells (data not shown). Distribution of $\alpha\beta$ and $\gamma\delta$ TCR expression in the T cell subpopulations was similar in HD (data not shown). In accordance with previous reports [35], CD4^{hi}CD8^{lo} DP T cells in RA do not express $\alpha\beta$ CD8 heterodimers but $\alpha\alpha$ homodimers, whereas CD8 SP cells are almost exclusively CD8$\alpha\beta$ positive (figure 2C).

DP T cells in HD have been described to partially belong to a population of T cells with NK phenotype, called NKT cells. [4]

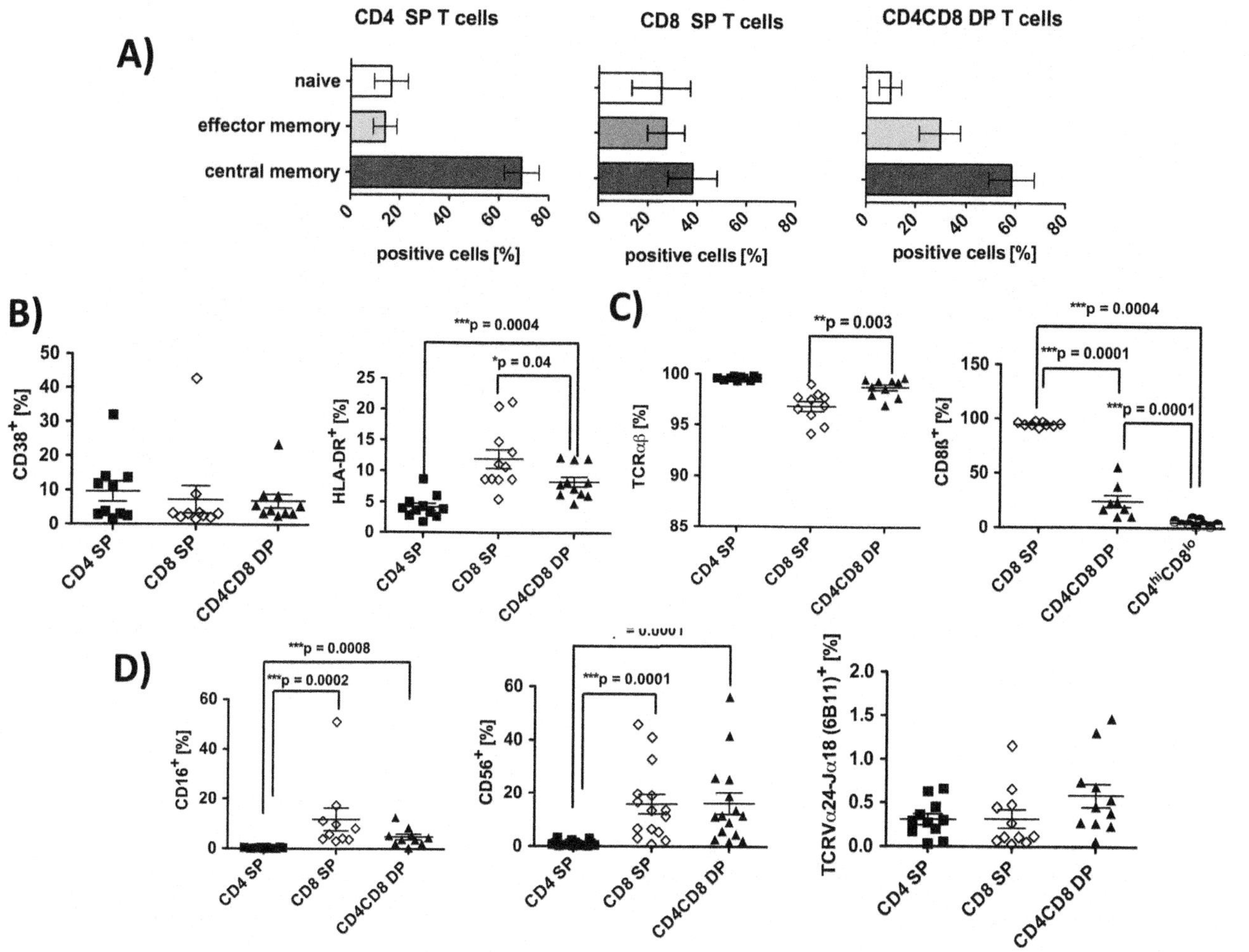

Figure 2. Phenotypic characterization of CD4CD8 DP T cells in RA patients. PBMC from RA patients were isolated and FACS analyses from live cells were performed (PI staining used for exclusion of dead cells). CD3 pregated cells were further gated on CD4 single, CD8 single and on CD4CD8 double positive T cells. **A)** Distribution of CD45RO$^-$CCR7$^+$ (naive) CD45RO$^+$CCR7$^-$ (effector memory) and CD45RO$^+$CCR7$^+$ (central memory) cells in the cell populations indicated. n = 5 5 **B)** Percentage of T cells positive for CD38 (n = 10) and HLA-DR (n = 11). **C)** Percentage of cells bearing a TCR alpha-beta (n = 10) and cells positive for CD8β (n = 9) in the T cell populations indicated. **(D)** Percentage of cells positive for CD16 (n = 10), CD56 (n = 15) and for TCRVα24-Jα18 (n = 11, marker for iNKT) in the T cell populations indicated. In all graphs, lines represent means and SEM. Significance as given, *p<0.05, **p<0.01, ***p<0.001.

To determine a possible NKT cell phenotype of DP T cells in RA, we used an antibody recognizing the TCRVα24-Jα18:Vβ11, described for invariant iNKT cells, and a combination of anti-CD16 together with anti-CD56 to check for non-invariant NKT cells. The frequency of iNKT cells was not significantly increased in the DP fraction (0.59%±0.13) when compared to CD4 SP or CD8 SP cells (0.31% vs. 0.32%) (figure 2D). Frequencies of CD16$^+$ cells were low but were significantly increased in DP T cells (4.8%±1.1) when compared to CD4 SP cells (figure 2D). Co-staining of CD56 and CD16 on DP T cells revealed the presence of some infrequent (2.4%±0.47) CD16$^+$CD56$^+$ cells which possibly fall into the category of non-invariant NKT cells (data not shown).

To investigate the TCR repertoire used by DP T cells of RA patients, we performed FACS analysis using 24 different antibodies recognizing a broad range of TCR BV chains. The BV usage within DP T cells of 10 RA patients is divers and does not differ significantly from CD4 SP or CD8 SP. (figure 3A) 5 patients showed a substantial overrepresentation of individual BV elements (BV2, BV17 and/or BV21.3) (representative examples given in figure 3B), possibly indicating antigen-driven clonal expansion.

DP T cells are Present in the Synovial Tissue and Display Features of T helper Cells

The target organ in rheumatoid arthritis is the synovium. Therefore we were interested in identifying DP T cells in the synovium of inflamed joints. As demonstrated in figure 4A we do find CD4CD8 double positive T cells (pregated on CD3$^+$ T cells) in the synovium (mean: 2.5%). Of note, the same RA patients also showed CD19$^+$ B cells in the synovium (figure 3A).

To explore the potential of CD4CD8 DP T cells to provide B cell help, the CXCR5 expression was analyzed, since this chemokine receptor has been described to be present on several subpopulation of T follicular helper (Tfh) cells, although with varying support for antibody secretion [20]. The results showed that DP T cells from RA patients can express CXCR5, although the fraction of CXCR5 positive cells is higher in CD4 SP than in CD4CD8DP cells (mean: 9.5% vs. 4.1.%, p = 0.03, figure 4B).

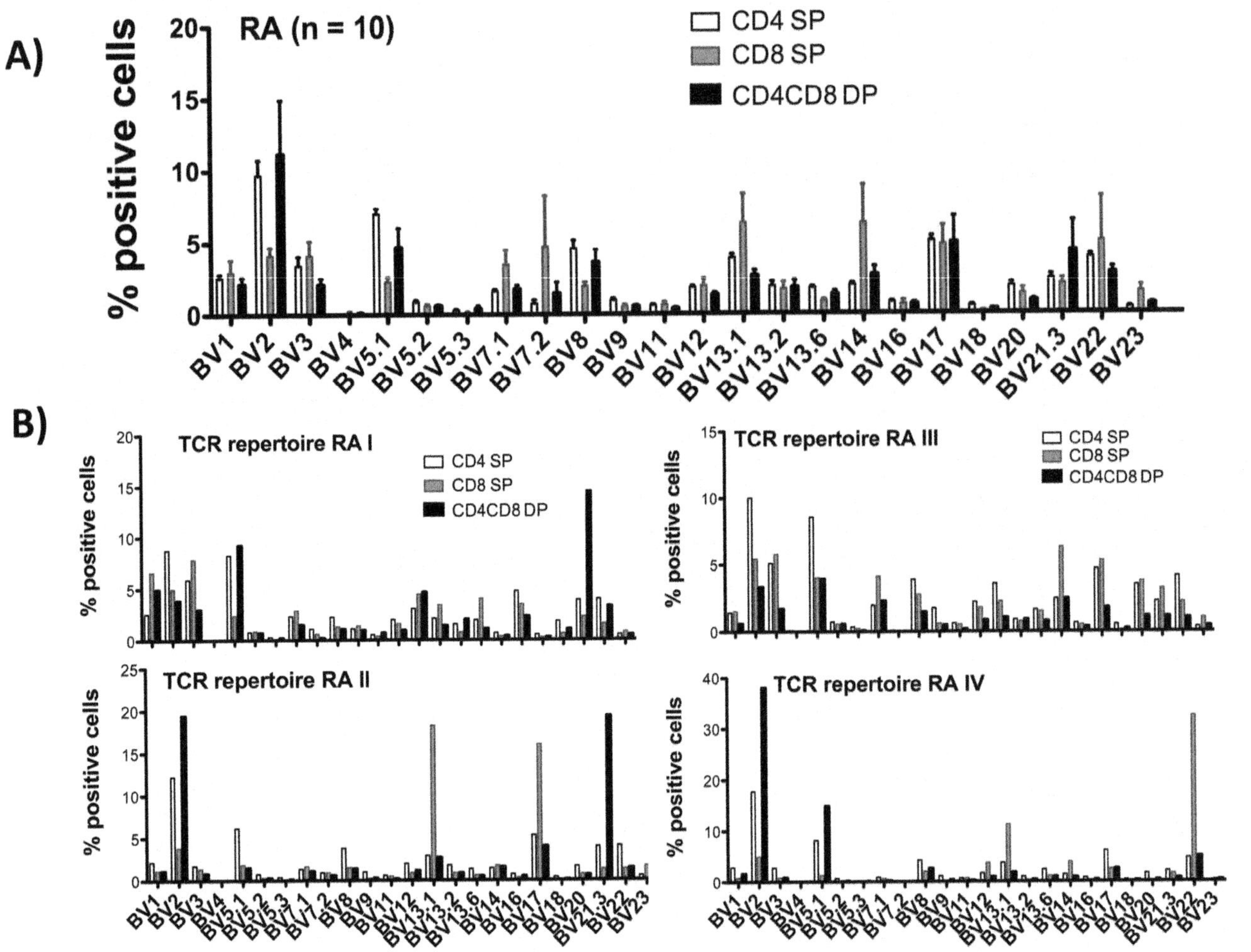

Figure 3. TCR BV distribution in CD4CD8 double positive T cells of RA patients. PBMC from RA patients were isolated and FACS analyses from live cells were performed (PI staining used for exclusion of dead cells). CD3 pre-gated cells were further gated on CD4 single, CD8 single and on CD4CD8 double positive T cells. Bar charts depict the percentage of cells positive for each BV element in the indicated T cell subpopulations investigated. **A)** Mean distribution of 24 TCR BV elements in peripheral blood T cells from 10 RA patients. **B)** Examples of the individual distribution of 24 TCR BV elements in 4 RA patients.

Similar frequencies were found in DP T cells from healthy individuals (mean 5.1%, data not shown).

As functional and possibly more specific markers of Tfh cells, the ability to secrete IL-4 and IL-21 following restimulation in vitro was determined, since both cytokines are required for B cell help [20,21]. Determination of IL-4 secretion of DP T cells upon in vitro short term restimulation with Cytostim showed a substantial fraction of them to produce IL-4 (figure 4C). Importantly, this percentage of IL-4 producers was significantly higher in RA patients than in healthy controls (mean: 1.99% vs. 0.71%, $p = 0.0006$).

Most importantly, however, a large fraction of DP cells (15–19%) was found to produce IL-21, compared to only 2% of CD4 SP T cells (figure 4D). No difference between the IL-21 production of DP T cells from healthy donors compared to those from RA patients was detectable (figure 4D).

DP T cells in RA Preferentially Produce IFNγ but not IL-17

Several abnormal T cell subpopulations are pathogenetically relevant in RA, among them Th17 cells and IFNγ producers [22–24]. Using cytokine secretion assays as well as intracellular FACS analysis, IFNγ and IL17 expression was determined in vitro after short term restimulation with the MHC-TCR crosslinker Cytostim (IFNγ) or with PMA/Ionomycin (IL-17). Frequencies of cytokine producers were calculated as percentage of total CD4CD8 DP T cells, since cytokine expression was not restricted to a particular subpopulation ($CD4^{hi}CD8^{lo}$ or $CD4^{lo}CD8^{hi}$) of DP T cells.

In RA patients, significantly more DP T cells produced IFNγ than CD4 SP or CD8 SP T cells (mean 21.1% vs. 3.9% or 12.7%, $p = 0.0001$ and $p = 0.012$, respectively) (figure 5A). In HD, in contrast, there was no significant difference in the percentage of IFNγ producers between the 3 different T cell populations (CD4 or CD8 SP and DP T cells, data not shown). Most importantly, the frequency of IFNγ producing DP T cells in RA patients significantly exceeds the frequency found in HD (11.4%) (figure 5A).

Results for IL-17 were less conclusive. IL-17 was mainly produced by CD4 SP T cells, and not by CD8 SP or DP positive T cells (figure 5B). Nevertheless, a trend towards higher IL-17 production was seen in CD4 SP T cells from RA patients compared to CD4 SP from HD T cells (figure 5B).

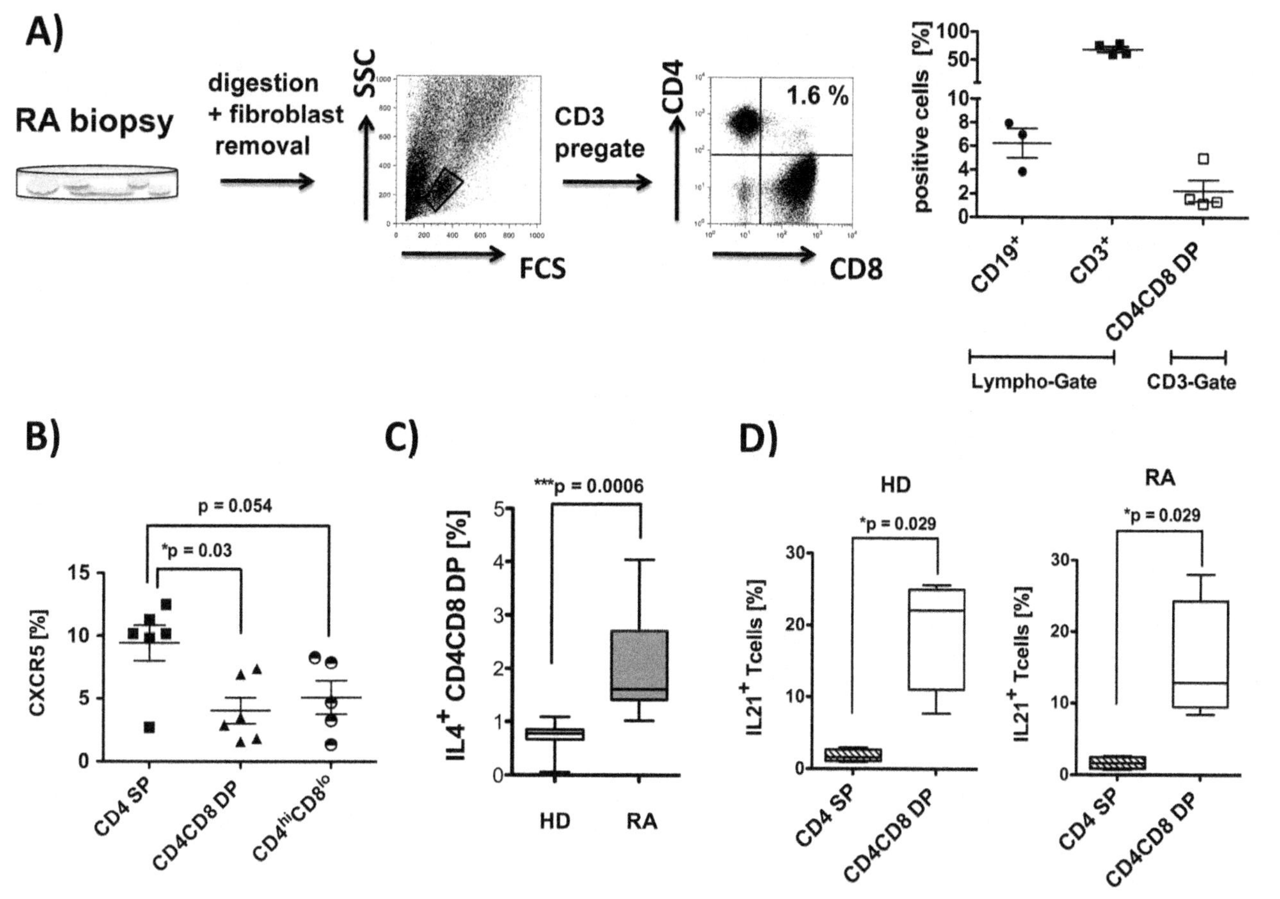

Figure 4. CD4CD8 double positive T cells are present in the synovium of RA patients and produce T helper 2 like cytokines. A) Single cell suspensions were prepared from synovial biopsies from RA patients (n = 4) and analyzed by flow cytometry using anti-CD19, anti-CD3, anti-CD4 and anti-CD8 monoclonal antibodies (PI staining used for exclusion of dead cells). Representative FACS plots are depicted. Each data point represents one experiment. **B)** PBMCs from RA patients (n = 6) were isolated and FACS analysis from live cells were performed (PI staining used for exclusion of dead cells). Cells were pre-gated on CD3^{+} T cells, and CXCR5 expression was analyzed in the subpopulation indicated. **C)** PBMC were stimulated in vitro for 4 hrs with Cytostim. Subsequently, an IL-4 specific secretion assay was performed, and expression of CD4 and CD8 was determined in vital cells (PI staining used for exclusion of dead cells) pre-gated on CD3. Percentage of IL-4 producing CD4CD8 double positive T cells in HD (n = 7) and RA patients (n = 8) is given. **D)** PBMCs from HD (n = 4) and RA (n = 4) were stimulated with PMA/Iono for 4 hrs, and intracellular staining for IL-21 was performed. Cells are counterstained with anti-CD3, anti-CD4 and anti-CD8. Depicted is the percentage of cytokine producers in total CD4CD8 DP T cells and in CD4 SP cells. Box plots in C) and D) show median, interquartile range, and 10–90 percentiles. Significance as given, *$p<0.05$.

DP T cells are more Frequent in Latent CMV Infection and Correlate with the Occurrence of CMV Specific Cytokine Producers

Latent CMV infection in rheumatoid arthritis is associated with a more severe cause of joint destruction, as published recently by our group and others [1,17]. This association was limited to ACPA positive RA. Based on the observed increase of DP T cells in ACPA positive RA, which are readily able to produce IFNγ in response to polyclonal stimuli, we decided to stratify the patients according to the presence or absence of anti-CMV IgG antibodies in the serum. The results showed significantly higher frequencies of CD4^{hi}CD8^{lo} DP positive T cells, in anti-CMV IgG positive RA patients compared to CMV^{-} patients (mean 1.81% vs 0.71%, p = 0.007, figure 6A). This difference remained significant, if the analysis was restricted to ACPA positive patients only (mean 2.27% vs. 1.55%, p = 0.039). Interestingly, the highest frequencies of CD4CD8 DP T cells (mean%: 2.27) were found in patients simultaneously positive for anti-CMV IgG and ACPA (data not shown).

CD4^{+}CD28^{null} T cells are increased in RA patients and associated with a more severe course of the disease [13,25]. In addition, they are known to occur in the course of a latent CMV infection both in RA patients and in healthy controls. Therefore, the frequency of CD4^{+}CD28^{null}T cells was determined in the RA patients and found to correlated with the percentages of total CD4CD8 DP T cells (figure 6B). This correlation was restricted to ACPA^{+} RA patients and was not present in ACPA negative patients. Furthermore, DP T cells were found to preferentially have lost CD28 expression (mean%: 19,4, n = 13) in ACPA positive RA patients when compared to CD4 SP (mean%: 1.97) T cells, while the frequency of CD28 negative cells was even higher in CD8 SP (mean%: 33) T cells (figure 6B).

Finally, in order to investigate the CMV response, we restimulated (4 hrs) PBMC from anti-CMV IgG seropositive RA patients with CMV lysate or control lysate and determined the CMV specific IFNγ production of CD4 SP T cells and CD4CD8 DP T cells by cytokine secretion assay. The frequency of CMV specific IFNγ producers was found to correlate with the frequencies of total CD4CD8 DP T cells in CMV^{+} RA patients

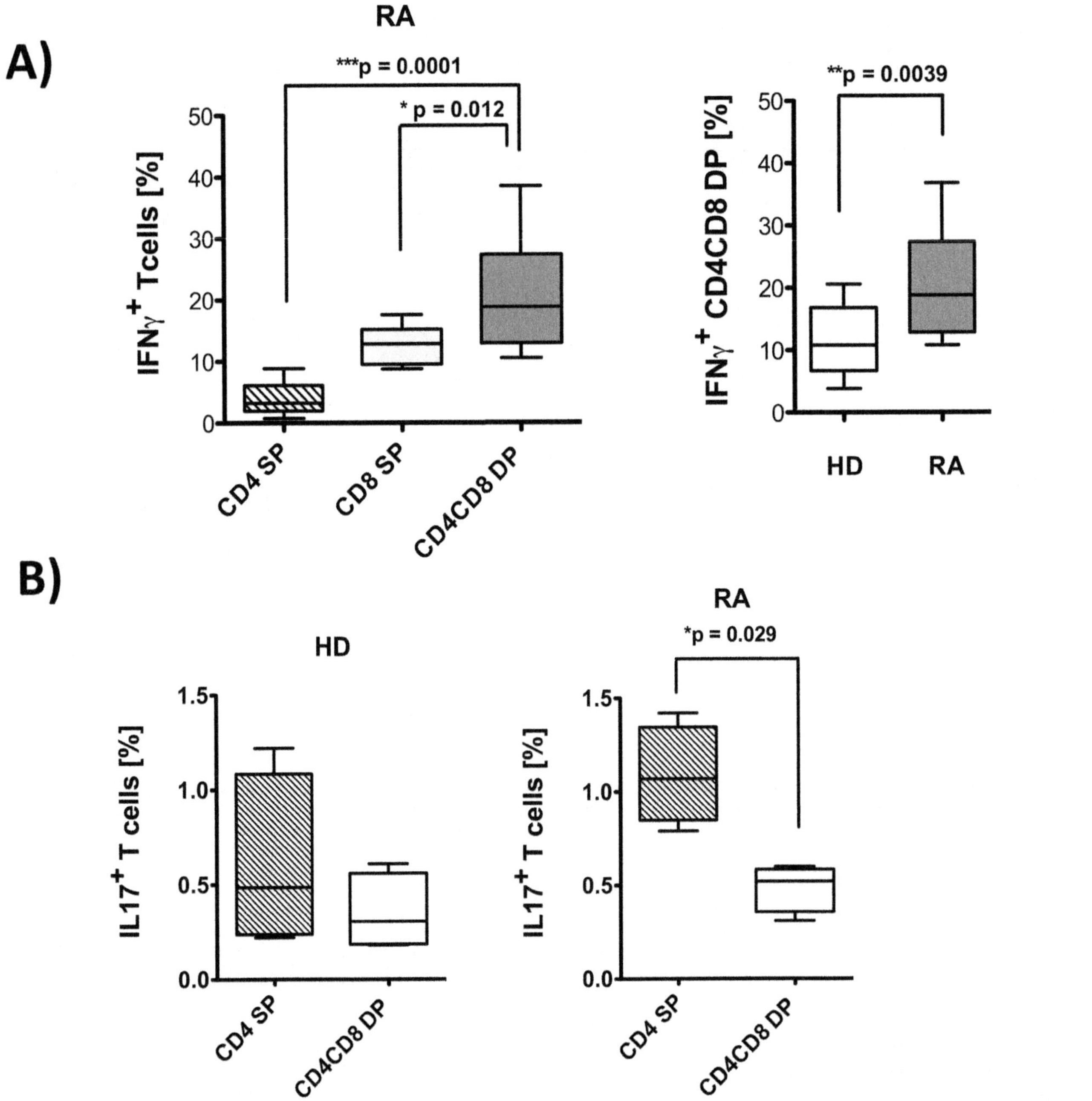

Figure 5. CD4CD8 double positive T cells from RA patients produce inflammatory IFNγ. PBMC from RA and HD were stimulated in vitro for 4 hrs with Cytostim (A) or PMA/Iono (B). Subsequently, cytokine specific secretion assays (A) or intracellular stainings (B) were performed and cells were counterstained with anti-CD3, anti-CD4 and anti-CD8. Flow cytometric cytokine analysis were performed on live cells for IFNγ secretion (PI staining used for exclusion of dead cells) or on fixed cells for intra-cellular staining for IL-17, in each case after pre-gating on $CD3^+$ T cells. **A)** Percentage of IFNγ producing T cells in samples from rheumatoid arthritis patients (n = 12, left panel and grey box in the right panel) and healthy donors (n = 13, clear box in the right panel) among CD4 SP, CD8 SP and CD4CD8 DP T cells. **B)** Percentage of IL-17 producing CD4 SP and CD4CD8 double positive T cells from RA patients (n = 4) and HD (n = 4). Presented box plots show median, interquartile range, and 10–90 percentiles. Significance as given, $*p<0.05$, $**p<0.01$, $***p<0.001$.

(figure 6C). Interestingly, the CMV specific IFNγ response of CD4CD8 DP T cells from RA patients was significantly higher (2.09) than in HD (0.67) (figure 6D). The antigen-induced, CMV specific proliferation of CD4 SP T cells, in contrast, did not correlate with the frequency of DP T cells (figure 6E).

Discussion

The study was conducted to investigate a possible role for peripheral CD4CD8 double positive T cells in the pathogenesis of rheumatoid arthritis.

The results show, that in RA patients, a significant number of mature T cells are indeed double positive for both co-receptors,

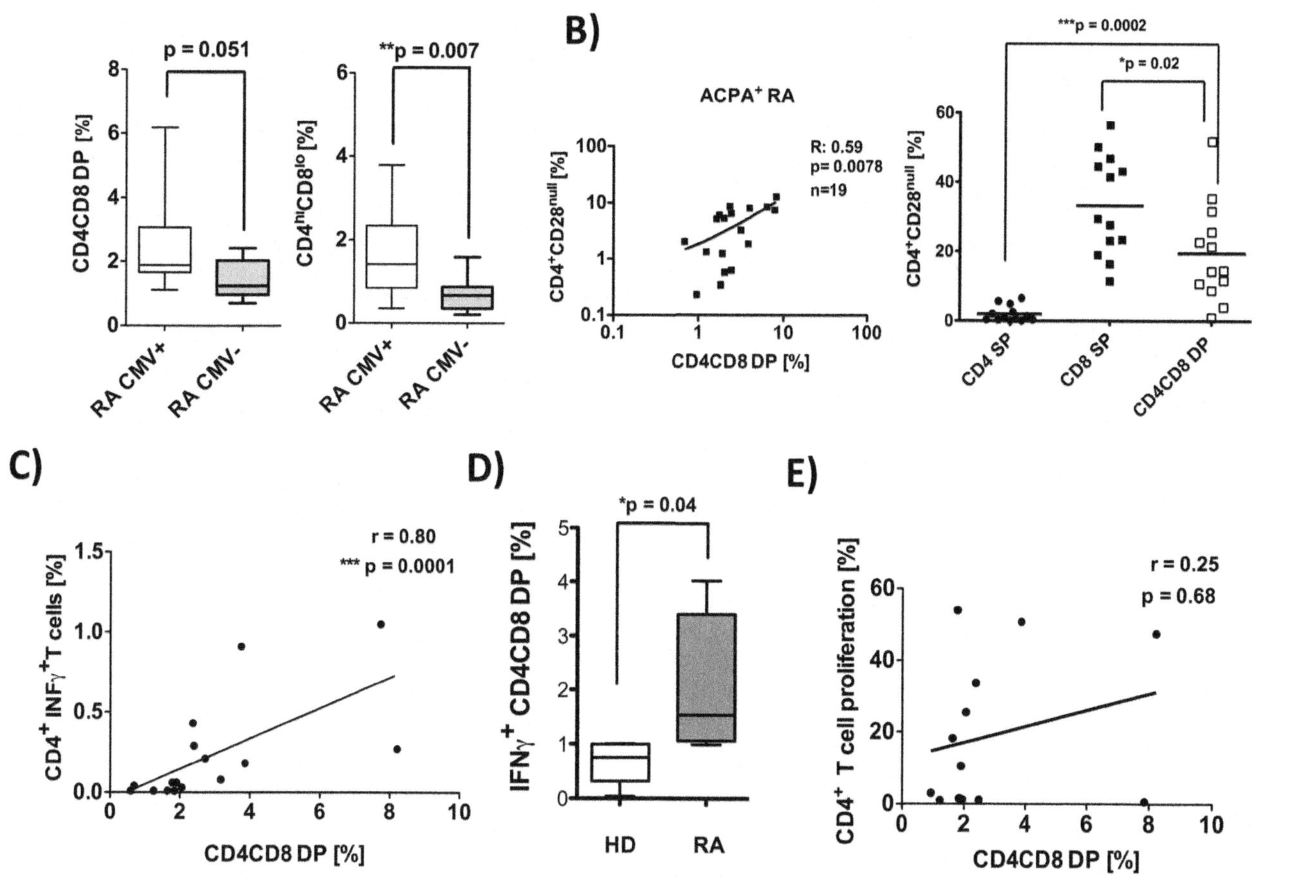

Figure 6. Frequencies of CD4CD8 double positive T cells are increased in CMV positive RA patients and correlate with CMV specific INFγ producers. A) PBMC were isolated from CMV$^+$ RA patients (n = 28) and CMV$^-$ RA patients (n = 12) and analyzed by flow cytometry using anti-CD19, anti-CD3, anti-CD4 and anti-CD8 monoclonal antibodies (PI staining used for exclusion of dead cells). **B)** Correlation of the frequency of total double positive T cells with CD4$^+$CD28^{null} T cells in ACPA$^+$ RA patients (left graph) and comparison of frequencies of CD28^{null} cells among CD4 SP, CD8 SP and total DP T cells (right graph). **C–D)** PBMCs were restimulated with CMV-lysate for 4 hrs in vitro. Subsequently, an INFγ specific secretion assay was performed and cells were counterstained with aCD3, aCD4 and aCD8. Flow cytometric cytokine analyses were performed on live cells (PI staining used for exclusion of dead cells) pre-gated on CD3$^+$ T cells. **C)** Depicted is the correlation of CMV specific INFγ producing CD4 T cells with the frequencies of CD4CD8 DP cells from the same donor (n = 16). **D)** CMV specific INFγ producing CD4CD8 DP T cells from RA (n = 5) and HD (n = 5) are shown. **E)** PBMCs were labeled with CFDA-SE and restimulated with CMV-lysat (n = 13) for 7 d in vitro. Depicted is the correlation of CMV specific CD4 T cell proliferation with the frequencies of CD4CD8 DP cells from the same donor. Presented box plots show median, interquartile range, and 10–90 percentiles. Significance as given, *p<0.05, **p<0.01, ***p<0.001.

CD4 and CD8. Those cells, which can also be found in healthy individuals – although in significantly lower numbers – preferentially display a memory phenotype, and have been reported to bear no markers of naïve T cells or recent thymic emigrants [3] which makes it unlikely that they escaped from the thymus as double positive cells.

Instead, their co-receptor expression pattern with higher CD4 than CD8 expression, and the fact that CD4^{hi}CD8^{lo} are the most prominent DP T cell subpopulation, as well as the generally presumed pivotal role of CD4+ MHC class II restricted T lymphocytes in RA, suggests that those cells were originally CD4 SP T cells, which gained expression of the second co-receptor CD8. De novo CD8 expression in CD4$^+$ T cells under the influence of cytokines like IL-4 has already been described decades ago [26], but the paucity of IL-4 typically found in RA, makes such cytokine driven CD8 expression as an explanation for the emergence of DP T cells in RA less likely. Nevertheless, the increased IL-4 production of DP T cells in RA may sustain their CD8 expression in an autocrine manner.

Two new studies published very recently offer an alternative explanation, since they have identified defined transcription programs which can initiate CD8 gene expression in CD4 SP T cells, for example the silencing of the transcription factor Thpok [27,28] The precise mechanism underlying the emergence of DP T cells in RA remains to be determined, however.

Increased numbers of double positive T cells were detectable only in ACPA positive and not in ACPA negative RA patients. This suggests their involvement in the autoreactive T cell help provided for auto-reactive, antibody producing B cells in this disease. In line with this, a fraction of the double positive T cells was found to express the typical marker of T follicular helper cells, CXCR5. The percentage of CXCR5 positive cells amongst double-positive T cells was lower, however, than their percentage amongst CD4 SP T cells, which argues against a preferential role of DP T cells as TfH cells. Nevertheless, a proportion of DP T cells might provide B cell help, especially by their production of cytokines with a role in T-B cell collaboration, in particular of IL-21. The site for this B cell help could be non classical follicular centers, which are found in the synovium of a sizable fraction of RA patients. [29,30].

RA patients with ACPA positive disease have a more severe course of the disease with extra-articular manifestations and increased subclinical arteriosclerosis compared to ACPA- patients [17]. The increased frequency of CD4CD8 DP T cells in our study in ACPA positive RA might reflect the more pronounced immune deviations in those patients and indicates that those cells might be involved in the destructive immune response in this disease.

Phenotypic characterization of DP T cells in RA reveals them to be $\alpha\beta$ T cells of a memory phenotype. Similar characteristics have been published for DP T cells in healthy donors [3].

NK T cells have received increasing attention in autoimmunity research recently. DP T cells in RA are not invariant NKT cells, but a small fraction was positive for markers for non-invariant NKT cells. This is in contrast to published data [4] for HD and might indicate a pathogenetically relevant, disease specific role of DP T cell subpopulations in RA. Furthermore, TCR BV analysis reveals an overrepresentation of individual BV elements (BV2, BV17 and/or BV21.3) in DP T cells of some RA patients, possibly indicating antigen-driven clonal expansion.

DP T cells are present in the rheumatoid synovium. In addition, our results show that a high percentage of DP T cells have lost expression of the ubiquitous costimulatory molecule CD28, and that their frequency is increased in CMV^{+} RA patients. $CD4^{+}CD28^{null}$ SP T cells are found in 25–70% of RA patients and are associated with a more severe course of the disease [13,25,31]. Recently, we reported CMV^{+} RA to be associated with a more severe course of joint destruction [1], and latent CMV infection is known to lead to an expansion of $CD4^{+}CD28^{null}$ T cells both in RA patients and in healthy individuals.

The present study showed enhanced frequencies of DP T cells in CMV^{+} RA. Recently, we reported an increased CMV specific IFNγ production in RA compared to CMV^{+} healthy controls. [1] Furthermore, the frequency of DP T cells in the present study was found to correlate with the frequency of $CD4^{+}$ CMV specific IFNγ producers. Interestingly, a low but significant fraction of CD4 SP T cells, and even higher frequencies of the DP T cells in RA do produce CMV specific IFNγ, more frequently though than T cells from HD. This is in line with virus specific DP T cells described in HIV patients [7]. Taken together, those results suggests that DP T cells are at least in part the results of the same RA specific, CMV triggered perturbation in the peripheral T cell pool, which also leads to the occurrence of $CD4^{+}CD28^{null}$ T cells. A CMV specific enhanced effector response for DP T cells has already been found in HD [8] and DP T cells are therefore likely also to be involved in the enhanced CMV response in RA.

Independently of CMV specificity, we found DP T cells to produce high amounts of IFNγ, but no IL-17, upon polyclonal stimulation. IFNγ is a key cytokine driving the autoimmune response in RA [23,32]. DP T cells in healthy, aging individuals are known to be capable of producing IFNγ upon polyclonal restimulation [33]. CD28 negative Th cells in RA have also been shown to secrete IFNγ upon autoreactive stimulation, and in line with this, the DP T cells in RA are also preferentially CD28 negative. Therefore, CD4CD8 DP T cells in RA seem to be part of the pathological T cell pool characterized by replicative exhaustion, aberrant IFNγ production and phenotypic alterations including the loss of the ubiquitous co-stimulatory molecule CD28. DP T cells might be the result of a differentiation program set in place in terminally differentiated memory Th cells, that is switched on under conditions associated with immunosenescence, including the memory inflation observed in latent CMV infection or the chronic autoimmune response in rheumatoid arthritis.

Conclusion

In summary, we are the first to demonstrate increased frequencies of peripheral CD4CD8 double positive T cells in ACPA positive RA.

DP T cells are present in the inflamed synovium. These cells display features of T helper cells by the production of IL-4 and IL-21. Furthermore, the production of IFNγ, loss of CD28 and the association with CMV positive RA imply a functional contribution to the pathogenesis of the disease.

Author Contributions

Conceived and designed the experiments: DQ UW. Performed the experiments: DQ KR. Analyzed the data: DQ KR. Contributed reagents/materials/analysis tools: RS CB. Wrote the paper: DQ UW.

References

1. Pierer M, Rothe K, Quandt D, Schulz A, Rossol M et al. (2012) Association of anticytomegalovirus seropositivity with more severe joint destruction and more frequent joint surgery in rheumatoid arthritis. Arthritis Rheum 64(6): 1740–1749.
2. Nascimbeni M, Shin EC, Chiriboga L, Kleiner DE, Rehermann B et al. (2004) Peripheral CD4(+)CD8(+) T cells are differentiated effector memory cells with antiviral functions. Blood 104(2): 478–486.
3. Parel Y, Chizzolini C (2004) CD4+ CD8+ double positive (DP) T cells in health and disease. Autoimmun Rev 3(3): 215–220.
4. Zloza A, Al-Harthi L (2006) Multiple populations of T lymphocytes are distinguished by the level of CD4 and CD8 coexpression and require individual consideration. J Leukoc Biol 79(1): 4–6.
5. Desfrancois J, Moreau-Aubry A, Vignard V, Godet Y, Khammari A et al. (2010) Double positive CD4CD8 alphabeta T cells: a new tumor-reactive population in human melanomas. PLoS One 5(1): e8437.
6. Parel Y, Aurrand-Lions M, Scheja A, Dayer JM, Roosnek E, et al. (2007) Presence of CD4+CD8+ double-positive T cells with very high interleukin-4 production potential in lesional skin of patients with systemic sclerosis. Arthritis Rheum 56(10): 3459–3467.
7. Frahm MA, Picking RA, Kuruc JD, McGee KS, Gay CL et al. (2012) CD4+ CD8+ T cells represent a significant portion of the anti-HIV T cell response to acute HIV infection. J Immunol 188(9): 4289–4296.
8. Suni MA, Ghanekar SA, Houck DW, Maecker HT, Wormsley SB et al. (2001) CD4(+)CD8(dim) T lymphocytes exhibit enhanced cytokine expression, proliferation and cytotoxic activity in response to HCMV and HIV-1 antigens. Eur J Immunol 31(8): 2512–2520.
9. Scheerens H, Su Z, Irving B, Townsend MJ, Zheng Y et al. (2011) MTRX1011A, a humanized anti-CD4 monoclonal antibody, in the treatment of patients with rheumatoid arthritis: a phase I randomized, double-blind, placebo-controlled study incorporating pharmacodynamic biomarker assessments. Arthritis Res Ther 13(5): R177.
10. Maxwell LJ, Singh JA (2010) Abatacept for rheumatoid arthritis: a Cochrane systematic review. J Rheumatol 37(2): 234–245.
11. Horneff G, Burmester GR, Emmrich F, Kalden JR (1991) Treatment of rheumatoid arthritis with an anti-CD4 monoclonal antibody. Arthritis Rheum 34(2): 129–140.
12. Klareskog L, Catrina AI, Paget S (2009) Rheumatoid arthritis. Lancet 373(9664): 659–672.
13. Wagner U, Pierer M, Kaltenhauser S, Wilke B, Seidel W et al. (2003) Clonally expanded CD4+CD28null T cells in rheumatoid arthritis use distinct combinations of T cell receptor BV and BJ elements. Eur J Immunol 33(1): 79–84.
14. Dorner T, Radbruch A, Burmester GR (2009) B-cell-directed therapies for autoimmune disease. Nat Rev Rheumatol 5(8): 433–441.
15. Durie FH, Foy TM, Masters SR, Laman JD, Noelle RJ (1994) The role of CD40 in the regulation of humoral and cell-mediated immunity. Immunol Today 15(9): 406–411.
16. Daridon C, Burmester GR, Dorner T (2009) Anticytokine therapy impacting on B cells in autoimmune diseases. Curr Opin Rheumatol 21(3): 205–210.
17. Gerli R, Bartoloni Bocci E, Sherer Y, Vaudo G, Moscatelli S et al. (2008) Association of anti-cyclic citrullinated peptide antibodies with subclinical atherosclerosis in patients with rheumatoid arthritis. Ann Rheum Dis 67(5): 724–725.
18. Ghia P, Prato G, Stella S, Scielzo C, Geuna M et al. (2007) Age-dependent accumulation of monoclonal CD4+CD8+ double positive T lymphocytes in the peripheral blood of the elderly. Br J Haematol 139(5): 780–790.

19. Holling TM, van der Stoep N, Quinten E, van den Elsen PJ (2002) Activated human T cells accomplish MHC class II expression through T cell-specific occupation of class II transactivator promoter III. J Immunol 168(2): 763–770.
20. Morita R, Schmitt N, Bentebibel SE, Ranganathan R, Bourdery L et al (2011) Human blood CXCR5(+)CD4(+) T cells are counterparts of T follicular cells and contain specific subsets that differentially support antibody secretion. Immunity 34(1): 108–121.
21. O'Shea JJ, Paul WE (2010) Mechanisms underlying lineage commitment and plasticity of helper CD4+ T cells. Science 327(5969): 1098–1102.
22. Cho BA, Sim JH, Park JA, Kim HW, Yoo WH et al. (2012) Characterization of Effector Memory CD8(+) T Cells in the Synovial Fluid of Rheumatoid Arthritis. J Clin Immunol 32 (4): 709–720.
23. McInnes IB, Schett G (2007) Cytokines in the pathogenesis of rheumatoid arthritis. Nat Rev Immunol 7(6): 429–442.
24. Raza K, Falciani F, Curnow SJ, Ross EJ, Lee CY et al. (2005) Early rheumatoid arthritis is characterized by a distinct and transient synovial fluid cytokine profile of T cell and stromal cell origin. Arthritis Res Ther 7(4): R784–795.
25. Schmidt D, Martens PB, Weyand CM, Goronzy JJ (1996) The repertoire of CD4+ CD28- T cells in rheumatoid arthritis. Mol Med 2(5): 608–618.
26. Paliard X, Malefijt RW, de Vries JE, Spits H (1988) Interleukin-4 mediates CD8 induction on human CD4+ T-cell clones. Nature 335(6191): 642–644.
27. Mucida D, Husain MM, Muroi S, van Wijk F, Shinnakasu R et al. (2013) Transcriptional reprogramming of mature CD4(+) helper T cells generates distinct MHC class II-restricted cytotoxic T lymphocytes. Nat Immunol 14(3): 281–289.
28. Reis BS, Rogoz A, Costa-Pinto FA, Taniuchi I, Mucida D (2013) Mutual expression of the transcription factors Runx3 and ThPOK regulates intestinal CD4(+) T cell immunity. Nat Immunol 14(3): 271–280.
29. Humby F, Bombardieri M, Manzo A, Kelly S, Blades MC et al. (2009) Ectopic lymphoid structures support ongoing production of class-switched autoantibodies in rheumatoid synovium. PLoS Med 6(1): e1.
30. MacLennan IC, Toellner KM, Cunningham AF, Serre K, Sze DM et al. (2003) Extrafollicular antibody responses. Immunol Rev 194: 8–18.
31. Gerli R, Vaudo G, Bocci EB, Schillaci G, Bistoni O, et al. (2009) Different roles for anti-cyclic citrullinated peptide antibodies and CD4+CD28null cells in the acceleration of atherosclerosis in rheumatoid arthritis: comment on the article by Farragher et al. Arthritis Rheum 60(2): 631–632.
32. Miossec P, Kolls JK (2012) Targeting IL-17 and TH17 cells in chronic inflammation. Nat Rev Drug Discov 11(10): 763–776.
33. Franceschi C, Bonafe M, Valensin S, Olivieri F, De Luca M et al. (2000) Inflamm-aging. An evolutionary perspective on immunosenescence. Ann N Y Acad Sci 908: 244–254.
34. Kelly-Rogers J, Madrigal-Estebas L, O'Connor T, Doherty DG (2006) Activation-induced expression of CD56 by T cells is associated with a reprogramming of cytolytic activity and cytokine secretion profile in vitro. Hum Immunol 67: 863–873.
35. Lambert C, Ibrahim M, Iobagiu C, Genin C (2005) Significance of unconventional peripheral CD4+CD8dim T cell subsets. J Clin Immunol 25(5): 418–427.

22

Systemic but No Local Effects of Combined Zoledronate and Parathyroid Hormone Treatment in Experimental Autoimmune Arthritis

Kresten Krarup Keller[1]*, Jesper Skovhus Thomsen[2], Kristian Stengaard-Pedersen[1], Ellen-Margrethe Hauge[1]

1 Department of Rheumatology, Aarhus University Hospital, Aarhus, Denmark, **2** Department of Biomedicine – Anatomy, Aarhus University, Aarhus, Denmark

Abstract

Introduction: Local bone erosions and osteoporosis in rheumatoid arthritis (RA) are the result of a more pronounced bone resorption than bone formation. Present treatment strategies for RA inhibit inflammation, but do not directly target bone erosions. The aim of the study was in experimental arthritis to investigate the juxtaarticular and systemic effects of simultaneous osteoclast inhibition with zoledronate (ZLN) and osteoblast stimulation with parathyroid hormone (PTH).

Methods: Arthritis was induced in 36 SKG mice. The mice were randomized to three treatment groups and an untreated group: ZLN, PTH, PTH+ZLN, and untreated. Arthritis score and ankle width measurements were performed. Histological sections were cut from the right hind paw, and design-based stereological estimators were used to quantify histological variables of bone volume and bone formation and resorption. The femora were DXA- and μCT-scanned, and the bone strength was determined at the femoral neck and mid-diaphysis.

Results: Locally, we found no differences in arthritis score or ankle width throughout the study. Similarly, none of the treatments inhibited bone erosions or stimulated bone formation in the paw. Systemically, all treatments improved bone mineral density, strength of the femoral neck and mid-diaphysis, and μCT parameters of both cortical and trabecular bone. In addition, there was an additive effect of combination treatment compared with single treatments for most trabecular parameters including bone mineral density and bone volume fraction.

Conclusions: No local effect on bone was found by the combined action of inhibiting bone resorption and stimulating bone formation. However, a clear systemic effect of the combination treatment was demonstrated.

Editor: Dominique Heymann, Faculté de médecine de Nantes, France

Funding: This work was supported by the Danish Rheumatism Association, The A.P. Møller Foundation for the Advancement of Medical Science, Aase and Ejnar Danielsens Foundation, the Hørslev Foundation, Clinical Institute Aarhus University, Peter Ryholts Grant and the Hede Nielsens Family Foundation. The μCT scanner was donated by the Velux Foundation. The funders had no role in study design, data collection and analysis, decision to publish, or preparation of the manuscript.

Competing Interests: The authors have declared that no competing interests exist.

* E-mail: kresten@ana.au.dk.

Introduction

It is well known that patients with rheumatoid arthritis (RA) develop both local bone erosions and systemic osteoporosis. Local bone erosion in RA is mediated through bone resorption by the osteoclast at the cartilage-pannus junction [1]. Studies indicate that the bone formation is less pronounced in RA compared to the bone resorption [2,3], and impact of RA on the Wnt signaling pathway is probably crucial to this process [4]. However, healing of erosions can be seen, but most often in patients with remission [5]. Osteoporosis in RA is mainly mediated by inflammation [6], resulting in an increased fracture risk independently of glucocorticoid use [7]. Treatment of RA has improved considerably over the last decade, but even with the best current therapies, a number of patients still have progression of erosive bone changes in the joints [8]. Present treatment strategies for RA inhibit inflammation, but do not directly target bone erosions. Consequently, treatment strategies that directly target bone are relevant.

Bisphosphonates are inhibitors of bone resorption, which are mainly used for treatment of osteoporosis [9]. The most powerful bisphosphonate is zoledronate (ZLN), and the effect on osteoporosis is well documented [10]. Parathyroid hormone (PTH) given intermittently is a powerful bone anabolic drug, which stimulates bone formation through the activation and maturation of cells of the osteoblast-line. Treatment with intermittent PTH increases BMD and decreases fracture risk in osteoporosis [11]. Inhibiting bone resorption with ZLN combined with stimulation of bone formation with PTH may inhibit development of erosions in the joints of RA patients, and in addition the combination may heal erosions. In clinical or experimental arthritis, no study has yet investigated the combined effect of ZLN and PTH.

The SKG mouse model for RA is characterized by symmetrical affection of peripheral joints (ankle, tarsal, and finger joints in all

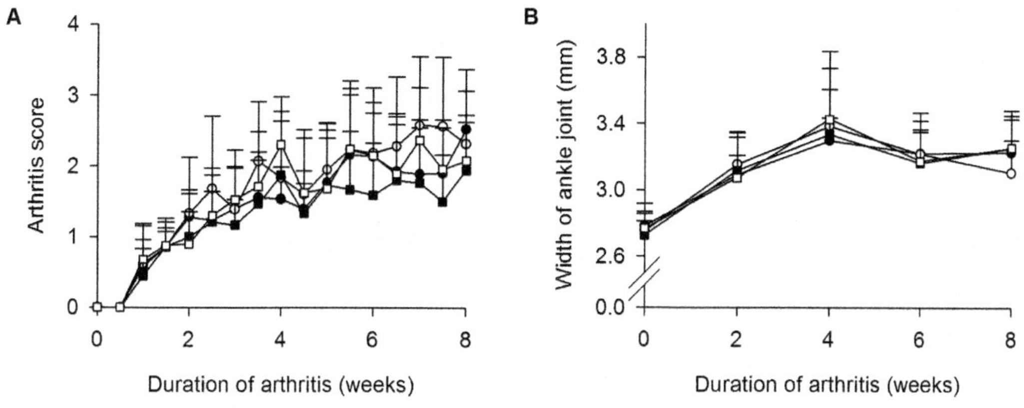

Figure 1. Similar severity of arthritis in the different groups. Arthritis score (**A**) and mean width of hind limb ankle joints (**B**). Untreated (□), PTH (■), ZLN (○), and ZLN+PTH (●). Values are mean plus standard deviations. N = 9 mice per group.

four limbs), rheumatoid factor, elevated cytokines (IL-1, Il-6, TNF-α, and Il-17), and systemic manifestations such as inflammation of the lungs and skin [12–15]. This model is also characterized by both local and systemic bone loss [16–18], and recently we demonstrated that systemic bone loss is present early after arthritis induction [19]. Consequently, the SKG model is suitable for studying the effect of bone targeting therapies in experimental chronic arthritis.

We hypothesize that stimulation of bone formation and inhibition of bone resorption may represent an effective future treatment strategy, for both local and systemic bone loss in RA. Hence, the objective of the present study was to investigate the juxtaarticular and systemic effects of simultaneous osteoclast inhibition with ZLN and osteoblast stimulation with PTH in the SKG mouse model of RA.

Methods

Animals, arthritis induction, and assessment of arthritis

The study comprised 36 8- to 10-week-old female SKG mice housed as previously described in detail [18]. Arthritis was induced with an intraperitoneal (i.p.) injection of 20 mg mannan suspended in 0.2 ml PBS, which induces the arthritis through the complement system [20].

Arthritis was scored twice weekly in accordance to the SKG scale [12]. In addition, the hind limb ankle width was measured every other week with an electronic sliding caliper, and the mean width of the right and left ankle joint was calculated. Both evaluations were performed by an observer blinded for the group distribution.

Calcein (Sigma-Aldrich, St Louis, MO, USA) 15 mg/kg and tetracycline (Sigma-Aldrich) 30 mg/kg fluorochrome labels was administered i.p. 8 and 4 days before the end of the study respectively. Eight weeks after arthritis induction (i.e. when the mice were 16- to 18-week-old), the mice were anesthetized with isoflurane (IsoFlo vet, Abbot Laboratories Ltd. Kent, UK) and euthanized by cervical dislocation.

Ethics statement

The principles of laboratory animal care recommended by the US National Institute of Health were followed. The study was approved by the Danish Animal Experiments Inspectorate (permit number 2011/561-64).

Treatment

Treatment was initiated 11 days after arthritis induction with mannan. The mice were assigned to 4 treatment groups ($n = 9$ per group): placebo+placebo (untreated), ZLN+placebo (ZLN), placebo+PTH (PTH), and ZLN+PTH. Human PTH (1–34) (Bachem, Bubendorf, Switzerland) or placebo were dissolved in saline and 2% mouse serum and subsequently injected subcutaneously (s.c.) at 80 μg/kg 5 times a week for 6 weeks and 3 days [21]. ZLN (Novartis, Basel, Switzerland) or placebo were injected s.c. at 100 μg/kg 5 times a week for 6 weeks and 3 days [22]. One mouse in the ZLN group had to be euthanized after 7 weeks due to a misplaced injection.

Histological preparation of paws

After euthanization the right hind paw was cut 0.5 cm above the ankle joint and across the middle of the metatarsal bones, fixed in 70% ethanol, and subsequently embedded undecalcified in methylmethacrylate [23]. Tissue blocks were rotated randomly around a vertical axis through the longitudinal axis of the paw and 7-μm-thick sections were cut exhaustively on a microtome (Reichert Jung GmbH, Heidelberg, Germany) using the principles of vertical sectioning [24]. Approximately 10 levels each comprising 12 sections were acquired for each paw using the principles of systematic, uniform random sampling [25]. Finally, the sections were stained with Masson-Goldner trichrome, for tartrate-resistant acid phosphatase (TRAP), or left unstained for epifluorescent microscopy.

Evaluation of histological sections

The microscope (Nikon ECLIPSE 80i, Tokyo, Japan) was equipped with a motorized Proscan 11 stage (Prior, Cambridge, UK), a MT1201 microcator (Heidenhain, Traunreit, Germany), a DP72 digital camera (Olympus, Tokyo, Japan), and a fluorescence illuminator (Prior, Cambridge, UK). The microscope system was connected to a PC with the stereological software newCAST (version 4.2.1.0, Visiopharm, Hørsholm, Denmark).

All parameters were evaluated in the tarsus at a total magnification of ×457. The tarsus was defined as all tarsal bones excluding the tibial and the metatarsal bones. Absolute bone volume (BV) was estimated using a point grid with an area per point of 36712 μm^2. For absolute mineralizing surfaces (MS) and osteoclast-covered bone surfaces (Oc.S) a line grid with an area per length of 29.9 μm was used. These parameters were estimated

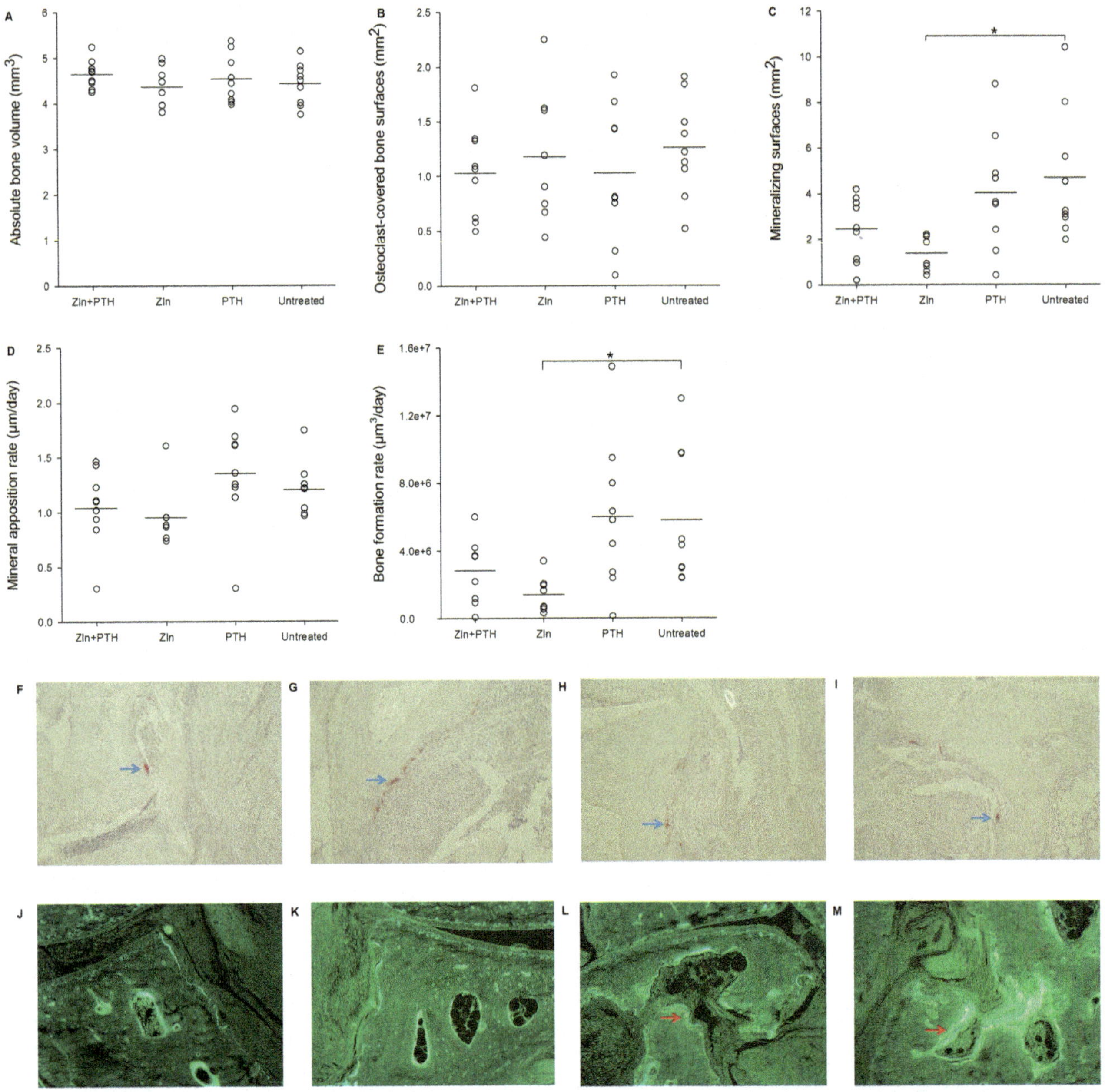

Figure 2. Bone changes in mouse paws evaluated with stereology of the right hind paw. Horizontal lines indicate mean values. N = 8–9 mice per group and * $= p<0.01$. Representative pictures of are demonstrated (total magnification ×457): PTH+ZLN (**F and J**), ZLN (**G and K**), PTH (**H and L**) and Untreated (**I and M**). Red cells indicate osteoclasts in the TRAP stained sections (blue arrows) (**F–I**). Tetracycline (yellow) and calcein (green) labels are demonstrated in unstained sections (red arrows) (**J–M**).

according to stereological estimators as previously described in detail [18].

The mineralizing surfaces were defined as the number of intercepts with fluorochrome double labels plus half the number of intercepts with single labels. Mineral apposition rate (MAR) and bone formation rate (BFR) were estimated using the principles described by Dempster et al. [26]. Briefly, MAR was calculated as the mean of the interlabel width (iL.Wi) multiplied by the correction coefficient ($\pi/4$) and divided by the interlabel time. When double labels were absent a MAR value of 0.3 µm/day was used [27]. Subsequently, BFR was estimated as MS multiplied by MAR.

The average coefficient of error (CE) for the bone volume estimates was determined as earlier described to 2.5% [18]. CE for surface parameters could not be estimated, because the formula for CE of a surface is not valid due to the large variation in size between different sections of a mouse paw.

Dual Energy X-ray Absorptiometry

After euthanization the right femora was exarticulated at the hip and the knee joint and stored in Ringer's solution at −20°C. The femora were thawed, dissected free of soft connective tissue, and placed in a standardized way in a peripheral DXA scanner (Sabre XL, Norland Stratec, Pforzheim, Germany) and scanned with a

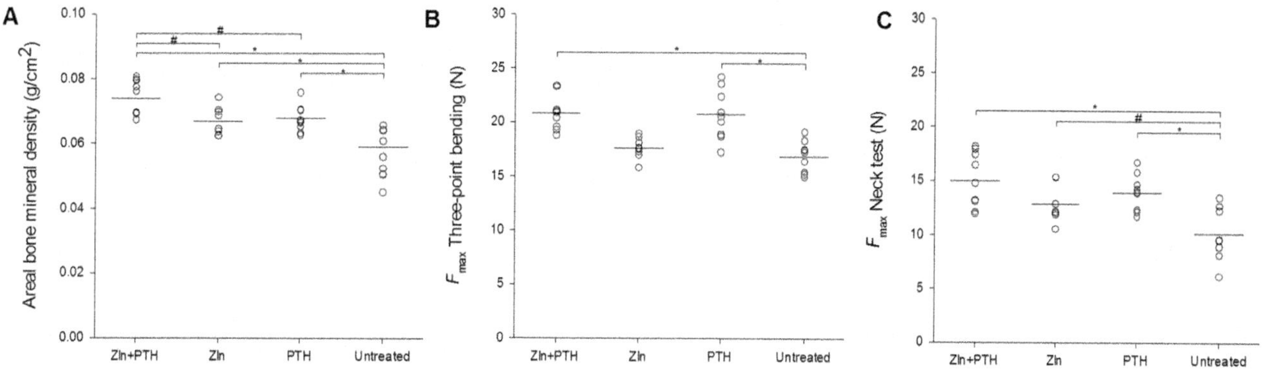

Figure 3. Area bone mineral density evaluated by DEXA and bone strength of the right femur. Area bone mineral density of the total femur in the different groups (**A**). Bone strength was measured in the mid-diaphysis with three-point bending (**B**) and in the femoral neck with compression testing (**C**). N = 7–9 mice per group. * $=p<0.01$ and # $=p<0.05$.

pixel size of 0.1 mm ×0.1 mm at a velocity of 2 mm/s. The areal bone mineral density (aBMD) was determined using the software provided with the scanner.

Mechanical testing

After the DXA-scans, the maximum load of the mid-femoral diaphysis was determined by three-point bending test in a materials-testing machine (5566; Instron, High Wycombe, UK) as previously described in detail [19]. After the three-points bending test the proximal half of the femur was placed in a custom-made device for standardized fixation [28]. The fixation device was placed in the materials testing machine and compressive load was placed on the top of the femoral head at a constant velocity of 2 mm/min until fracture of the femoral neck. The measured data included the maximum load (F_{max}) given in Newton (N).

Micro Computed Tomography (μCT)

Before the three-point bending test, the cortical bone of the femoral mid-diaphysis was scanned in a desktop μCT scanner (Scanco μCT 35, Scanco Medical AG, Brüttiselen, Switzerland). A 0.82 mm high volume of interest (VOI) was scanned in high resolution mode (1000 projections/180°) with a spatial resolution of 3.5×3.5×3.5 μm^3, an X-ray tube voltage of 55 kVp and current of 145 μA, and an integration time of 800 ms. The data sets were low-pass filtered using a Gaussian filter ($\sigma = 0.8$, support = 1) and segmented with a fixed threshold filter (618.0 mgHA/cm^3). The threshold was found as the midpoint between the peaks representing bone and marrow in the attenuation histogram [29]. The structural evaluation was performed with the software provided with the scanner (IPL, version 5.11, Scanco Medical AG, Brüttisellen, Switzerland). The measured data included: Cortical bone area (Ct.Ar) and average cortical thickness (Ct.Th).

After the three point bending test, the distal half of the femur was placed in the μCT scanner and the distal femur was scanned with the same scanning parameters as the femoral mid-diaphysis. A 700-μm-high VOI was demarcated in the distal femoral metaphysis starting 950 μm beneath the lowest point of the hyaline cartilage in the epiphyseal growth plate thereby excluding the primary spongiosa from the analysis. The data sets were low-pass filtered using a Gaussian filter ($\sigma = 1.3$, support = 2) and segmented with a fixed threshold filter (589.6 mgHA/cm^3). The threshold was found in the same way as for cortical bone. Measured data included: volumetric bone mineral density (vBMD), trabecular thickness (Tb.Th*), trabecular separation (Tb.Sp*), trabecular number (Tb.N*), structure model index (SMI), and bone volume fraction (BV/TV) [29,30].

Statistics

Data were analyzed using STATA (version 11, Statacorp, College station, USA). Groups were compared with one-way ANOVA. Normality was checked with QQ-plots. If the hypothesis of equal means in the groups were rejected, pair wise comparisons between groups were made. All treatment groups were compared with untreated animals and if the hypothesis of no difference was rejected it was tested whether the hypothesis of no difference between combination treatment and the two other treatment groups could be rejected. If data were not normally distributed, Kruskal-Wallis test was performed, followed by the two sample Wilcoxon rank-sum test (Mann Whitney's U test). P-values below 0.05 were considered statistically significant.

Results

Arthritis score and ankle width

Arthritis score was similar for all groups throughout the study (Figure 1A). Likewise, the mean width of the hind limb ankle increased in all groups with time, but no differences were detected between the groups at any time point throughout the study (Figure 1B).

Histological evaluation of bone in mouse paws

The BV of the tarsus, evaluated with stereological estimators, did not differ between the groups (Figure 2A). Likewise, Oc.S did not differ between the groups indicating similar bone resorption in the different groups (Figure 2B). MS was significantly lower in the ZLN group than in the untreated group ($p<0.01$) (Figure 2C). Furthermore, MAR did not differ between the groups, whereas BFR was significantly lower in the ZLN group than in the untreated group ($p<0.01$) (Figure 2 D&E). Representative pictures of histological sections are supplied in Figure 2.

DXA and mechanical testing of the femora

The aBMD of the total femur was significantly higher in all treatment groups than in the untreated group ($p<0.01$). In addition, the aBMD was significantly higher in the PTH+ZLN group than in both the ZLN and the PTH group ($p<0.05$) (Figure 3A).

The fracture strength of the femoral mid-diaphysis was significantly higher in the groups treated with PTH than in the

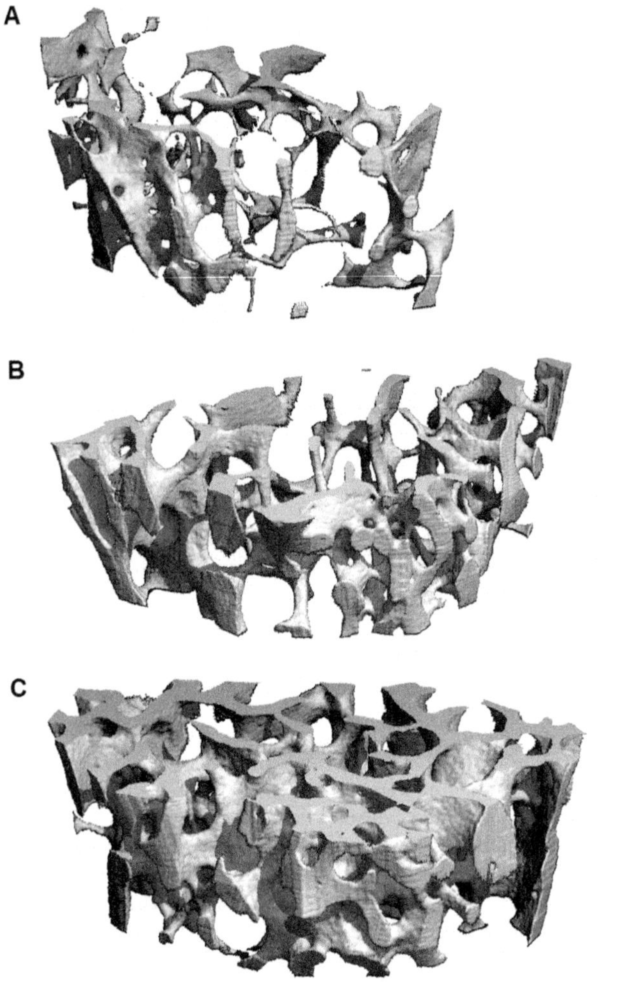

Figure 4. μCT pictures of trabecular bone. Representative μCT pictures of trabecular bone in the femur metaphysis. Untreated (**A**), PTH (**B**), ZLN (**C**) and PTH+ZLN (**D**) treated mice are demonstrated.

untreated group ($p<0.01$) (Figure 3B). In addition, the femoral neck was significantly stronger in all treatment groups than in the untreated group ($p<0.01$ and $p<0.05$). However, at the femoral neck the combination treatment did not result in significantly stronger bone than the single treatments (Figure 3C).

μCT of femoral trabecular bone

Trabecular bone was evaluated in the distal femoral metaphysis, and as illustrated in Figure 4, substantial differences between groups were demonstrated. The vBMD of the distal femoral metaphysis was significantly higher for all treatment groups than for the untreated group. In addition, the vBMD for the combination group was significantly greater than for the two single treatment groups ($p<0.01$) (Figure 5A). The results for BV/TV were similar (Figure 5B). SMI was significantly lower in the treatment groups than in the untreated group indicating that the trabeculae in the treated animals were more plate-like. Moreover, there was an additive effect of combination treatment compared to single treatments ($p<0.01$) (Figure 5 C). Trabecular thickness Tb.Th* was higher in the treatment groups than in the untreated group, and in addition Tb.Th* was higher in the combination group than in the two single treatment groups ($p<0.01$) (Figure 5D). Finally, Tb.Sp* was lower and Tb.N* was higher in the treatment groups than in the untreated group ($p<0.01$ and $p<0.05$) (Figure 5E&F).

μCT of femoral cortical bone

Cortical thickness Ct.Th at the femoral mid-diaphysis was greater in all treatment groups than in the untreated group, but there was no additive effect of the combination treatment ($p<0.01$ or $p<0.05$) (Figure 6A). Likewise, the cross sectional cortical bone area Ct.Ar was higher in the treatment groups than in the untreated group ($p<0.01$ or $p<0.05$) (Figure 6B).

Discussion

During the last decades, treatment of RA has improved considerably, but local bone erosions and osteoporosis are not prevented in all patients. Currently, treatment is mainly focused on inhibition of the inflammation, whereas bone loss is not directly targeted. In the present study we investigated the combined effect of the bone anti-resorptive zoledronate (ZLN) treatment and the bone anabolic intermittent parathyroid hormone (PTH) treatment.

The systemic effect of ZLN for osteoporosis is well known and documented [10]. Previous experimental [22,31] and clinical studies [32] have found that ZLN is also an effective drug against inflammation-induced bone loss in RA. A finding, which has been confirmed by the present study, as we showed that femoral neck fracture strength, femoral aBMD, and femoral cortical and trabecular μCT parameters improved compared with the untreated group. In contrast, there was no improvement of the fracture strength of the femoral mid-diaphysis, which is probably due to the lack of remodeling in cortical bone in rodents.

In the present study ZLN did not prevent the development of local bone erosions. Bone volume and resorption were unchanged, and actually a suppression of bone formation was seen. This is at variance with previous animal studies, where a clear preventive effect of ZLN on bone erosions was demonstrated [22,31,33]. There may be several explanations for the conflicting results. In the studies various animal models were used. The SKG model results in a chronic RA-like arthritis, whereas e.g. the collagen arthritis model used in some of the other studies are more acute and burns out after a short time. In addition, in the present study we performed stereology, whereas histomorphometry was performed in the previous studies. Stereology based quantitative histology is free of assumptions concerning shape of the tissue and orientation, and it gives quantities in absolute volume, area, length, or numbers. On the other hand conventional histomorphometry is based on assumptions of shape and orientation and reports data in 2D-terms such as area and perimeter. Finally, the dose of ZLN was not exactly the same in all studies. ZLN has been used in one randomized controlled trial with RA patients [32]. In that study no difference between the treatment groups were found

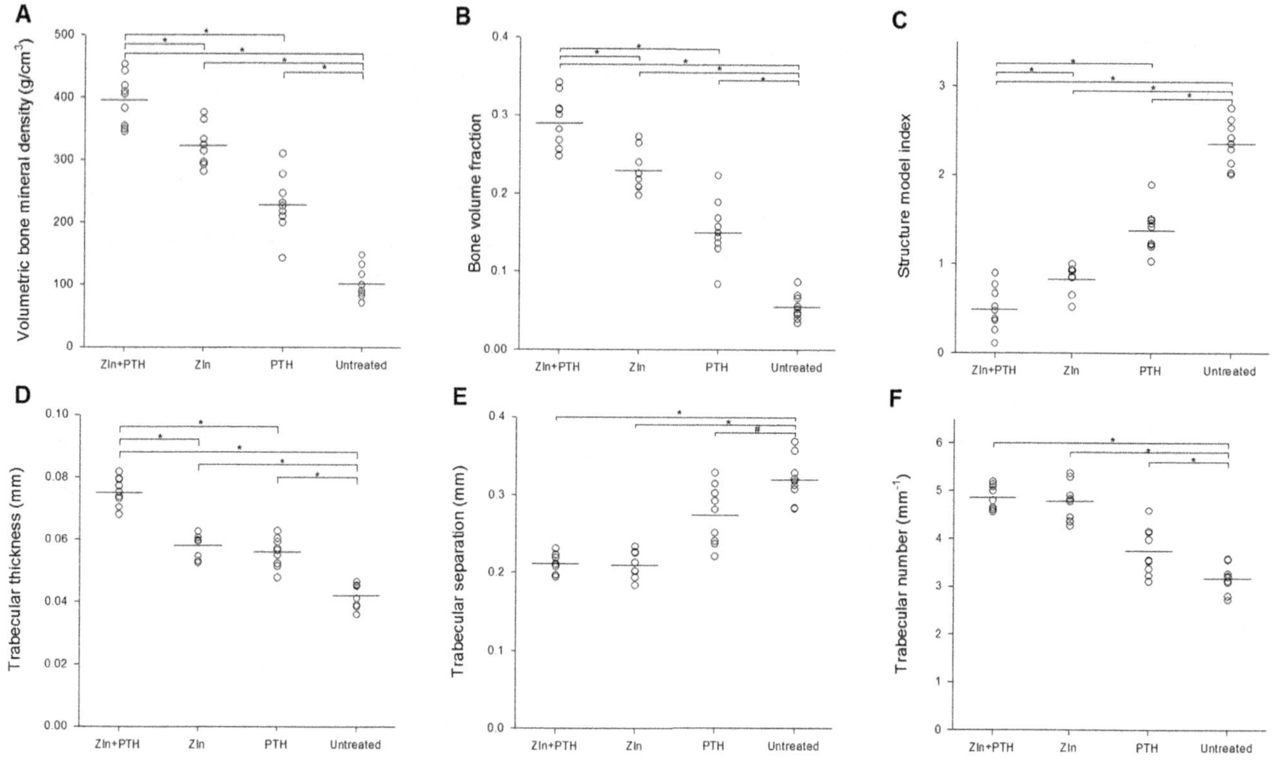

Figure 5. μCT parameters from trabecular bone. Results from μCT evaluation of trabecular bone in the femoral metaphysis of the right femora. N = 8–9 mice per group. * = $p<0.01$ and # = $p<0.05$.

in the primary endpoint of erosions visualized by magnetic resonance imaging (MRI). In general, human studies of RA treatment with bisphosphonates have been disappointing concerning the effect on joint erosions [34,35]. A reason may be that ZLN inhibit osteoclasts directly, but do not inhibit the recruitment of osteoclasts through the receptor activator of nuclear factor κB ligand (RANKL) [36]. It is conceivable that the inflammatory signal for osteoclastogenesis locally in the joint is so powerful that it can outweigh the osteoclasts killed by the ZLN treatment. Blocking of the osteoclast recruitment may therefore inhibit local bone erosions. This view is supported by a clinical study of the RANKL inhibitor denosumab in RA, which was able to arrest the progression of erosions as assessed by both MRI and conventional radiographs [37]. Consequently, it would be interesting to study inhibition of both the inflammation and the osteoclasts in a future study. In summary, our results illustrates that ZLN may not effectively inhibit osteoclastic resorption in joints with arthritis, and thus not inhibit local bone erosions. Moreover, ZLN may be potentially harmful, because bone formation is further inhibited, which could hamper the healing of existing joint erosions in RA.

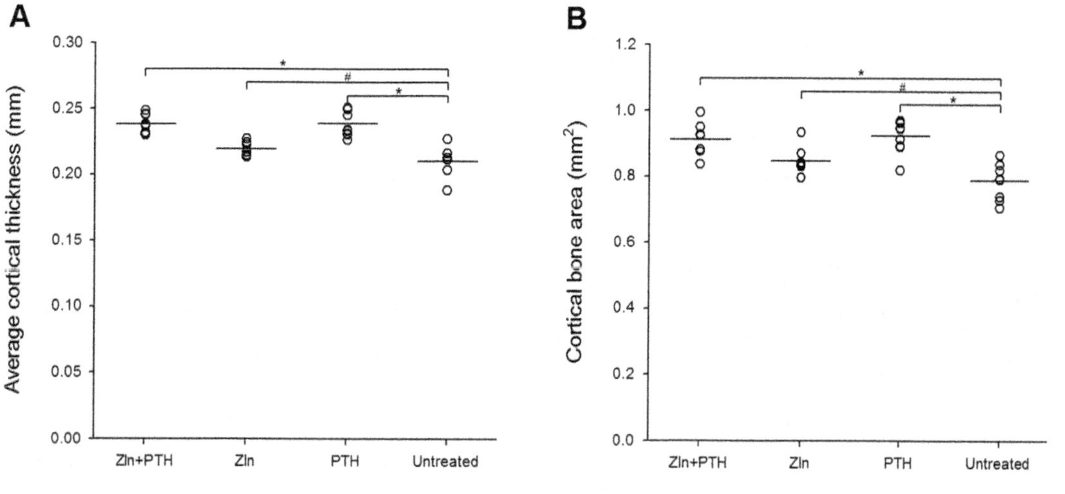

Figure 6. μCT parameters from cortical bone. Results from μCT evaluation of cortical bone in the mid-diaphysis of the femur. N = 8–9 mice per group. * = $p<0.01$ and # = $p<0.05$.

Intermittent PTH is an effective bone anabolic treatment regimen for postmenopausal osteoporosis [11]. We evaluated the systemic effect of intermittent PTH on inflammation-induced bone loss, and found a clear effect. Femoral neck and mid-diaphyseal bone strength, aBMD, and cortical as well as trabecular μCT parameters improved compared with the untreated group. Our study confirms the experimental results published by others [21,38]. However, the effect in clinical trials with RA patients remains to be seen.

We were not able to demonstrate an effect of PTH locally in the joint, and this result is consistent with other studies. One group found no local effect of PTH in collagen-induced arthritis (CIA) in rats [38]. Another group found no effect of PTH alone on bone erosion in the TNF-transgenic mouse model, whereas a combination with anti-TNF was effective [21]. Furthermore, the same researchers demonstrated no effect on local erosions using the CIA and the adjuvant-induced arthritis model in rats, but found a clear effect if PTH was combined with either inhibition of RANKL or TNF [39]. These results indicate that directly or indirectly inhibition of osteoclast differentiation and maturation may be important for the local effect of PTH in arthritis. Therefore, PTH may potentially heal bone erosions in RA, but should be combined with inhibition of osteoclast differentiation.

In the present study the main objective was to investigate the combined effect of osteoblast stimulation by PTH and osteoclast inhibition by ZLN. The combination therapy was not effective on the inflammation as ascertained by arthritis score. This finding was expected because neither of the two single therapies improved inflammation. In fact, ZLN may even enhance inflammation [33], although we did not find evidence for this in our study. We also investigated the effect of combination therapy on local bone changes and were only able to demonstrate an inhibition of bone formation. RA is characterized by an increased osteoclastic bone resorption and an inhibition of bone formation, and we hypothesized that targeting both, would reduce the presence of bone erosions. However, as discussed above, ZLN inhibited bone formation and a potential positive effect of PTH on bone formation was simply not able to reverse this inhibition. In contrast, there was an effect of the combination treatment on systemic bone loss. Thus, we found an additive effect of the combination therapy, which improved trabecular bone structure, but did not translate into an additive effect on bone strength. There was no additional effect of combination therapy on cortical parameters. Again, the reason may be the lack of effect of ZLN, because of absent cortical bone remodeling in rodents. The effect of stimulating bone formation and inhibiting bone erosions varied locally and systemically in our study. Thus, the mechanisms for inducing local and systemic bone loss are probably very different and the strong inflammatory drive on the local bone resorption and formation compared with the systemic bone remodelling is probably crucial. The local bone loss is influenced by local cytokines in the joint such as TNF-alpha and IL-1 modulating Wnt signalling in osteoblasts leading to inhibited bone formation as well as stimulated bone resorption through RANKL [4,40,41]. Synovial fibroblasts and local glucocorticoid synthesis may play a role in the different local bone response to inflammation [42].

Our study is the first to investigate and demonstrate the combined effect of PTH and a bisphosphonate in arthritis. In clinical osteoporosis research the effect of this combination is still under debate. One research group did not find an effect of combining alendronate and PTH in a clinical trial [43]. Another group found an effect on BMD if PTH was added to alendronate treatment [44] and an early increase in BMD in combination treatment with PTH and ZLN compared to single treatment [45]. Recently a significant effect was demonstrated by adding PTH to ibandronate [46].

There are limitations to our study. Systemic bone loss was investigated in the femur and not in the spine, which is a typical site for studying systemic bone loss. However, arthritis in SKG mice does not affect the knee joint [12]. Hence, the observed femoral bone changes are indeed caused by a systemic and not a local effect of arthritis.

In conclusion, we demonstrated that combination treatment with ZLN and PTH was effective on systemic but not on local bone loss in a mouse model of RA. Therefore, this combination treatment may represent an effective strategy to prevent osteoporosis in RA, whereas local bone erosions should be treated in a different manner, probably by targeting the osteoclast differentiation or combining osteoclast inhibition with inhibition of inflammation. Hence, different mechanisms may influence local and systemic bone loss in arthritis.

Acknowledgments

The authors are grateful for the skillful technical assistance of Jette Barlach and Helle Christiansen.

Author Contributions

Conceived and designed the experiments: KKK JST KSP EMH. Performed the experiments: KKK JST. Analyzed the data: KKK JST KSP EMH. Contributed reagents/materials/analysis tools: KKK JST KSP EMH. Wrote the paper: KKK. Corrected the manuscript: JST KSP EMH.

References

1. Gravallese EM, Harada Y, Wang JT, Gorn AH, Thornhill TS, et al. (1998) Identification of cell types responsible for bone resorption in rheumatoid arthritis and juvenile rheumatoid arthritis. Am J Pathol 152(4): 943–951.
2. Walsh NC, Reinwald S, Manning CA, Condon KW, Iwata K, et al. (2009) Osteoblast function is compromised at sites of focal bone erosion in inflammatory arthritis. J Bone Miner Res 24(9): 1572–1585.
3. Keller KK, Thomsen JS, Stengaard-Pedersen K, Dagnaes-Hansen F, Nyengaard JR, et al. (2012) Bone formation and resorption are both increased in experimental autoimmune arthritis. PLoS One 7(12): e53034.
4. Diarra D, Stolina M, Polzer K, Zwerina J, Ominsky MS, et al. (2007) Dickkopf-1 is a master regulator of joint remodeling. Nat Med 13(2): 156–163.
5. Rau R. (2006) Is remission in rheumatoid arthritis associated with radiographic healing? Clin Exp Rheumatol 24(6 Suppl 43): S-41–4.
6. Roux C. (2011) Osteoporosis in inflammatory joint diseases. Osteoporos Int 22(2): 421–433.
7. van Staa TP, Geusens P, Bijlsma JW, Leufkens HG, Cooper C. (2006) Clinical assessment of the long-term risk of fracture in patients with rheumatoid arthritis. Arthritis Rheum 54(10): 3104–3112.
8. Graudal N, Jurgens G. (2010) Similar effects of disease-modifying antirheumatic drugs, glucocorticoids, and biologic agents on radiographic progression in rheumatoid arthritis: Meta-analysis of 70 randomized placebo-controlled or drug-controlled studies, including 112 comparisons. Arthritis Rheum 62(10): 2852–2863.
9. Khosla S, Bilezikian JP, Dempster DW, Lewiecki EM, Miller PD, et al. (2012) Benefits and risks of bisphosphonate therapy for osteoporosis. J Clin Endocrinol Metab 97(7): 2272–2282.
10. Recknor C. (2011) Zoledronic acid for prevention and treatment of osteoporosis. Expert Opin Pharmacother 12(5): 807–815.
11. Cosman F. (2008) Parathyroid hormone treatment for osteoporosis. Curr Opin Endocrinol Diabetes Obes 15(6): 495–501.
12. Sakaguchi N, Takahashi T, Hata H, Nomura T, Tagami T, et al. (2003) Altered thymic T-cell selection due to a mutation of the ZAP-70 gene causes autoimmune arthritis in mice. Nature 426(6965): 454–460.
13. Hata H, Sakaguchi N, Yoshitomi H, Iwakura Y, Sekikawa K, et al. (2004) Distinct contribution of IL-6, TNF-alpha, IL-1, and IL-10 to T cell-mediated spontaneous autoimmune arthritis in mice. J Clin Invest 114(4): 582–588.

14. Hirota K, Hashimoto M, Yoshitomi H, Tanaka S, Nomura T, et al. (2007) T cell self-reactivity forms a cytokine milieu for spontaneous development of IL-17+ th cells that cause autoimmune arthritis. J Exp Med 204(1): 41–47.
15. Kobayashi K, Suda T, Nan-Ya K, Sakaguchi N, Sakaguchi S, et al. (2006) Cytokine production profile of splenocytes derived from zymosan A-treated SKG mice developing arthritis. Inflamm Res 55(8): 335–341.
16. Caetano-Lopes J, Nery AM, Henriques R, Canhao H, Duarte J, et al. (2009) Chronic arthritis directly induces quantitative and qualitative bone disturbances leading to compromised biomechanical properties. Clin Exp Rheumatol 27(3): 475–482.
17. Caetano-Lopes J, Nery AM, Canhao H, Duarte J, Cascao R, et al. (2010) Chronic arthritis leads to disturbances in the bone collagen network. Arthritis Res Ther 12(1): R9.
18. Keller KK, Stengaard-Pedersen K, Dagnaes-Hansen F, Nyengaard JR, Sakaguchi S, et al. (2011) Histological changes in chronic autoimmune SKG-arthritis evaluated by quantitative three-dimensional stereological estimators. Clin Exp Rheumatol 29(3): 536–543.
19. Keller KK, Lindgaard LM, Wogensen L, Dagnaes-Hansen F, Thomsen JS, et al. (2013) SKG arthritis as a model for evaluating therapies in rheumatoid arthritis with special focus on bone changes. Rheumatol Int 33(5): 1127–1133.
20. Hashimoto M, Hirota K, Yoshitomi H, Maeda S, Teradaira S, et al. (2010) Complement drives Th17 cell differentiation and triggers autoimmune arthritis. J Exp Med 207(6): 1135–1143.
21. Redlich K, Gortz B, Hayer S, Zwerina J, Doerr N, et al. (2004) Repair of local bone erosions and reversal of systemic bone loss upon therapy with anti-tumor necrosis factor in combination with osteoprotegerin or parathyroid hormone in tumor necrosis factor-mediated arthritis. Am J Pathol 164(2): 543–555.
22. Herrak P, Gortz B, Hayer S, Redlich K, Reiter E, et al. (2004) Zoledronic acid protects against local and systemic bone loss in tumor necrosis factor-mediated arthritis. Arthritis Rheum 50(7): 2327–2337.
23. Erben RG. (1996) Trabecular and endocortical bone surfaces in the rat: Modeling or remodeling? Anat Rec 246(1): 39–46.
24. Baddeley AJ, Gundersen HJ, Cruz-Orive LM. (1986) Estimation of surface area from vertical sections. J Microsc 142(Pt 3): 259–276.
25. Gundersen HJ, Jensen EB. (1987) The efficiency of systematic sampling in stereology and its prediction. J Microsc 147(Pt 3): 229–263.
26. Dempster DW, Compston JE, Drezner MK, Glorieux FH, Kanis JA, et al. (2013) Standardized nomenclature, symbols, and units for bone histomorphometry: A 2012 update of the report of the ASBMR histomorphometry nomenclature committee. J Bone Miner Res 28(1): 2–17.
27. Hauge E, Mosekilde L, Melsen F. (1999) Missing observations in bone histomorphometry on osteoporosis: Implications and suggestions for an approach. Bone 25(4): 389–395.
28. Mosekilde L, Thomsen JS, Orhii PB, McCarter RJ, Mejia W, et al. (1999) Additive effect of voluntary exercise and growth hormone treatment on bone strength assessed at four different skeletal sites in an aged rat model. Bone 24(2): 71–80.
29. Bouxsein ML, Boyd SK, Christiansen BA, Guldberg RE, Jepsen KJ, et al. (2010) Guidelines for assessment of bone microstructure in rodents using micro-computed tomography. J Bone Miner Res 25(7): 1468–1486.
30. Thomsen JS, Laib A, Koller B, Prohaska S, Mosekilde L, et al. (2005) Stereological measures of trabecular bone structure: Comparison of 3D micro computed tomography with 2D histological sections in human proximal tibial bone biopsies. J Microsc 218(Pt 2): 171–179.
31. Le Goff B, Soltner E, Charrier C, Maugars Y, Redini F, et al. (2009) A combination of methotrexate and zoledronic acid prevents bone erosions and systemic bone mass loss in collagen induced arthritis. Arthritis Res Ther 11(6): R185.
32. Jarrett SJ, Conaghan PG, Sloan VS, Papanastasiou P, Ortmann CE, et al. (2006) Preliminary evidence for a structural benefit of the new bisphosphonate zoledronic acid in early rheumatoid arthritis. Arthritis Rheum 54(5): 1410–1414.
33. Sims NA, Green JR, Glatt M, Schlict S, Martin TJ, et al. (2004) Targeting osteoclasts with zoledronic acid prevents bone destruction in collagen-induced arthritis. Arthritis Rheum 50(7): 2338–2346.
34. Breuil V, Euller-Ziegler L. (2006) Bisphosphonate therapy in rheumatoid arthritis. Joint Bone Spine 73(4): 349–354. 10.1016/j.jbspin.2005.10.019.
35. Valleala H, Laasonen L, Koivula MK, Risteli J, Konttinen YT. (2012) Effect of oral clodronate on structural damage and bone turnover in rheumatoid arthritis. Clin Exp Rheumatol 30(1): 114–117.
36. Romas E. (2005) Bone loss in inflammatory arthritis: Mechanisms and therapeutic approaches with bisphosphonates. Best Pract Res Clin Rheumatol 19(6): 1065–1079.
37. Cohen SB, Dore RK, Lane NE, Ory PA, Peterfy CG, et al. (2008) Denosumab treatment effects on structural damage, bone mineral density, and bone turnover in rheumatoid arthritis: A twelve-month, multicenter, randomized, double-blind, placebo-controlled, phase II clinical trial. Arthritis Rheum 58(5): 1299–1309.
38. Fukata S, Hagino H, Okano T, Yamane I, Kameyama Y, et al. (2004) Effect of intermittent administration of human parathyroid hormone on bone mineral density and arthritis in rats with collagen-induced arthritis. Arthritis Rheum 50(12): 4060–4069.
39. Schett G, Middleton S, Bolon B, Stolina M, Brown H, et al. (2005) Additive bone-protective effects of anabolic treatment when used in conjunction with RANKL and tumor necrosis factor inhibition in two rat arthritis models. Arthritis Rheum 52(5): 1604–1611.
40. Gravallese EM, Manning C, Tsay A, Naito A, Pan C, et al. (2000) Synovial tissue in rheumatoid arthritis is a source of osteoclast differentiation factor. Arthritis Rheum 43(2): 250–258.
41. Pettit AR, Ji H, von Stechow D, Muller R, Goldring SR, et al. (2001) TRANCE/RANKL knockout mice are protected from bone erosion in a serum transfer model of arthritis. Am J Pathol 159(5): 1689–1699.
42. Hardy R, Juarez M, Naylor A, Tu J, Rabbitt EH, et al. (2012) Synovial DKK1 expression is regulated by local glucocorticoid metabolism in inflammatory arthritis. Arthritis Res Ther 14(5): R226.
43. Black DM, Greenspan SL, Ensrud KE, Palermo L, McGowan JA, et al. (2003) The effects of parathyroid hormone and alendronate alone or in combination in postmenopausal osteoporosis. N Engl J Med 349(13): 1207–1215.
44. Cosman F, Wermers RA, Recknor C, Mauck KF, Xie L, et al. (2009) Effects of teriparatide in postmenopausal women with osteoporosis on prior alendronate or raloxifene: Differences between stopping and continuing the antiresorptive agent. J Clin Endocrinol Metab 94(10): 3772–3780.
45. Cosman F, Eriksen EF, Recknor C, Miller PD, Guanabens N, et al. (2011) Effects of intravenous zoledronic acid plus subcutaneous teriparatide [rhPTH(1–34)] in postmenopausal osteoporosis. J Bone Miner Res 26(3): 503–511.
46. Schafer AL, Sellmeyer DE, Palermo L, Hietpas J, Eastell R, et al. (2012) Six months of parathyroid hormone (1–84) administered concurrently versus sequentially with monthly ibandronate over two years: The PTH and ibandronate combination study (PICS) randomized trial. J Clin Endocrinol Metab 97(10): 3522–3529.

23

Sphingolipids in Human Synovial Fluid - A Lipidomic Study

Marta Krystyna Kosinska[1], Gerhard Liebisch[2], Guenter Lochnit[3], Jochen Wilhelm[4], Heiko Klein[1], Ulrich Kaesser[5], Gabriele Lasczkowski[6], Markus Rickert[1], Gerd Schmitz[2], Juergen Steinmeyer[1]*

1 Department of Orthopedics, Justus-Liebig-University Giessen, Giessen, Germany, **2** Department of Clinical Chemistry and Laboratory Medicine, University Hospital Regensburg, Regensburg, Germany, **3** Department of Biochemistry, Justus-Liebig-University Giessen, Giessen, Germany, **4** Medical Clinic II/IV, Justus-Liebig-University Giessen, Giessen, Germany, **5** Internistisches Praxiszentrum am Krankenhaus Balserische Stiftung, Giessen, Germany, **6** Institute of Forensic Medicine, Justus-Liebig-University Giessen, Giessen, Germany

Abstract

Articular synovial fluid (SF) is a complex mixture of components that regulate nutrition, communication, shock absorption, and lubrication. Alterations in its composition can be pathogenic. This lipidomic investigation aims to quantify the composition of sphingolipids (sphingomyelins, ceramides, and hexosyl- and dihexosylceramides) and minor glycerophospholipid species, including (lyso)phosphatidic acid, (lyso)phosphatidylglycerol, and bis(monoacylglycero)phosphate species, in the SF of knee joints from unaffected controls and from patients with early (eOA) and late (lOA) stages of osteoarthritis (OA), and rheumatoid arthritis (RA). SF without cells and cellular debris from 9 postmortem donors (control), 18 RA, 17 eOA, and 13 lOA patients were extracted to measure lipid species using electrospray ionization tandem mass spectrometry - directly or coupled with hydrophilic interaction liquid chromatography. We provide a novel, detailed overview of sphingolipid and minor glycerophospholipid species in human SF. A total of 41, 48, and 50 lipid species were significantly increased in eOA, lOA, and RA SF, respectively when compared with normal SF. The level of 21 lipid species differed in eOA SF versus SF from lOA, an observation that can be used to develop biomarkers. Sphingolipids can alter synovial inflammation and the repair responses of damaged joints. Thus, our lipidomic study provides the foundation for studying the biosynthesis and function of lipid species in health and most prevalent joint diseases.

Editor: Paul Proost, University of Leuven, Rega Institute, Belgium

Funding: This work was supported in part by a grant of the DRB foundation and by the "LipidomicNet" project, funded within the Seventh Framework Programme of the European Union (Grant agreement number 202272). The funders had no role in study design, data collection and analysis, decision to publish, or preparation of the manuscript. No additional external funding was received for this study.

Competing Interests: The authors have declared that no competing interests exist.

* E-mail: juergen.steinmeyer@ortho.med.uni-giessen.de

Introduction

Synovial fluid (SF) can be viewed as an ultrafiltrate of plasma that contains locally synthesized factors, such as cytokines; growth factors; and lubricating compounds, such as lubricin, hyaluronic acid, and phospholipids. The chief functions of SF are shock absorption; load bearing; lubrication of articular surfaces, such as those of cartilage, the meniscus, tendons, and ligaments; and nutrition and communication medium of joints.

Altered composition or concentrations of SF components are linked to osteoarthritis (OA) and rheumatoid arthritis (RA) [1–3]. A precise profile of the chemical composition of SF during disease-related alterations will increase our knowledge about the pathogenesis and possible options to treat these joint diseases.

Sphingolipids (SLs) are a class of lipids that include ceramide (Cer) species, sphingomyelins (SMs) and more complex glycosphingolipids. A common constituent of all SLs is the sphingoid base, which is an organic aliphatic amino alcohol sphingosine (SPH) or a structurally similar compound [4]. The metabolic pathways of SLs form complex networks of reactions that involve many enzymes and intermediate metabolites that are needed for the biosynthesis, degradation, and remodeling of individual SLs [4–6].

SLs are structural components of plasma membranes and bioactive molecules that have significant functions in proliferation and growth as well as differentiation, cellular signal transduction, and apoptosis in many mammalian cells for instance fibroblast-like synoviocytes (FLSs) and neural cells [7–11]. The function of SLs depends on their acyl chain length and degree of saturation.

The balance between levels of individual SLs is critical. For instance, sphingosine-1-phosphate (S1P) antagonizes Cer-mediated apoptosis [9]. Exogenous Cer in turn was reported to regulate proliferation in human FLSs from OA and RA patients [7]. Treatment of FLSs with micromolar concentrations of C6-Cer inhibits proliferation through G_o/G_1 arrest, similar to what has been observed after serum starvation [7].

Cardiolipins (CLs) are tetra-acylated glycerophospholipids that are part of the inner mitochondrial membranes in eukaryotic cells. CLs regulate energy production [12,13], whereas free radical oxidation products of CLs are important mediators of mitochondria-dependent apoptosis [14–16]. Altered levels and composition of CLs are linked to diseases, such as diabetes [13], heart failure [13,17], Parkinson disease [18], and a rare cardiomyopathy, known as Barth syndrome [19].

Bis(monoacylglycero)phosphate (BMP) is an acidic phospholipid and an isomer of phosphatidylglycerol (PG). BMPs are formed on the surface of intralysosomal vesicles during the degradation of PGs and CLs and stimulate the enzymatic hydrolysis of membrane-bound SLs. The highest levels of negatively charged BMPs are found in the internal vesicles of lysosomes, and the concentration of BMPs increases as late endosomes convert into lysosomes [20]. BMPs are important for endosomal and lysosomal function, and altered levels of BMP species have been reported in a group of diseases, known as lysosomal storage disorders, in which lysosomal dysfunction leads to the accumulation of secondary metabolites, as observed in Gaucher disease, Fabry disease, mucopolysaccharidosis, Pompe disease, and drug-induced phospholipidosis [20,21].

Phosphatidic acid (PA) is a biosynthetic precursor of lipids, like PGs, CLs, and BMPs. There are two lipids that are chemically similar to PA: lysophosphatidic acid (LPA) and cyclic PA (cPA). LPA has an identical chemical structure to PA, except that it contains a single fatty acid (FA). LPA regulates many physiological and pathophysiological responses and is one of the most active naturally occurring lipids [22]. cPA act as a lipid mediator with several biological activities. Notably, cPA was recently reported to possess some antiinflammatory and chondroprotective activities in a rabbit model of OA [23].

The normal use of articular joints may damage cells found within SF which may be thus an additional source of many components of SF, including intracellular lipids that are not actively secreted into the SF. Chondrocytes, synovial lining cells, leukocytes (predominantly T cells), and cells from the meniscus, tendon, and ligaments are normally found at the borderline of SF or in SF. In addition, SF is an ultrafiltrate of the plasma so that lipids might also derive from the blood.

The levels, composition, and functions of SL, CL, LPA, PA, BMP, PG and lysophosphatidylglycerol (LPG) species in SF are unknown. Thus, we aimed to identify and quantify SL, CL, LPA, PA, LPG, PG, and BMP species. In particular, we wanted to investigate whether these lipid species are related to the health status of synovial joints using SF from normal donors as well as from patients with RA, early (eOA) or with late stages (lOA) of OA.

Materials and Methods

Inclusion and Exclusion Criteria

The SF originated from 9 deceased donors, 18 patients with RA and 30 patients with OA (Table 1). The present study was approved by the Ethical Review Committee of the Faculty of Medicine (Justus-Liebig-University of Giessen, Germany), and all patients provided written informed consent to donor samples for research. The Ethical Review Committee (protocol #62/06) waived the need for consent to be obtained from relatives of deceased donors since a judicial order to perform autopsy existed and, furthermore, to avoid additional emotional drain on relatives.

We used the Outerbridge classification scale (OU) to subcategorise the osteoarthritic changes in the joints as early (eOA) and late (lOA) stages of the disease [24]. For this, the 6 cartilage surfaces of the patella, trochlea and the medial and lateral sides of the femoral condyles and the tibia were macroscopically evaluated and the resulting cumulative OU score was divided by six in order to obtain an average score valid for the entire joint. Early osteoarthritic disease stages were defined as those which showed an average score ≤2, while late stages of the disease were defined as those with an OU score >2. Patients with RA were classified as described in the guidelines of the American College of Rheumatology [25]. SF was removed during autopsies of knee healthy donors at the Institute of Forensic Medicine, University of Giessen at the times after death described in Figure 1.

The SF was withdrawn into a syringe either during an arthroscopy (eOA) or during an otherwise necessary knee puncture (RA). In contrast, the SF of patients with late stage disease (lOA) was obtained during a knee prosthetic implantation.

Processing of the Synovial Fluid

The SF was processed as described elsewhere [26]. Briefly, SF was macroscopically evaluated, pressed through a 1.2 micron filter, and then 10% (v/v) inhibitors were added in order to inhibit proteases and phospholipases. This was followed by centrifugation of the SF for 45 min at 16,100×g and RT in order to pellet the cellular debris [26,27]. Finally, the supernatant was frozen at −86°C for further lipid analysis.

Extraction of Sphingolipids and Phospholipids

The cell and cellular debris-free supernatant was extracted in the presence of internal lipid standards (Avanti Polar Lipids, Alabaster, AL, USA) in order to specifically quantify extracellular SMs and Cer species [26,28]. In addition, aliquots of the SF supernatant were extracted with butanol in order to determine hexosylceramide (HexCer) species, dihexosylceramide (Hex_2Cer) species, sphingoid bases, sphingosylphosphorylcholine (SPC) [29], S1P, LPAs, CLs, BMPs, PGs, and PAs [30,31]. In brief, SF was first buffered with 400 μl 30 mM citric acid and 40 mM disodium hydrogen phosphate. Lipids were then extracted with 1-butanol, dried, and redissolved in 50 μl ethanol.

Mass Spectrometric Quantification of Lipid Species

As already described the SM and Cer species were determined using electrospray ionisation mass spectrometry (ESI-MS/MS) [28,32]. In addition, we used MS/MS after liquid chromatographic separation (LC-MS/MS) to determine HexCer species, Hex_2Cer species, sphingoid bases, SPC [29], S1P, LPAs [30], CLs, BMPs, PGs and PAs [31]. Lipid species were annotated as published [33].

Data Analysis

A possible dilution of SF by a joint effusion would result in a clearly reduced concentration of certain lipids as determined by ESI-MS/MS. The liver produces urea which is not synthesized or metabolized in articular joints. Urea diffuses without any restriction across the synovium and can therefore be used to evaluate unknown dilution. The dilution effect was corrected by the method described by Kraus *et al* [26,34]. For this purpose, the concentration of urea was first measured in both SF and serum so that a dilution factor for the SF according to Kraus *et al* [34] could be calculated. Urea was determined using a commercially available kit (BioAssay Systems, Hayward, CA, USA).

Statistical Analysis of the Measured Values Obtained

In our exploratory study, a non-Gaussian distribution of the measured values was assumed so that a non-parametric statistical analysis was carried out. The Kruskal-Wallis test was used to identify statistically significant differences in the levels of lipid species between different cohorts. The false discovery rate was controlled at 5% (Benjamini-Hochberg adjustment).. For the selected species, the Steel-Dwass multiple comparisons was applied to determine statistically significant differences in lipid concentrations between individual cohorts (control, eOA, lOA, RA) while controlling the family-wise error-rate at 5%.

Table 1. Characteristics of synovial fluid donors.

	Postmortem donors. n = 9	Patients with eOA. n = 17	Patients with lOA. n = 13	Patients with RA. n = 18
Age	22 (21–25)	36 (25–49)	70 (67–74)	64 (49–71)
female/male	1/8	6/11	7/6	14/4
BMI	24.8 (20.8–25.2)	24.7 (22.6–26.9)	27.7 (25.8–30.1)	29.5 (24.8–32.8)
CRP	nd	0.5 (0.5–1.0)	1.6 (1.13–1.85)	13.2 (5.3–38.8)
No. of cells/μl SF	nd	nd	nd	6100 (2588–12,925)
DAS28	nd	nd	nd	3.48 (3.32–4.56)

Inclusion criteria: both genders, age 18–85 years inclusive, BMI<40, CRP≤3 mg/L, and all CRP levels for RA. Exclusion criteria: joint infection; severe liver or kidney disease; any surgery within the last 3 months; knee joint surgery within the last 6 months; diabetes mellitus (OA); drug abuse; intraarticular treatment with hyaluronate; or corticosteroid treatment within the last 3 months; HIV infection; tumor/cancer.

We used the statistical software "R" version 2.14.0 to perform the Kruskal-Wallis test, Benjamini-Hochberg adjustment as well as the Steel-Dwass tests. The data obtained are presented as medians with interquartile ranges for the box plots. The values quoted in the text represent the median together with the interquartile range in brackets.

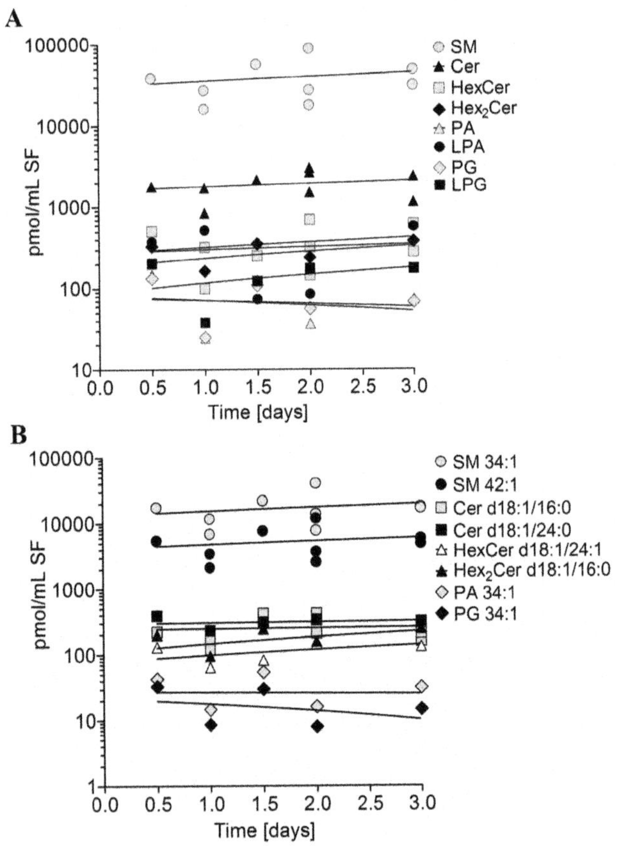

Figure 1. Postmortem stability of lipids extracted from human synovial fluid of healthy knee joints used as controls. Lipids were determined by electrospray ionization tandem mass spectrometry (ESI-MS/MS) or liquid chromatography coupled with tandem mass spectrometry (LC-MS/MS) as outlined in *Material and Methods.* Values are displayed as a scatterplot of the concentration of each lipid class and species by postmortem time. (**A**): Lipid classes, (**B**): Lipid species. SM-sphingomyelin, Cer-ceramide, HexCer-hexosylceramide (most likely glucosylceramide), Hex_2Cer-dihexosylceramide (most likely lactosylceramide), PA-phospatidic acid, LPA-lysophosphatidic acid, PG-phosphatidylglycerol, LPG-lysophosphatidylglycerol.

Results

Sphingomyelin Molecular Species

Using established ESI-MS/MS method the changes in the concentrations of SM species were examined (28). Of the SL classes that we examined, SMs were the most abundant in SF. The concentration of total SMs in control SF was 39 nmol/ml, multiplying 2.4-fold in eOA (92 nmol/ml; $p<0.05$), 4.4-fold in lOA (172 nmol/ml; $p\leq0.001$), and 3.2-fold in RA (126 nmol/ml; $p\leq0.001$). Nineteen SM species, based on the length and saturation of the attached FAs, were identified in human SF as shown in Figure 2. SM 34:1 was the predominant species among SMs, accounting for 38% to 44% of total SMs in all cohorts (Figure 2). In addition, versus control SF, 19 SM species were elevated by 2.4-fold (2.2–2.8-fold; $p<0.05$) in eOA, 4.8fold (4.1–5.4-fold; $p\leq0.001$) in lOA, and in RA SF 3.5-fold (2.8–4.2-fold; $p\leq0.001$). Notably, all SM species had risen approximately 2-fold in SF from eOA to lOA ($p\leq0.05$, Figure 2).

Ceramide Molecular Species

In order to quantify Cer species, ESI-MS/MS analysis was used. Furthermore, LC-MS/MS method was performed to quantify HexCer and Hex_2Cer species. Within analysed SLs, the second most prominent group of SLs in human SF was Cer species. The concentration of total Cer species was 1.4 nmol/ml in SF from controls, elevated 2-fold in SF from eOA (2.8 nmol/ml; n.s.), 3.9-fold in lOA SF (5.5 nmol/ml; $p\leq0.01$), and 3-fold in SF from RA (4.2 nmol/ml; $p\leq0.001$). Six Cer species were identified; Cer d18:0/24:0 was the predominant species (Figure 3A). As expected, the level of most Cer species was higher in lOA and RA SF, such as Cer d18:1/16:0, Cer d18:1/22:0, Cer d18:1/23:0, and Cer d18:1/24:1. Notably, most Cer species contained saturated FAs, constituting 68.9% to 74.9% of total Cer species in all cohorts (Figure 3A).

Further, the molecular species of HexCer and Hex_2Cer were quantified. Five HexCer species and 5 Hex_2Cer species were detected in human SF (Figure 3B and 4A). The percentage distribution of these species differed slightly between all cohorts, except for Hex_2Cer d18:1/24:0 which was high in eOA, and Hex_2Cer d18:1/24:1, which was low in eOA (Figure 4A). HexCer species and Hex_2Cer species were low in control SF but higher in the SF of all other cohorts. In comparison with control SF, the concentrations of HexCer species increased by 3.9-fold (3.4–4.2-fold; $p\leq0.001$) in eOA, 5.8-fold (4.8–6.1-fold; $p\leq0.01$) in lOA,

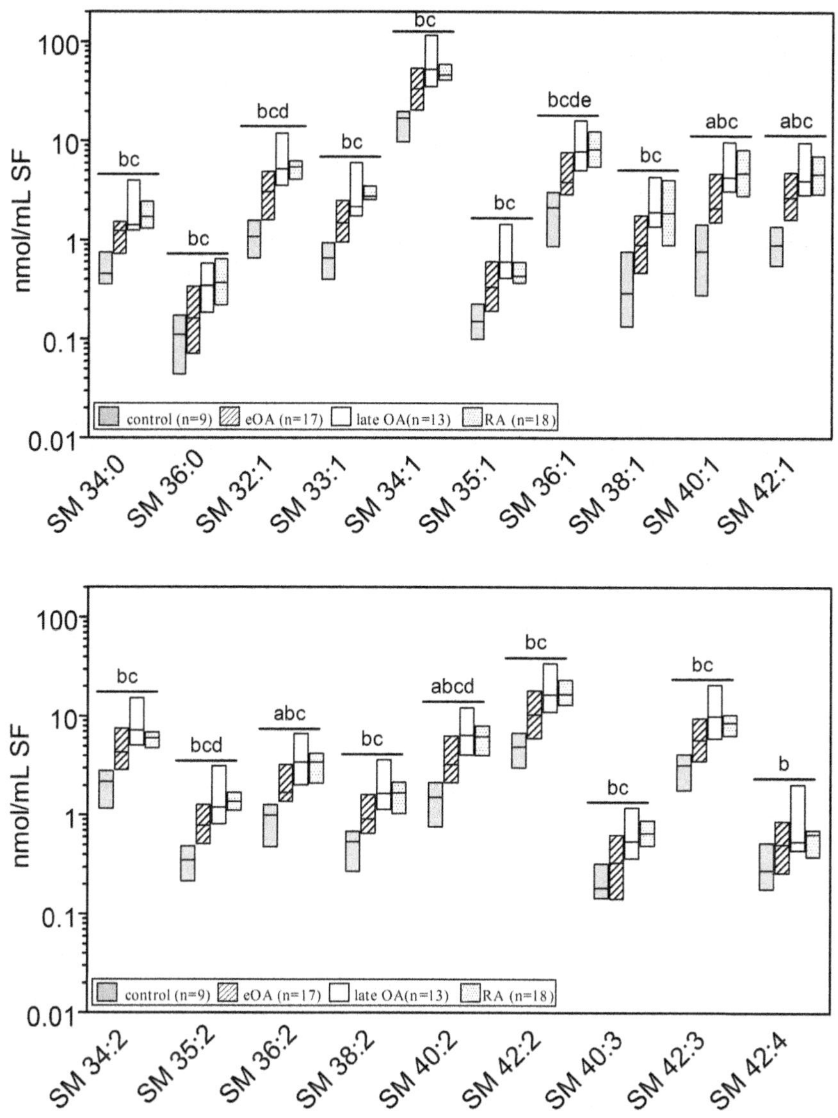

Figure 2. Concentrations of sphingomyelin species in human knee synovial fluid. Synovial fluid was obtained from donors serving as controls and from patients with early osteoarthritis (eOA), late OA (lOA), and rheumatoid arthritis (RA). SM species were determined by electrospray ionization tandem mass spectrometry as outlined in *Material and Methods*. Species annotation is based on the notion that 2 hydroxyl groups are linked to a sphingoid base. Values are presented as median and interquartile range. Significance was considered in the following way: a: p≤0.05: control vs eOA; b: p≤0.05: control vs lOA; c: p≤0.05: control vs RA; d: p≤0.05: eOA vs lOA; and e: p≤0.05: eOA vs RA. SM- sphingomyelin.

and in RA SF 5.8-fold (5.3–6.1-fold; p≤0.001) (Figure 3B), whereas Hex_2Cer species rose by 3.4-fold (3.2–5.5-fold; p≤0.001) in eOA, 4.5-fold (4.4–5.2-fold; p≤0.05) in lOA, and in RA SF 6.9-fold (6.9–7.3-fold; p≤0.001) (Figure 3B).

Lysosphingolipids and Their Phosphates

The values for S1P and sphinganine-1-phosphate in SF were below the limit of detection (6 pmol/ml for undiluted samples). We identified the following species in RA SF: SPH d18:0 [11.3 pmol/ml (0.0–21.2 pmol/ml)], SPH d18:1 [20.0 pmol/ml (15.2–24.8 pmol/ml)], SPC d18:0 [1.0 pmol/ml (0.0–1.8 pmol/ml)], and SPC d18:1 [16.1 pmol/ml (10.8–31.2 pmol/ml)]. Only 2 SL species in OA SF [SPH d18:1, 5.2 pmol/ml (0.0–16.9 pmol/ml) and SPC d18:1, 10.1 pmol/ml (4.6–19.5 pmol/ml)] were detected.

Molecular Species of Cardiolipins and BMPs

CLs possess a unique dimeric structure, bearing phosphatidyl moieties that are linked by a bridging glycerol, to which 4 FAs are attached. Our mass spectrometric analysis only enabled us to measure the sum of double bounds and carbon atoms in each of the 2 phosphatidyl moieties. The CL species concentrations were below the limit of detection, except for CL 36:4/36:4, which was elevated in RA SF.

Only 2 BMP species (BMP 18:1/18:1 and BMP 18:2/18:1) were above the limit of detection (Table 2). The highest levels of these species were observed in RA SF. In comparison with control SF, the levels of these BMP species rose by 1.6-fold (1.4–1.7-fold; ns) in all other cohorts.

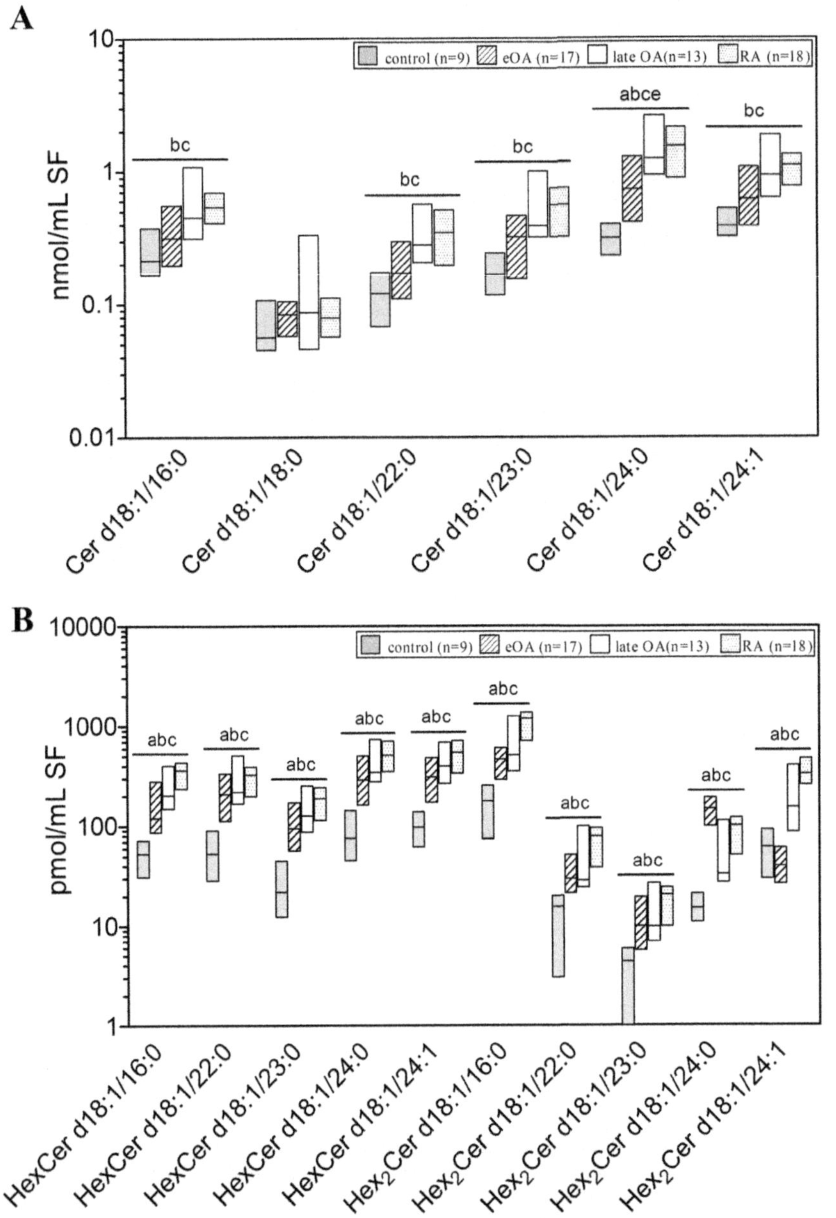

Figure 3. Concentrations of ceramide species in human knee synovial fluid. Synovial fluid was obtained from donors serving as controls and from patients with early osteoarthritis (eOA), late OA (lOA), and rheumatoid arthritis (RA). Cer species were determined by electrospray ionization tandem mass spectrometry as outlined in *Material and Methods*. Values are presented as median and interquartile range. Significance was considered in the following way: a: p≤0.05: control vs eOA; b: p≤0.05: control vs lOA; c: p≤0.05: control vs RA; d: p≤0.05: eOA vs lOA; and e: p≤0.05: eOA vs RA. (**A**): Cer species, (**B**): HexCer and Hex$_2$Cer species. Cer- ceramide, HexCer- hexosylceramide (most likely glucosylceramide), Hex$_2$Cer- dihexosylceramide (most likely lactosylceramide).

Molecular Species of PA, PG, and Lysophospholipids (LPA, LPG)

As a class, PAs and PGs contain 2 FA chains. Our mass spectrometric analysis allowed us only to determine the sum of double bonds as well as carbon atoms in the FAs, as shown in Figure 5A and 6.

Four PA and 5 LPA species, based on the number of double bounds and chain length, were detected in human SF (Figure 4B and 5). The relative distribution of these species was similar in all cohorts, except for high levels of LPA 18:0 in eOA and low levels of LPA 18:2 in eOA (Figure 4B). Notably, the concentrations of all PA and LPA species were similar in eOA, lOA, and RA SF. However, in comparison with control SF, the levels of all PA species increased 3.0-fold (2.3–3.8-fold; p≤0.05) in eOA, 4.5-fold (3.9–4.9; p≤0.05) in lOA, and in RA SF 6.7-fold (6.0–7.5; p≤0.001) (Figure 5A). Similarly, versus control SF, the levels of all LPA species rose by 2.7-fold (2.4–3.2-fold; p≤0.01) in eOA, 4.0-fold (3.6–4.4; p≤0.01) in lOA, and in RA SF 3.6-fold (3.2–4.1; p≤0.001) (Figure 5B).

The relative distribution of PG and LPG species did not differ between cohorts (Figure 5C). The major PG species in human SF were those with 34 and 36 C-atoms (PG 34:1, PG 36:1, and PG

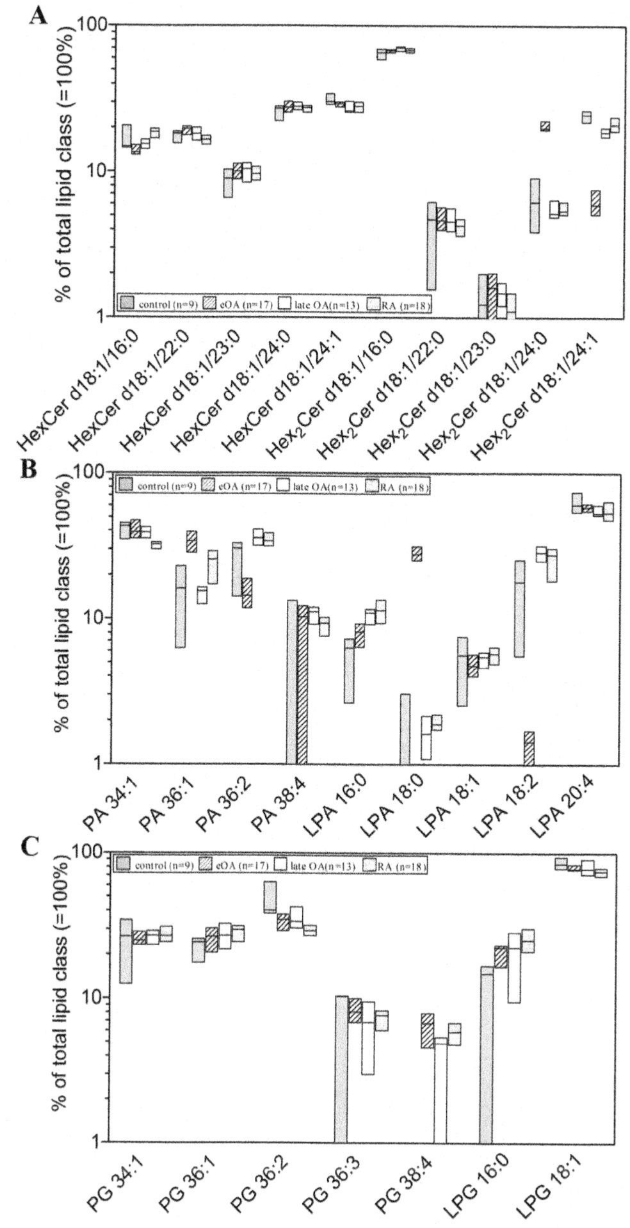

Figure 4. Relative distribution of HexCer and Hex_2Cer, PA, LPA, PG and LPG species in in human knee synovial fluid. Synovial fluid was obtained from donors serving as controls and from patients with early osteoarthritis (eOA), late OA (lOA), and rheumatoid arthritis (RA). The data show the percentage of the lipid species from the total corresponding lipid class (= 100%). Values are presented as median and interquartile range. (**A**): HexCer and Hex_2Cer species, (**B**): PA and LPA species, (**C**): PG and LPG species. HexCer- hexosylceramide (most likely glucosylceramide), Hex_2Cer- dihexosylceramide (most likely lactosylceramide), PA- phosphatidic acid, LPA- lysophosphatidic acid, PG- phosphatidylglycerol, LPG- lysophosphatidylglycerol.

36:2 with concentrations between 0.062 and 3.07 pmol/ml; Figure 6). Five PG and 2 LPG (LPG 16:0 and LPG 18:1) species were found in human SF at concentrations of 0.1–5.0 pmol/ml (Figure 6). Notably, in comparison with control SF, the levels of all PG and LPG species were elevated by 3.5-fold (2.5–5.6-fold; $p \leq 0.01$) in eOA, 3.6-fold (2.8–4.6; $p \leq 0.05$) in lOA, and in RA SF 2.9-fold (1.9–4.5; $p \leq 0.01$). However, the levels of PG and LPG species did not differ between eOA and lOA SF.

Post Mortem Stability of Sphingolipids in SF

The 9 postmortem donors died of intoxication (4×), multiple trauma (2×), cardiomyopathy (1×), pulmonary embolism (1×), and craniocerebral trauma (1×). The SF was obtained with a syringe during the autopsy of 9 adult donors without any known joint disease within a window of several hours to up to 5 days after the time-point of death. Since the stability of sphingolipids in SF as a function of the post-mortem time after time of death is unknown, the concentrations of several lipid species that exist at high levels in the SF (SM 34:1, SM 42:2, Cer d18: 1/24: 0) were plotted against the time between death and autopsy. Figure 6 show that no relevant changes occur in the level of sphingolipids within the time frame of sample collection. Furthermore, no discordant values is obvious in Figure 1 indicating that the cause of death appears to have no impact on the level of lipid species. However, the numbers of investigated SF per cause of death is too low to generalize this observation.

In order to confirm the stability of the lipid species mathematically, a linear regression of the data was obtained, and the slope of the line was calculated together with the 95% confidence interval. None of the slopes differed from 0 (values not shown).

Sphingolipids and Age of Donors

It is not known whether the level of sphingolipids in SF may be also dependent on the age of donors. Furthermore, the four cohorts of our study differ from each other with respect of their average age. Therefore the concentration of investigated lipid classes and species was plotted against the age of each donor within each cohort. Figure 7 as well as Figures S1, S2, S3 shows that the age of donors had no impact on the concentrations of lipids within the four investigated cohorts. Also, a linear regression of the data was calculated together with the slope and the 95% confidence interval revealing, that none of the slopes differed significantly from 0 (values not shown).

Adjustment of Data

The adjusted values were obtained from there corresponding nonadjusted concentrations by multiplying with a dilution factor [34] and resulting data are shown both for classes (Table 3) and individual species (Table S1). During OA water SF might be diluted by water due to inflammation-induced effusion. Therefore, the concentrations of lipid species were corrected for possible dilution. The concentrations of urea were determined within serum and SF in order to calculate a dilution factor for SF; this procedure was formerly developed to adjust for the dilution introduced by lavage during some biomarker studies. Compared with the level of lipids in SF of controls, eOA, lOA, and RA had elevated concentrations of most lipid species independent of whether they were adjusted or nonadjusted. However, the differences between most lipid species in eOA and lOA were more obvious using the adjusted values (Table S1)

Discussion

Lipids such as SLs, PAs, LPAs, LPGs, and BMPs and other groups of lipids are known to be bioactive molecules, but their location and function in SF of articular joints remain to be discovered. The lack of knowledge on the profile, quantity, and function of these lipids in human SF underscore the need for detailed studies in this area. Changes in the composition and

Table 2. Concentrations of bis(monoacylglycero)phosphate (BMP) species.

Concentration [pmol/ml]				
BMP-specie	**control (n = 9)**	**eOA (n = 17)**	**lOA (n = 13)**	**RA (n = 18)**
BMP 18:1/18:1	27.8 (17.5–46.8)	23.1 (15.4–37.9)	36.7 (22.9–74.7)	24.2 (19.8–30.9)
BMP 18:2/18:1	15.6 (9.27–20.0)	16.8 (11.5–25.5)	25.4 (15.9–46.3)	18.8 (13.9–23.6)

Concentrations of bis(monoacylglycero)phosphate (BMP) species in knee synovial fluid obtained from donors serving as controls and from patients with early osteoarthritis (eOA), late OA (lOA), and rheumatoid arthritis (RA). BMP species were determined by electrospray ionization tandem mass spectrometry as outlined in *Material and Methods*. Values are presented as median and interquartile range in the brackets. BMP-Bis(monoacylglycero)phosphate, eOA-early osteoarthritis, lOA-late osteoarthritis, RA-rheumatoid arthritis.

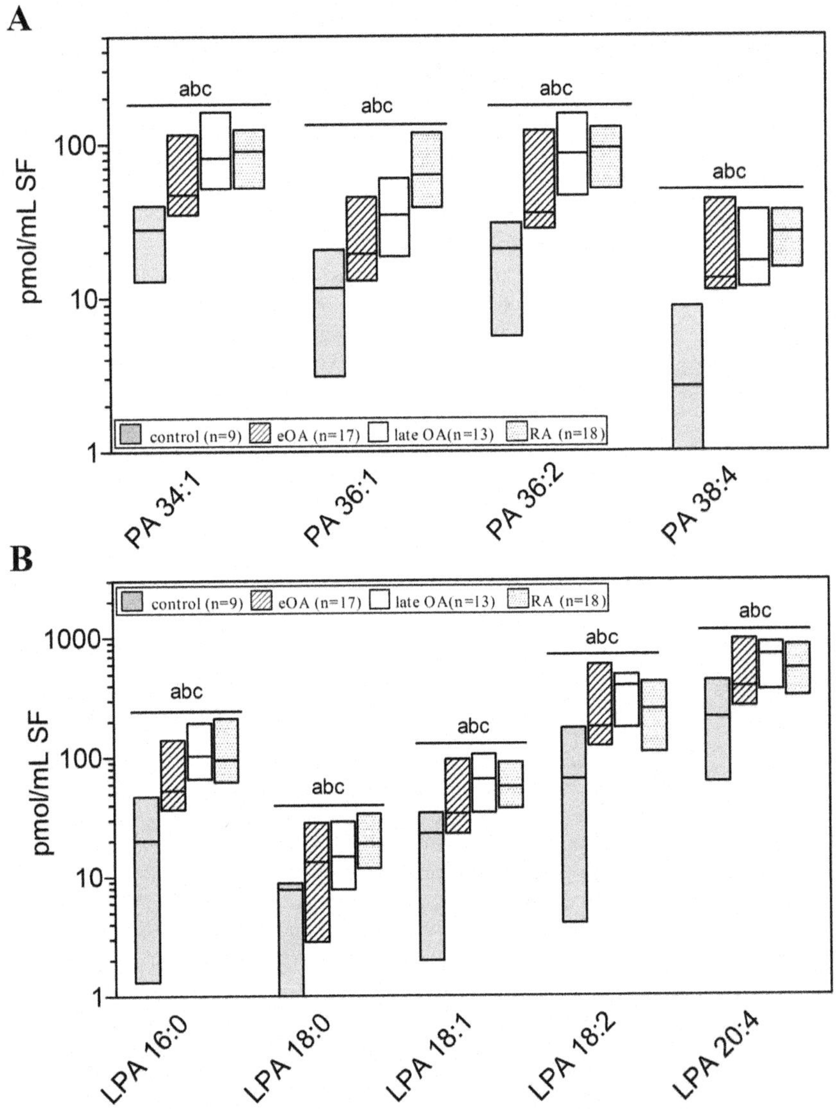

Figure 5. Concentrations of phosphatidic acid (PA) and lysophosphatidic acid (LPA) species in human knee synovial fluid. Synovial fluid was obtained from donors serving as controls and from patients with early osteoarthritis (eOA), late OA (lOA), and rheumatoid arthritis (RA). PA and LPA species were determined liquid chromatography coupled with tandem mass spectrometry as outlined in *Material and Methods*. Species annotation is based on the notion that only ester bonds are present. Values are presented as median and interquartile range. Significance was considered in the following way: a: p≤0.05: control vs eOA; b: p≤0.05: control vs lOA; and c: p≤0.05: control vs RA. (**A**): PA species, (**B**): LPA species. PA- phosphatidic acid, LPA- lysophosphatidic acid.

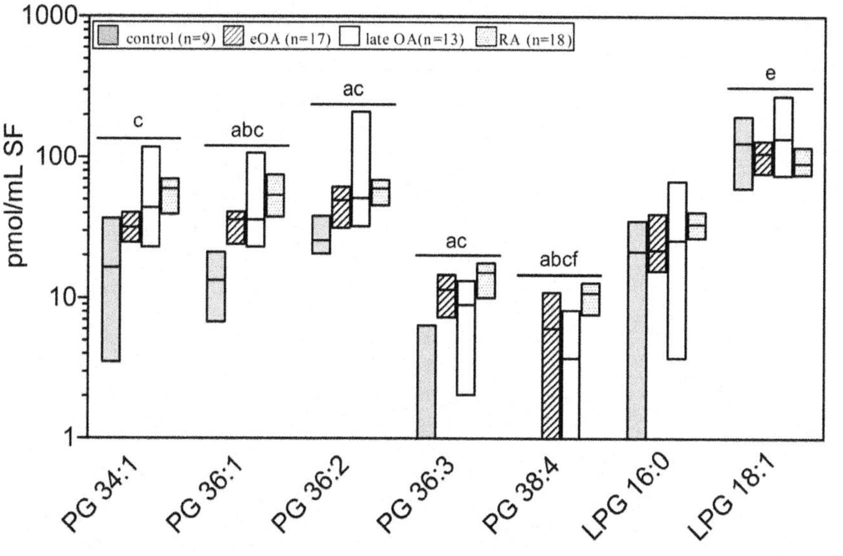

Figure 6. Concentrations of phosphatidylglycerol (PG) and lysophosphatidylglycerol (LPG) species in human knee synovial fluid. Synovial fluid was obtained from donors serving as controls and from patients with early osteoarthritis (eOA), late OA (lOA), and rheumatoid arthritis (RA). PG and LPG species were determined by liquid chromatography coupled with tandem mass spectrometry as outlined in *Material and Methods.* Species annotation is based on the notion that only ester bonds are present. Values are presented as median and interquartile range. Significance was considered in the following way: a: $p \leq 0.05$: control vs eOA; b: $p \leq 0.05$: control vs lOA; c: $p \leq 0.05$: control vs RA; d: $p \leq 0.05$: eOA vs lOA; e: $p \leq 0.05$: eOA vs RA; and f: $p \leq 0.05$: lOA vs RA. PG- phosphatidylglycerol, LPG- lysophosphatidylglycerol.

concentrations of various lipids have been already linked with several human disorders [19,26].

We have reported that concentrations of phospholipids species increase in SF of RA and OA compared with SF obtained from donors used as controls [26]. The principle finding of our current study is that a broad spectrum of SL species, their precursors, and intermediate metabolites was found in human SF. Moreover, the concentrations of 41 lipids in eOA SF, 48 species in lOA SF, and 50 species in RA SF increase significantly in comparison with control SF. Notably, the levels of 21 lipid species were altered between eOA and lOA SF, indicating that the lipid composition of SF reflects the severity of OA disease. Thus, our findings may be used to develop biomarkers to discriminate eOA from lOA, and eOA from healthy joints.

Until recently, there have been no sensitive methods to detect these species at low concentrations in biological materials. The lipidomic methods that we used in this study [28–32], allowed us to identify and quantify many lipid species that have not been reported in SF. This is why our lipidomic investigation reports for the first time about the composition of SL and minor glycerophospholipids species in human SF.

SMs and Cer species regulate many processes, including stress responses, proliferation and differentiation, apoptosis, and senescence [35–37]. Using chondrocytes and explants from rabbit articular cartilage, exogenous cell-permeable C2-Cer at concentrations over 25 μM were noted to induce apoptosis, up regulate MMP-1, -3, and -13, and ultimately induce articular cartilage matrix degradation by collagen type II cleavage and proteoglycan loss from cartilage [38–41]. Further, Cer species are reported to be mediators that induce proinflammatory cytokine production and possibly apoptosis in cultured human RA FLS [7,11] as well as cultured chondrocytes [38]. *In vitro* administration of synthetic exogenous C2- or C6-Cer at concentrations below 25 μM did not affect apoptosis but inhibited the proliferation of FLS in OA and RA [7]. However, intraarticular injection of 34.5 μg C2-Cer into the ankle joints of mice increased the population of apoptotic synovial cells [11].

We observed higher concentrations of several Cer species in SF from RA and lOA compared with control SF indicating that Cer species may be involved in the progression of OA and RA. However, the exact function of extracellular SM and Cer species, alone and in combination, in synovial joints is unknown. Further studies are needed to show whether Cer species are synthesized *de novo* or are the result of higher sphingomyelinase activity.

CLs are nearly exclusively a constituent of the mitochondrial inner membrane: extracellular CLs in body fluids have not been reported. We detected CLs only in RA SF. Thus, we speculate that the presence of CLs in SF is a hallmark of RA and that CLs can be used to develop a novel diagnostic tool for RA. However, it is unknown whether CLs in SF have functions. The source of CLs in RA SF is not known and further studies are needed to identify where the CLs come from. One possible source are the cells that are enriched in RA SF compared with OA and control SF and which can be damaged by normal joint movement so that mitochondrial lipids like CLs are released. Although we removed cells and cellular debris from SF by centrifugation and filtration, these techniques are unable to eliminate molecular micelles.

LPAs can promote the proliferation of many cell types. *In vitro* stimulation with 1 or 5 μM exogenous LPA stimulates the proliferation of rat primary chondrocytes [42,43]. Moreover, the expression of six G-protein-coupled LPA receptors increases in RA FLS. Thus, LPAs appear to function as lipid mediators between cells displaying growth factor-like activities [44]. We noted elevated levels of all PA and LPA species in SF of RA and OA compared with control SF, consistent with previous findings [45]. The higher concentration of LPAs is likely attributed to increased secretion and activity of enzymes for example phospholipase A_2 [46] and may point to a possible repair response. However, further studies need to evaluate the functions of LPA species as intercellular lipid mediators that induce cell proliferation and have growth factor-like activities in damaged articular cartilage.

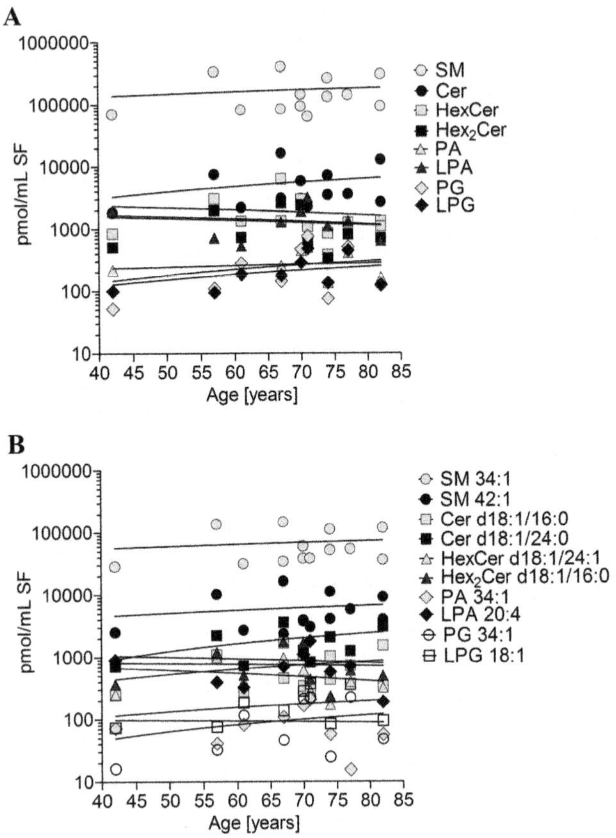

Figure 7. Concentrations of lipids in human synovial fluid as a function of the age of patients with late stage osteoarthritis. Lipids were determined by electrospray ionization tandem mass spectrometry (ESI-MS/MS) or liquid chromatography coupled with tandem mass spectrometry (LC-MS/MS) as outlined in *Material and Methods*. Values are displayed as a scatterplot of the concentration of each lipid class and species by age of donors. (**A**): Lipid classes, (**B**): Lipid species. SM-sphingomyelin, Cer-ceramide, HexCer-hexosylceramide (most likely glucosylceramide), Hex_2Cer-dihexosylceramide (most likely lactosylceramide), PA-phospatidic acid, LPA-lysophosphatidic acid, PG-phosphatidylglycerol, LPG-lysophosphatidylglycerol.

Recently, cPA was reported to stimulate the production of HA in human OA articular chondrocytes and to provide some anti-inflammatory and chondroprotective activities in a rabbit model of OA [23]. However, our methods applied did not allow us to quantify cPA in SF.

This study is the first to report about PG species in SF. PGs are important components of the pulmonary surfactant system [47]. Thus, we hypothesize that PG species have similar functions in synovial joints. However, our study demonstrates that PG species exist at low concentrations in human SF. Moreover, the PG species in human SF are also found in human plasma; albeit, human plasma appears to have more PG species than SF [20,48]. In, contrast to human plasma, in which only saturated LPG species (LPG16:0 and LPG 18:0) have been reported [49], human SF contains a high proportion of monounsaturated LPG 18:1. Notably, versus control SF, the concentrations of all PG species were significantly elevated in eOA, lOA, and RA SF. BMP, a structural isomer of PG, was also detected in SF at low levels, and 2 BMP species were identified. However, the function and source of extracellular PG, LPG, and BMP species are unknown.

Table 3. Impact of dilution factor on the concentrations of lipid classes.

Lipid class	eOA (n = 17) [%]	lOA (n = 13) [%]	RA (n = 18) [%]
SM	118.2 (110.5–123.8)	157.1 (146.5–173.5)	88.1 (83.4–89.2)
Cer	130.7 (122.6–132.9)	157.7 (154.9–164.1)	81.2 (78.4–87.3)
HexCer	110.1 (110.1–111.6)	153.1 (152.7–158.6)	86.0 (82.8–88.5)
Hex_2Cer	103.9 (99.8–105.4)	138.4 (135.5–139.8)	81.2 (77.5–81.9)
PA	103.3 (98.9–106.8)	180.0 (165.7–185.7)	82.8 (79.1–85.6)
LPA	109.9 (108.3–113.3)	176.3 (152.6–190.6)	84.2 (80.1–88.3)
PG	100.0 (98.9–108.5)	123.9 (121.1–126.4)	84.2 (80.8–86.4)
LPG	107.6 (101.9–113.3)	143.2 (133.0–153.4)	82.9 (81.9–83.9)
BMP	97.3 (95.4–99.3)	165.0 (165.0–165.0)	79.6 (77.9–81.2)

Impact of dilution factor on the concentrations of lipid classes as expressed as percentage of uncorrected values (= 100%). Lipids were determined by electrospray ionization tandem mass spectrometry or liquid chromatography coupled with tandem mass spectrometry, and corrected for possible dilution as outlined in *Material and Methods*. Values are median and interquartile range. eOA-early osteoarthritis, lOA-late osteoarthritis, RA-rheumatoid arthritis, SM-sphingomyelin, Cer-ceramide, HexCer-hexosylceramide (most likely glucosylceramide), Hex_2Cer-dihexosylceramide (most likely lactosylceramide), PA-phosphatidic acid, LPA-lysophosphatidic acid, PG-phosphatidylglycerol, LPG-lysophosphatidylglycerol, BMP-bis(monoglycero)phosphate.

In conclusion, this lipidomic investigation presents for the first time a comprehensive survey of SLs and minor glycerophospholipids in human SF. Our mass spectrometric analysis of lipids in SF from patients with eOA, lOA, and RA knee joints indicate disease and stage-dependent differences. Certain species of SM and Cer may, at least in part, be involved in the pathogenesis of OA and RA. The paucity of detailed data on the functions of lipid species in RA and OA underscore the necessity for further studies. Our study lays the foundation for addressing specific questions regarding the biosynthesis and function of lipid species in SF.

Supporting Information

Figure S1 Concentrations of lipids in human synovial fluid as a function of the age of donors used as controls. Synovial fluid was obtained post mortem from donors with healthy knee joints. Lipids were determined by electrospray ionization tandem mass spectrometry (ESI-MS/MS) or liquid chromatography coupled with tandem mass spectrometry (LC-MS/MS) as outlined in *Material and Methods*. Values are displayed as a scatterplot of the concentration of each lipid class and species by age of donors. (**A**): Lipid classes, (**B**): Lipid species. SM-sphingomyelin, Cer-ceramide, HexCer-hexosylceramide (most likely glucosylceramide), Hex_2Cer-dihexosylceramide (most likely lactosylceramide), PA-phospatidic acid, LPA-lysophosphatidic acid, PG-phosphatidylglycerol, LPG-lysophosphatidylglycerol.

Figure S2 Concentrations of lipids in human synovial fluid as a function of the age of patients with early stage osteoarthritis. Lipids were determined by electrospray ionization tandem mass spectrometry (ESI-MS/MS) or liquid chromatography coupled with tandem mass spectrometry (LC-MS/MS) as outlined in *Material and Methods*. Values are displayed as a scatterplot of the concentration of each lipid class and species by age of donors. (**A**): Lipid classes, (**B**): Lipid species. SM-sphingomyelin, Cer-ceramide, HexCer-hexosylceramide (most likely glucosylceramide), Hex_2Cer-dihexosylceramide (most likely lactosylceramide), PA-phospatidic acid, LPA-lysophosphatidic acid, PG-phosphatidylglycerol, LPG-lysophosphatidylglycerol.

Figure S3 Concentrations of lipids in human synovial fluid as a function of the age of patients with rheumatoid arthritis. Lipids were determined by electrospray ionization tandem mass spectrometry (ESI-MS/MS) or liquid chromatography coupled with tandem mass spectrometry (LC-MS/MS) as outlined in *Material and Methods*. Values are displayed as a scatterplot of the concentration of each lipid class and species by age of donors. (**A**): Lipid classes, (**B**): Lipid species. SM-sphingomyelin, Cer-ceramide, HexCer-hexosylceramide (most likely glucosylceramide), Hex_2Cer-dihexosylceramide (most likely lactosylceramide), PA-phospatidic acid, LPA-lysophosphatidic acid, PG-phosphatidylglycerol, LPG-lysophosphatidylglycerol.

Table S1 Concentrations of lipid species presented in Figure 1–7. Lipids were determined by electrospray ionization tandem mass spectrometry or liquid chromatography coupled with tandem mass spectrometry as outlined in *Material and Methods*. Data (nmol/ml or pmol/ml) obtained were either uncorrected (normal font) or corrected with the dilution factor per Kraus *et al.* (34, bold font). Values are median and interquartile range. The concentrations of urea were determined within serum and SF to calculate a dilution factor for SF; this procedure was formerly developed to adjust for the dilution introduced by lavage during some biomarker studies. eOA-early osteoarthritis, lOA-late osteoarthritis, RA-rheumatoid arthritis, SM-sphingomyelin, Cer-ceramide, HexCer-hexosylceramide (most likely glucosylceramide), Hex_2-Cer-dihexosylceramide (most likely lactosylceramide), PA-phospatidic acid, LPA-lysophosphatidic acid, PG-phosphatidylglycerol, LPG-lysophosphatidylglycerol, SPH-sphingosine, SPC-sphingosylphosphorylcholine, CL-cardiolipin, BMP-bis(monoglycero)phosphate.

Acknowledgments

The authors thank Magdalena Singer, Christiane Hild, and Simone Düchtel for excellent technical support and Manuela Döller for assistance with the study organization.

Author Contributions

Conceived and designed the experiments: MKK GS G. Lochnit JS. Performed the experiments: MKK G. Liebisch G. Lochnit JW HK UK G. Lasczkowski MR. Analyzed the data: MKK G. Liebisch GS JW JS. Contributed reagents/materials/analysis tools: G. Liebisch G. Lochnit JW HK UK G. Lasczkowski MR. Wrote the paper: MKK JS. Involved in drafting the article or revising it critically for important intellectual content, and approving the final version to be published: GLI GLO JW HK UK GL GS MR.

References

1. Bellamy N, Campbell J, Robinson V, Gee T, Bourne R, et al. (2006) Viscosupplementation for the treatment of osteoarthritis of the knee. Cochrane Database Syst Rev: CD005321.
2. Ludwig TE, McAllister JR, Lun V, Wiley JP, Schmidt TA (2012) Diminished cartilage-lubricating ability of human osteoarthritic synovial fluid deficient in proteoglycan 4: Restoration through proteoglycan 4 supplementation. Arthritis Rheum 64: 3963–3971.
3. Schmidt TA, Gastelum NS, Nguyen QT, Schumacher BL, Sah RL (2007) Boundary lubrication of articular cartilage: role of synovial fluid constituents. Arthritis Rheum 56: 882–891.
4. Lahiri S, Futerman AH (2007) The metabolism and function of sphingolipids and glycosphingolipids. Cell Mol Life Sci 64: 2270–2284.
5. Merrill AH Jr (2011) Sphingolipid and glycosphingolipid metabolic pathways in the era of sphingolipidomics. Chem Rev 111: 6387–6422.
6. Marchesini N, Hannun YA (2004) Acid and neutral sphingomyelinases: roles and mechanisms of regulation. Biochem Cell Biol 82: 27–44.
7. Gerritsen ME, Shen CP, Perry CA (1998) Synovial fibroblasts and the sphingomyelinase pathway: sphingomyelin turnover and ceramide generation are not signaling mechanisms for the actions of tumor necrosis factor-alpha. Am J Pathol 152: 505–512.
8. Cutler RG, Mattson MP (2001) Sphingomyelin and ceramide as regulators of development and lifespan. Mech Ageing Dev 122: 895–908.
9. Spiegel S, Milstien S (2003) Sphingosine-1-phosphate: an enigmatic signalling lipid. Nat Rev Mol Cell Biol 4: 397–407.
10. Luberto C, Kraveka JM, Hannun YA (2002) Ceramide regulation of apoptosis versus differentiation: a walk on a fine line. Lessons from neurobiology. Neurochem Res 27: 609–617.
11. Ichinose Y, Eguchi K, Migita K, Kawabe Y, Tsukada T, et al. (1998) Apoptosis induction in synovial fibroblasts by ceramide: in vitro and in vivo effects. J Lab Clin Med 131: 410–416.
12. Schlame M, Ren M (2009) The role of cardiolipin in the structural organization of mitochondrial membranes. Biochim Biophys Acta 1788: 2080–2083.
13. Houtkooper RH, Vaz FM (2008) Cardiolipin, the heart of mitochondrial metabolism. Cell Mol Life Sci 65: 2493–2506.
14. Schug ZT, Gottlieb E (2009) Cardiolipin acts as a mitochondrial signalling platform to launch apoptosis. Biochim Biophys Acta 1788: 2022–2031.
15. Yin H, Zhu M (2012) Free radical oxidation of cardiolipin: chemical mechanisms, detection and implication in apoptosis, mitochondrial dysfunction and human diseases. Free Radic Res 46: 959–974.
16. Ji J, Kline AE, Amoscato A, Samhan-Arias AK, Sparvero LJ, et al. (2012) Lipidomics identifies cardiolipin oxidation as a mitochondrial target for redox therapy of brain injury. Nat Neurosci 15: 1407–1413.
17. Ventura-Clapier R, Garnier A, Veksler V (2004) Energy metabolism in heart failure. J Physiol 555: 1–13.
18. Ellis CE, Murphy EJ, Mitchell DC, Golovko MY, Scaglia F, et al. (2005) Mitochondrial lipid abnormality and electron transport chain impairment in mice lacking alpha-synuclein. Mol Cell Biol 25: 10190–10201.
19. Schlame M, Ren M (2006) Barth syndrome, a human disorder of cardiolipin metabolism. FEBS Lett 580: 5450–5455.
20. Meikle PJ, Duplock S, Blacklock D, Whitfield PD, Macintosh G, et al. (2008) Effect of lysosomal storage on bis(monoacylglycero)phosphate. Biochem J 411: 71–78.
21. Hullin-Matsuda F, Luquain-Costaz C, Bouvier J, Delton-Vandenbroucke I (2009) Bis(monoacylglycero)phosphate, a peculiar phospholipid to control the fate of cholesterol: Implications in pathology. Prostaglandins Leukot Essent Fatty Acids 81: 313–324.
22. Tokumura A (2002) Physiological and pathophysiological roles of lysophosphatidic acids produced by secretory lysophospholipase D in body fluids. Biochim Biophys Acta 1582: 18–25.
23. Masuda I, Okada K, Momohara S (2013) Cyclic phosphatidic acid (CPA) stimulates the production of hyaluronic acid (HA) in human osteoarthritic articular chondrocytes, and intraarticular administration of CPA supresses pain, swelling, and cartilage destruction in rabbit experimental osteoarthritis. Osteoarthritis Cartilage 21: Abstracts:S296–S297.
24. Outerbridge RE (1961) The etiology of chondromalacia patellae. J Bone Joint Surg Br 43-B: 752–757.
25. Arnett FC, Edworthy SM, Bloch DA, McShane DJ, Fries JF, et al. (1988) The American Rheumatism Association 1987 revised criteria for the classification of rheumatoid arthritis. Arthritis Rheum 31: 315–324.
26. Kosinska MK, Liebisch G, Lochnit G, Wilhelm J, Klein H, et al. (2013) A lipidomic study of phospholipid classes and species in human synovial fluid. Arthritis Rheum 65: 2323–2333.
27. Berckmans RJ, Nieuwland R, Kraan MC, Schaap MC, Pots D, et al. (2005) Synovial microparticles from arthritic patients modulate chemokine and cytokine release by synoviocytes. Arthritis Res Ther 7: R536–544.
28. Liebisch G, Lieser B, Rathenberg J, Drobnik W, Schmitz G (2004) High-throughput quantification of phosphatidylcholine and sphingomyelin by electrospray ionization tandem mass spectrometry coupled with isotope correction algorithm. Biochim Biophys Acta 1686: 108–117.
29. Scherer M, Leuthauser-Jaschinski K, Ecker J, Schmitz G, Liebisch G (2010) A rapid and quantitative LC-MS/MS method to profile sphingolipids. J Lipid Res 51: 2001–2011.
30. Scherer M, Schmitz G, Liebisch G (2009) High-throughput analysis of sphingosine 1-phosphate, sphinganine 1-phosphate, and lysophosphatidic acid in plasma samples by liquid chromatography-tandem mass spectrometry. Clin Chem 55: 1218–1222.
31. Scherer M, Schmitz G, Liebisch G (2010) Simultaneous quantification of cardiolipin, bis(monoacylglycero)phosphate and their precursors by hydrophilic interaction LC-MS/MS including correction of isotopic overlap. Anal Chem 82: 8794–8799.
32. Liebisch G, Drobnik W, Reil M, Trumbach B, Arnecke R, et al. (1999) Quantitative measurement of different ceramide species from crude cellular extracts by electrospray ionization tandem mass spectrometry (ESI-MS/MS). J Lipid Res 40: 1539–1546.

33. Liebisch G, Vizcaino JA, Kofeler H, Trotzmuller M, Griffiths WJ, et al. (2013) Shorthand notation for lipid structures derived from mass spectrometry. J Lipid Res 54: 1523–1530.
34. Kraus VB, Huebner JL, Fink C, King JB, Brown S, et al. (2002) Urea as a passive transport marker for arthritis biomarker studies. Arthritis Rheum 46: 420–427.
35. Niemela PS, Hyvonen MT, Vattulainen I (2006) Influence of chain length and unsaturation on sphingomyelin bilayers. Biophys J 90: 851–863.
36. Drobnik W, Liebisch G, Audebert FX, Frohlich D, Gluck T, et al. (2003) Plasma ceramide and lysophosphatidylcholine inversely correlate with mortality in sepsis patients. J Lipid Res 44: 754–761.
37. Mizushima N, Kohsaka H, Miyasaka N (1998) Ceramide, a mediator of interleukin 1, tumour necrosis factor alpha, as well as Fas receptor signalling, induces apoptosis of rheumatoid arthritis synovial cells. Ann Rheum Dis 57: 495–499.
38. Sabatini M, Rolland G, Leonce S, Thomas M, Lesur C, et al. (2000) Effects of ceramide on apoptosis, proteoglycan degradation, and matrix metalloproteinase expression in rabbit articular cartilage. Biochem Biophys Res Commun 267: 438–444.
39. Sabatini M, Thomas M, Deschamps C, Lesur C, Rolland G, et al. (2001) Effects of ceramide on aggrecanase activity in rabbit articular cartilage. Biochem Biophys Res Commun 283: 1105–1110.
40. Tetlow LC, Adlam DJ, Woolley DE (2001) Matrix metalloproteinase and proinflammatory cytokine production by chondrocytes of human osteoarthritic cartilage: associations with degenerative changes. Arthritis Rheum 44: 585–594.
41. Colosimo M, McCarthy N, Jayasinghe R, Morton J, Taylor K, et al. (2000) Diagnosis and management of subdural haematoma complicating bone marrow transplantation. Bone Marrow Transplant 25: 549–552.
42. Kim MK, Lee HY, Park KS, Shin EH, Jo SH, et al. (2005) Lysophosphatidic acid stimulates cell proliferation in rat chondrocytes. Biochem Pharmacol 70: 1764–1771.
43. Hurst-Kennedy J, Boyan BD, Schwartz Z (2009) Lysophosphatidic acid signaling promotes proliferation, differentiation, and cell survival in rat growth plate chondrocytes. Biochim Biophys Acta 1793: 836–846.
44. Orosa B, Gonzalez A, Mera A, Gomez-Reino JJ, Conde C (2012) Lysophosphatidic acid receptor 1 suppression sensitizes rheumatoid fibroblast-like synoviocytes to tumor necrosis factor-induced apoptosis. Arthritis Rheum 64: 2460–2470.
45. Song HY, Lee MJ, Kim MY, Kim KH, Lee IH, et al. (2010) Lysophosphatidic acid mediates migration of human mesenchymal stem cells stimulated by synovial fluid of patients with rheumatoid arthritis. Biochim Biophys Acta 1801: 23–30.
46. Pruzanski W, Keystone EC, Sternby B, Bombardier C, Snow KM, et al. (1988) Serum phospholipase A2 correlates with disease activity in rheumatoid arthritis. J Rheumatol 15: 1351–1355.
47. Agassandian M, Mallampalli RK (2013) Surfactant phospholipid metabolism. Biochim Biophys Acta 1831: 612–625.
48. Quehenberger O, Armando AM, Brown AH, Milne SB, Myers DS, et al. (2010) Lipidomics reveals a remarkable diversity of lipids in human plasma. J Lipid Res 51: 3299–3305.
49. Lee JY, Min HK, Moon MH (2011) Simultaneous profiling of lysophospholipids and phospholipids from human plasma by nanoflow liquid chromatography-tandem mass spectrometry. Anal Bioanal Chem 400: 2953–2961.

Risk of Multiple Myeloma in Rheumatoid Arthritis: A Meta-Analysis of Case-Control and Cohort Studies

Kaini Shen[1]✤, Gufeng Xu[2]✤, Qing Wu[3], Daobin Zhou[1], Jian Li[1]*

1 Department of Hematology, Peking Union Medical College Hospital, Chinese Academy of Medical Sciences and Peking Union Medical College, Beijing, People's Republic of China, **2** Zhejiang University, School of Medicine, Hangzhou, Zhejiang, People's Republic of China, **3** Division of Health Sciences Research, Mayo Clinic, Scottsdale, Arizona, United States of America

Abstract

Objectives: multiple myeloma is a malignant neoplasm of plasma cells mainly affecting elderly patients. Despite the wealth of information available on therapeutic strategies, the etiology and pathogenesis of myeloma remain unclear. In the current study, a meta-analysis was conducted to assess the possible association between rheumatoid arthritis and myeloma.

Methods: a literature search was conducted with PubMed, EMBASE and Web of Science for relevant studies published by December 25, 2013. Additionally, we searched annual meeting abstracts of the American Society of Hematology from 2004 to 2013. Only original studies that investigated the association between rheumatoid arthritis and myeloma were included. In total, 8 case-control and 10 cohort studies were identified for analysis.

Results: the meta-estimate of the association between rheumatoid arthritis and myeloma was 1.14 (95% CI, 0.97–1.33) overall, with significant heterogeneity among studies. The relationship between myeloma and other autoimmune diseases was additionally examined from available data. Our results showed that myeloma risk is increased 1.31 to 1.65-fold in pernicious anemia and 1.36 to 2.30-fold in ankylosing spondylitis patients.

Conclusion: Rheumatoid arthritis does not appear to alter the risk of myeloma, while between-study heterogeneity analyses suggest caution in the interpretation of results. Pernicious anemia and ankylosing spondylitis may be potential risk factors for myeloma development. Future large-scale epidemiological studies with reliable exposure biomarkers are necessary to establish the possible contribution of autoimmune disorders to multiple myeloma.

Editor: Riccardo Dolcetti, IRCCS National Cancer Institute, Italy

Funding: This work was supported by National Public Health Grand Research Foundation (No. 201202017). The funders had no role in study design, data collection and analysis, decision to publish, or preparation of the manuscript.

Competing Interests: The authors have declared that no competing interests exist.

* E-mail: lijian@pumch.cn

✤ These authors contributed equally to this work.

Introduction

Multiple myeloma (MM) is one of the most common hematologic malignancies with poor prognosis, characterized by neoplastic proliferation of monoclonal plasma cells. The incidence of MM in developed countries is about 5–7 cases per 100 000 individuals [1]. Despite extensive research efforts over the last two decades, the risk factors of MM remain to be established. Numerous case-control and cohort studies to date have suggested that several environmental factors may be associated with the risk of MM, such as ionizing radiation [2], benzene [3] and agricultural occupation [4]. The relationship between autoimmune disease and hematopoietic malignancies was initially postulated in 1964 [5]. However, the issue of whether autoimmune diseases increase the incidence of MM remains controversial.

On the basis of animal models of MM, it is suggested that repeated antigenic stimulation of the immune system plays an important role in MM development [6,7]. A number of studies have confirmed an association of lymphoma with autoimmune conditions [8–12], including rheumatoid arthritis (RA), systemic lupus erythematosus (SLE), and autoimmune hemolytic anemia, although the underlying pathogenesis is unclear. Similarly, the relationship between MM and autoimmune disease has been a long-term subject of investigation, but inconsistent results have been obtained to date.

The main aim of this meta-analysis was to estimate the comparative risk of developing MM in RA patients versus the general population. Two additional goals were (1) to explore the variation in the association of RA and MM among subgroups of interest and (2) to investigate if there is an association between MM and other autoimmune diseases.

Methods

Search Strategy

A literature search was conducted with PubMed (from January 1, 1951), EMBASE (from January 1, 1955) and Web of Science (from January 1, 1970) using the following search terms: rheumatoid arthritis, autoimmune disease, etiology, epidemiology,

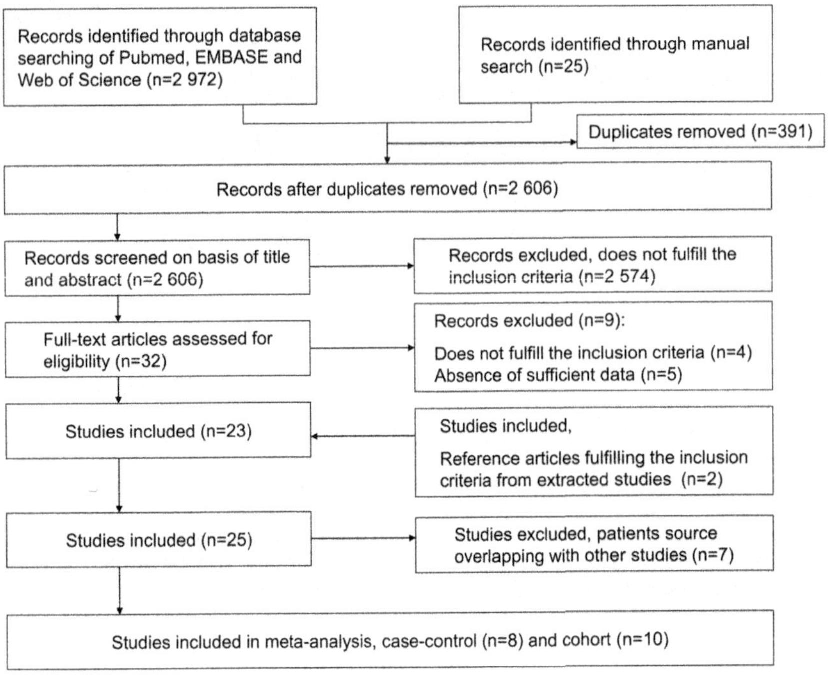

Figure 1. Flow diagram depicting the identification and selection of eligible case-control and cohort studies.

risk factors, multiple myeloma, cancer, malignancy. The final search strategy in PubMed was attached as appendix. The last literature search was performed on December 25, 2013. We also searched annual meeting abstracts of the American Society of Hematology from 2004 to 2013 to identify eligible unpublished data. All references cited in the retrieved articles were additionally reviewed to indentify additional eligible studies. Inclusion criteria were as follows: human participants without limitation of sex or geographic location, case-control or cohort studies, prior medical history of RA as exposure, MM as outcome, studies that reported relative risk (RR), standardized incidence ratio (SIR) or odds ratio (OR) of MM patients with prior history of RA, publication in English. In addition, the selection of cohort studies for inclusion was made regardless of specific RA management strategies. When duplicate reports for the same population and data source were eligible, we chose the original reports with the largest sample size. Case series, case reports, in vitro and animal studies were excluded. Eligibility assessment was performed independently by two reviewers, and disagreements resolved by consensus.

Data Extraction

Two authors performed data extraction independently, and any discrepancies were addressed by discussion and re-evaluation. We obtained information on the author, year of publication, country of origin, source of case, control and cohort, controlled factors, diagnosis criteria and treatment regimen for RA. Cohort size, number of cases, cohort duration, SIR and 95% confidence intervals (CIs) or sufficient data to allow calculation of these numbers were additionally necessary for cohort studies. For case-control studies, the exact numbers of cases and controls by RA, OR and 95% CIs were required. For the purpose of ascertaining the relationship between MM and other autoimmune diseases, related data were recorded, where available, according to the above extraction principles.

The Newcastle-Ottawa Scale (NOS), developed for evaluating the quality of nonrandomized studies [13], was used by two independent reviewers to assess the methodological quality of each study, and the scores subsequently used in subgroup analysis. A score of ≤5 was considered as relative low quality [14].

Statistical Analyses

In case-control studies, OR and 95% CIs for MM risk factors were directly extracted from original research papers or calculated when not provided. The primary outcome for cohort studies was SIR and corresponding 95% CI. In cases where SIRs were not specifically reported, calculations were made from the number of observed MM divided by the number of expected cases in the general population provided by authors, and 95% CI determined using the standard error of the natural logarithm of SIR, estimated from the inverse of the square root of the observed number of cases. The measure of interest was RR, estimated from ORs in case-control studies and SIRs in cohort studies. Since the incidence of MM is low, SIR and OR produce similar estimate of RR, thus we present all results as RR for simplicity [15–17]. Between-study heterogeneity was examined using a chi-square test of heterogeneity and I^2 measure of inconsistency. P-values less than 0.1 or the I^2 statistic greater than 50% were considered statistically significant [18]. Under these conditions, data were pooled based on the method of Dersimonian and Laird under a random effects model otherwise under fixed effects model. Two-tailed $p \leq 0.05$ was considered statistically significant for all analyses.

To evaluate publication bias, we constructed a funnel plot and applied Begg's test. Trim and Fill analysis was used to estimate the number of missing studies and their potential effects on outcomes. Sensitivity analyses were additionally conducted to ascertain the robustness of our findings. The influence of RA was examined by excluding studies restricted to elderly patients (≥65 years) or

Table 1. Characteristics of case-control studies enrolled in the meta-analysis.

Author	Year	Country	Sex	Controls	Cases		Controls		OR (95% CI)	Controlled Factors
					RA	Non-RA	RA	Non-RA		
Pearce NE	1986	New Zealand	M	Population	4	72	7	308	2.30 (0.60–8.00)	Age, registration year
Cohen HJ	1987	USA	M+F	Hospital	62	91	203	210	0.70 (0.48–1.03)	Age, gender, race, disease status
Boffetta P	1989	USA	M+F	Population	39	89	164	348	0.90 (0.60–1.50)	Age, gender, race, residence
Lewis DR	1994	USA	M+F	Population	64	509	241	1 890	0.80 (0.60–1.10)	Age, gender, race
Vlajinac HD	2003	Yugoslavia	M+F	Hospital	12	85	5	95	2.60 (0.90–7.60)	Age, gender, residence
Landgren O	2006	USA	F	Population	7	172	9	682	2.30 (0.80–6.50)	none
Anderson LA	2009	USA	M+F	Population	263	9 211	3 289	119 242	1.00 (0.90–1.10)	Gender, year of diagnosis, age at diagnosis
Lindqvist EK	2011	Sweden	M+F	Population	111	19 001	567	74 841	0.80 (0.60–0.90)	Age, gender, residence

Abbreviations: RA, rheumatoid arthritis; OR, odds ratio; CI, confidence intervals; M, male; F, female.

Table 2. Characteristics of cohort studies enrolled in the meta-analysis.

Author	Year	Country	Sex	Cohort Size	Number of MM	SIR (95% CI)	Follow-up Duration (PY)
Isomaki HA	1982	Finland	M+F	46 101	28	2.20 (1.52–3.19)	213 911
Mellemkjaer L	1996	Denmark	M+F	20 699	21	1.10 (0.70–1.70)	144 421
Kauppi M	1997	Finland	M+F	9 469	8	1.20 (0.50–2.30)	65 391
Thomas E	2000	England	M+F	26 623	38	1.66 (1.21–2.28)	151 987
Setoguchi S	2006	USA	M+F	7 830	19	2.00 (1.26–3.12)	33 410
Herrinton LJ	2008	USA	M+F	2 982	2	2.36 (0.28–8.50)	7 791
Brown LM	2008	USA	M	–	94	1.17 (0.94–1.45)	27 years
Parikh-Patel A	2009	USA	M+F	84 475	64	0.90 (0.70–1.15)	405 540
Hemminki K	2012	Sweden	M+F	72 309	81	0.88 (0.70–1.09)	731 954
Dreyer L	2013	Denmark	M+F	7 159	4	1.76 (0.66–4.69)	24 811

Abbreviations: M, male; F, female; MM, multiple myeloma; SIR, standardized incidence ratio; CI, confidence intervals; PY, person years.
–: Not mentioned.

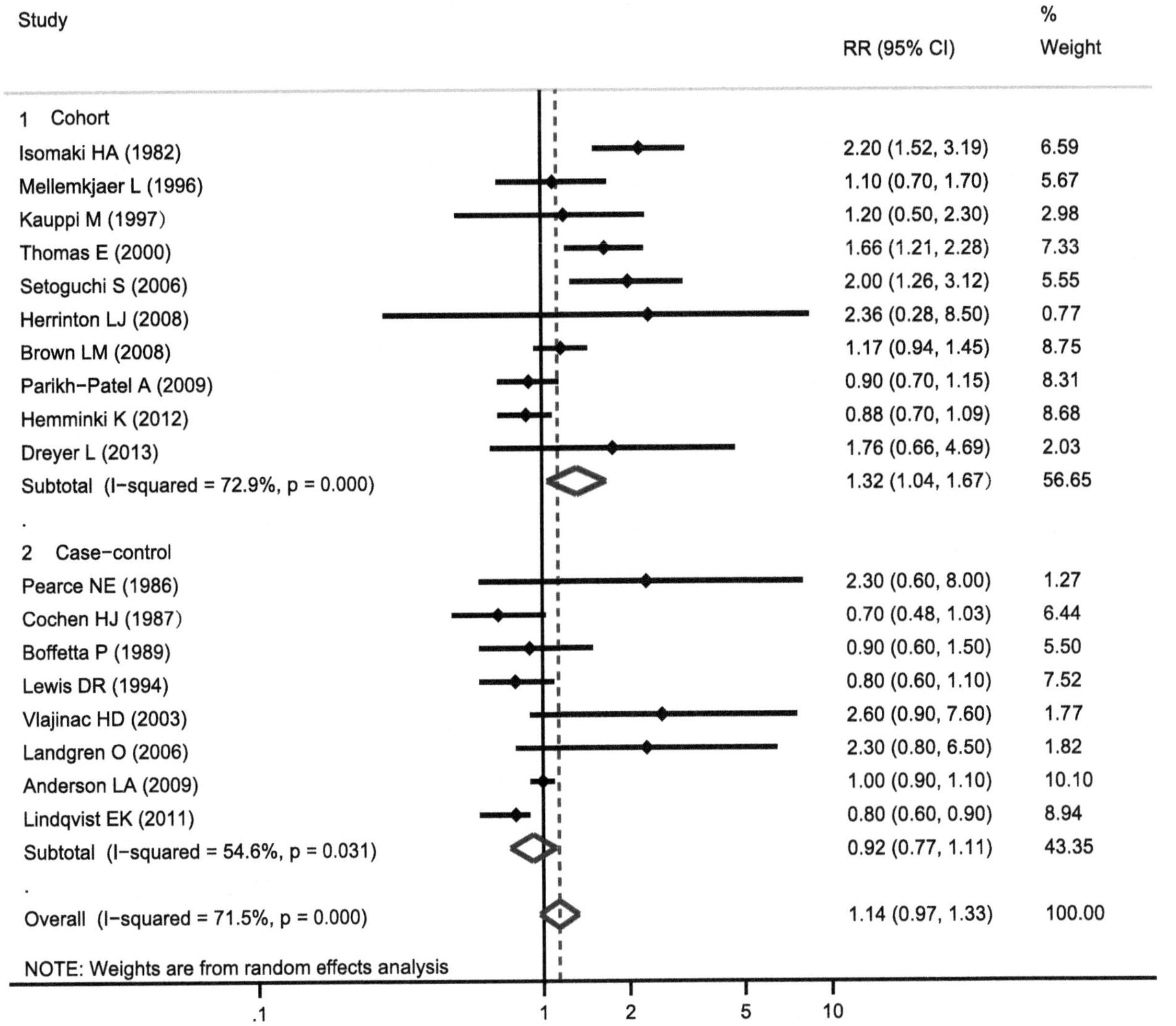

Figure 2. Forest plot of studies on multiple myeloma development risk in rheumatoid arthritis.

single-sex participants and those that failed to control important confounders. All meta-analyses were conducted with Stata 12.0.

Results

Abstract evaluation yielded thirty-two potential studies for analysis (Figure 1), of which five [19–23] were excluded, since they

Table 3. Sensitivity analysis of the association between multiple myeloma and rheumatoid arthritis according to different exclusion criteria.

Studies included	Studies (N)	RR (95% CI)	p value	I^2 (%)
All studies	18	1.14 (0.97–1.33)	<0.001	71.5
Studies without age restriction of participants[a]	17	1.09 (0.94–1.27)	<0.001	68.7
Studies with both male and female participants[b]	15	1.11 (0.94–1.32)	<0.001	74.1
Studies that controlled for important confounding factors[c]	16	1.11 (0.95–1.30)	<0.001	73.1

[a]Excludes the study by the group of Setoguchi [41].
[b]Excludes studies by the groups of Pearce [25], Landgren [36] and Brown [45].
[c]Excludes studies by the groups of Pearce [25] and Landgren [36].
Abbreviations: N, number; RR, relative risk; NS, not significant; CI, confidence interval.

Table 4. Meta-analysis of multiple myeloma incidence by subgroup.

	Subgroup	Analyses (N)	RR (95% CI)	p-value	I^2 (%)
Overall	Study design	Cohort (10)	1.32 (1.04–1.67)	<0.001	72.9
		Case-control (8)	0.92 (0.77–1.11)	0.031	54.6
	Publication year	Before 2000 (7)	1.10 (0.77–1.59)	<0.001	75.7
		After 2000 (11)	1.15 (0.96–1.37)	<0.001	71.3
	Study quality	NOS≤5 (13)	1.29 (1.02–1.64)	<0.001	72.7
		NOS>5 (5)	0.95 (0.79–1.14)	0.024	64.3
	Region[a]	USA (9)	1.02 (0.86–1.22)	0.008	61.4
		Europe (8)	1.30 (0.93–1.79)	<0.001	80.9
Cohort	Publication year	Before 2000 (3)	1.48 (0.90–2.45)	0.047	67.3
		After 2000 (7)	1.25 (0.96–1.61)	0.002	72.0
	Study quality	NOS≤5 (9)	1.36 (1.02–1.81)	<0.001	75.9
		NOS>5 (1)	1.17 (0.94–1.45)	–	–
	Region	USA (4)	1.25 (0.89–1.77)	0.017	70.4
		Europe (6)	1.37 (0.95–1.97)	<0.001	77.7
	Mean follow-up[b]	<5 years (5)	1.63 (0.97–2.74)	<0.001	80.4
		≥5 years (4)	1.17 (0.82–1.66)	0.015	71.2
Case-control	Publication year	Before 2000 (4)	0.81 (0.65–1.02)	0.352	8.1
		After 2000 (4)	1.02 (0.77–1.36)	0.021	69.1
	Study quality	NOS≤5 (4)	1.14 (0.71–1.83)	0.060	59.5
		NOS>5 (4)	0.88 (0.71–1.10)	0.046	62.5
	Region[a]	USA (5)	0.91 (0.74–1.11)	0.116	45.9
		Europe (2)	1.28 (0.41–3.96)	0.033	77.9
	Control type	Population (6)	0.92 (0.78–1.10)	0.088	47.8
		Hospital (2)	1.22 (0.34–4.36)	0.023	80.6

Abbreviations: N, number; M, male; F, female; RR, relative risk; NOS, Newcastle-Ottawa Scale.
[a]One case-control study conducted in New Zealand was excluded from analysis.
[b]One study with unknown mean follow-up duration was excluded from analysis.
–: Cannot be calculated.

failed to provide sufficient data for calculation. Twenty-three case-control and cohort studies were included after full text assessment. Another two publications [24,25] were incorporated after examining references from the extracted articles. Among the 25 studies, seven [12,26–31] were subsequently excluded for overlap in case or cohort resources. Consequently, our meta-analysis consisted of eight [24,25,32–37] case-control and ten [10,38–46] cohort studies.

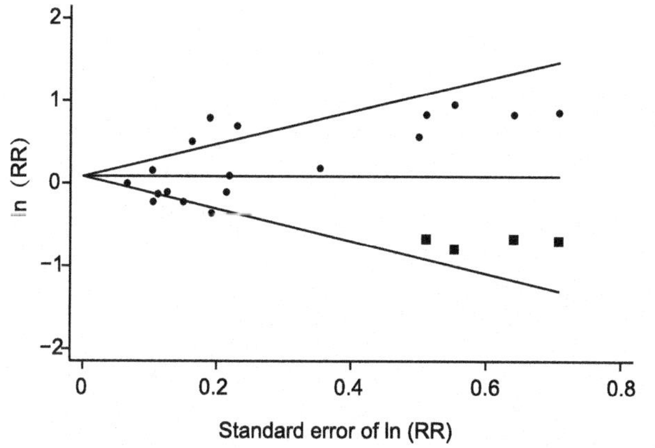

Figure 3. Funnel plot for case-control and cohort studies (dots: original data; squares: filled data).

All the studies published from 1982 to 2013 were performed in USA or Europe, except one case- control study from New Zealand [25]. There was slight overlap in the patient populations of two studies [38,40] from Finland. Landgren et al. [36] limited the study subjects to women, while the groups of Pearce [25] and Brown [45] mainly focused on the role of prior autoimmune disorders in male MM. The NOS scores varied from 5 to 7 in all case-control studies, with the exception of the reported score of 3 by Landgren and co-workers [36] as a result of unsatisfactory comparability. Since almost all the cohort studies used the expected cancer incidence calculated from national cancer rates as a comparison instead of the non-exposed cohort, NOS scores were relatively low, ranging from 4 to 5.

In the eight case-control studies, OR was all obtained from the published articles or calculated from the numbers of cases and controls by RA. In four cohort studies [10,38,43,44], the SIRs and 95% CIs were estimated from the number of observed MM and expected MM incidence provided by authors, while others were directly extracted from the original article. Only three studies [41,42,44] reported the type of treatment for RA before MM diagnosis. All important information is presented in Tables 1 and 2.

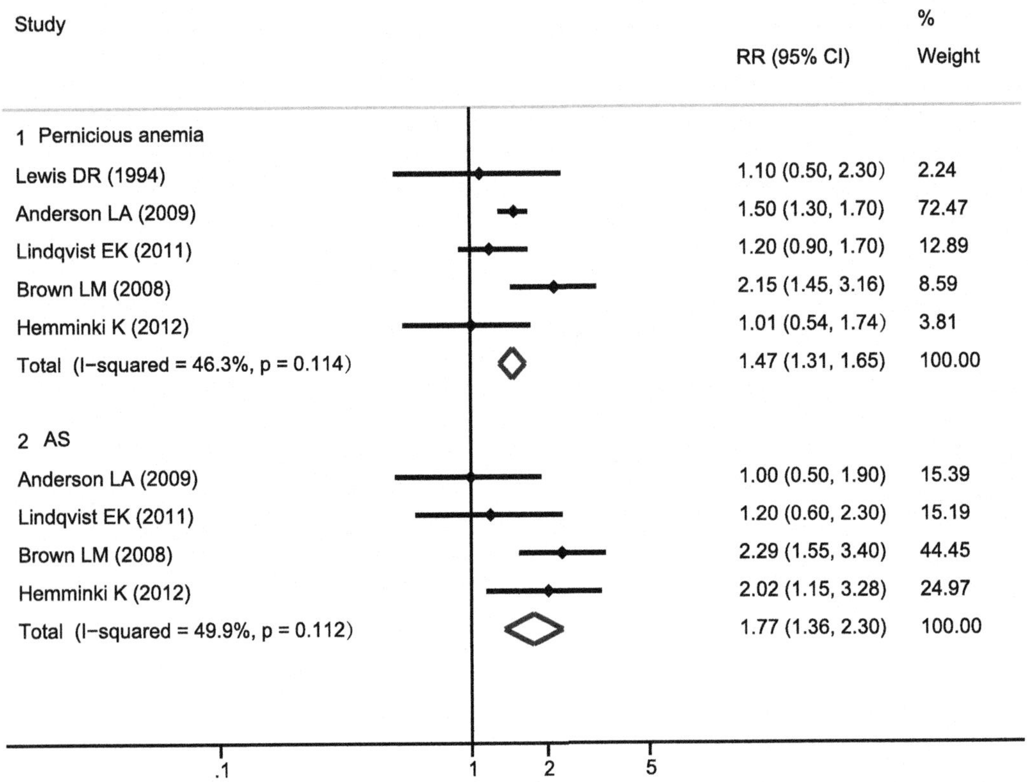

Figure 4. Forest plot of studies on multiple myeloma development risk in pernicious anemia and AS.

The RRs of MM for RA versus non-RA patients overall and by study design was presented (Figure 2). The random-effects pooled RRs for MM were 1.32 (95% CI, 1.04–1.67) for cohort studies and 0.92 (95% CI, 0.77–1.11) for case-control studies. Compared with non-RA patients, RA patients showed an RR of 1.14 (95% CI, 0.97–1.33) regardless of study type, possibly suggesting lack of association between RA and MM. However, overall analysis revealed significant between-study heterogeneity ($p<0.1$; $I^2 = 71.5\%$).

Sensitivity analysis was presented in Table 3. After excluding studies restricted to elderly patients (≥65 years) or single-sex participants and those that failed to adjust important factors, overall RR decreased slightly to 1.09, 1.11 and 1.11, respectively.

To investigate the source of heterogeneity, subset analysis by study design, publication year, study quality, geographic region, control type and average follow-up duration was conducted. Statistical association between RA and MM was only found to be significant in studies with relatively low quality (RR = 1.29, 95% CI, 1.02–1.64) and cohort studies with relatively low quality (RR = 1.36, 95% CI, 1.02–1.81). Overall, in studies with relatively higher quality according to NOS, as well as those published after 2000, RA was not associated with increase in MM risk (RR = 0.95, 95% CI, 0.79–1.14 and RR = 1.15, 95% CI 0.96–1.37, respectively). Notably, subgroup analyses failed to define the reason for heterogeneity (Table 4).

Publication bias in this meta-analysis was suspected as indicated from the funnel plot and Begg's test (p = 0.081). However, RR values remained similar after Trim and Fill correction for possible missing data (RR = 1.14, 95% CI 0.97–1.33 before Trim and Fill versus RR = 1.09, 95% CI 0.93–1.27 after Trim and Fill) (Figure 3).

The reported relevance of other autoimmune diseases, including pernicious anemia and ankylosing spondylitis (AS), in MM incidence is presented (Figure 4). Patients with pernicious anemia and AS displayed a 1.31- to 1.65-fold and 1.36- to 2.30-fold increase in MM risk, respectively. In contrast, MM development appeared to be unrelated to prior medical history of psoriasis (RR = 0.91, 95% CI, 0.78–1.05), SLE (RR = 1.18, 95% CI, 0.88–1.60), Sjögren syndrome (SS) (RR = 1.22, 95% CI 0.83–1.78) or polymyositis/dermatomyositis (RR = 1.37, 95% CI 0.86–2.17). The between-study heterogeneity analyses were all not statistically significant.

Discussion

Our meta-analysis results suggest that MM seems not more common in patients with a past history of RA, consistent with our sensitivity data. However, subgroup analysis revealed that RA patients are more likely to suffer from subsequent MM in cohort studies (RR = 1.32, 95% CI 1.04–1.67). Information on prior autoimmune diseases in case-control studies was mostly obtained from self-reports through interviews or questionnaires, while in cohort studies, investigators relied mainly on linkage records, which probably attributed to the differences between the two types of studies. Notably, subset analysis confirmed that statistical association between RA and MM was only significant in studies with NOS score≤5, further indicating that RA might not act as risk factor for MM.

A number of studies have explored whether repeated or chronic antigenic stimulation leads to hematopoietic malignancies. Some researchers [31] reported elevated risk for MM in patients with RA, while others [47,48] reached different conclusions. An antigenic stimulation hypothesis was proposed to explain the excessive risk of MM in patients with autoimmune diseases. Chronic immune stimulation resulting from autoimmune disorders, with its associated lymphocyte activation, tends to induce uncontrolled proliferation of malignant plasma cells, leading to MM [49]. Since no biologic marker has been developed that can effectively measure lifetime immune stimulation, this theory remains controversial. Meanwhile, evidence from previous studies indicates that increased risk could be a consequence of therapy, rather than the disease itself. For instance, higher risk of non-Hodgkin's lymphoma and MM has been reported following use of steroids [36,50], which are important for autoimmune disease treatment. Similarly, cytotoxic and immunosuppressive drugs may suppress immunodefense against malignant cells and lead to oncogenesis [51]. Moreover, there may be a common genetic or environmental susceptibility in autoimmune diseases and plasma cell tumors, or undiagnosed MM may manifest with clinical features that mimic connective tissue diseases. Taking our current results and the above studies into account, the credibility of the antigenic stimulation hypothesis is called into question.

Only one cohort study [39] investigated the effect of the duration of follow-up on the risk of MM and determined that the borderline excess of MM was confined to the early 4-year follow-up. Thomas [10] proposed that although increased risk of MM persisted for hematopoietic cancers throughout the follow-up period, the greatest excess was within the first 3 months after hospitalization. These findings could possibly indicate a common etiologic factor for RA and MM, or further prove the association confirmed in above two studies might be resulted from detection bias. With the current common application of anti-TNF drugs, concern has been raised about the risk of developing malignancy related with their use [52]. However, as implied from two studies mentioned earlier [41,44], there was no significant increase in the risk of MM among anti-TNF users. Considering the small number of reports available, further studies are warranted to account for this potential confounder when examining the relationship of autoimmune diseases and MM.

Meta-analysis results revealed that pernicious anemia is another risk factor for MM, consistent with several prior epidemiologic studies [53,54]. The related pathogenesis may involve immune alterations or chromosome abnormalities in the bone marrow of patients with pernicious anemia [54]. On the other hand, vitamin B12 deficiency caused by pernicious anemia may promote MM development by disrupting normal homeostasis for one-carbon metabolism [55]. The lack of association of MM with psoriasis, SLE, SS, and polymyositis/dermatomyositis raises the question of whether oncogenesis is dependent on the type of autoimmune disease. A number of studies evaluating the risk of MM in AS [45] and polymyalgia rheumatic [37] patients have reported positive associations, similar to our assessment of AS and MM. Assumptions such as whether an autoimmune disease resulting in MM is associated with disease activity, amount of autoantibody, and the extent of organ involvement should be examined. Although the current meta-analysis presents a more precise estimate of MM risk in RA patients than individual studies, significant heterogeneity remains a primary limitation of our study. Subgroup analyses failed to determine the source of heterogeneity. The diversity of subject sources and study methodologies may have led to inconsistencies. One such example is the study by Boffetta [33] including 282 patients that died from MM, meaning that they were likely to suffer from more severe diseases and past medical history obtained from their family members was possibly incomplete. Similarly, another study [41] was restricted to subjects older than 65 years whose disease spectrum may be distinct from that of the general population. The variable proportions of races in different studies may additionally contribute to significant heterogeneity. Moreover, misclassification of patients may have occurred in case-control studies, since no consistent diagnosis criteria were applied by investigators and most enrollments were dependent on reports and certificates, rather than specific laboratory data, similar to enrollment in cohort studies. As indicated in cohort studies, RA patients may develop MM after more than 20 years, in which case recall bias may exist in case-control studies.

Another limitation of this study is that certain articles had to be excluded, since no data on MM and RA were available, although their relationship was evaluated. Exclusion of such studies may have led to results bias. In spite of this, the possible bias might not be so evident, since why these data were not reported mostly lied in that authors found no specific association between RA and MM. Although publication bias was borderline significant as indicated by Begg's test, adjustment for possibly missing manuscripts yielded similar results, strongly supporting the robustness of our analyses.

Conclusion

Despite its limitations, our meta-analysis provides novel evidence for increased MM development risk in AS and pernicious anemia, although the underlying pathogenesis remains controversial. Notably, RA does not appear to alter the risk of MM, while between-study heterogeneity suggested caution in the interpretation of results. Further large-scale longitudinal studies containing details of risk factors and treatment information are necessary to determine the pathophysiological mechanism linking autoimmune diseases and MM. Moreover, identification of reliable exposure biomarkers of immune stimulation would be significantly beneficial.

Author Contributions

Conceived and designed the experiments: KNS GFX QW DBZ JL. Performed the experiments: KNS GFX QW JL. Analyzed the data: KNS GFX QW JL. Contributed reagents/materials/analysis tools: JL. Wrote the paper: KNS GFX QW.

References

1. Kyle RA, Therneau TM, Rajkumar SV, Larson DR, Plevak MF, et al. (2004) Incidence of multiple myeloma in Olmsted County, Minnesota - Trend over 6 decades. Cancer 101: 2667–2674.
2. Cuzick J (1981) Radiation-Induced Myelomatosis. New England Journal of Medicine 304: 204–210.
3. Infante PF (2006) Benzene exposure and multiple myeloma - A detailed meta-analysis of benzene cohort studies. Living In a Chemical World: Framing the Future In Light Of the Past 1076: 90–109.
4. Blair A, Zahm SH, Pearce NE, Heineman EF, Fraumeni JF (1992) Clues to Cancer Etiology from Studies of Farmers. Scandinavian Journal of Work Environment & Health 18: 209–215.

5. Lea AJ (1964) An association between the rheumatic diseases and the reticuloses. Ann Rheum Dis: 480–484.
6. Potter M (1986) Plasmacytomas in Mice. Seminars in Oncology 13: 275–281.
7. Radl J, Croese JW, Zurcher C, Van den Enden-Vieveen MH, de Leeuw AM (1988) Animal model of human disease. Multiple myeloma. Am J Pathol 132: 593–597.
8. Smedby KE, Vajdic CM, Falster M, Engels EA, Martinez-Maza O, et al. (2008) Autoimmune disorders and risk of non-Hodgkin lymphoma subtypes: a pooled analysis within the InterLymph consortium. Blood 111: 4029–4038.
9. Mellemkjaer L, Pfeiffer RM, Engels EA, Gridley G, Wheeler W, et al. (2008) Autoimmune disease in individuals and close family members and susceptibility to non-Hodgkin's lymphoma. Arthritis and Rheumatism 58: 657–666.
10. Thomas E, Brewster DH, Black RJ, Macfarlane GJ (2000) Risk of malignancy among patients with rheumatic conditions. International Journal of Cancer 88: 497–502.
11. Landgren O, Engels EA, Pfeiffer RM, Gridley G, Mellemkjaer L, et al. (2006) Autoimmunity and susceptibility to Hodgkin lymphoma: A population-based case-control study in Scandinavia. Journal of the National Cancer Institute 98: 1321–1330.
12. Gridley G, McLaughlin JK, Ekbom A, Klareskog L, Adami HO, et al. (1993) Incidence of Cancer among Patients with Rheumatoid-Arthritis. Journal of the National Cancer Institute 85: 307–311.
13. Wells G, Shea B, O'Connell D, Peterson J, Welch V, et al. (2011) The Newcastle-Ottawa Scale (NOS) for assessing the quality of nonrandomized studies in meta analyses. Ottawa, ON, Canada: Ottawa Hospital Research Institute. Available: http://www.ohri.ca/programs/clinical_epidemiology/oxford.asp. Accessed 28 December 2013.
14. Beranger R, Le Cornet C, Schuz J, Fervers B (2013) Occupational and Environmental Exposures Associated with Testicular Germ Cell Tumours: Systematic Review of Prenatal and Life-Long Exposures. Plos One 8.
15. Greenland S (1987) Quantitative Methods In the Review Of Epidemiologic Literature. Epidemiologic Reviews 9: 1–30.
16. Siristatidis C, Sergentanis TN, Kanavidis P, Trivella M, Sotiraki M, et al. (2013) Controlled ovarian hyperstimulation for IVF: impact on ovarian, endometrial and cervical cancer-a systematic review and meta-analysis. Human Reproduction Update 19: 105–123.
17. Larsson SC, Mantzoros CS, Wolk A (2007) Diabetes mellitus and risk of breast cancer: A meta-analysis. International Journal Of Cancer 121: 856–862.
18. Higgins JPT, Thompson SG, Deeks JJ, Altman DG (2003) Measuring inconsistency in meta-analyses. British Medical Journal 327: 557–560.
19. Doody MM, Linet MS, Glass AG, Friedman GD, Pottern LM, et al. (1992) Leukemia, lymphoma, and multiple myeloma following selected medical conditions. Cancer Causes Control 3: 449–456.
20. Bourguet CC, Logue EE (1993) Antigenic stimulation and multiple myeloma. A prospective study. Cancer 72: 2148–2154.
21. Prior P, Symmons DPM, Hawkins CF, Scott DL, Brown R (1984) Cancer Morbidity in Rheumatoid-Arthritis. Annals of the Rheumatic Diseases 43: 128–131.
22. Buchbinder R, Barber M, Heuzenroeder L, Wluka AE, Giles G, et al. (2008) Incidence of melanoma and other malignancies among rheumatoid arthritis patients treated with methotrexate. Arthritis & Rheumatism-Arthritis Care & Research 59: 794–799.
23. Chen YJ, Chang YT, Wang CB, Wu CY (2011) The Risk of Cancer in Patients With Rheumatoid Arthritis A Nationwide Cohort Study in Taiwan. Arthritis and Rheumatism 63: 352–358.
24. Anderson LA, Gadalla S, Morton LM, Landgren O, Pfeiffer R, et al. (2009) Population-based study of autoimmune conditions and the risk of specific lymphoid malignancies. International Journal of Cancer 125: 398–405.
25. Pearce NE, Smith AH, Howard JK, Sheppard RA, Giles HJ, et al. (1986) Case-Control Study of Multiple-Myeloma and Farming. British Journal of Cancer 54: 493–500.
26. Eriksson M (1993) Rheumatoid arthritis as a risk factor for multiple myeloma: a case-control study. Eur J Cancer 29A: 259–263.
27. Landgren O, Linet MS, McMaster ML, Gridley G, Hemminki K, et al. (2006) Familial characteristics of autoimmune and hematologic disorders in 8,406 multiple myeloma patients: A population-based case-control study. International Journal of Cancer 118: 3095–3098.
28. Askling J, Fored CM, Baecklund E, Brandt L, Backlin C, et al. (2005) Haematopoietic malignancies in rheumatoid arthritis: lymphoma risk and characteristics after exposure to tumour necrosis factor antagonists. Annals of the Rheumatic Diseases 64: 1414–1420.
29. Hemminki K, Li X, Sundquist K, Sundquist J (2008) Cancer risk in hospitalized rheumatoid arthritis patients. Rheumatology 47: 698–701.
30. Isomaki HA, Hakulinen T, Joutsenlahti U (1978) Excess risk of lymphomas, leukemia and myeloma in patients with rheumatoid arthritis. J Chronic Dis 31: 691–696.
31. Hakulinen T, Isomaki H, Knekt P (1985) Rheumatoid-Arthritis and Cancer Studies Based on Linking Nationwide Registries in Finland. American Journal of Medicine 78: 29–32.
32. Cohen HJ, Bernstein RJ, Grufferman S (1987) Role of Immune Stimulation in the Etiology of Multiple-Myeloma - a Case Control Study. American Journal of Hematology 24: 119–126.
33. Boffetta P, Stellman SD, Garfinkel L (1989) A Case-Control Study of Multiple-Myeloma Nested in the American-Cancer-Society Prospective-Study. International Journal of Cancer 43: 554–559.
34. Lewis DR, Pottern LM, Brown LM, Silverman DT, Hayes RB, et al. (1994) Multiple-Myeloma among Blacks and Whites in the United-States - the Role of Chronic Antigenic-Stimulation. Cancer Causes & Control 5: 529–539.
35. Vlajinac HD, Pekmezovic TD, Adanja BJ, Marinkovic JM, Kanazir MS, et al. (2003) Case-control study of multiple myeloma with special reference to diet as risk factor. Neoplasma 50: 79–83.
36. Landgren O, Zhang YW, Zahm SH, Inskip P, Zheng TZ, et al. (2006) Risk of multiple myeloma following medication use and medical conditions: A case-control study in Connecticut women. Cancer Epidemiology Biomarkers & Prevention 15: 2342–2347.
37. Lindqvist EK, Goldin LR, Landgren O, Blimark C, Mellqvist UH, et al. (2011) Personal and family history of immune-related conditions increase the risk of plasma cell disorders: a population-based study. Blood 118: 6284–6291.
38. Isomaki HA, Hakulinen T, Joutsenlahti U (1982) Excess risk of lymphomas, leukemia and myeloma in patients with rheumatoid arthritis. Annals of the Rheumatic Diseases 41: 34–36.
39. Mellemkjaer L, Linet MS, Gridley G, Frisch M, Moller H, et al. (1996) Rheumatoid arthritis and cancer risk. Eur J Cancer 32A: 1753–1757.
40. Kauppi M, Pukkala E, Isomaki H (1997) Elevated incidence of hematologic malignancies in patients with Sjogren's syndrome compared with patients with rheumatoid arthritis (Finland). Cancer Causes Control 8: 201–204.
41. Setoguchi S, Solomon DH, Weinblatt ME, Katz JN, Avorn J, et al. (2006) Tumor necrosis factor alpha antagonist use and cancer in patients with rheumatoid arthritis. Arthritis Rheum 54: 2757–2764.
42. Herrinton LJ, Liu L, Shoor S, Mines D (2008) Risk of lymphoproliferative cancer among patients with severe rheumatoid arthritis, 1996–2002. Ann Rheum Dis 67: 574–575.
43. Parikh-Patel A, White RH, Allen M, Cress R (2009) Risk of cancer among rheumatoid arthritis patients in California. Cancer Causes Control 20: 1001–1010.
44. Dreyer L, Mellemkjaer L, Andersen AR, Bennett P, Poulsen UE, et al. (2013) Incidences of overall and site specific cancers in TNF alpha inhibitor treated patients with rheumatoid arthritis and other arthritides - a follow-up study from the DANBIO Registry. Annals of the Rheumatic Diseases 72: 79–82.
45. Brown LM, Gridley G, Check D, Landgren O (2008) Risk of multiple myeloma and monoclonal gammopathy of undetermined significance among white and black male United States veterans with prior autoimmune, infectious, inflammatory, and allergic disorders. Blood 111: 3388–3394.
46. Hemminki K, Liu XD, Forsti A, Ji JG, Sundquist J, et al. (2012) Effect of autoimmune diseases on incidence and survival in subsequent multiple myeloma. Journal of Hematology & Oncology 5.
47. Gramenzi A, Buttino I, Davanzo B, Negri E, Franceschi S, et al. (1991) Medical History and the Risk of Multiple-Myeloma. British Journal of Cancer 63: 769–772.
48. Cuzick J, Destavola BL (1989) Autoimmune Disorders and Multiple-Myeloma. International Journal of Epidemiology 18: 283–283.
49. Symmons DPM (1988) Neoplasia in Rheumatoid-Arthritis. Journal of Rheumatology 15: 1319–1322.
50. Holly EA, Bracci PM (2003) Population-based study of non-Hodgkin lymphoma, histology, and medical history among human immunodeficiency virus-negative participants in San Francisco. American Journal of Epidemiology 158: 316–327.
51. Bachman TR, Sawitzke AD, Perkins SL, Ward JH, Cannon GW (1996) Methotrexate-associated lymphoma in patients with rheumatoid arthritis - Report of two cases. Arthritis and Rheumatism 39: 325–329.
52. Bongartz T, Sutton AJ, Sweeting MJ, Buchan I, Matteson EL, et al. (2006) Anti-TNF antibody therapy in rheumatoid arthritis and the risk of serious infections and malignancies: Systematic review and meta-analysis of rare harmful effects in randomized controlled trials (vol 295, pg 2275, 2006). Jama-Journal Of the American Medical Association 295: 2482–2482.
53. Hsing AW, Hansson LE, Mclaughlin JK, Nyren O, Blot WJ, et al. (1993) Pernicious-Anemia and Subsequent Cancer - a Population-Based Cohort Study. Cancer 71: 745–750.
54. Brinton LA, Gridley G, Hrubec Z, Hoover R, Fraumeni JF (1989) Cancer Risk Following Pernicious-Anemia. British Journal of Cancer 59: 810–813.
55. Friso S, Choi SW (2005) The potential cocarcinogenic effect of vitamin B12 deficiency. Clin Chem Lab Med 43: 1158–1163.

Retinol Binding Protein 4 Concentrations Relate to Enhanced Atherosclerosis in Obese Patients with Rheumatoid Arthritis

Patrick H. Dessein[1]*, Linda Tsang[2], Gavin R. Norton[1], Angela J. Woodiwiss[1], Ahmed Solomon[3]

1 Cardiovascular Pathophysiology and Genomics Research Unit, School of Physiology, Faculty of Health Sciences, University of the Witwatersrand, Johannesburg, South Africa, **2** Milpark Hospital, Johannesburg, South Africa, **3** Department of Rheumatology, Charlotte Maxeke Johannesburg Academic Hospital, Faculty of Health Sciences, University of the Witwatersrand, Johannesburg, South Africa

Abstract

Background: Retinol binding protein 4 (RBP) enhances metabolic risk and atherogenesis. Whether RBP4 contributes to cardiovascular risk in rheumatoid arthritis (RA) is unknown.

Methods: We assessed RBP4 concentrations and those of endothelial activation molecules including E-selectin, vascular cell adhesion molecule-1, intercellular adhesion molecule-1 and monocyte chemoattractant protein-1 by ELISA, and the common carotid artery intima-media thickness (cIMT) and carotid artery plaque by ultrasound in 217 (112 black and 105 white) patients with RA. Relationships were identified in potential confounder and mediator adjusted mixed regression models.

Results: RBP4 concentrations were associated with systolic and mean blood pressure, and those of glucose and E-selectin (partial $R = -0.207$ ($p = 0.003$), -0.195 ($p = 0.006$), -0.155 ($p = 0.03$) and -0.191 ($p = 0.007$), respectively in all patients); these RBP4-cardiovascular risk relations were mostly reproduced in patients with but not without adverse traditional or non-traditional cardiovascular risk profiles. RBP4 concentrations were not associated with atherosclerosis in all patients, but related independently to cIMT (partial $R = 0.297$, $p = 0.03$) and plaque (OR (95%CI) = 2.95 (1.31–6.68), $p = 0.008$) in those with generalized obesity, as well as with plaque in those with abdominal obesity (OR (95%CI) = 1.95 (1.12–3.42), $p = 0.01$).

Conclusion: In the present study, RBP4 concentrations were inversely associated with metabolic risk and endothelial activation in RA. This requires further investigation. RBP4 concentrations were related to enhanced atherosclerosis in patients with generalized or/and abdominal obesity.

Editor: Marià Alemany, University of Barcelona, Faculty of Biology, Spain

Funding: The study was supported by the South African Medical Research Council, grant number MRC2008_DES, and the National Research Foundation. The funders had no role in the study design, data collection and analysis, decision to publish, or preparation of the manauscript.

Competing Interests: The authors have declared that no competing interests exist.

* E-mail: Dessein@telkomsa.net

Introduction

Retinol binding protein 4 (RBP4) was characterized in 1968 for its transporting role of retinol from storage sites in the liver to extrahepatic tissues [1]. During the beginning of this century, RBP4 was discovered to be an adipokine in that it is produced by adipocytes, induces gluconeogenesis by stimulating phosphoenolpyruvate carboxykinase in the liver and impairs peripheral and hepatic insulin sensitivity [2–5]. Several RBP4 gene variants are associated with adiposity, the predisposition to visceral accumulation of adipose tissue, insulin secretion or/and insulin resistance and type 2 diabetes [5,6]. Visceral obesity [7] and liver fat content [8] is associated with high circulating RBP4 concentrations, which relate to metabolic risk factors [3,5].

A recent cellular study showed that RBP4 consistently stimulates the expression of inflammatory molecules in human retinal capillary and umbilical vein endothelial cells [9]. High RBP4 concentrations are associated with increased atherosclerosis [10] and incident coronary event rates [11].

Several adipokines other than RBP4 and including adiponectin [12], leptin [13] and resistin [14] can participate importantly in the pathophysiology of rheumatoid arthritis (RA), a prototypic inflammatory disease. In this regard, RBP4 concentrations are also associated with those of inflammatory markers, and successful lifestyle intervention in obese subjects results in reduced RBP4 concentrations that are closely related not only to decreased insulin resistance, triacylglycerol levels and blood pressure but also reduced systemic inflammation [15]. A recent investigation revealed that treatment with tumor necrosis factor-α blockade reduces RBP4 concentrations in ankylosing spondylitis, another inflammatory disorder [16].

Patients with RA sustain a markedly enhanced risk of cardiovascular disease (CVD) that is effectuated by adverse conventional cardiovascular risk factors, high-grade inflammation and genetic determinants [17–20]. Nevertheless, atherogenesis in

RA remains inadequately elucidated and current recommendations on CVD risk stratification reportedly have important limitations [18,21,22]. It is in this context that the need for identifying novel biomarkers of enhanced cardiovascular risk in RA has been raised [18,21].

The presence of rheumatic disease can impact on the production as well as the relationships of adipokines with cardiometabolic risk and atherogenesis [23–25]. Lupus alters the effects of leptin on lipid metabolism and atherogenesis [23]. Whereas adiponectin is well recognized for its protective effects against cardiovascular risk in the population at large, adiponectin concentrations associate independently and paradoxically with high blood pressure in black Africans with but not without RA [24,25]. A paradoxically positive adiponectin-endothelial activation relationship was also documented in white patients with RA [25]. The potential role of RBP4 in atherogenesis and CVD risk stratification in RA has, to our knowledge, not been investigated.

In the present study, we measured RBP4 concentrations, surrogate markers of enhanced early atherogenesis comprising E-selectin, vascular cell adhesion molecule-1 (VCAM-1), intercellular adhesion molecule-1 (ICAM-1) and monocyte chemoattractant protein-1 (MCP-1), and common carotid artery intima-media thickness and carotid artery plaque by ultrasound in both black and white patients with RA. We examined the independent relationships of RBP4 concentrations with cardiometabolic risk, endothelial activation and carotid atherosclerosis.

Materials and Methods

Patients

The present study was conducted according to the principles outlined in the Helsinki declaration. The Human Research Ethics Committee (Medical) from the University of the Witwatersrand in Johannesburg, South Africa approved the protocol (approval number: M06-07-33). Participants gave informed, written consent. This investigation forms part of an ongoing study on cardiovascular risk in RA as previously reported [26–28]. Two hundred and seventeen consecutive African patients (112 black and 105 white) that met the 1988 American College of Rheumatology and 2010 American College of Rheumatology/European League Against Rheumatism criteria for RA [29,30] were enrolled. All invited participants agreed to participate. Each patient used disease modifying agents for rheumatic disease (DMARD) at the time of the study. The mean (SD) number of DMARD employed was 2.4 (0.9) and these included methotrexate, chloroquine, leflunomide, sulphasalazine, azathioprine, tetracycline, cyclophosphamide, penicillamine, tumor necrosis factor-α inhibitors and rituximab in 84.8, 66.8, 29.5, 20.3, 14.8, 10.6, 3.7, 2.8, 3.7 and 1.2% of patients respectively. Prednisone was used by only 2.3% of participants. Data were missing in fewer than 5% of any of the recorded characteristics.

Assessments

We recorded demographic features and lifestyle factors. Height, weight and waist and hip circumference were measured using standard approaches. The body mass index (BMI) was calculated and abdominal obesity and fat distribution were estimated by waist circumference and waist-height ratio, and waist-hip ratio respectively. For the purpose of this study, generalized and abdominal obesity were diagnosed in patients with a BMI of >29.9 kg/m2 and National Cholesterol Education Program metabolic syndrome waist circumference criterion [31], respectively. We recorded disease duration and rheumatoid factor status. Disease activity was assessed by the Clinical Disease Activity Index (CDAI) [32]. Extra-articular manifestations included the current or previously recorded (hospital record review) presence of pericarditis, pleuritis, Felty's syndrome, cutaneous vasculitis, neuropathy, scleritis or episcleritis, retinal vasculitis, glomerulonephritis, vasculitis affecting other organs, amyloidosis, keratoconjunctivitis sicca, xerostomia, Sjogren's syndrome, pulmonary fibrosis, bronchiolitis obliterans organizing pneumonia, cervical myelopathy, subcutaneous nodules and rheumatoid nodules in other locations [33]. C-reactive protein concentrations were determined using immunoturbidimetric methods. Standard laboratory blood tests of erythrocyte sedimentation rate, renal and liver function, hematological parameters, lipids and glucose were performed. The glomerular filtration rate was estimated using the Modification of Diet in Renal Disease equation [34]. Cardiovascular drugs included antihypertensive agents and glucose and lipid lowering drugs.

Recorded metabolic risk factors included systolic, diastolic and mean blood pressure, lipid concentrations and ratios, and glucose levels. Hypertension was defined as an average systolic blood pressure ≥140 or/and diastolic blood pressure ≥90 mmHg or/and current use of antihypertensive medications. Dyslipidemia was diagnosed when the atherogenic index, i.e. the cholesterol-HDL cholesterol ratio was >4 and proatherogenic non-HDL cholesterol concentrations were calculated by subtracting HDL cholesterol from total cholesterol concentrations [35,36]. Diabetes was identified as the use of glucose lowering agents or a fasting plasma glucose ≥7 mmol/l, and raised fasting glucose when the respective concentrations was ≥5.6 mmol/l [31]. As reported previously, we also measured interleukin-6 (IL-6) concentrations [37] and those of 3 other adipokines including adiponectin that comprises different isoforms [25], resistin [26] and leptin [27].

We measured endothelial activation molecule concentrations including those of soluble E-selectin, VCAM-1, ICAM-1 and MCP-1 using a solid-phase sHS, R & D Systems, Inc., Minneapolis, MN, USA). Their lower detection limits were 0.009 ng/l, 0.6 ng/l, 0.096 ng/l and 5.0 pg/ml respectively; their inter- and intra-assay coefficients of variation were 7.9 and 5.8, 7.0 and 3.1, 5.5 and 4.6 and 5.7 and 5.8 respectively.

BAS (see acknowledgement) and AS performed the carotid artery ultrasound measurements in private and public healthcare patients, respectively. Both operators obtained images of at least 1 cm length of the distal common carotid arteries for measurement of the intima-media thickness of the far wall from an optimal angle of incidence defined as the longitudinal angle of approach where both branches of the internal and external carotid artery are visualized simultaneously [38] and with high resolution B-mode ultrasound (Image Point, Hewlett Packard, Andover, MA, USA and SonoCalc IMT, Sonosite Inc, Bothell, Wash, USA used by BAS and AS, respectively) employing linear array 7.5 MHz probes. The details of the methodology used by BAS were reported previously [39]. The equipment used by AS involves the application of a unique semi-automated border detection program that was previously found to provide highly reproducible results [38]. The intima-media thicknesses in the left and right common carotid artery were measured and the cIMT was defined as the mean of these. Carotid artery plaque was defined as a focal structure that encroaches into the arterial lumen of at least 0.5 mm or 50% of the surrounding intima-media thickness value, or demonstrates a thickness of >1.5 mm as measured from the media-adventitia interface to the intima-lumen interface [40]. Both operators were blinded to the cardiovascular risk profiles of the patients. Repeat ultrasound examinations by both operators on 23 patients revealed Spearman correlations between repeat cIMT measurements of 0.983 and 0.956 for BAS and AS, respectively, and the correlation between measurements made by BAS and AS was 0.926. Both operators identified carotid artery bulb or/and internal carotid artery plaque in 11 of these 23 patients with full agreement.

RBP4 concentrations were measured in serum using a solid-phase sandwich ELISA (Quantikine HS, R&D Systems, Inc., Minneapolis, MN, USA). The lower detection limit was 0.048 mM/l and the inter- and intra-assay coefficients of variation were 7.2 and 6.9% respectively.

Data analysis

Dichotomous variables are expressed as proportions and continuous variables as mean (SD) or median (interquartile range) when non-normally distributed. Non-normally distributed characteristics were also logarithmically transformed prior to their inclusion in multivariable statistical analysis.

Associations of age at disease onset or at the time of the study and sex and population grouping with RBP4 concentrations were assessed by entering the respective characteristics together in single mixed regression models. Associations of other baseline characteristics with RBP4 concentrations were evaluated in models with adjustment for demographic characteristics that included age at the time of the study and not age at disease onset since the latter was less strongly related to RBP4 concentrations.

The independent relations of RBP4 concentrations with metabolic risk factors were assessed in demographic characteristic, alcohol use, glomerular filtration rate (potential confounders or/ and determinants identified in previous analysis) and cardiovascular drug use adjusted mixed linear regression models; waist-hip ratio was additionally forced into these models. The independent relations of RBP4 concentrations with endothelial activation and cIMT and plaque were determined in Framingham score (calculated from age, sex and major conventional risk factors), race, alcohol use, waist-hip ratio glomerular filtration rate, and systemic inflammation (C-reactive protein and interleukin-6 concentrations) adjusted mixed (linear or logistic as appropriate) regression models.

Patients with RA that experience conventional major risk factors or severe disease are reportedly at high risk of cardiovascular disease. Inflammation also directly increases cardiovascular risk and contributes to the atherogenic effects of conventional cardiovascular risk factors. Additionally, age is an established independent risk factor for RA as well as cardiovascular disease, and obesity contributes significantly to an increased 10-year cardiovascular disease event probability in RA patients [41]. Obesity also influences RBP4 production in non-RA subjects. For these reasons together with our recent experience with adipokine metabolism in RA [42], additional sensitivity analysis was performed with re-evaluation of the respective associations in various subgroups. When appropriate, patients were categorized in subgroups based on median values; accordingly, as only 27 patients had diabetes. In view of the small number of patients that were male or rheumatoid factor positive or had extra-articular features, sensitivity analysis in subgroups based on the presence or absence of these characteristics was not performed. Also, with regard to acute phase responses, as the erythrocyte sedimentation rate is more closely associated to cardiovascular disease than C-reactive protein concentrations in RA, patients were stratified based on their erythrocyte sedimentation rate.

Statistical computations were made using the GB Stat program (Dynamic Microsystems, Inc, Silverspring, Maryland, USA) and SAS software, version 9.1 (The SAS Institute, Cary, NC). Significance was set at $p<0.05$.

Results

Patient Characteristics

The demographic features, lifestyle factors, anthropometric measures, RA characteristics, systemic inflammatory markers including C-reactive protein and interleukin-6 concentrations and leukocyte counts, glomerular filtration rate and use of antirheumatic and cardiovascular agents in the present cohort were previously reported. The median (interquartile range) erythrocyte sedimentation rate, and alanine transferase and aspartate transferase concentrations were 13 (5–28) mm/hr, and 22 (17–28) and 25 (20–30) u/l, respectively. Conventional metabolic risk factors, adipokine and endothelial activation molecule concentrations, and cIMT and plaque prevalence are shown in Table 1. Generalized and abdominal obesity were present in 58.7 and 34.3, and 43.9 and 16.3 and % of black and white patients, respectively. Only 7 patients had previously diagnosed established cardiovascular disease that included cerebrovascular disease, myocardial infarction and peripheral arterial disease in 5, 1 and 1 of the cases, respectively.

Associations between Baseline Characteristics and RBP4 Concentrations

As given in Table 2, age at the time of the study as well as age at RA onset and alcohol use were associated with high, and black ethnicity and the glomerular filtration rate with low RBP4 concentrations. In univariate analysis, the mean (SD) RBP4 concentrations were 1.47 (0.88) and 2.13 (0.92) mM/l in black and white patients with RA ($p<0.0001$).

Independent associations of RBP4 concentrations with metabolic risk

Table 3 shows that RBP4 concentrations were independently and inversely associated with systolic and mean blood pressure, and glucose concentrations. RBP4 concentrations were not related to lipid values, levels of other adipokines and the leptin-adiponectin ratio.

Table 4 gives findings in sensitivity analysis. RBP4 concentrations were associated with systolic and mean blood pressure in hypertensive but not in normotensive patients with RA. In patients with raised fasting glucose [31], the RBP4-glucose relation was numerically stronger than in the whole group (partial $R=-0.184$ versus -0.155 (see Table 3), but this was not nevertheless significant, possibly because of the small number of patients in this group ($n=34$). RBP4 concentrations were not associated with those of glucose in patients with normal fasting glucose levels.

Independent relationships of RBP4 concentrations with endothelial activation and carotid atherosclerosis

As shown in Table 5, RBP4 concentrations were independently and inversely related to those of E-selectin; the positive relation between RBP4 and MCP-1 did not reach significance ($p=0.06$). RBP4 concentrations were not associated with cIMT and plaque.

Table 6 gives the results obtained in sensitivity analysis. The inverse RBP4 - E-selectin relation was reproduced in patients aged ≤55 but not > 55 years, and in those with but not without ≥2 major traditional cardiovascular risk factors, a Framingham score of ≥2, overall and abdominal obesity, an RA duration of >10 years, absent or mild disease activity, an erythrocyte sedimentation rate of >12 mm/hr and black ethnicity; RBP4 concentrations were not significantly associated with those of E-selectin in patients with and without carotid artery plaque. The extent of effect of RBP4 concentrations on those of E-selectin was larger in those

Table 1. Conventional metabolic risk factors, adipokines, endothelial activation and carotid atherosclerosis in activation and carotid atherosclerosis in 217 RA patients.

Conventional metabolic risk factors	
Hypertension (%)	62.2
Total cholesterol-HDL cholesterol ratio>4	18.4
Diabetes (%)	12.4
Blood pressure values	
Systolic blood pressure (mmHg)	135 (22)
Diastolic blood pressure (mmHg)	83 (13)
Mean blood pressure (mmHg)	118 (18)
Lipid values	
Total cholesterol (mM)	4.8 (1.0)
HDL cholesterol (mM)	1.54 (1.30–1.89)
Total cholesterol-HDL cholesterol ratio	3.2 (1.0)
LDL cholesterol (mM)	2.7 (0.8)
Non HDL cholesterol (mM)	3.1 (2.6–3.8)
Triacylglycerols (mM)	1.0 (0.8–1.4)
Triacylglycerol-HDL cholesterol ratio	0.7 (0.5–1.0)
Glucose (mM)	4.8 (4.5–5.2)
Adipokines	
Leptin (pM)	638 (342–1159)
Adiponectin (μg/ml)	7.36 (4.82–12.19)
Leptin-adiponectin ratio	86.7 (70.9–95.1)
Resistin (nM)	2.71 (1.82–4.25)
Retinol binding protein 4 (μM)	1.78 (0.09)
Endothelial activation	
E-selectin (ng/ml)	39.0 (18.6)
VCAM (ng/ml)	833 (668–1041)
ICAM-1 (ng/ml)	274 (211–352)
MCP-1 (pg/ml)	424 (265–679)
Carotid atherosclerosis	
cIMT (mm)	0.709 (0.109)
Plaque (%)	40.6

Mean (standard deviation (SD)), median and interquartile range or proportions are shown. HDL = high density lipoprotein, LDL = low density lipoprotein, VCAM = vascular cell adhesion molecule, ICAM = intercellular adhesion molecule, MCP = monocyte chemoattractant protein, cIMT = common carotid artery intima-media thickness.

with compared to those without ≥2 major cardiovascular risk factors (standardized β (SE) = −0.534 (0.174) versus −0.151 (0.081), p = 0.04).

As also shown in Table 6, RBP4 concentrations were associated with cIMT and plaque in patients with but not without overall obesity, and with plaque in those with but not without abdominal obesity. Further, RBP4 concentrations were independently related to plaque in black but not white patients with RA.

When RA characteristics were additionally adjusted for in the models in Tables 5 and 6, the results were materially unaltered (data not shown).

The mean (SD) RBP4 concentrations were numerically but not significantly higher in those with and without established cardiovascular disease (2.39 (1.28) versus 1.77 (0.94) uM/l, p = 0.1). In view of the small number of patients with the respective outcome characteristic, multivariable analysis was not performed.

Table 2. Associations of baseline characteristics with retinol binding protein 4 concentrations.

Characteristics	Partial R	p
Age at disease onset	**0.157**	**0.02**
Age at study time	0.169	0.01
Female	0.025	0.7
Race (white = 1; black = 2)	**−0.330**	**<0.0001**
Smoking current	0.109	0.1
Exercise	−0.079	0.3
Alcohol use	**0.160**	**0.02**
Body mass index	0.027	0.7
Waist circumference	−0.013	0.9
Waist-hip ratio*	0.061	0.4
RA duration	−0.050	0.5
Rheumatoid factor positive	−0.032	0.6
CDAI*	0.066	0.3
Deformed joints*	−0.076	0.3
Prednisone use	0.072	0.3
Erythrocyte sedimentation rate*	−0.066	0.4
C-reactive protein*	0.082	0.2
Interleukin-6*	0.067	0.3
Leukocytes*	0.001	1.0
Alanine aminotransferase*	0.043	0.5
Aspartate aminotransferase*	0.011	0.9
Glomerular filtration rate*	**−0.134**	**0.05**

Data were analyzed in mixed regression models in which sex and race, age at study time and race, age at study time and sex, and all 3 demographic characteristics were adjusted for in the 1st and 2nd, 3rd, 4th and the remaining models, respectively. Significant associations are shown in bold type. RA = rheumatoid arthritis, CDAI = Clinical Disease Activity Score.
*Logarithmically transformed variables.

Discussion

In this RA study, adiposity was not associated with RBP4 concentrations. However, obesity adversely influenced the impact of this adipokine on atherosclerosis. Indeed, RBP4 concentrations were independently related to increased carotid atherosclerosis only in patients with overall and abdominal obesity. Further, although RBP4 concentrations were lower in black compared to white patients, they were associated with atherosclerosis in the former but not the latter. This was possibly due to the far larger prevalence of excess adiposity in black compared to white patients. Consideration of RBP4 concentrations may improve cardiovascular risk stratification in RA [18].

Paradoxical adipokine - CVD risk associations as we found between RBP4 concentrations and metabolic risk and endothelial activation, were previously reported [25,43]. Such relations are thought to represent a compensatory change in adipokine production in the presence of chronic vascular disease and aimed at reducing metabolic risk [43]. However, we found that the presence of plaque did not influence the impact of RBP4 concentrations on cardiovascular risk. By contrast, the inverse RBP4 - CVD risk associations were mostly reproduced only in

Table 3. Independent relationships of retinol binding protein 4 concentrations with metabolic risk factors.

Characteristics	Partial R	p
Conventional metabolic risk factors		
Blood pressure value		
Systolic blood pressure	**−0.207**	**0.003**
Diastolic blood pressure	−0.102	0.2
Mean blood pressure	**−0.195**	**0.006**
Lipid values		
Total cholesterol	0.090	0.2
HDL cholesterol*	−0.002	1.0
Total cholesterol-HDL cholesterol ratio	0.060	0.2
LDL cholesterol	0.089	0.2
Non HDL cholesterol	0.099	0.2
Triacylglycerols*	−0.031	0.7
Triacylglycerols-HDL cholesterol ratio*	−0.022	0.8
Glucose*	**−0.155**	**0.03**
Adipokines		
Leptin*	0.052	0.5
Adiponectin*	−0.044	0.6
Leptin-adiponectin ratio*	0.043	0.6
Resistin	0.024	0.7

Data were analyzed in mixed regression models in which demographic characteristics, alcohol use, the waist-hip ratio, the glomerular filtration rate and cardiovascular drugs were adjusted for. Significant associations are shown in bold type. HDL = high-density lipoprotein, LDL = low-density lipoprotein, VCAM = vascular adhesion molecule, ICAM = intercellular adhesion molecule, MCP = monocyte chemoattractant protein. *Logarithmically transformed variables.

patients with adverse traditional or nontraditional cardiovascular risk profiles. Our cross-sectional study design precludes drawing inferences on the direction of causality. Additionally, our findings on the associations of RBP4 concentrations with metabolic risk factors and endothelial activation differ and in fact contrast to those previously reported in non-RA subjects [5,9]. Therefore, these relations need further study.

Table 5. Independent relationships of retinol binding protein 4 concentrations with endothelial activation and atherosclerosis.

Characteristics	Partial R	p
Endothelial activation molecules		
E-selectin	**−0.191**	**0.007**
VCAM-1*	0.012	0.9
ICAM-1*	−0.039	0.6
MCP-1*	0.135	0.06
Carotid atherosclerosis		
Intima-media thickness	−0.000	1.0
	OR (95% CI)	**p**
Plaque	1.18 (0.86–1.61)	0.3

Retinol binding protein 4-endothelial activation and retinol binding protein 4-atherosclerosis relations were assessed in mixed regression models with adjustment for the log Framingham score (calculated from age, sex and major conventional risk factors), race, alcohol use, waist-hip ratio, glomerular filtration rate, and systemic inflammation (C-reactive protein and interleukin-6 concentrations). Significant association is shown in bold type.
VCAM = vascular cell adhesion molecule, ICAM = intercellular adhesion molecule, OR = odds ratio, CI = confidence interval.
*Characteristics that were non-normally distributed and were logarithmically transformed prior to entering them in linear regression models.

RBP4 induces insulin resistance [44]. We did not directly assess this metabolic risk factor. RBP4 concentrations were nonetheless not associated with the triacylglycerols-HDL cholesterol and leptin-adiponectin ratios, which are surrogate markers of insulin resistance [45,46]. Future studies on the potential impact of RBP4 on metabolic risk in RA should include markers of insulin resistance such as the homeostasis model assessment of insulin resistance.

Our finding of lower RBP4 concentrations in black compared to white patients with RA is congruent with an earlier investigation

Table 4. Independent relationships of retinol binding protein 4 concentrations with systolic and mean blood pressure, and glucose levels amongst subgroups.

Relationship	Subgroups	Partial R	p
Retinol binding protein 4 versus			
Systolic blood pressure			
	Hypertensives (n = 135)	**−0.213**	**0.02**
	Normotensives (n = 82)	−0.028	0.8
Mean blood pressure			
	Hypertensives (n = 135)	**−0.209**	**0.02**
	Normotensives (n = 82)	0.011	0.9
Glucose*			
	Glucose ≥5.6 mmol/l (n = 31)	−0.184	0.4
	Glucose <5.6 mmol/l (n = 181)	−0.026	0.8
	Missing data (n = 5)		

Data were analyzed in adjusted mixed regression models as in Table 3. Significant differences amongst relations are shown in bold type. *Logarithmically transformed variable.

Table 6. Independent relationships of retinol binding protein 4 concentrations with those of E-selectin and atherosclerosis amongst subgroups.

	E-selectin		cIMT		Plaque	
Subgroups	**Partial R**	**p**	**Partial R**	**p**	**OR (95% CI)**	**p**
Age >55						
Yes (n = 127)	−0.140	0.1	−0.067	0.5	0.89 (0.61–1.29)	0.5
No (n = 90)	**−0.246**	**0.03**	−0.016	0.9	0.89 (0.45–1.75)	0.7
≥2 major traditional CV risk factor						
Yes (n = 58)	**−0.440**	**0.004**	0.125	0.4	1.55 (0.66–3.65)	0.3
No (n = 151)	−0.154	0.07	−0.030	0.7	1.09 (0.75–1.57)	0.7
Missing data (n = 8)						
Framingham score >2						
Yes (n = 121)	**−0.258**	**0.006**	−0.036	0.7	1.07 (0.71–1.60)	0.7
No (n = 88)	−0.115	0.3	−0.154	0.2	0.89 (0.49–1.59)	0.7
Missing data (n = 8)						
Carotid artery plaque						
Yes (n = 88)	−0.178	0.1	0.108	0.4	....	....
No (n = 129)	−0.181	0.054	−0.060	0.5	....	....
Obesity						
Yes (n = 107)	**−0.282**	**0.04**	**0.297**	**0.03**	**2.95 (1.31–6.68)**	**0.008**
No (n = 104)	−0.108	0.2	−0.113	0.2	0.71 (0.48–1.05)	0.08
Missing (n = 6)						
MetS waist						
Present (n = 100)	**−0.231**	**0.03**	0.016	0.9	**1.95 (1.12–3.42)**	**0.01**
Absent (n = 114)	−0.181	0.07	−0.048	0.6	0.65 (0.42–1.01)	0.06
Missing data (n = 3)						
RA duration >10 years						
Yes (n = 116)	**−0.236**	**0.01**	−0.015	0.9	1.09 (0.72–1.66)	0.7
No (n = 100)	−0.133	0.3	0.063	0.6	1.04 (0.60–1.83)	0.9
Missing data (n = 1)						
CDAI >10						
Yes (n = 92)	**−0.247**	**0.02**	0.093	0.4	1.01 (0.64–1.62)	0.9
No (n = 125)	−0.158	0.1	0.008	0.9	1.05 (0.69–1.60)	0.8
Erythrocyte sedimentation rate >12 mm/hr						
Yes (n = 112)	**−0.220**	**0.03**	−0.045	0.7	1.32 (0.86–2.03)	0.2
No (n = 99)	−0.170	0.1	0.002	1.0	0.78 (0.44–1.41)	0.4
Missing data (n = 6)						
Population						
Black (n = 112)	**−0.228**	**0.02**	0.149	0.1	**1.74 (1.06–2.86)**	**0.02**
White (n = 105)	−0.170	0.09	−0.145	0.2	0.85 (0.52–1.40)	0.5

Data were analyzed in adjusted mixed regression models as in Table 5. Significant association is shown in bold type. cIMT = carotid intima-media thickness, OR = odds ratio, CI = confidence intervals, CV = cardiovascular, MetS = metabolic syndrome, RA = rheumatoid arthritis, CDAI = Clinical Disease Activity Score.

that showed disparities in RBP4 gene polymorphisms amongst black and white Americans [6]. Although increased liver fat content [8] is associated with increased RBP4 concentrations, we are unaware of a reported relation of alcohol consumption with levels of this adipokine, as shown by us in RA. Importantly also in this context, none of the reported independent associations between RBP4 concentrations and other recorded characteristics in the present study were altered upon further adjustment for alanine and aspartate aminotransferase concentrations (data not shown). Aminotransferase levels were previously shown to independently relate to metabolic risk and atherosclerosis in RA [47].

We assessed the production of 4 endothelial activation molecules that mediate the initial stages of atherosclerosis. Endothelial activation is strongly up-regulated and associated with prevalent and incident atherosclerosis in RA [48,49]. We comprehensively adjusted for a wide range of confounders including the anthropometric measure of waist-hip circumference that is associated with RBP4 concentrations and cardiovascular events in non-RA subjects. Anthropometric measures are also related to atherosclerosis in RA [35]. This study has however additional limitations. Retinol and iron status are further potential confounders in the present context and were not evaluated [5]. Micronutrient deficiencies exist in urbanized South Africans from which our participants originated [50]. In a recent national survey on 3229 adult South Africans (79% black), retinol intake was documented to be adequate and iron intake inadequate [50]. Also, the effects of RBP4 on endothelial activation occur independently of retinol [9]. As was done in the original study by Graham and colleagues [3] as well as in many other reported investigations that followed, RBP4 concentrations were measured by ELISA, which can undervalue RBP4 concentrations in insulin resistant persons [5,51]. Quantitative western blotting standardized to full-length RBP4 protein is suggested to be the most reliable method to measure RBP4 levels [5,51]. Nevertheless, in an investigation by von Eynatten and colleagues [52], RBP4 concentrations quantified by ELISA were strongly associated with those measured by western blotting (R = 0.70 to 0.92). Finally, circulating RBP4 concentrations do not necessarily represent its tissue concentrations [5].

Conclusion

The present study reveals that RBP4 concentrations are inversely related to metabolic risk and endothelial activation in RA. These findings require further elucidation. RBP4 concentrations were independently associated with enhanced atherosclerosis in RA patients with generalized or/and abdominal obesity.

Author Contributions

Conceived and designed the experiments: PHD LT AS. Performed the experiments: PHD AS. Analyzed the data: PHD LT AJW GRN. Contributed reagents/materials/analysis tools: PHD LT GRN AJW AS. Wrote the paper: PHD LT. Revised the paper critically for important intellectual content: PHD LT GRN AJW AS. Gave final approval of the version to be published: PHD LT GRN AJW AS.

References

1. Kanai M Raz A, Goodman DS (1968) Retinol-binding protein: the transport protein for vitamin A in human plasma. J Clin Invest 47: 2025–2044.
2. Abel ED, Peroni O, Kim JK, Kim YB, Boss O, et al. (2001) Adipose-selective targeting of the *GLUT4* gene impairs insulin action in muscle and liver. Nature 409: 729–733.
3. Graham TE, Yang Q, Bluher M, Hammarstedt A, Ciaraldi TP, et al. (2006) Retinol-binding protein 4 and insulin resistance in lean, obese, and diabetic subject. N Engl J Med 354: 2552–2263.
4. Yang Q, Graham TE, Mody N, Preitner F, Peroni OD, et al. (2005) Serum retinol binding protein 4 contributes to insulin resistance in obesity and type 2 diabetes. Nature 436: 356–362.
5. Kotnik P, Fischer-Posovszky P, Wabitsch (2011) RPB4: a controversial adipokine. Eur J Endocrinol 165: 703–711.
6. Craig RL, Chu WS, Elbein SC (2007) Retinol binding protein 4 as a candidate gene for type 2 diabetes and prediabetic intermediate trails. Mole Genet Metab 90: 338–344.
7. Kloting N, Graham TE, Berndt J, Kralisch S, Kovacs P, et al. (2007) Serum retinol-binding protein is more highly expressed in visceral than in subcutaneous adipose tissue and is a marker of intra-abdominal fat mass. Cell Metab 6: 79–87.
8. Stefan N, Hennige AM, Staiger H, Machann J, Schick F, et al. (2007) High circulating retinol-binding protein 4 is associated with elevated liver fat but not with total, subcutaneous, visceral, or intramyocellular fat in humans. Diabetes Care 30: 1173–1178.
9. Farjo KM, Farjo RA, Halsey S, Moiseyev G, Ma J-x (2012) Retinol-binding protein 4 induces inflammation in human endothelial cells by an NADPH oxidase- and nuclear factor kappa B-dependent and retinol-independent mechanism. Cole Cell Biol 32: 5103–5115.
10. Bobbert T, Raila J, Schwarz F, Mai K, Henze A, et al. (2010) Relation between retinol, retinol-binding protein 4, transthyretin and carotid intima media thickness. Atherosclerosis 213: 549–551.
11. Mallat Z, Simon T, Benessiano J, Clement K, Taleb S, et al. (2009) Retinol-binding protein 4 and prediction of incident coronary events in healthy men and women. J Clin Endocrinol Metab 94: 255–260.
12. Frommer KW, Zimmermann B, Meier FM, Schroder D, Heil M, et al. (2010) Adiponectin-mediated changes in effector cells involved in the pathophysiology of rheumatoid arthritis. Arthritis Rheum 62:2886–2899.
13. Tong KM, Shieh DC, Chen CP, Tzeng CY, Wang SP, et al. (2008) Leptin induces IL-8 expression via leptin receptor IRS-1, P13K, Akt cascade and promotion of NF-κB/p300 binding in human synovial fibroblasts. Cell Signal 20:1478–1488.
14. Bokarewa M, Nagaev I, Dahlberg L, Smith U, Tarkowski A, et al. (2005) Resistin, an adipokine with potent proinflammatory properties. J Immunol 174:5789–95.
15. Balagopal P, Graham TE, Kahn BB, Altomare A, Funanage V, et al. (2007) Reduction of elevated serum retinol binding protein in obese children by lifestyle intervention: association with subclinical inflammation. J Clin Endocrinol Metab 92: 1971–1974.
16. Genre F, Lopez-Mejias R, Miranda-Filloy JA, Ubilla B, Carnero-Lopez B, et al. (2013) Antitumour necrosis factor-α treatment reduces retinol-binding protein 4 serum levels in non-diabetic ankylosing spondylitis patients. Ann Rheum Dis. doi: 10.1136/annrheumdis-2013-204484.
17. Gabriel SE, Crowson CS (2012) Risk factors for cardiovascular disease in rheumatoid arthritis. Curr Opin Rheumatol 24:171–176.
18. Dessein PH, Semb AG (2013) Could cardiovascular disease risk stratification and management in rheumatoid arthritis be enhanced? Ann Rheum Dis 72:1743–1746.
19. Dessein PH, Joffe BI (2006) When is a patient with rheumatoid arthritis at risk for cardiovascular disease? J Rheumatol 33:201–203.
20. Garcia-Bermudez M, Lopez-Mejias R, Genre F, Castaneda S, Gonzalez-Gay C, et al. (2013) SMAD3 rs12228212 gene polymorphism is associated with reduced risk to cerebrovascular accidents and subclinical atherosclerosis in anti-CCP negative Spanish rheumatoid arthritis patients. PLoS One 8: E77695. doi: 10.1371/journal.pone.0077695.
21. Crowson CS, Gabriel SE (2011) Towards improving cardiovascular risk management in patients with rheumatoid arthritis: the need for accurate risk assessment. Ann Rheum Dis 70:719–21.
22. Corrales A, Gonzalez-Juanatey C, Peiro ME, Blanco R, Llorca J, et al. (2013) Carotid ultrasound is useful for the cardiovascular risk stratification of patients with rheumatoid arthritis: results of a population-based study. Ann Rheum Dis. doi: 10.1136/annrheumdis-2012-203101].
23. Hahn BH, Lourencco EV, McMahon M, Skaggs B, Le E, et al. (2010) Pro-inflammatory high-density lipoproteins and atherosclerosis are induced in lupus-prone mice by a high-fat diet and leptin. Lupus 19:913–917.
24. Dessein PH, Norton GR, Badenhorst M, Woodiwiss AJ, Solomon A (2013) Rheumatoid arthritis impacts on the independent relationships between circulating adiponectin concentrations and cardiovascular metabolic risk. Mediators Inflamm. doi: 10.1155/2013/461849.
25. Dessein PH, Woodiwiss AJ, Norton GR, Tsang L, Solomon A (2013) Independent associations of total and high molecular weight adiponectin with cardiometabolic risk and surrogate markers of enhanced early atherogenesis in black and white patients with rheumatoid arthritis: a cross-sectional study. Arthritis Res Ther 15: R128.
26. Dessein PH, Norton GR, Woodiwiss AJ, Solomon A (2013) Independent relationship between circulating resistin concentrations and endothelial activation in rheumatoid arthritis. Ann Rheum Dis 72: 1586–1588.
27. Dessein PH, Norton GR, Woodiwiss AJ, Tsang L, Solomon A (2014) Age impacts on the independent relationships of leptin with cardiometabolic risk and surrogate markers of enhanced early atherogenesis in black and white patients with rheumatoid arthritis: a cross-sectional study. Rheumatol Int (in press).
28. Dessein PH, Norton GR, Joffe BI, Abdool-Carrim AT, Woodiwiss AJ, et al. (2013) Metabolic cardiovascular risk burden and atherosclerosis in African black and Caucasian women with rheumatoid arthritis: a cross-section study. Clin Exp Rheumatol 31: 53–61.
29. Arnett FC, Edworthy SM, Bloch DA, Mcshane DJ, Fries JF, et al. (1988) The American Rheumatism Association 1987 revised criteria for the classification of rheumatoid arthritis. Arthritis Rheum 31:315–324.
30. Aletaha D, Neogi T, Silman AJ, Funovits J, Felson DT, et al (2010) 2010 rheumatoid arthritis classification criteria: an American College of Rheumatology/European League Against Rheumatism collaborative initiative. Ann Rheum Dis 69:1580–1588.
31. Grundy SM, Hansen B, Smith SC, Cleeman JI, Kahn RA (2004) Clinical mamagement of metabolic syndrome: report of the American Heart Association/National Heart, Lung, and Blood Institute/American Diabetes Association Conference on Scientific Issues Related to Management. Circulation 109:551–556.
32. Gulfe A, Aletaha D, Saxne T, Geborek P (2009) Disease activity level, remission and response in established rheumatoid arthritis: Performance of various criteria sets in an observational cohort, treated with anti-TNF agents. BMC Musculoskelet Discord 10:41.
33. Myasoedova E, Crowson CS, Turesson C, Gabriel SE, Matteson EL (2011) Incidence of extraarticular rheumatoid arthritis in Olmsted County, Minnesota, in 1995-2007 versus 1985-1994: a population-based study. J Rheumatol 38:983–989.

34. Levey AS, Coresh J, Balk E, Kausz AT, Levin A, et al. (2003) National Kidney Foundation practice guidelines for chronic kidney disease: evaluation, classification, and stratification. Ann Intern Med 139:137–147.
35. Solomon A, Norton GR, Woodiwiss AJ, Dessein PH (2012) Obesity and carotid atherosclerosis in African black and Caucasian women with established rheumatoid arthritis: a cross-sectional study. Arthritis Res Ther 14:R67.
36. Dessein PH, Christian BF, Solomon A (2009) Which are the determinants of dyslipidemia in rheumatoid arthritis and does socioeconomic status matter in this regard? J Rheumatol 36:1357–1361.
37. Dessein PH, Solomon A, Woodiwiss AJ, Norton GR, Tsang L, et al. (2013) Marked independent relationship between circulating interleukin-6 concentrations and endothelial activation in rheumatoid arthritis. Mediators Inflamm. doi: 10.1155/2013/510243.
38. Gepner AD, Korcarz CE, Aeschlimann SE, LeCaire TJ, Palta M, et al. (2006) Validation of a carotid intima-media thickness border detection program for use in an office setting. J Am Soc Echocardiogr 19:223–8.
39. Dessein PH, Joffe BI, Veller MG, Stevens BA, Tobias M, et al. (2005) Traditional and nontraditional cardiovascular risk factors are associated with atherosclerosis in rheumatoid arthritis. J Rheumatol 32:435–42.
40. Touboul PJ, Hennerici MG, Meairs S, Adams H, Amarenco P, et al. (2007) Mannheim carotid intima-media thickness consensus (2004-2006). An update on behalf of the Advisory Board of the 3rd and 4th Watching the Risk Symposium, 13th and 15th European Stroke Conferences, Mannheim, Germany, 2004, and Brussels, Belgium, 2006. Cerebrovasc Dis 23:75–80.
41. Maradit Kremers H, Crowson Cs, Therneau TM, Roger VL, Gabriel S (2008) High ten-year risk of cardiovascular disease in newly diagnosed rheumatoid arthritis. Arthritis Rheum 58: 2268–2274.
42. Dessein PH, Solomon A (2014) Towards the elucidation of the true impact of adipocytokines on cardiovascular risk in rheumatoid arthritis. Arthritis Res Ther (in press).
43. Sattar N, Nelson SM (2008) Adiponectin, diabetes, and coronary heart disease in older persons: unraveling the paradox. J Clin Endocrinol Metab 93: 3299–3301.
44. Takashima N, Tomoike H, Iwai N (2006) Retinol-binding protein 4 and insulin resistance. N Engl J Med 355: 1392–1395.
45. Dessein PH, Joffe BI, Stanwix AE (2004) Subclinical hypothyroidism is associated with insulin resistance in rheumatoid arthritis. Thyroid 14: 443–446.
46. Finucane FM, Luan J, Wareham NJ, Sharp SJ, O'Rahilly S, et al. (2009) Correlation of the leptin:adiponectin ratio with measures of insulin resistance in non-diabetic individuals. Diabetologia 52: 2345–2349.
47. Dessein PH, Woodiwiss AJ, Joffe BI, Norton GR (2007) Aminotransferases are associated with insulin resistance and atherosclerosis in rheumatoid arthritis. BMC Cardiovasc Disord 7: 31.
48. Dessein PH, Joffe BI, Singh S (2005) Biomarkers of endothelial dysfunction, cardiovascular risk factors and atherosclerosis in rheumatoid arthritis. Arthritis Res Ther 7:R634–643.
49. Sodergren A, Karp K, Boman K, Eriksson C, Lundstrom E, et al. (2010) Atherosclerosis in early rheumatoid arthritis: very early endothelial activation and rapid progression of intima media thickness. Arthritis Res Ther 12:R158.
50. Steyn NP, Wolmarans P, Nel JH, Bourne LT (2007) National fortification of staple food can make a significant contribution to micronutrient intake of South African adults. Public Health Nutr 11:307–313.
51. Graham TE, Wason CJ, Bluher M, Kahn BB (2007) Shortcomings in methodology complicate measurements of serum retinol binding protein (RBP$) in insulin-resistant human subjects. Diabetologia 50: 814–823.
52. von Eynatten M, Lepper PM, Liu D, Lang K, Baumann M, et al. (2007) Retinol-binding protein 4 is associated with components of the metabolic syndrome, but not with insulin resistance, in men with type 2 diabetes or coronary artery disease. Diabetologia 50: 1930–1937.

Calibration of the PROMIS Physical Function Item Bank in Dutch Patients with Rheumatoid Arthritis

Martijn A. H. Oude Voshaar[1]*, Peter M. ten Klooster[1], Cees A. W. Glas[2], Harald E. Vonkeman[1,3], Erik Taal[1], Eswar Krishnan[4], Hein J. Bernelot Moens[5], Maarten Boers[6], Caroline B. Terwee[6], Piet L. C. M. van Riel[7], Mart A. F. J. van de Laar[1,3]

1 Arthritis Center Twente and Psychology, Health & Technology, University of Twente, Enschede, The Netherlands, **2** Department of Research Methodology, Measurement and Data Analysis, University of Twente, Enschede, The Netherlands, **3** Department of Rheumatology and Clinical Immunology, Medisch Spectrum Twente, Enschede, The Netherlands, **4** Arthritis, Rheumatism, and Aging Medical Information System Program, Stanford University School of Medicine, Palo Alto, California, United States of America, **5** Department of Rheumatology and Clinical Immunology, Ziekenhuisgroep Twente, Almelo, The Netherlands, **6** Department of Epidemiology and Biostatistics, Vrije Universiteit Medical Center, Amsterdam, The Netherlands, **7** Department of Rheumatic Diseases, Radboud University Medical Centre, Nijmegen, The Netherlands

Abstract

Objective: To calibrate the Dutch-Flemish version of the PROMIS physical function (PF) item bank in patients with rheumatoid arthritis (RA) and to evaluate cross-cultural measurement equivalence with US general population and RA data.

Methods: Data were collected from RA patients enrolled in the Dutch DREAM registry. An incomplete longitudinal anchored design was used where patients completed all 121 items of the item bank over the course of three waves of data collection. Item responses were fit to a generalized partial credit model adapted for longitudinal data and the item parameters were examined for differential item functioning (DIF) across country, age, and sex.

Results: In total, 690 patients participated in the study at time point 1 (T2, N = 489; T3, N = 311). The item bank could be successfully fitted to a generalized partial credit model, with the number of misfitting items falling within acceptable limits. Seven items demonstrated DIF for sex, while 5 items showed DIF for age in the Dutch RA sample. Twenty-five (20%) items were flagged for cross-cultural DIF compared to the US general population. However, the impact of observed DIF on total physical function estimates was negligible.

Discussion: The results of this study showed that the PROMIS PF item bank adequately fit a unidimensional IRT model which provides support for applications that require invariant estimates of physical function, such as computer adaptive testing and targeted short forms. More studies are needed to further investigate the cross-cultural applicability of the US-based PROMIS calibration and standardized metric.

Editor: Amr H. Sawalha, University of Michigan, United States of America

Funding: This study was funded by the Dutch Arthritis Association, project number 11-1-203; http://www.reumafonds.nl/. The funders had no role in study design, data collection and analysis, decision to publish, or preparation of the manuscript.

Competing Interests: The authors have declared that no competing interests exist.

* E-mail: A.H.Oudevoshaar@utwente.nl

Introduction

Rheumatoid arthritis (RA) is one of the most prevalent rheumatic diseases, characterized by pain and swelling of the joints which may lead to significant disability. Patient-reported physical function is a core outcome domain in RA research [1,2]. Physical function is typically assessed using standard, fixed-length questionnaires. Although often extensively validated, key limitations of these traditional questionnaires remain their static nature and limited measurement range and measurement precision, frequently leading to ceiling and floor effects and limited sensitivity to change [3–8]. Recent studies have suggested that these shortcomings may be overcome by item response theory (IRT) based item banking [9,10]. IRT calibrated item banks can serve as a platform for tailored assessment of patient-reported outcomes, through developing targeted short forms or computerized adaptive tests (CATs). Both methods of assessment ensure that patients respond to questions that are more relevant to their specific level of disability and that only minimal questions need to be answered, while retaining or surpassing the measurement precision of fixed-length instruments.

The Patient-Reported Outcomes Measurement Information System (PROMIS) initiative has developed and calibrated item banks for assessing several important domains of health status, including physical function, across a wide variety of chronic diseases and conditions and the general population in the US [11]. Using data from the general population and several clinical samples in the US, all items in the item banks are calibrated on a common, standardized metric. Potentially, the PROMIS physical function (PF) item bank could also lead to improved assessment of physical function in clinical or comparative studies in RA. Indeed, recent studies have already shown a 20-item PROMIS PF short form to be more precise and more responsive to change than traditional questionnaires in RA [12]. Recently, the PROMIS PF item bank has been translated and culturally adapted for use among Dutch and Flemish populations. Pretesting of the translated items revealed that the items were understood by patients as intended and culturally appropriate for use in Dutch populations with arthritis [13,14]. Before an item bank can be used in a new population, however, it should be demonstrated that data collected from that population can be fit to an appropriate IRT model. If this is the case, a latent metric specific for this population can be created that allows invariant estimates of the item parameters and physical function levels to be obtained (e.g., item parameters that are independent of the physical function level of the respondents used to calibrate the item bank) [15]. As a result, physical function estimates on a common scale may be obtained from any number and combination of items in the item bank and applications such as CATs and targeted short forms become possible. A second question that needs to be addressed is whether the relationship between observed physical function scores and the physical function trait measured by the item bank is equivalent to this relationship for the original population. If this is the case, this would provide evidence that the model parameters can be expressed on a common scale [16]. In case of the PROMIS PF item bank, this would mean that data from the specific population can be scored using the US-based PROMIS calibration and standardized metric, making scores directly comparable between populations.

The aims of the current study were to calibrate the Dutch-Flemish PROMIS PF item bank in a prospective cohort of Dutch patients with RA and to evaluate its measurement equivalence with data from the total PROMIS wave 1 calibration sample in the US and a smaller subset of US RA patients.

Methods

Patients

Data for this study were collected within the Dutch Rheumatoid Arthritis Monitoring (DREAM) registry. The DREAM registry is an observational multicenter cohort study that monitors the course of unselected RA patients in the Netherlands. Both patient-reported and clinical outcomes are collected and monitored using a web-based data acquisition and storage system. Patient-reported outcomes, including the Health Assessment Questionnaire disability index (HAQ-DI) and the SF-36 health survey, are completed preceding every visit to the outpatient clinic. Between September 2012 and September 2013, all participating patients from three DREAM hospitals were informed about the study and invited to participate upon logging on to their patient portals preceding their visit to the clinic.

Data collection designs

Dutch DREAM data. To optimize data quality and minimize patient burden, an incomplete longitudinal design was used for calibrating the Dutch-Flemish item bank in the Dutch RA patients, in which different subsets of items (booklets) were administered to different patients. The booklets were linked using common items, making it possible to place all items on a single scale [17]. Since previous research has found that the number of common items within booklets improves the stability of IRT models estimated from incomplete calibration designs, [18] the item responses on the HAQ-DI and the SF-36 physical functioning scale (PF-10), the two most widely used measures of physical function in RA, were added to the calibration design. A graphical overview of the calibration design is presented in Figure 1.

Upon consenting to participate, patients were allocated randomly to one of six booklets. Besides the HAQ-DI and PF-10, each booklet contained two sets of approximately 20 of the 121 PROMIS PF items and each of the six sets featured in two booklets in such a way that half of the items in each booklet overlapped with the previous booklet and half with the next. On successive participations, patients were allocated to booklet N+2 (for N = 1,2,3,4) or N−4 (for N = 5,6), where N is the booklet that was administered at the preceding participation, so that patients completed the full item bank after three participations. The sample sizes of the six groups were approximately equal so that all items received an approximately equal number of responses.

From historical log data of physical function items in the DREAM registry, it was estimated that the majority of patients would need no more than 10 minutes to complete each booklet of approximately 40 items. An effort was made to balance the relative difficulty of the items in each booklet by ordering the items according to their peak statistical information on the latent IRT metric according to the US PROMIS wave 1 calibration results. As 20% of the PROMIS PF items has a different stem (i.e., 'does your health now limit you…' rather 'than are you able to…') and associated set of response options, each booklet contained a proportional number of these items.

US PROMIS wave 1 data. PROMIS wave 1 data for 14 candidate item pools, including three pools of physical function items, were collected between July 2006 to March 2007 from over 21,000 participants selected from both the US general population and specific clinical populations [19]. The data collection design of the wave 1 data consisted of both so-called 'full bank administrations', where participants were administered two sets of 56 items from only one or two item pools, and 'block administrations' where participants completed 14 blocks of seven items from all item pools. To avoid complicating the calibration design and analyses, we chose to model only the available full bank data from the general population sample and the block data available from the clinical sample of RA patients.

The full bank arm of the data collection design for physical function in the general population consisted of two booklets that were completed by two independent samples of 942 and 995 respondents, respectively. The booklets were complementary in that each PF item featured in only one booklet and together the booklets contained all 121 final items of the PROMIS PF item bank. Besides the PROMIS PF items, respondents completed the HAQ-DI or PF-10 or both. The HAQ-DI and PF-10 data were included in the calibrations in order to obtain a linked structure so that the US item parameters could be placed on a common latent scale, despite the lack of overlapping PROMIS PF items between the two booklets. Additionally, two clinical samples of 273 and 280 RA patients completed a booklet with a selection of seven items from each of the three PF item pools. Twenty-four of these 42 administered items were calibrated in the final US PROMIS PF item bank (13 and 11 items from each booklet, respectively).

Measures

PROMIS physical function (PF) item bank. The PROMIS PF item bank measures self-reported, current capability to carry out activities that require physical actions, ranging from self-care (activities of daily living) to more complex activities that require a combination of skills, often within a social context. The final calibrated item bank contains 121 questions assessing the functioning of the upper extremities (dexterity), lower extremities (walking or mobility), and central regions (neck, back), as well as

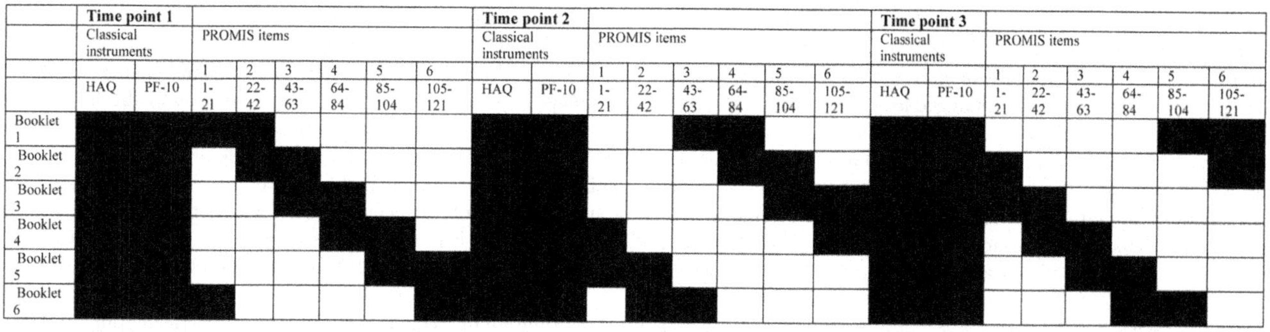

Figure 1. Sampling design of the Dutch calibration study.

instrumental activities of daily living, such as running errands [19]. Each item is scored on a 5 point rating scale, with higher scores indicating better functioning. The Dutch-Flemish translation of the item bank was developed according to the universal PROMIS translation approach (http://www.nihpromis.org/measures/translations), which included extensive forward-back translation procedures, expert reviews, and cognitive debriefing interviews among Dutch and Flemish participants [20].

Health Assessment Questionnaire disability index (HAQ-DI). The HAQ-DI contains 20 items measuring physical disabilities over the past week in eight categories of daily living: dressing and grooming, rising, eating, walking, hygiene, reach, grip, and activities [21]. Each item is scored on a 4-point rating scale from 0 (without any difficulty) to 3 (unable to do). Disability scores were calculated according to the alternative scoring rule, which does not account for the use of aids and help from others [22]. Category scores are averaged to produce a total score between 0 and 3, with higher values indicating more disability. The Dutch consensus version of the HAQ-DI was used in the DREAM data collection.

SF-36 Health Survey physical functioning scale (PF-10). The PF-10 is one of the eight scales of the SF-36 Health Survey and consists of 10 items measuring perceived current limitations in a variety of physical activities on a 3-point response scale from 1 (yes, limited a lot) to 3 (no, not limited at all). Scores of the PF-10 items are summed and linearly transformed to range between 0 and 100, with higher scores indicating better physical functioning [23]. The Dutch version of the SF-36v2 was used in the DREAM study [24].

Additional patient-reported and clinical measures. The Dutch DREAM registry additionally collected patient-reported general health, disease activity, fatigue, and pain in the past week on 0–100 visual analog scales (VASs), with higher scores indicating worse status. Clinical data were collected during visits to the outpatient clinic, including a 28-tender joint count, 28-swollen joint count, and erythrocyte sedimentation rate. Together with the VAS general health, these measures were combined into a single index of clinical disease activity (DAS28) [25].

Statistical analysis

All IRT analyses were performed with the MIRT software package [26]. The marginal maximum likelihood estimation procedure was utilized to estimate the model parameters and the latent physical function levels of patients were estimated using the expected a posteriori (EAP) method throughout all analyses. Latent physical function scores are expressed on a scale with a mean of 0 and SD of 1. A multidimensional generalization of the two-parameter generalized partial credit model (GPCM), suitable for the analysis of longitudinal, polytomous data [27], was used to model the Dutch data. In this model, the item parameters pertain to time point specific latent dimensions and the dependency between item responses at different time points is modeled by the correlation between the dimensions. The model allows patients' levels of physical function to change over time but item parameters are constrained to be equal across time points. To evaluate whether the item parameters were stable over time, the presence of longitudinal differential item functioning (DIF) was evaluated using regression analysis as proposed by Te Marvelde & Glas [28]. To this end, unidimensional GPCM estimates of the Dutch PROMIS data were obtained for each time point separately. The resulting threshold parameters were regressed on the threshold parameters emanating from one of the other two models in a series of univariate regression models. Individual items were considered to display statistically significant longitudinal DIF in case an item's 99% confidence interval did not intersect the regression line [28].

Fit of the longitudinal IRT model was assessed using Lagrange multiplier (LM) statistics, which evaluate whether observed item scores correspond to those expected by the item characteristic function [29]. To evaluate the magnitude of model violation of significant LM tests, effect size statistics (ES) were also obtained. These effect sizes are differences between average observed and expected scores across 3 total-score level groups. To compute these effect sizes, the patients were divided in 3 groups of approximately equal size obtaining low, intermediate, and high scores. The observed and expected scores were divided by the maximum attainable item score, such that a difference of, say, 0.10 indicated that the observed average score was 10% different from its expectation under the model. Items were considered to lack fit in case Ps<0.05 and ES statistics were >0.10 [30]. We first evaluated fit within time points by estimating the unidimensional GPCM 3 times, once for each time point. Subsequently, fit of the total multidimensional model, with item parameters constrained to be equal across time points and which includes the covariance matrix between time points, was evaluated. The Dutch data was evaluated for DIF across age (median split at 58 years) and sex. To this end the baseline model was extended by partitioning the booklets further according to age or sex and DIF was evaluated across two marginal distributions of physical function of males vs. females and younger vs. older patients, respectively. DIF across the marginal distributions was evaluated with an LM test for DIF [31].

Cross-cultural equivalence with the original US data was investigated first using the wave 1 general population data. The analysis was subsequently repeated on the independent subset of 25 items administered to the US RA patients [19]. US item parameters were obtained from a unidimensional GPCM and analysis of cross-cultural DIF was again performed with the regression analysis method outlined above [28]. To examine the impact of any observed DIF, US and Dutch baseline data were jointly modeled in a unidimensional GPCM with country-specific item parameters for those items flagged for cross-cultural DIF. The resulting EAP estimates were compared to those emanating from a model without country-specific item parameters. In both models, the mean was set to zero for US respondents (SD = 1). The agreement between the resulting latent EAP estimates was evaluated by calculating intraclass correlation coefficients (ICCs, model A,1) and the limits of agreement according to the Bland-Altman method [32]. Two independent data sets were available of US RA patients. The first sample (Stanford sample) contained 14 items administered to 273 patients and the second sample (Polimetrix sample) contained 10 items administered to 280 patients. To evaluate RA-related DIF, the baseline model of Dutch RA-patients was extended to incorporate these data. DIF was subsequently evaluated across three marginal distributions (Dutch, Stanford, and Polimetrix) using the LM test approach outlined above.

Results

Participant characteristics

Baseline data of 690 Dutch RA patients was available for analysis (Table 1). Of these, 489 and 311 patients completed booklets at T2 and T3, respectively. Average time between participations was 6.0 months (SD = 2.5) for T1 to T2 and 4. months (SD = 1.8) for T2 and T3. On average, Dutch patients had relatively low disease activity and high levels of physical function at baseline. Whereas the US general population and the combined RA samples had a balanced sex distribution, 64% of the Dutch RA patients were female, reflecting the greater prevalence of RA among women. The average level of physical function of US general population respondents was higher than that of Dutch RA patients according to the HAQ-DI and the average age of US general population respondents was lower.

Evaluation of the longitudinal IRT model in the Dutch data

Table 2 presents an overview of the LM tests and the average observed and average expected item scores across three total score level groups for the PROMIS PF items administered in the odd booklets at T1 (see Figure 1). Results were similar for the even booklets and the other time points. The items are organized according to the point on the latent scale where they provide their optimum information, as an indication of the relative difficulty of the activities they refer to. As expected, more 'easy' items referred to simple activities of daily living, such as eating or getting up from a chair, while items involving increasingly higher levels of cardiopulmonary function were clustered around the higher end of the latent metric. For most items, average observed scores were quite high considering the 1–5 rating scale of the PROMIS items, reflecting the relatively high level of physical function of the sample. Item scores expected by the IRT model tended to be close to the observed item scores across total score groups, leading to an acceptable average ES of 0.01 for time point 1.

The number of items exhibiting lack of fit was very low for all three time points. For T1, T2 and T3 respectively, only 14 (3%), 12 (3%) and 5 (1%) items demonstrated misfit according to the LM test. Moreover, ESs exceeded 0.10 only for two items, both at T3 (PFA9, ES = 0.10 and PFA15, ES = 0.11) The item parameters were stable over time, with all correlations between threshold parameters at different time points exceeding 0.90 and all of the 99% confidence intervals intersecting the regression line in the three univariate regression analyses.

In the subsequent evaluation of the longitudinal (multidimensional) model, 6.3% of item level fit statistics showed lack of fit to the model, which corresponds approximately to the level of significant item tests expected based on chance. None of the items showed lack of fit in both or, in case of the HAQ-DI and PF-10 items, all booklets that it was included in, nor did any item show misfit across time points. The multidimensional IRT model provides estimates of the correlation of PF over the three different time points. The correlation between between latent PF levels across the three time points ranged from 0.73 between T1 and T3 to 0.87 between T1 and T2, indicating that physical function levels were quite stable over time. The overall conclusion was that model fit was acceptable.

DIF across age and gender

Seven items demonstrated DIF for sex, while five items showed DIF for age in the Dutch RA sample at baseline (Table 3). For all items flagged for sex DIF, men reported slightly higher scores than expected by the IRT model, whereas women reported lower scores than expected, indicating that the activities were easier for male RA patients. Likewise, all items flagged for age DIF, except item PFA53 ('Are you able to run errands and shop?') were more easily endorsed by younger rather than older patients.

Equivalence with PROMIS wave 1 data

To evaluate measurement equivalence, US item parameters were obtained and compared with the Dutch item parameters

Table 1. Sample characteristics.

	Dutch RA patients (N = 690)	US RA patients (N = 557)	US general population (N = 1937)
Female, N (%)	371 (63.6%)	293 (52.6%)	1004 (51.8)
Age, M (SD)	56.8 (11.8)	56.66 (10.9)	50.5 (18.3)
DAS28, M (SD)	2.1 (1.1)	-	-
VAS General health, M (SD)	25.1 (23.6)	-	-
VAS Disease activity, M (SD)	28.2 (23.4)	-	-
VAS Fatigue, M (SD)	33.1 (29.8)	-	-
VAS Pain, M (SD)	27.6 (22.7)	-	-
HAQ-ADI, M (SD)	0.5 (0.6)	-	0.2 (0.4)

VAS = Visual analog scale; DAS28 = 28-joint disease activity score.

Table 2. Evaluation of item fit for PROMIS items in the odd booklets at time 1.

Item code	Item stem	LM	P	ES	Score group					
					1		2		3	
					Obs	Exp	Obs	Exp	Obs	Exp
PFC53	Are you able to get in and out of bed?	0.53	0.77	0.02	3.91	3.86	4.54	4.50	4.86	4.95
PFB48	Does your health now limit you in taking a shower?	0.35	0.84	0.01	3.97	4.03	4.71	4.72	4.95	4.96
PFA15	Are you able to stand up from an armless straight chair?	1.13	0.57	0.01	3.88	3.77	4.76	4.72	5.00	4.99
PFC6	**Are you able to walk a block (about 100 m) on flat ground? ***	3.12	0.21	0.01	4.23	4.25	4.97	4.92	5.00	4.99
PFB26	Are you able to shampoo your hair?	0.14	0.93	<0.01	3.97	3.98	4.85	4.83	5.00	4.99
PFA45	Are you able to get out of bed into a chair?	1.26	0.53	0.01	4.40	4.32	4.80	4.85	5.00	4.99
PFA51	Are you able to sit on the edge of a bed?	0.01	0.99	<0.01	4.65	4.64	4.94	4.94	5.00	5.00
PFA30	Are you able to step up and down curbs?	1.46	0.48	0.01	4.13	4.24	4.84	4.89	5.00	4.99
PFC47	Are you able to be out of bed most of the day?	1.13	0.57	0.01	4.57	4.56	4.81	4.91	5.00	4.98
PFB18	Are you able to shave your face or apply makeup?	0.27	0.87	0.01	4.23	4.24	4.85	4.89	5.00	4.99
PFC46	Are you able to transfer from a bed to a chair and back?	2.85	0.24	0.02	4.28	4.14	4.84	4.90	5.00	4.99
PFA40	Are you able to turn a key in a lock?	2.34	0.31	0.02	3.83	3.98	4.71	4.64	4.97	4.97
PFB16	Are you able to press with your index finger (for example ringing a doorbell)?	2.41	0.30	0.01	4.40	4.40	4.92	4.84	5.00	4.99
PFC39	Are you able to stand without losing your balance for several minutes?	7.77	0.02	0.03	3.97	4.19	4.89	4.74	4.95	4.96
PFC51	Are you able to wipe yourself after using the toilet?	0.16	0.92	0.01	4.20	4.18	4.80	4.77	5.00	4.98
PFA54	Are you able to button your shirt?	0.27	0.88	0.01	3.86	3.79	4.59	4.60	4.89	4.91
PFB31	Are you able to open car doors?	2.00	0.37	0.02	4.19	4.03	4.65	4.67	4.98	4.97
PFB29	Are you able to lift a full cup or glass to your mouth?	1.93	0.38	0.01	4.28	4.35	4.93	4.87	5.00	4.99
PFA50	Are you able to brush your teeth?	1.79	0.41	0.01	4.32	4.36	4.93	4.88	5.00	4.99
PFC45	**Are you able to sit on and get up from the toilet? †**	2.88	0.24	0.01	3.98	4.02	4.90	4.83	5.00	4.99
PFB27	Are you able to tie a knot or a bow?	7.91	0.02	0.05	3.26	3.62	4.66	4.49	4.89	4.94
PFB20	Are you able to cut a piece of paper with scissors?	3.24	0.20	0.02	3.91	4.05	4.77	4.69	5.00	4.97
PFA44	Are you able to put on a shirt or blouse?	5.81	0.05	0.03	3.83	3.96	4.80	4.66	4.94	4.97
PFA35	Are you able to open and close a zipper?	3.76	0.15	0.02	3.88	3.99	4.89	4.80	5.00	4.99
PFB22	Are you able to hold a plate full of food?	1.34	0.51	0.01	4.03	4.03	4.66	4.79	4.97	4.97
PFA16	Are you able to dress yourself, including tying shoelaces and buttoning your clothes?	1.88	0.39	0.01	3.60	3.65	4.76	4.66	4.95	4.96
PFA38	Are you able to stand for short periods of time?	0.23	0.89	0.01	3.77	3.73	4.50	4.50	4.95	4.96
PFA48	Are you able to peel fruit?	1.96	0.38	0.02	3.69	3.75	4.65	4.53	4.93	4.92
PFB15	Are you able to change the bulb in a table lamp?	0.12	0.94	0.01	4.00	3.97	4.78	4.80	4.98	4.98
PFC49	**Are you able to water a house plant? †**	2.75	0.25	0.02	4.26	4.42	4.95	4.93	5.00	5.00
PFB33	Are you able to remove something from your back pocket?	2.95	0.23	0.03	3.83	4.05	4.83	4.78	4.97	4.98
PFB21	Are you able to pick up coins from a table top?	0.68	0.71	0.02	3.97	3.89	4.63	4.57	4.89	4.92
PFB10	Are you able to climb up five steps?	0.12	0.94	0.01	3.76	3.81	4.66	4.64	5.00	4.97
PFB19	Are you able to squeeze a new tube of toothpaste?	0.49	0.78	0.01	4.18	4.10	4.84	4.85	5.00	4.98
PFB36	Are you able to put on a pullover sweater?	0.73	0.70	0.01	4.17	4.09	4.76	4.80	4.95	4.96
PFC29	Are you able to walk up and down two steps?	0.97	0.61	0.02	3.89	3.77	4.59	4.71	4.92	4.91
PFA56	Are you able to get in and out of a car?	0.24	0.89	0.01	3.89	3.89	4.55	4.51	4.95	4.95
PFA36	**Are you able to put on and take off a coat or jacket? †**	1.51	0.47	0.02	3.74	3.83	4.58	4.50	4.98	4.95
PFA32	**Are you able to stand with your knees straight?**	2.44	0.30	0.02	4.20	4.10	4.90	4.84	5.00	4.99
PFA43	Are you able to write with a pen or pencil?	0.32	0.85	0.01	3.89	3.85	4.71	4.67	4.97	4.97
PFB49	Does your health now limit you in going for a short walk (less than 15 minutes)?	0.03	0.98	0.01	3.34	3.32	4.24	4.26	4.86	4.88
PFA22	Are you able to open previously opened jars?	1.09	0.58	0.01	3.78	3.68	4.49	4.50	4.88	4.88
PFB25	Are you able to push open a door after turning the knob?	1.65	0.44	0.02	4.42	4.32	4.82	4.87	5.00	4.98
PFB41	Are you able to trim your fingernails?	3.30	0.19	0.03	4.03	3.81	4.67	4.72	4.92	4.96
PFB23	Are you able to pour liquid from a bottle into a glass?	1.40	0.50	0.01	4.43	4.40	4.84	4.91	5.00	4.99
PFA52	Are you able to tie your shoelaces?	4.11	0.13	0.02	3.48	3.58	4.64	4.49	4.98	4.95

Table 2. Cont.

Item code	Item stem	LM	P	ES	Score group 1 Obs	Score group 1 Exp	Score group 2 Obs	Score group 2 Exp	Score group 3 Obs	Score group 3 Exp
PFA49	**Are you able to bend or twist your back? ***	0.29	0.86	0.01	3.77	3.84	4.52	4.55	4.91	4.93
PFB3	**Does your health now limit you in putting a trash bag outside? †**	2.27	0.32	0.03	3.19	3.08	3.82	3.97	4.82	4.88
PFA9	Are you able to bend down and pick up clothing from the floor?	1.13	0.57	0.02	3.85	3.72	4.55	4.54	4.90	4.94
PFA37	Are you able to stand for short periods of time?	2.04	0.36	0.02	4.00	3.88	4.74	4.66	5.00	4.95
PFA17	Are you able to reach into a high cupboard?	1.98	0.37	0.02	3.31	3.24	4.34	4.22	4.89	4.88
PFB43	Does your health now limit you in taking care of your personal needs (dress, comb hair, toilet, eat, bathe)?	0.09	0.95	0.01	3.63	3.59	4.42	4.42	4.92	4.95
PFC31	Are you able to reach into a low cupboard?	0.64	0.73	0.01	3.43	3.44	4.50	4.39	4.92	4.91
PFB11	Are you able to wash dishes, pots, and utensils by hand while standing at a sink?	0.13	0.94	0.01	3.88	3.88	4.71	4.67	4.97	4.97
PFA18	Are you able to use a hammer to pound a nail?	0.10	0.95	0.01	3.45	3.43	4.58	4.60	4.92	4.94
PFB37	Are you able to turn faucets on and off?	0.67	0.72	0.01	3.80	3.78	4.78	4.73	4.92	4.96
PFB56	Are you able to lift one pound (0.5 kg) to shoulder level without bending your elbow?	0.47	0.79	0.01	3.47	3.47	4.68	4.62	4.92	4.93
PFC43	**Are you able to use your hands, such as for turning faucets, using kitchen gadgets, or sewing? †**	0.80	0.67	0.02	3.44	3.54	4.21	4.26	4.83	4.88
PFC52	Are you able to turn from side to side in bed?	2.25	0.32	0.02	3.45	3.59	4.63	4.55	4.90	4.95
PFB32	Are you able to stand unsupported for 10 minutes?	1.17	0.56	0.03	3.34	3.50	4.50	4.38	4.95	4.87
PFA53	Are you able to run errands and shop?	0.96	0.62	0.02	3.39	3.28	4.37	4.32	4.92	4.95
PFB17	Are you able to put on and take off your socks?	0.96	0.62	0.01	3.87	3.76	4.71	4.70	4.97	4.96
PFA28	Are you able to open a can with a hand can opener?	2.45	0.29	0.02	3.19	3.09	4.15	4.30	4.85	4.84
PFA21	**Are you able to go up and down stairs at a normal pace? ***	0.55	0.76	0.02	3.17	3.22	4.21	4.14	4.83	4.88
PFB13	**Are you able to carry a shopping bag or briefcase? †**	0.06	0.97	<0.01	3.30	3.31	4.12	4.14	4.91	4.90
PFA34	Are you able to wash your back?	2.38	0.30	0.02	3.15	3.13	4.37	4.22	4.80	4.85
PFC41	Are you able to sit down in and stand up from a low, soft couch?	3.48	0.18	0.03	2.89	3.11	4.06	3.93	4.73	4.70
PFC38	Are you able to walk at a normal speed?	0.09	0.95	0.01	3.23	3.17	4.31	4.31	4.91	4.91
PFB40	Are you able to stand up on tiptoes?	0.14	0.93	0.01	3.24	3.20	4.50	4.47	4.89	4.85
PFA25	**Are you able to do yard work like raking leaves, weeding, or pushing a lawn mower? ***	0.68	0.71	0.02	2.79	2.69	3.58	3.55	4.68	4.65
PFA29	**Are you able to pull heavy objects (10 pounds/ 5 kg) towards yourself? †**	0.46	0.79	0.01	2.74	2.74	3.74	3.68	4.77	4.70
PFA47	**Are you able to pull on trousers? †**	0.96	0.62	0.01	3.95	3.88	4.78	4.81	5.00	5.00
PFC56	Does your health now limit you in walking about the house?	2.21	0.33	0.02	3.54	3.78	4.56	4.54	4.95	4.96
PFA12	**Are you able to push open a heavy door? †**	0.59	0.75	0.01	2.97	2.89	4.03	4.06	4.79	4.79
PFA8	Are you able to move a chair from one room to another?	1.83	0.40	0.02	2.84	3.03	4.37	4.35	4.95	4.90
PFB54	Does your health now limit you in going OUTSIDE the home, for example to shop or visit a doctor's office?	0.16	0.92	0.01	3.73	3.76	4.79	4.77	5.00	4.97
PFC32	**Are you able to climb up 5 flights of stairs? ***	0.39	0.82	0.02	3.08	3.15	4.20	4.27	4.80	4.84
PFA42	**Are you able to carry a laundry basket up a flight of stairs? ***	4.66	0.10	0.04	2.74	2.71	3.70	3.99	4.91	4.81
PFB39	Are you able to reach and get down a 5 pound (2 kg) object from above your head?	2.72	0.26	0.04	2.34	2.59	3.57	3.62	4.51	4.65
PFA23	Are you able to go for a walk of at least 15 minutes?	0.52	0.77	0.02	3.41	3.28	4.37	4.36	4.92	4.90
PFA11	Are you able to do chores such as vacuuming or yard work?	0.57	0.75	0.02	2.94	2.88	3.71	3.79	4.83	4.70
PFB34	Are you able to change a light bulb overhead?	0.29	0.86	0.01	2.89	2.88	4.18	4.25	4.85	4.84
PFA6	Does your health now limit you in bathing or dressing yourself?	0.32	0.85	0.01	3.43	3.48	4.34	4.33	4.93	4.95
PFA55	**Are you able to wash and dry your body? †**	2.31	0.31	0.01	3.62	3.62	4.56	4.70	5.00	4.99
PFB14	Are you able to take a tub bath?	2.53	0.28	0.04	3.25	2.96	4.38	4.48	4.97	4.87
PFB12	Are you able to make a bed, including spreading and tucking in bed sheets?	2.42	0.30	0.03	2.69	2.84	4.03	4.17	4.92	4.82
PFA14	Are you able to carry a heavy object (over 10 pounds/5 kg)?	0.27	0.88	0.01	2.72	2.65	3.63	3.62	4.64	4.59
PFA31	Are you able to get up from the floor from lying on your back without help?	1.52	0.47	0.03	2.88	2.70	3.61	3.66	4.78	4.70
PFC40	Are you able to kneel on the floor?	1.60	0.45	0.03	2.54	2.50	3.37	3.62	4.60	4.56
PFB42	Are you able to stand unsupported for 30 minutes?	0.65	0.72	0.02	2.69	2.59	3.91	3.79	4.71	4.70

Table 2. Cont.

Item code	Item stem	LM	P	ES	Score group					
					1		2		3	
					Obs	Exp	Obs	Exp	Obs	Exp
PFC37	**Does your health now limit you in climbing one flight of stairs? ***	0.49	0.78	0.01	3.18	3.25	4.35	4.40	4.90	4.93
PFB28	**Are you able to lift 10 pounds (5 kg) above your shoulder?**	6.43	0.04	0.05	2.68	2.26	3.59	3.69	4.69	4.65
PFC54	Does your health now limit you in getting in and out of the bathtub?	7.25	0.03	0.05	3.05	2.66	3.65	3.70	4.91	4.81
PFB8	Are you able to carry two bags filled with groceries 100 yards (100 m)?	3.58	0.17	0.04	2.15	2.05	3.43	3.08	4.44	4.41
PFA41	Are you able to squat and get up?	0.93	0.63	0.02	2.79	2.66	3.65	3.61	4.67	4.62
PFA10	Are you able to stand for one hour?	2.83	0.24	0.04	2.43	2.36	3.74	3.49	4.69	4.49
PFB9	Are you able to jump up and down?	0.58	0.75	0.02	2.62	2.51	4.16	4.10	4.85	4.80
PFA5	Does your health now limit you in lifting or carrying groceries?	1.22	0.54	0.02	2.45	2.55	3.43	3.32	4.51	4.53
PFA13	Are you able to exercise for an hour?	4.52	0.10	0.04	2.33	2.40	3.58	3.25	4.44	4.35
PFB24	Are you able to run a short distance, such as to catch a bus?	0.83	0.66	0.02	2.39	2.34	3.63	3.76	4.67	4.65
PFC10	**Does your health now limit you in climbing several flights of stairs? ***	3.02	0.22	0.04	3.22	2.96	4.14	4.19	4.95	4.84
PFC36	Does your health now limit you in walking more than a mile (1.6 km)?	0.76	0.68	0.02	2.77	2.77	4.27	4.14	4.73	4.81
PFB1	Does your health now limit you in doing moderate work around the house like vacuuming, sweeping floors or carrying in groceries?	2.15	0.34	0.03	2.35	2.42	3.43	3.25	4.50	4.57
PFB50	How much difficulty do you have doing your daily physical activities, because of your health?	0.51	0.78	0.01	2.74	2.76	3.59	3.52	4.56	4.59
PFB44	Does your health now limit you in doing moderate activities, such as moving a table, pushing a vacuum cleaner, bowling, or playing golf?	0.75	0.69	0.02	2.32	2.34	3.20	3.08	4.47	4.43
PFA33	Are you able to exercise hard for half an hour?	2.85	0.24	0.04	2.06	2.24	3.36	3.56	4.51	4.54
PFA3	Does your health now limit you in bending, kneeling, or stooping?	0.03	0.99	0.01	2.54	2.52	3.53	3.52	4.51	4.53
PFC13	Are you able to run 100 yards (100 m)?	4.63	0.10	0.04	1.89	1.89	3.08	3.52	4.50	4.55
PFB5	**Does your health now limit you in hiking a couple of miles (3 km) on uneven surfaces, including hills? ***	0.73	0.69	0.02	1.89	1.99	3.32	3.37	4.59	4.62
PFC12	Does your health now limit you in doing two hours of physical labor?	3.49	0.18	0.04	2.68	2.61	3.02	3.22	4.23	4.43
PFC35	Does your health now limit you in doing eight hours of physical labor?	4.17	0.12	0.04	1.33	1.52	2.50	2.62	4.03	4.15
PFA4	**Does your health now limit you in doing heavy work around the house like scrubbing floors, or lifting or moving heavy furniture? ***	0.11	0.95	0.01	1.59	1.58	2.47	2.51	4.23	4.13
PFB51	Does your health now limit you in participating in active sports such as swimming, tennis, or basketball?	3.41	0.18	0.05	2.23	2.01	2.45	2.64	4.02	3.85
PFA1	**Does your health now limit you in doing vigorous activities, such as running, lifting heavy objects, participating in strenuous sports? ***	1.48	0.48	0.04	1.56	1.44	1.95	2.05	3.69	3.47
PFB7	Does your health now limit you in doing strenuous activities such as backpacking, skiing, playing tennis, bicycling or jogging?	2.27	0.32	0.05	1.46	1.60	2.00	1.96	3.65	3.30
PFA19	Are you able to run or jog for two miles (3 km)?	2.12	0.35	0.02	1.29	1.26	1.25	1.40	2.59	2.57
PFA39	Are you able to run at a fast pace for two miles (3 km)?	3.27	0.19	0.03	1.25	1.35	1.45	1.60	2.51	2.60
PFC7	Are you able to run five miles (8 km)	2.16	0.34	0.03	1.16	1.14	1.23	1.38	2.67	2.49
PFC33	Are you able to run ten miles (16 km)?	99.00	1.00	0.02	1.09	1.07	1.00	1.06	1.59	1.46
PFB30	**Are you able to open a new milk carton? †**	1.07	0.58	0.02	2.85	3.01	3.97	3.93	4.71	4.75

LM = Lagrange multiplier statistic; ES = Effect size statistic; Obs = Average observed item score; Exp = Average expected item score; Items flagged for cross-cultural DIF are presented in bold. *Activity is relatively more difficult to perform for the US general population sample; †Activity is relatively more easy to perform for US general population sample.

using the regression analysis approach. Twenty-five items showed at least some level of uniform DIF in the regression analysis. For 11 of these items, Dutch patients were more likely to endorse lower response options according to the item response curves, indicating that these activities were relatively more difficult for them compared to the US general population. All these items involved the use of the hand or arms (see Table 2). Twelve items were more difficult for US respondents, of which five involved climbing stairs. Consequently, all items referring to climbing stairs were more precise at lower levels of overall physical function in the Dutch RA patients, whereas items involving dexterity tended to have better measurement precision at higher levels of function, as illustrated by two typical item information curves in Figure 2.

In the analysis of cross-cultural DIF in Dutch and US RA patients, the mean was set to zero for the Polimetrix sample and the latent means of the Dutch and Stanford sample were respectively -0.07 and 0.09, indicating that physical function

Table 3. Differential item functioning (DIF) across age and sex in the Dutch RA sample.

Item code	Item stem	LM	P	ES	Obs	Exp	Obs	Exp
Sex					**Female**		**Male**	
PFB28	Are you able to lift 10 pounds (5 kg) above your shoulder?	13.60	<0.01	0.31	3.10	3.39	4.09	3.74
PFA12	Are you able to push open a heavy door?	8.38	<0.01	0.19	3.60	3.76	4.29	4.06
PFA14	Are you able to carry a heavy object (over 10 pounds/5 kg)?	9.56	<0.01	0.28	3.37	3.56	4.17	3.81
PFB39	Are you able to reach and get down a 5 pound (2 kg) object from above your head?	5.51	0.02	0.20	3.45	3.64	4.07	3.84
PFB14	Are you able to take a tub bath?	4.53	0.03	0.16	3.89	4.08	4.35	4.22
PFC45	Are you able to sit on and get up from the toilet?	5.00	0.03	0.10	4.64	4.56	4.61	4.72
PFA29	Are you able to pull heavy objects (10 pounds/ 5 kg) towards yourself?	4.32	0.04	0.18	3.54	3.66	4.16	3.92
					Older		Younger	
PFC13	Are you able to run 100 yards (100 m)?	10.42	<0.01	0.25	2.93	3.27	3.64	3.45
PFC35	Does your health now limit you in doing eight hours of physical labor?	6.32	0.01	0.22	2.37	2.60	3.01	2.79
PFC12	Does your health now limit you in doing two hours of physical labor?	5.07	0.02	0.14	3.25	3.42	3.62	3.50
PFA53	Are you able to run errands and shop?	5.84	0.02	0.11	4.30	4.16	4.21	4.29
PFA4	Does your health now limit you in doing heavy work around the house like scrubbing floors, or lifting or moving heavy furniture?	4.45	0.03	0.14	2.46	2.60	3.01	2.87

LM = Lagrange multiplier statistic; ES= Effect size statistic; Obs = Average observed item score; Exp = Average expected item score.

levels were comparable between the samples. Seven out of 24 items showed significant DIF in the analysis (table 4).

Impact of cross-cultural DIF

In the joint calibration of the Dutch RA data and the US general population data, with country-specific item parameters for the 25 DIF items, the mean of the latent physical function scores was set to 0 (SD = 1) for the US sample and the mean for Dutch RA patients was −1.18 (SD = 1.21), illustrating the considerably lower level of physical function of the Dutch RA patients. This estimate was very close to that observed in the original model without country-specific item parameters (M = −1.01, SD = 1.08), suggesting that the observed item DIF had little impact influence on the average total estimate obtained from all administered items. Moreover, agreement between total estimates was high (ICC = 0.99) and the limits of agreement were narrow, ranging from −0.23 to 0.25 in the Dutch data and from −0.20 to 0.18 in the US data.

Discussion

This study presents the preliminary calibration and cross-cultural evaluation of the Dutch-Flemish translation of the PROMIS physical function (PF) item bank for Dutch patients with RA. The findings of the study indicate that the PROMIS PF item bank is a promising tool for applications such as CAT and tailored short forms in RA patients. However, some concerns remain regarding its cross-cultural measurement equivalence. Using the US-based standardized PROMIS calibration and metric requires further study.

The first principal finding of the current study was that the item bank could be successfully calibrated in a sample of Dutch patients with RA using an appropriate IRT model. To our knowledge, this is the first study to actually demonstrate that the full PROMIS PF item bank can be fitted to an appropriate IRT model in an RA sample. Therefore the current study provides support for the validity of applications of the item bank that require invariant estimates of the item and person parameters, such as CAT or short forms using a metric specific to Dutch patients with RA.

As a general rule, the stability of item parameters increases with more data. In that sense, the item parameters obtained in the current study should be considered preliminary and data that will be collected in future studies with the item bank in Dutch RA patients can be used to update the calibrations. Several ongoing studies in the Netherlands are evaluating the item bank in other patient groups. Future studies should evaluate the equivalence of the resulting item parameters across conditions to evaluate whether a common Dutch metric can be created.

The second principal finding of the study was that 25 of the PROMIS items (20%) showed substantial cross-cultural uniform DIF. The relatively high number of DIF items was not unexpected given that many items assess similar content (e.g. climbing stairs). Moreover, similar percentages of items with cross-cultural DIF are generally identified in scales with fewer items [30,33]. Interestingly, all the PROMIS physical function item bank items that involve climbing stairs were more difficult for the US general population sample, compared to Dutch RA patients. This replicates findings in an earlier study we performed on the cross-cultural equivalence of HAQ-II in US and Dutch RA patients [30]. One speculative explanation for this repeated finding could be that Europeans are more accustomed to climbing stairs, since stairs are more prevalent

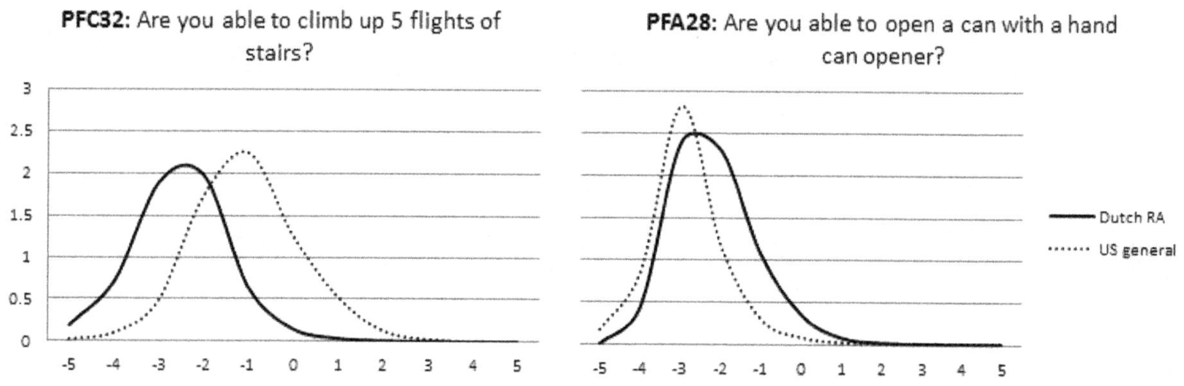

Figure 2. Country specific local measurement precision of two culturally biased items.

in Europe, both in domestic and communal settings. However the US and Dutch sample might have also differed on key variables that might explain the observed DIF. For example body mass index has been linked to stair climbing in previous studies [34]. It would be interesting for future studies to evaluate the presence of body mass index related DIF in the PROMIS physical function items. By contrast, most items that were found to be more difficult for Dutch RA patients refer to activities involving the hands or the arms. This was not a surprising result, considering that disability of particularly the hands is a well-known clinical feature in RA. In fact, we had anticipated to find more DIF items between RA and the general population sample for items measuring dexterity. However, it should be noted that DREAM registry includes patients upon diagnosis with very early RA and these patients are treated aggressively. This is reflected in the average level of disease activity being below the commonly used DAS28 remission criterion of 2.6 and the low levels of disability observed, compared with international benchmarks in RA [35,36]. Therefore, typical

Table 4. Differential item functioning (DIF) across Dutch and US RA patients.

		LM	P	ES	OBS	EXP	OBS	EXP
					Dutch		US	
PFB27	Are you able to tie a knot or a bow?	7.49	0.01	0.11	4.37	4.49	4.72	4.62
PFB20	Are you able to cut a piece of paper with scissors?	2.55	0.11	0.05	4.58	4.63	4.83	4.78
PFA17	Are you able to reach into a high cupboard?	1.07	0.30	0.04	4.13	4.17	4.49	4.46
PFB16	Are you able to press with your index finger (for example ringing a doorbell)?	0.30	0.58	0.02	4.75	4.76	4.89	4.87
PFA19	Are you able to run or jog for two miles (3 km)?	3.67	0.06	0.07	1.74	1.85	2.03	2.01
PFB21	Are you able to pick up coins from a table top?	0.41	0.52	0.03	4.49	4.52	4.73	4.71
PFA23	Are you able to go for a walk of at least 15 minutes?	12.71	<0.01	0.19	4.21	3.98	4.05	4.20
PFA22	Are you able to open previously opened jars?	5.39	0.02	0.09	4.35	4.44	4.56	4.48
PFB25	Are you able to push open a door after turning the knob?	<0.01	0.95	<0.01	4.71	4.71	4.75	4.74
PFB17	Are you able to put on and take off your socks?	0.36	0.55	0.02	4.45	4.47	4.62	4.60
PFB19	Are you able to squeeze a new tube of toothpaste?	4.41	0.04	0.07	4.63	4.70	4.86	4.80
PFB22	Are you able to hold a plate full of food?	1.32	0.25	0.04	4.57	4.61	4.69	4.65
PFA28	Are you able to open a can with a hand can opener?	7.23	0.01	0.13	4.05	4.19	4.35	4.24
PFB24	Are you able to run a short distance, such as to catch a bus?	4.97	0.03	0.13	3.53	3.40	3.30	3.42
PFA18	Are you able to use a hammer to pound a nail?	2.04	0.15	0.06	4.28	4.35	4.58	4.53
PFA16	Are you able to dress yourself, including tying shoelaces and buttoning your clothes?	1.49	0.22	0.03	4.41	4.45	4.59	4.56
PFA20	Are you able to cut your food using eating utensils?	8.65	<0.01	0.10	4.51	4.62	4.81	4.73
PFB23	Are you able to pour liquid from a bottle into a glass?	0.06	0.80	0.01	4.74	4.74	4.75	4.76
PFA21	Are you able to go up and down stairs at a normal pace?	30.32	<0.01	0.24	4.12	3.87	3.89	4.12
PFA25	Are you able to do yard work like raking leaves, weeding, or pushing a lawn mower?	7.77	0.01	0.12	3.67	3.55	3.53	3.64
PFB26	Are you able to shampoo your hair?	1.89	0.17	0.04	4.64	4.68	4.78	4.75
PFA15	Are you able to stand up from an armless straight chair?	35.86	<0.01	0.19	4.51	4.31	4.32	4.50
PFB15	Are you able to change the bulb in a table lamp?	1.44	0.23	0.04	4.62	4.66	4.83	4.79
PFB18	Are you able to shave your face or apply makeup?	0.95	0.33	0.03	4.72	4.75	4.88	4.85

manifestations of RA-related disability may have been absent for many patients in the current study. Moreover, all items with collapsed response options involved measuring disability of the hands and these items showed severe distributional problems, even in the Dutch RA data with very few patients endorsing the lower response options. These two factors limit the sensitivity of the analyses with respect to RA-related DIF, and therefore studies in RA populations with more pronounced disease are desirable.

The results of the DIF analyses suggest that the Dutch RA data is not strictly equivalent to US general population data at the level of individual items, which was also observed in a previous study evaluating a Spanish language version of the item bank [37]. A limitation of the study design is that it cannot be definitively concluded whether observed differences in response probabilities conditional on overall level of function occurred because of disease characteristics or cross-cultural differences, since not all items were administered to US RA patients and no general population Dutch data is yet available. However, previous studies have generally shown European versions of physical function instruments to be equivalent to US versions in arthritis populations [30,33], while substantial DIF has been observed across rheumatic conditions in one previous study [38]. It also seems unlikely that observed DIF occurred as a result of translation errors, given the rigorous approach in translating and that all items refer to everyday activities that are very common in both US and The Netherlands. For these reasons, more studies are needed before firm conclusions regarding the measurement equivalence can be made. If such studies consistently identify certain items to exhibit DIF, their item parameters can still be expressed on a common metric by assigning group-specific item parameters to biased items. This allows cross-cultural comparison even in the presence of significantly biased items and physical function levels to be expressed on the PROMIS standardized metric if this is desired. In the mean time we recommend that those interested in expressing physical function levels of Dutch RA patients on the PROMIS standardized metric to select only items that were not flagged for DIF in the current study.

In the analysis of impact of DIF on total EAP estimates of physical function, we observed that biased items appeared to have a negligible influence on total physical function estimates from all items that were administered to patients at baseline. It should be stressed though that patients were administered between 48 and 72 items which is likely to be greater than the number of items that will be administered in practical applications of the item bank. In a recent validation study of a PROMIS PF CAT only four items were administered on average to obtain physical function estimates [39]. The impact of DIF on physical function estimates is likely to be greater in such situations, provided that the item characteristics of biased items make them likely to be selected in such an application. Future studies should further evaluate the impact on physical function estimates in situations were fewer items are administered.

In the current study we used different methods to identify DIF. Whenever possible, DIF was evaluated using LM statistics. An advantage of this method is that violations of model assumptions can be investigated within a framework that directly pertains to the observed scores. As a result, the magnitude and direction of DIF can also be directly inferred from a weighted difference between average observed and average expected scores. In the regression analysis the direction of DIF had to be inferred indirectly by inspecting the response curves and item information functions visually. A limitation of the DIF analysis is therefore that no qualifications regarding the magnitude of DIF could be given in the current study of equivalence with the PROMIS wave 1 general population data. The reason we resorted to the regression analysis in the analysis of cross-cultural equivalence was that the US general population data suffered from severe ceiling effects, with the majority of respondents endorsing the higher response options. Consequently, insufficient variability was present within total score level groups for the LM test to produce interpretable results. For this reason also, no indication of model fit could be given for the US data. The longitudinal DIF analysis could not be performed with the LM test since the test compares scores on individual items between two groups, but in the longitudinal design, each item was presented to each patient only once.

In summary, the results of this study show that the PROMIS physical function item bank could be fitted to an IRT model that assumes physical function to be a unidimensional trait. However, a substantial number of its items showed statistically significant DIF compared to the US general population wave 1 data. Although the impact of observed DIF on physical function estimates was minimal in this study, more studies are needed to evaluate the validity of the PROMIS standardized metric in RA patients in the Netherlands.

Author Contributions

Conceived and designed the experiments: MOV CG PTK MVDL EK. Performed the experiments: MOV CG. Analyzed the data: MOV CG PTK CBT. Contributed reagents/materials/analysis tools: HV ET EK HM MVDL PVR CBT MB. Wrote the paper: MOV PTK CG HV ET EK HM MB CBT PVR MVDL.

References

1. Felson DT, Anderson JJ, Boers M, Bombardier C, Chernoff M, et al. (1993) The American College of Rheumatology preliminary core set of disease activity measures for rheumatoid arthritis clinical trials. The Committee on Outcome Measures in Rheumatoid Arthritis Clinical Trials. Arthritis Rheum 36: 729–740.
2. Wolfe F, Lassere M, van der Heijde D, Stucki G, Suarez-Almazor M, et al. (1999) Preliminary core set of domains and reporting requirements for longitudinal observational studies in rheumatology. J Rheumatol 26: 484–489.
3. Pincus T, Summey JA, Soraci SA, Jr., Wallston KA, Hummon NP (1983) Assessment of patient satisfaction in activities of daily living using a modified Stanford Health Assessment Questionnaire. Arthritis Rheum 26: 1346–1353.
4. Stucki G, Stucki S, Bruhlmann P, Michel BA (1995) Ceiling effects of the Health Assessment Questionnaire and its modified version in some ambulatory rheumatoid arthritis patients. Ann Rheum Dis 54: 461–465.
5. Pincus T, Swearingen C, Wolfe F (1999) Toward a multidimensional Health Assessment Questionnaire (MDHAQ): assessment of advanced activities of daily living and psychological status in the patient-friendly health assessment questionnaire format. Arthritis Rheum 42: 2220–2230.
6. Wolfe F, Michaud K, Pincus T (2004) Development and validation of the health assessment questionnaire II: a revised version of the health assessment questionnaire. Arthritis Rheum 50: 3296–3305.
7. Pincus T, Sokka T, Kautiainen H (2005) Further development of a physical function scale on a MDHAQ [corrected] for standard care of patients with rheumatic diseases. J Rheumatol 32: 1432–1439.
8. Oude Voshaar MA, Ten Klooster PM, Taal E, van de Laar MA (2011) Measurement properties of physical function scales validated for use in patients with rheumatoid arthritis: A systematic review of the literature. Health Qual Life Outcomes 9: 99.
9. Fries JF, Cella D, Rose M, Krishnan E, Bruce B (2009) Progress in assessing physical function in arthritis: PROMIS short forms and computerized adaptive testing. J Rheumatol 36: 2061–2066.
10. Rose M, Bjorner JB, Becker J, Fries JF, Ware JE (2008) Evaluation of a preliminary physical function item bank supported the expected advantages of the Patient-Reported Outcomes Measurement Information System (PROMIS). J Clin Epidemiol 61: 17–33.
11. Cella D, Yount S, Rothrock N, Gershon R, Cook K, et al. (2007) The Patient-Reported Outcomes Measurement Information System (PROMIS): progress of an NIH Roadmap cooperative group during its first two years. Med Care 45: S3–S11.
12. Hays RD, Spritzer KL, Fries JF, Krishnan E (2013) Responsiveness and minimally important difference for the Patient-Reported Outcomes Measure-

ment Information System (PROMIS) 20-item physical functioning short form in a prospective observational study of rheumatoid arthritis. Ann Rheum Dis.
13. Terwee CB, Roorda LD, de Vet HC, Dekker J, Westhovens R, et al. (2014) Dutch-Flemish translation of 17 item banks from the Patient-Reported Outcomes Measurement Information System (PROMIS). Qual Life Res.
14. Oude Voshaar MA, Ten Klooster PM, Taal E, Krishnan E, van de Laar MA (2012) Dutch translation and cross-cultural adaptation of the PROMIS(R) physical function item bank and cognitive pre-test in Dutch arthritis patients. Arthritis Res Ther 14: R47.
15. Hambleton RK, Swaminathan H, Rogers HJ (1991) Fundamentals of item response theory: Sage.
16. Ellis BB (1989) Differential item functioning: Implications for test translations. Journal of Applied Psychology 74: 912.
17. Holman R, Lindeboom R, Glas CA, Vermeulen M, de Haan RJ (2003) Constructing an item bank using item response theory: the AMC Linear Disability Score project. Health Services and Outcomes Research Methodology 4: 19–33.
18. Kim S-H, Cohen AS (2002) A comparison of linking and concurrent calibration under the graded response model. Applied Psychological Measurement 26: 25–41.
19. Cella D, Riley W, Stone A, Rothrock N, Reeve B, et al. (2010) The Patient-Reported Outcomes Measurement Information System (PROMIS) developed and tested its first wave of adult self-reported health outcome item banks: 2005–2008. J Clin Epidemiol 63: 1179–1194.
20. Terwee CB, Roorda LD, De Vet HC, Dekker J, Westhovens R, et al. (submitted for publication) Dutch-Flemish translation of 17 item banks from the Patient Reported Outcomes Measurement Information System (PROMIS).
21. Fries JF, Spitz P, Kraines RG, Holman HR (1980) Measurement of patient outcome in arthritis. Arthritis Rheum 23: 137–145.
22. Fries JF (2009) The Health Assessment Questionnaire (HAQ) and the Improved HAQ. Stanford: Stanford University School of Medicine, Division of Immunology & Rheumatology.
23. Ware JE, Jr., Sherbourne CD (1992) The MOS 36-item short-form health survey (SF-36). I. Conceptual framework and item selection. Med Care 30: 473–483.
24. ten Klooster PM, Vonkeman HE, Taal E, Siemons L, Hendriks L, et al. (2013) Performance of the Dutch SF-36 version 2 as a measure of health-related quality of life in patients with rheumatoid arthritis. Health Qual Life Outcomes 11: 77.
25. Prevoo ML, van 't Hof MA, Kuper HH, van Leeuwen MA, van de Putte LB, et al. (1995) Modified disease activity scores that include twenty-eight-joint counts. Development and validation in a prospective longitudinal study of patients with rheumatoid arthritis. Arthritis Rheum 38: 44–48.
26. Glas CA (2010) Preliminary manual of the software program Multidimensional Item Response Theory (MIRT). University of Twente, Enschede, The Netherlands.
27. Muraki E (1992) A generalized partial credit model: Application of an EM algorithm. Appl Psychol Meas 16: 159–176.
28. te Marvelde JM, Glas CA, Van Landeghem G, Van Damme J (2006) Application of multidimensional item response theory models to longitudinal data. Educational and Psychological Measurement 66: 5–34.
29. Glas CAW (1999) Modification indices for the 2-PL and the nominal response model. Psychometrika 64: 273–294.
30. Oude Voshaar MA, Glas CA, Ten Klooster PM, Taal E, Wolfe F, et al. (2013) Crosscultural Measurement Equivalence of the Health Assessment Questionnaire II. Arthritis Care Res (Hoboken) 65: 1000–1004.
31. Glas CAW (1998) Detection of differential item functioning using Lagrange multiplier tests. Statistica Sinica 8: 647–668.
32. Bland JM, Altman DG (1986) Statistical methods for assessing agreement between two methods of clinical measurement. Lancet 1: 307–310.
33. Roorda L, Jones C, Waltz M, Lankhorst G, Bouter L, et al. (2004) Satisfactory cross cultural equivalence of the Dutch WOMAC in patients with hip osteoarthritis waiting for arthroplasty. Annals of the rheumatic diseases 63: 36.
34. Vincent HK, Vincent KR, Lamb KM (2010) Obesity and mobility disability in the older adult. Obes Rev 11: 568–579.
35. Krishnan E, Tugwell P, Fries JF (2004) Percentile benchmarks in patients with rheumatoid arthritis: Health Assessment Questionnaire as a quality indicator (QI). Arthritis Res Ther 6: R505–513.
36. van Riel PL, van Gestel AM (2000) Clinical outcome measures in rheumatoid arthritis. Ann Rheum Dis 59 Suppl 1: i28–31.
37. Paz SH, Spritzer KL, Morales LS, Hays RD (2013) Evaluation of the Patient-Reported Outcomes Information System (PROMIS((R))) Spanish-language physical functioning items. Qual Life Res 22: 1819–1830.
38. van Groen MM, ten Klooster PM, Taal E, van de Laar MA, Glas CA (2010) Application of the health assessment questionnaire disability index to various rheumatic diseases. Qual Life Res 19: 1255–1263.
39. Hung M, Baumhauer JF, Latt LD, Saltzman CL, Soohoo NF, et al. (2013) Validation of PROMIS Physical Function Computerized Adaptive Tests for Orthopaedic Foot and Ankle Outcome Research. Clin Orthop Relat Res 471: 3466–3474.

27

Anti-Cyclic Citrullinated Peptide Antibody Is Associated with Interstitial Lung Disease in Patients with Rheumatoid Arthritis

Yufeng Yin[1☉], **Di Liang**[1☉], **Lidan Zhao**[1], **Yang Li**[1], **Wei Liu**[2], **Yan Ren**[1], **Yongzhe Li**[1], **Xiaofeng Zeng**[1], **Fengchun Zhang**[1], **Fulin Tang**[1], **Guangliang Shan**[3], **Xuan Zhang**[1*]

1 Department of Rheumatology, Peking Union Medical College Hospital, Chinese Academy of Medical Sciences and Peking Union Medical College, Beijing, China, 2 Department of Radiology, Peking Union Medical College Hospital, Chinese Academy of Medical Sciences and Peking Union Medical College, Beijing, China, 3 Department of Epidemiology, Institute of Basic Medical Sciences, Chinese Academy of Medical Sciences and Peking Union Medical College, Beijing, China

Abstract

Objective: Patients with rheumatoid arthritis (RA) are at risk to develop RA-associated interstitial lung disease (RA-ILD). This retrospective study aimed to investigate the potential association of the positivity of serum anti-cyclic citrullinated peptide antibody (anti-CCP2) and rheumatoid factor (RF) with RA-ILD in RA patients.

Methods: A total of 285 RA patients were recruited at the inpatient service of Peking Union Medical College Hospital in China between 2004 and 2013. Individual patients were evaluated for the evidence of ILD. The concentrations of serum anti-CCP2 and RF in individual patients were measured. The potential risk factors for ILD in RA patients were assessed by univariate and multivariate models.

Results: There were 71 RA patients with RA-ILD, accounting for 24.9% in this population. The positive rates of anti-CCP2 and RF in the patients with RA-ILD were significantly higher than that in the patients with RA-only (88.7% vs. 67.3%, $p<0.001$; 84.5% vs. 70.6%, $p=0.02$, respectively). Univariate and multivariate logistic regression analysis revealed that RA patients with positive serum anti-CCP2, but not RF, were associated with an increased risk of ILD (crude odds ratio [cOR] 3.83, 95% confidence interval [CI] 1.74–8.43, $p<0.001$; adjusted odds ratio [aOR] 3.50, 95% CI 1.52–8.04, $p<0.001$).

Conclusion: Our findings suggest that positive serum anti-CCP2, but not RF, may be associated with RA-ILD in RA patients.

Editor: Song Guo Zheng, Penn State University, United States of America

Funding: This study is supported by the grants of the National Natural Science Foundation of China (30972731, 81172859, 81273312, 81302594), the National High Technology Research and Development Project of China (2011AA020111, 2012AA02A513), the National Major Scientific and Technological Special Project (2012ZX09303006-002), the Research Special Fund for Public Welfare Industry of Health (201202004), the Capital Health Research and Development of Special (2011-4001-02), and the National laboratory Special Fund (2060204). The funders had no role in study design, data collection and analysis, decision to publish, or preparation of the manuscript.

Competing Interests: The authors have declared that no competing interests exist.

* E-mail: zxpumch2003@sina.com

☉ These authors contributed equally to this work.

Introduction

Patients with rheumatoid arthritis (RA) display high levels of autoantibodies as well as extra-articular manifestations, such as interstitial lung disease (ILD) [1–3]. The RA-related interstitial lung disease (RA-ILD) occurs in nearly 7–10% of the RA patients, and often is associated with a poor prognosis [4,5]. Therefore, the discovery of risk factors contributing to the development of ILD will be of great significance in the prevention and intervention of patients with RA-ILD.

Autoantibodies are valuable biomarkers for the diagnosis of RA and extra-articular manifestations. Antibodies against cyclic citrullinated peptides (anti-CCP2) and rheumatoid factor (RF) have been identified in patients with RA [6]. Previous studies have shown that the specificity and sensitivity of anti-CCP2 detection for the diagnosis of RA are 96–99% and 47–88% respectively, dependent on the characteristics of the RA population [6,7]. Anti-CCP2 antibodies may be implicated in the pathogenesis of RA and are valuable for evaluating the erosive or non-erosive progression of articular injury in RA patients [8,9]. In addition, anti-CCP2 antibodies have been shown to be highly specific or independently associated with the development of extra-articular manifestations, including ischemic heart disease [10], type 1 diabetes mellitus [11], serositis [12], and subclinical atherosclerosis in patients with RA [13]. RF is another autoantibody most commonly detected in RA [1,14]. Detection of both anti-CCP2 and RF has additional values for the early diagnosis of RA, particularly for those with RA at early stage of the disease process [15].

However, the potential association of anti-CCP2 and RF with the development of ILD in RA patients remains controversial [16–18]. There is little information about whether anti-CCP2 antibodies or RF are associated with ILD in RA patients. In this study, we tested the levels of serum anti-CCP2 and RF in 285 patients with RA and analyzed the potential factors that were correlated with ILD in this population.

Methods

Ethics statement

The experimental protocol was approved by the Institute Review Board of Peking Union Medical College Hospital. All patients provide their written informed consent to participate in this study.

Study population

This study was approved by the Institute Review Board of Peking Union Medical College Hospital. A total of 285 patients with RA were recruited at the inpatient service of the Department of Rheumatology of Peking Union Medical College Hospital from January 2004 to October 2013. All patients fulfilled the criteria for the diagnosis of RA revised by the American College of Rheumatology (ACR) in 1987 [1]. Patients with RA-ILD were diagnosed by the presence of typical features in the lung by high-resolution computerized tomography (HRCT). The chest HRCT scans were evaluated by an expert radiologist in a blinded manner. According to the consensus for idiopathic interstitial pneumonias of the American Thoracic Society/European Respiratory Society (ATS/ERS) [19], the features of HRCT included irregular linear or reticular opacities, ground-glass opacities, consolidation, honeycombing, septal thickening, and traction bronchiectasis or bronchiolectasis. The disease activity of individual patients was evaluated by disease activity score in 28 joints (DAS28) [20,21]. Individuals were excluded if she/he had a history of ILD before the diagnosis of RA, other chronic lung diseases or incomplete medical record.

Clinical assessment

The demographic and clinical data of individual patients were retrospectively reviewed. These data included age, gender, disease duration, and cigarette smoking, co-existent autoimmune diseases, such as systemic lupus erythematosus (SLE), polymyositis/dermatomyositis (PM/DM), systemic sclerosis (SSc) and Sjögren's syndrome. The disease duration was defined from the onset of joint swelling and/or tenderness. Individuals with previous history of treatment with biological or general disease-modifying anti-rheumatic drugs (DMARDs) and corticosteroids for more than three months were recorded.

Blood samples were obtained from individual patients when they first visited to our institution. The positivity for serum anti-CCP2 (≥25 U/ml) and RF (≥15 IU/ml) in these patients was determined by enzyme linked immunosorbent assay (ELISA) using the specific kit (Euroimmun, Lübeck, Germany) and nephelometry method (Behring, Germany), respectively. The concentrations of serum C-reactive protein (CRP) as well as the value of erythrocyte sedimentation rate (ESR) in individual patients were routinely examined.

Statistical analyses

All values are expressed as the mean ± SD or median with interquartile range (IQR) for normally and non-normally distributed data, respectively. The difference in individual variables between the RA-ILD and RA-only groups was analyzed by univariate model. Comparison of continuous data was performed using independent Student's t and Mann-Whitney non-parametric U test for normal and non-normal data respectively, and of categorical data using the Pearson Chi-square test or Fisher's exact test. The stratification analyses for age and disease duration were conducted by Cochran-Mantel-Haenszel Chi-square test. The relationship of individual variables with RA-ILD was analyzed using a multivariate logistic regression model with stepwise selected variables. The collinearity of variables was assessed and explained by variance inflation factor (VIF) greater than 4.0 and tolerance less than 0.25 [22]. All statistical analyses were performed using the SPSS software (version 17.0, SPSS Inc., Chicago, IL, USA) and a two-tailed P-value of less than 0.05 was considered statistically significant.

Results

Patients and clinical characteristics

To determine the potential risk factors associated with ILD, a total of 285 patients with RA were recruited. Their demographic and clinical characteristics are summarized in **Table 1**. There were 71 patients with ILD, accounting for 24.9% in this population. The RA-ILD patients were significantly older and had significantly longer duration than that of the RA-only group of patients. However, there was no significant difference in the distribution of gender and in the percentages of smokers between the RA-only and RA-ILD groups of patients.

There was no significant difference in the percentages of complications and treatment history between these two groups of patients. Both groups of patients had similar levels of disease severity, the concentrations of serum CRP and ESR. There were 61 (21.4%) patients who had at least one other connective tissue disease (CTD), including 7 patients with SSc, 41 Sjögren's Syndrome, 4 PM/DM, and 16 SLE. There were 234 (82.1%), 180 (63.2%), 38 (13.3%) and 227 (79.6%) of patients receiving medication of prednisone, methotrexate, biological DMARD, or chemical DMARD, respectively (**Table 1**).

HRCT features and anti-CCP2 and RF status

In 71 patients with RA-ILD, HRCT scans of the lung revealed 48 cases with irregular line or reticular opacities, 22 cases with ground-glass attenuation, 26 cases with basal consolidation, 10 patients with honey-combing, 27 patients with septal thickening and 12 patients with traction bronchiectasis or bronchiolectasis. However, these HRCT characteristics were not significantly associated with the positivity of anti-CCP2 and RF in these patients (**Table 2**).

The relationship between RA-ILD and anti-CCP2 or RF

Characterization of the levels of serum anti-CCP2 and RF revealed that 207 (72.6%) serum samples were positive for anti-CCP2 and 211 (74.0%) were positive for RF in this population. Both the positivity rates of anti-CCP2 and RF were significantly higher ($p<0.001$ and $p=0.02$ respectively) in the group of RA-ILD than RA-only (**Table 1**). Cochran-Mantel-Haenszel stratification analyses indicated that the percentages of anti-CCP2 positivity were significantly associated with older age and longer disease duration (OR_{M-H} 3.3, 95% CI 1.5–7.1, $p=0.003$ and OR_{M-H} 3.9, 95% CI 1.7–8.7, $p=0.001$, respectively) (**Table 3**).

Univariate and multivariate logistic regression analysis

Univariate logistic regression analysis revealed that age and disease duration were risk factors for RA-ILD (crude odds ratio [cOR] 1.06, 95% CI 1.03–1.09, $p<0.001$; and cOR 1.04, 95% CI 1.01–1.07, $p<0.001$ respectively). Treatment with methotrexate (MTX) or other chemical DMARDs was not significantly associated with RA-ILD (cOR 0.58, 95% CI 0.34–1.01,

Table 1. The demographic and clinical characteristics of patients.

Characteristics	All patients	RA-ILD	RA-only	p-value
Patients, n (%)	285 (100)	71 (24.9)	214 (75.1)	—
Age, mean (SD), years	51.7 (13.4)	58.3 (11.2)	49.5 (13.4)	<0.001
Female, n (%)	211 (74.0)	50 (70.4)	161 (75.2)	0.44
Disease duration, median (IQR), years	5.0 (1.0–12.0)	9.0 (2.0–18.0)	4.0 (1.0–10.1)	0.003
Cigarette smoking, n (%)	59 (20.7)	18 (25.4)	41 (19.2)	0.31
Complication With other CTD*, n (%)	61 (21.4)	15 (21.1)	46 (21.5)	1.0
Laboratory test				
Anti-CCP2, n (%)	207 (72.6)	63 (88.7)	144 (67.3)	<0.001
RF, n (%)	211 (74.0)	60 (84.5)	151 (70.6)	0.02
CRP, mean (SD), mg/dL	40.2 (56.3)	42.6 (75.4)	39.4 (48.5)	0.68
ESR, mean (SD), mm/h	56.2 (34.5)	56.6 (33.2)	56.1 (35.0)	0.93
DAS28, mean (SD)	5.4 (1.7)	5.2 (1.8)	5.5 (1.7)	0.13
Treatment history, n (%)				
Prednisone	234 (82.1)	58 (81.7)	176 (82.2)	1.0
Methotrexate	180 (63.2)	38 (53.5)	142 (66.4)	0.07
Biological DMARD	38 (13.3)	6 (8.5)	32 (15.0)	0.23
Chemical DMARD	227 (79.6)	52 (73.2)	175 (81.8)	0.13

RA-ILD: rheumatoid arthritis-associated interstitial lung disease; RA-only: rheumatoid arthritis without interstitial lung disease; IQR: interquartile range; CTD: autoimmune disease; CRP: C-reactive protein; ESR: erythrocyte sedimentation rate; DAS28: disease activity score with 28 joints;
*Other CTD included systemic lupus erythematosus, polymyositis/dermatomyositis, systemic scleroderma and Sjögren's syndrome.

p = 0.05, and cOR 0.61, 95% CI 0.32–1.14, p = 0.12; respectively). The positivity of anti-CCP2 and RF was significantly associated with ILD in RA patients (cOR 3.83; 95% CI 1.74–8.43, p<0.001; and cOR 2.28; 95% CI 1.12–4.61, p = 0.02 respectively). Further stratification of low, moderate and high levels of RF indicated that only high levels of serum RF (≥364.0 IU/ml) were associated with ILD in RA patients (p = 0.02). After adjustment of age and disease duration together with the absence of collinearity (VIF and tolerance were 1.03 and 0.97 respectively) and other related co-variables (**Table 4**), the positivity of anti-CCP2 remained a risk factor for ILD in RA patients (adjusted odds ratio [aOR] 3.50; 95% CI 1.52–8.04, p<0.001), regardless of the level of anti-CCP. However, after adjusting confounding factors including gender, age, disease duration, smoking, medications and other CTD complication, there was no significant association between any level of low, moderate and high positivity of RF and RA-ILD in this population (**Table 4**).

Discussion

The pulmonary manifestations in RA patients was firstly reported half a century ago [23] and affect 10 to 20% of RA patients, which is associated with increased mortality [24]. The ILD has been recognized as the most common complication in the lung of RA patients. In this retrospective study, we evaluated the potential factors that contributed to ILD in RA patients. We found that 24.9% RA patients suffered with ILD, which was higher than that reported [3,4]. The high rate of patients with ILD may be due to long disease duration in a large proportion of our RA patients. Indeed, we found that RA patients with ILD were significantly older and had longer duration than those patients without ILD in this population. Alternatively, the high rate of patients with ILD may stem from unique genetic background.

Some other risk factors for RA-ILD should also be considered in multivariate analysis of the associations of anti-CCP2 positivity with the RA-ILD. Firstly, a previous study has showed that ILD is a severe clinical entity presented in many

Table 2. The relationship between HRCT features and antibody status of anti-CCP2 and RF in patients with RA-ILD.

HRCT feature	Anti-CCP2 (+)	Anti-CCP2 (−)	p	RF (+)	RF (−)	p
Irregular line/reticular opacities, n (%)	43 (68.3)	5 (62.5)	0.71	39 (65.0)	9 (81.8)	0.49
Ground-glass attenuation, n (%)	21 (33.3)	1 (12.5)	0.42	20 (33.3)	2 (18.2)	0.48
Basal consolidation, n (%)	23 (36.5)	3 (37.5)	1.0	20 (33.3)	6 (54.5)	0.19
Honey-combing, n (%)	8 (12.7)	2 (25.0)	0.31	9 (15.0)	1 (9.1)	1.0
Septal thickening, n (%)	24 (38.1)	3 (37.5)	1.0	24 (40.0)	3 (27.3)	0.52
Traction bronchiectasis/bronchiolectasis, n (%)	9 (14.3)	3 (37.5)	0.13	10 (16.7)	2 (18.2)	1.0

Table 3. Stratification analyses of the association of anti-CCP2 with ILD in RA patients.

	RA-ILD	RA-only	OR_{M-H} (CI 95%)	p
Age				
<46 years, n (%)	14 (15.1)	79 (84.9)		
47–58 years, n (%)	19 (19.4)	79 (80.6)	3.3 (1.5–7.1)	0.003
>59 years, n (%)	38 (40.4)	56 (59.6)		
Disease duration				
<1.9 years, n (%)	17 (20.5)	66 (79.5)		
2.0–9.9 years, n (%)	19 (18.6)	83 (81.4)	3.9 (1.7–8.7)	0.001
>10.0 years, n (%)	35 (35.0)	65 (65.0)		

OR_{M-H}: Mantel-Haenszel odds ratio. 95% CI: 95% confidence interval. Age and disease duration of all patients were divided into three equal groups.

connective tissue diseases [25]. However, anti-CCP2 has been demonstrated to be extremely specific (96–98%) in patients with RA [26], but only 13.8% with SLE, 2.6% with SSc [27] and 7.5–9% with pSS [28,29]. In our study, 21.4% of patients had at least one other autoimmune disease besides RA and these patients distributed similarly in the RA-only and RA-ILD groups. Further univariate and multivariate analyses revealed that these comorbidities did not affect the significant association of the anti-CCP2 positivity with RA-ILD in this population. Secondly, we stratified patients, according to the radiologic features by HRCT and we found that there was no significant difference in the anti-CCP2 positivity among these subgroups of patients,which was in consistent with a previous report [16]. Thirdly, MTX has been considered as the standard therapy of DMARDs for RA patients. Although MTX has been considered as a low toxic drug, MTX treatment of patients with pre-existing RA-ILD can cause fatal complication [30]. In our study, we did not observe that treatment with MTX resulted in a fatal outcome. There was no significant difference in the anti-CCP2 positivity between the patients receiving MTX treatment and those without MTX treatment. Thus, MTX treatment may not affect the levels of serum anti-CCP2 in RA patients. Finally, we did not observe that regular smoking was associated with RA-ILD in this population of RA patients, which was in consistent with previous reports [31].

The positivity of anti-CCP2 and RF is valuable for the diagnosis of RA. We found that the percentages of patients with positive anti-CCP2 and/or RF in the RA-ILD group were significantly higher than that in the RA-only group. Further analysis revealed that the percentages of the older patients with anti-CCP2 positivity in the RA-ILD group were significantly higher than that in the RA-only group. The univariate model of logistic regression analyses indicated that the different levels of serum anti-CCP2, but only high levels of RF were associated with ILD in this population of RA patients. Further adjusting other covariates revealed that the positivity of anti-CCP2 was significantly correlated with ILD in RA patients. Our data were in consistent with recent reports in France [18] and Greece [12] and similar to that in Japan [32]. However, there was no significant difference in the positivity of anti-CCP2 between the RA patients with and without ILD in another Japanese population [16] and a Korean population [17]. The difference among these studies may come from difference in patient population, disease definition or methodology for detecting clinical parameters. The variable sensitivity and specificity of the methods for anti-CCP2 detection may also affect its value in evaluating the association with ILD. The significantly higher positivity in the RA-ILD patients indicated that the positivity of anti-CCP2 may be a good biomarker for the diagnosis of ILD in RA patients.

Table 4. Univariate and multivariate analyses of the associations of anti-CCP2 positivity with the RA-ILD.

	Univariate associations			Multivariate associations		
	β	cOR (95% CI)	p	β	aOR (95% CI)	p
Age	0.06	1.06 (1.03–1.09)	<0.001	0.05	1.06 (1.03–1.08)	<0.001
Disease duration	0.04	1.04 (1.01–1.07)	<0.001	0.04	1.04 (1.01–1.07)	0.02
Anti-CCP2						
Seropositive	1.34	3.83 (1.74–8.43)	<0.001	1.25	3.50 (1.52–8.04)	<0.001
Low positive	1.27	3.57 (1.46–8.76)	0.01	1.24	3.46 (1.35–8.89)	0.01
Moderate positive	1.54	4.67 (1.93–11.29)	0.00	1.44	4.22 (1.63–10.90)	0.003
High positive	1.20	3.32 (1.35–8.20)	0.01	1.08	2.96 (1.14–7.67)	0.03
RF						
Seropositive	0.82	2.28 (1.12–4.61)	0.02	−0.04	0.96 (0.38–2.44)	0.93
Low positive	0.74	2.10 (0.91–4.86)	0.08	0.38	1.46 (0.54–3.94)	0.45
Moderate positive	0.75	2.12 (0.93–4.82)	0.07	0.25	1.28 (0.45–3.66)	0.65
High positive	0.97	2.63 (1.16–5.93)	0.02	0.66	1.93 (0.68–5.47)	0.21

Univariate and multivariate associations of anti-CCP2 with the occurrence of RA-ILD was conducted by logistic regression with a backward stepwise model. Covariates in multivariate model included gender, age, disease duration, smoking, medication, and other CTD complication. β: partial regression coefficient; DMARDs: disease-modifying antirheumatic drugs; Anti-CCP2: anti-citrullinated peptide antibody; COR: crude odds ratio; AOR: adjusted odds ratio; 95% CI: 95% confidence interval. Three equal groups of low, moderate and high positive anti-CCP2 were defined as 25.0≤anti-CCP2<271.3 U/ml, 271.3≤anti-CCP2<941.2 U/ml and anti-CCP2≥941.2 U/ml, respectively. Three equal groups of low, moderate and high positive RF were defined as 15.0≤RF<114.0 IU/ml, 114.0≤RF<364.0 IU/ml and RF≥364.0 IU/ml, respectively.

We recognized that our study had limitations. We could not exclude the potential selection bias in our patients although individual patients were diagnosed as having ILD, according to the available diagnostic criteria [33]. Previous studies have estimated the prevalence of ILD in RA patients being about 3.7–33.0% in those without significant abnormal chest X-ray or respiratory symptoms [34–36]. It is possible that we may underestimate the prevalence of ILD in RA patients. In addition, we did exclude individual patients without complete medical records and those developed ILD prior to their RA diagnosis. Moreover, we had no complete medical records of all participants so that we were unable to evaluate whether a delay in treatment of patients with MTX and DMADRs can be a risk factor of ILD in RA patients. Finally, the small sample size in our study may interfere with some results, such as the lack of significant difference in the positivity of anti-CCP2 in different subtypes of ILD in this population. Furthermore, small sample size can lead to a false positive result and overestimate the magnitude of an association, particularly in a situation with multiple confounding variants. Therefore, further study in a bigger population is warranted to validate the value of anti-CCP2 positivity in evaluating the prognosis of ILD in RA patients.

In summary, we found significantly higher positivity of anti-CCP2 in RA patients with ILD than that in the RA alone patients. Our findings indicated that the positivity of anti-CCP2 is associated with ILD in RA patients.

Author Contributions

Conceived and designed the experiments: YY Yongzhe Li XZ FZ FT XZ. Performed the experiments: YY DL LZ Yang Li WL YR. Analyzed the data: YY DL GS. Contributed reagents/materials/analysis tools: Yongzhe Li XZ FZ FT XZ. Wrote the paper: YY DL.

References

1. Arnett FC, Edworthy SM, Bloch DA, McShane DJ, Fries JF, et al. (1988) The American Rheumatism Association 1987 revised criteria for the classification of rheumatoid arthritis. Arthritis Rheum 31: 315–324. PubMed: 3358796
2. Turesson C, O'Fallon WM, Crowson CS, Gabriel SE, Matteson EL (2003) Extra-articular disease manifestations in rheumatoid arthritis: incidence trends and risk factors over 46 years. Ann Rheum Dis 62: 722–727. PubMed: 12860726
3. Koduri G, Norton S, Young A, Cox N, Davies P, et al. (2010) Interstitial lung disease has a poor prognosis in rheumatoid arthritis: results from an inception cohort. Rheumatology (Oxford) 49: 1483–1489. PubMed: 20223814
4. Olson AL, Swigris JJ, Sprunger DB, Fischer A, Fernandez-Perez ER, et al. (2011) Rheumatoid arthritis-interstitial lung disease-associated mortality. Am J Respir Crit Care Med 183: 372–378. PubMed: 20851924
5. Turesson C, Matteson EL (2004) Management of extra-articular disease manifestations in rheumatoid arthritis. Curr Opin Rheumatol 16: 206–211. PubMed: 15103246
6. Zeng X, Ai M, Tian X, Gan X, Shi Y, et al. (2003) Diagnostic value of anti-cyclic citrullinated Peptide antibody in patients with rheumatoid arthritis. J Rheumatol 30: 1451–1455. PubMed: 12858440
7. Rodriguez-Mahou M, Lopez-Longo FJ, Sanchez-Ramon S, Estecha A, Garcia-Segovia A, et al. (2006) Association of anti-cyclic citrullinated peptide and anti-Sa/citrullinated vimentin autoantibodies in rheumatoid arthritis. Arthritis Rheum 55: 657–661. PubMed: 16874789
8. Rantapää-Dahlqvist S, de Jong BAW, Berglin E, Hallmans G, Wadell G, et al. (2003) Antibodies against cyclic citrullinated peptide and IgA rheumatoid factor predict the development of rheumatoid arthritis. Arthritis & Rheumatism 48: 2741–2749. PubMed: 14558078
9. Reparon-Schuijt CC, van Esch WJ, van Kooten C, Schellekens GA, de Jong BA, et al. (2001) Secretion of anti-citrulline-containing peptide antibody by B lymphocytes in rheumatoid arthritis. Arthritis Rheum 44: 41–47. PubMed: 11212174
10. Lopez-Longo FJ, Oliver-Minarro D, de la Torre I, Gonzalez-Diaz de Rabago E, Sanchez-Ramon S, et al. (2009) Association between anti-cyclic citrullinated peptide antibodies and ischemic heart disease in patients with rheumatoid arthritis. Arthritis Rheum 61: 419–424. PubMed: 19333979
11. Liao KP, Gunnarsson M, Kallberg H, Ding B, Plenge RM, et al. (2009) Specific association of type 1 diabetes mellitus with anti-cyclic citrullinated peptide-positive rheumatoid arthritis. Arthritis Rheum 60: 653–660. PubMed: 19248096
12. Alexiou I, Germenis A, Koutroumpas A, Kontogianni A, Theodoridou K, et al. (2008) Anti-cyclic citrullinated peptide-2 (CCP2) autoantibodies and extra-articular manifestations in Greek patients with rheumatoid arthritis. Clin Rheumatol 27: 511–513. PubMed: 18172572
13. Gerli R, Bartoloni Bocci E, Sherer Y, Vaudo G, Moscatelli S, et al. (2008) Association of anti-cyclic citrullinated peptide antibodies with subclinical atherosclerosis in patients with rheumatoid arthritis. Ann Rheum Dis 67: 724–725. PubMed: 18408112
14. Scott DL (2000) Prognostic factors in early rheumatoid arthritis. Rheumatology (Oxford) 39 Suppl 1: 24–29. PubMed: 11001376
15. Jansen AL, van der Horst-Bruinsma I, van Schaardenburg D, van de Stadt RJ, de Koning MH, et al. (2002) Rheumatoid factor and antibodies to cyclic citrullinated Peptide differentiate rheumatoid arthritis from undifferentiated polyarthritis in patients with early arthritis. J Rheumatol 29: 2074–2076. PubMed: 12375314
16. Inui N, Enomoto N, Suda T, Kageyama Y, Watanabe H, et al. (2008) Anti-cyclic citrullinated peptide antibodies in lung diseases associated with rheumatoid arthritis. Clin Biochem 41: 1074–1077. PubMed: 18638466
17. Jearn LH, Kim TY (2012) Level of anticitrullinated peptide/protein antibody is not associated with lung diseases in rheumatoid arthritis. J Rheumatol 39: 1493–1494. PubMed: 22753807
18. Aubart F, Crestani B, Nicaise-Roland P, Tubach F, Bollet C, et al. (2011) High levels of anti-cyclic citrullinated peptide autoantibodies are associated with co-occurrence of pulmonary diseases with rheumatoid arthritis. J Rheumatol 38: 979–982. PubMed: 21362759
19. American Thoracic Society, European Respiratory Society (2002) American Thoracic Society/European Respiratory Society International Multidisciplinary Consensus Classification of the Idiopathic Interstitial Pneumonias. This joint statement of the American Thoracic Society (ATS), and the European Respiratory Society (ERS) was adopted by the ATS board of directors, June 2001 and by the ERS Executive Committee, June 2001. Am J Respir Crit Care Med 165: 277–304. PubMed: 11790668
20. van der Heijde DM, van 't Hof MA, van Riel PL, Theunisse LA, Lubberts EW, et al. (1990) Judging disease activity in clinical practice in rheumatoid arthritis: first step in the development of a disease activity score. Ann Rheum Dis 49: 916–920. PubMed: 2256738
21. Zhang W, Shi Q, Zhao LD, Li Y, Tang FL, et al. (2010) The safety and effectiveness of a chloroform/methanol extract of Tripterygium wilfordii Hook F (T2) plus methotrexate in treating rheumatoid arthritis. J Clin Rheumatol 16: 375–378. PubMed: 21085018
22. Samouda H, Dutour A, Chaumoitre K, Panuel M, Dutour O, et al. (2013) VAT = TAAT-SAAT: innovative anthropometric model to predict visceral adipose tissue without resort to CT-Scan or DXA. Obesity (Silver Spring) 21: E41–50. PubMed: 23404678
23. Ellman P, Ball RE (1948) Rheumatoid disease with joint and pulmonary manifestations. Br Med J 2: 816–820. PubMed: 18890308
24. Brown KK (2007) Rheumatoid lung disease. Proc Am Thorac Soc 4: 443–448. PubMed: 17684286
25. Castelino FV, Varga J (2010) Interstitial lung disease in connective tissue diseases: evolving concepts of pathogenesis and management. Arthritis Res Ther 12: 213. PubMed: 20735863
26. van Noord C, Hooijkaas H, Dufour-van den Goorbergh BC, van Hagen PM, van Daele PL, et al. (2005) Diagnostic value of anti-cyclic citrullinated peptide antibodies to detect rheumatoid arthritis in patients with Sjogren's syndrome. Ann Rheum Dis 64: 160–162. PubMed: 15608321
27. Morita Y, Muro Y, Sugiura K, Tomita Y (2008) Anti-cyclic citrullinated peptide antibody in systemic sclerosis. Clin Exp Rheumatol 26: 542–547. PubMed: 18799082
28. Tobon GJ, Correa PA, Anaya JM (2005) Anti-cyclic citrullinated peptide antibodies in patients with primary Sjogren's syndrome. Ann Rheum Dis 64: 791–792. PubMed: 15834066
29. Gottenberg JE, Mignot S, Nicaise-Rolland P, Cohen-Solal J, Aucouturier F, et al. (2005) Prevalence of anti-cyclic citrullinated peptide and anti-keratin antibodies in patients with primary Sjogren's syndrome. Ann Rheum Dis 64: 114–117. PubMed: 15231509
30. Saravanan V, Kelly CA (2004) Reducing the risk of methotrexate pneumonitis in rheumatoid arthritis. Rheumatology (Oxford) 43: 143–147. PubMed: 12923285
31. Ayhan-Ardic FF, Oken O, Yorgancioglu ZR, Ustun N, Gokharman FD (2006) Pulmonary involvement in lifelong non-smoking patients with rheumatoid arthritis and ankylosing spondylitis without respiratory symptoms. Clin Rheumatol 25: 213–218. PubMed: 16091838
32. Mori S, Koga Y, Sugimoto M (2012) Different risk factors between interstitial lung disease and airway disease in rheumatoid arthritis. Respir Med 106: 1591–1599. PubMed: 22867979

33. Bongartz T, Nannini C, Medina-Velasquez YF, Achenbach SJ, Crowson CS, et al. (2010) Incidence and mortality of interstitial lung disease in rheumatoid arthritis: a population-based study. Arthritis Rheum 62: 1583–1591. PubMed: 20155830
34. Zrour SH, Touzi M, Bejia I, Golli M, Rouatbi N, et al. (2005) Correlations between high-resolution computed tomography of the chest and clinical function in patients with rheumatoid arthritis. Prospective study in 75 patients. Joint Bone Spine 72: 41–47. PubMed: 15681247
35. Gochuico BR, Avila NA, Chow CK, Novero LJ, Wu HP, et al. (2008) Progressive preclinical interstitial lung disease in rheumatoid arthritis. Arch Intern Med 168: 159–166. PubMed: 18227362
36. Brusselle G (2010) Rheumatoid arthritis and interstitial lung disease. Rheumatology (Oxford) 49: 1425–1426. PubMed: 20223815

Permissions

All chapters in this book were first published in PLOS ONE, by The Public Library of Science; hereby published with permission under the Creative Commons Attribution License or equivalent. Every chapter published in this book has been scrutinized by our experts. Their significance has been extensively debated. The topics covered herein carry significant findings which will fuel the growth of the discipline. They may even be implemented as practical applications or may be referred to as a beginning point for another development.

The contributors of this book come from diverse backgrounds, making this book a truly international effort. This book will bring forth new frontiers with its revolutionizing research information and detailed analysis of the nascent developments around the world.

We would like to thank all the contributing authors for lending their expertise to make the book truly unique. They have played a crucial role in the development of this book. Without their invaluable contributions this book wouldn't have been possible. They have made vital efforts to compile up to date information on the varied aspects of this subject to make this book a valuable addition to the collection of many professionals and students.

This book was conceptualized with the vision of imparting up-to-date information and advanced data in this field. To ensure the same, a matchless editorial board was set up. Every individual on the board went through rigorous rounds of assessment to prove their worth. After which they invested a large part of their time researching and compiling the most relevant data for our readers.

The editorial board has been involved in producing this book since its inception. They have spent rigorous hours researching and exploring the diverse topics which have resulted in the successful publishing of this book. They have passed on their knowledge of decades through this book. To expedite this challenging task, the publisher supported the team at every step. A small team of assistant editors was also appointed to further simplify the editing procedure and attain best results for the readers.

Apart from the editorial board, the designing team has also invested a significant amount of their time in understanding the subject and creating the most relevant covers. They scrutinized every image to scout for the most suitable representation of the subject and create an appropriate cover for the book.

The publishing team has been an ardent support to the editorial, designing and production team. Their endless efforts to recruit the best for this project, has resulted in the accomplishment of this book. They are a veteran in the field of academics and their pool of knowledge is as vast as their experience in printing. Their expertise and guidance has proved useful at every step. Their uncompromising quality standards have made this book an exceptional effort. Their encouragement from time to time has been an inspiration for everyone.

The publisher and the editorial board hope that this book will prove to be a valuable piece of knowledge for researchers, students, practitioners and scholars across the globe.

List of Contributors

Caifeng Xie, Liang Ma, Juan Liu, Xiuxia Li, Heying Pei, Mingli Xiang and Lijuan Chen
State Key Laboratory of Biotherapy, West China Medical School, Sichuan University, Chengdu, China

Ming-Wei Lin and Stephen Adelstein
Department of Clinical Immunology, Royal Prince Alfred Hospital, Sydney, New South Wales, Australia
Discipline of Medicine, Sydney Medical School, The University of Sydney, Sydney, New South Wales, Australia

Joshua W. K. Ho
Division of Genetics, Department of Medicine, Brigham and Women's Hospital, Harvard Medical School, Boston Massachusetts, United States of America

Leonard C. Harrison
The Walter and Eliza Hall Institute of Medical Research, Department of Clinical Immunology and Burnet Clinical Research Unit, The Royal Melbourne Hospital, Parkville, Victoria, Australia

Cristobal G. dos Remedios
Discipline of Anatomy, Bosch Institute, The University of Sydney, Sydney, New South Wales, Australia

Zhan-Chun Li, Jian-Wei Chen, Tao Ma, Guang-Qi Cheng, Yu-Qi Dong, Wei-li Wang and Zu-De Liu
Department of Orthopaedic Surgery, Ren Ji Hospital, School of Medicine, Shanghai Jiao Tong University, Shanghai, P. R. China

Jie Xiao
Department of Anesthesiology, Ren Ji Hospital, School of Medicine, Shanghai Jiao Tong University, Shanghai, P. R. China

Jin-Liang Peng
School of Biomedical Engineering/MED-X Research Institute, Shanghai Jiao Tong University, Shanghai, P. R. China

Marieke M. J. Herenius, Carla A. Wijbrandts, Daniëlle M. Gerlag and Paul P. Tak
Department of Clinical Immunology and Rheumatology, Academic Medical Center, University of Amsterdam, Amsterdam, The Netherlands

Winfried Häuser
Department of Psychosomatic Medicine and Psychotherapy Technische Universität München, Munich, Germany
Department Internal Medicine I, Klinikum Saarbrücken, Saarbrücken, Germany

Ana S. F. Oliveira and Maria C. Lebre
Department of Clinical Immunology and Rheumatology, Academic Medical Center, University of Amsterdam, Amsterdam, The Netherlands
Department of Experimental Immunology, Academic Medical Center, University of Amsterdam, Amsterdam, The Netherlands

Frederick Wolfe
National Data Bank for Rheumatic Diseases and University of Kansas School of Medicine, Wichita, Kansas, United States of America

Brian T. Walitt
Washington Hospital Center, Washington, D.C., United States of America

Robert S. Katz
Rush University Medical Center, Chicago, Illinois, United States of America

Paul Emery
Leeds Institute of Rheumatic and Musculoskeletal Medicine, University of Leeds, Leeds, United Kingdom
NIHR Leeds Musculoskeletal Biomedical Research Unit, Leeds Teaching Hospitals NHS Trust, Leeds, United Kingdom

William Rigby
The Geisel School of Medicine at Darthmouth, Lebanon, New Hampshire, United States of America

Paul P. Tak
The Geisel School of Medicine at Darthmouth, Lebanon, New Hampshire, United States of America
Academic Medical Centre, University of Amsterdam, Amsterdam, the Netherlands

Thomas Dörner
Charité University Hospitals and DRFZ, Berlin, Germany

Ewa Olech
University of Nevada School of Medicine, Las Vegas, Nevada, United States of America

Carmen Martin, Laurie Millar, Helen Travers and Elena Fisheleva
Roche Products, Ltd, Welwyn Garden City, United Kingdom

Yi-Ming Chen
Faculty of Medicine, National Yang-Ming University, Taipei, Taiwan, R.O.C
Division of Allergy, Immunology and Rheumatology, Taichung Veterans General Hospital, Taichung, Taiwan, R.O.C

Der-Yuan Chen
Faculty of Medicine, National Yang-Ming University, Taipei, Taiwan, R.O.C
Division of Allergy, Immunology and Rheumatology, Taichung Veterans General Hospital, Taichung, Taiwan, R.O.C
Institute of Biomedical Science, National Chung-Hsing University, Taichung, Taiwan, R.O.C
Institute of Microbiology and Immunology, Chung Shan Medical University, Taichung, Taiwan, R.O.C

Ling Yao
Division of Allergy, Immunology and Rheumatology, Taichung Veterans General Hospital, Taichung, Taiwan, R.O.C

Chi-Chen Lin
Institute of Biomedical Science, National Chung-Hsing University, Taichung, Taiwan, R.O.C

Kui-Chou Huang
Infection and Immunity Research Center, National Yang-Ming University, Taipei, Taiwan, R.O.C

Szu-Ting Chen
Department of Orthopedics and Traumatology, Taichung Veterans General Hospital, Taichung, Taiwan, R.O.C

Joung-Liang Lan
Faculty of Medicine, National Yang-Ming University, Taipei, Taiwan, R.O.C
Division of Allergy, Immunology and Rheumatology, Taichung Veterans General Hospital, Taichung, Taiwan, R.O.C
Division of Immunology and Rheumatology, China Medical University Hospital, Taichung, Taiwan, R.O.C
College of Chinese Medicine, China Medical University, Taichung, Taiwan, R.O.C

Shie-Liang Edmond Hsieh
Department of Orthopedics and Traumatology, Taichung Veterans General Hospital, Taichung, Taiwan, R.O.C
Institute of Clinical Medicine, National Yang-Ming University, Taipei City, Taiwan

Javier Rodríguez-Carrio, Banesa de Paz, Patricia López, Catuxa Prado and Ana Suárez
Area of Immunology, Department Of Functional Biology, Faculty Of Medicine, University Of Oviedo, Oviedo, Spain

Mercedes Alperi-López and Francisco Javier Ballina-García
Department of Rheumatology, Hospital Universitario Central De Asturias, Oviedo, Spain

Young-Sool Hah, Dong-Won Jeong and Hee Young Cho
Clinical Research Institute, Gyeongsang National University Hospital, Jinju, Republic of Korea

Yun-Hong Cheon, Hyun-Ok Kim, Sang-Il Lee and Hye Song Lim
Department of Internal Medicine and Institute of Health Science, Gyeongsang National University School of Medicine, Jinju, Republic of Korea

Byung-Hyun Park and Sun-O Ka
Department of Biochemistry, Chonbuk National University Medical School, Jeonju, Republic of Korea

Young-Rae Lee
Department of Oral b iochmistry, Wonkwang University School of Dentistry, Iksan, Republic of Korea

Myung-Kwan Han
Department of Microbiology, Chonbuk National University Medical School, Republic of Korea

Yukinori Okada
Division of Rheumatology, Immunology, and Allergy, Brigham and Women's Hospital, Harvard Medical School, Boston, Massachusetts, United States of America
Division of Genetics, Brigham and Women's Hospital, Harvard Medical School, Boston, Massachusetts, United States of America
Program in Medical and Population Genetics, Broad Institute, Cambridge, Massachusetts, United States of America
Department of Human Genetics and Disease Diversity, Tokyo Medical and Dental University Graduate School of Medical and Dental Sciences, Tokyo, Japan
Laboratory for Statistical Analysis, Center for Integrative Medical Sciences, RIKEN, Yokohama, Japan

Dorothee Diogo, Gosia Trynka and Robert M. Plenge
Division of Rheumatology, Immunology, and Allergy, Brigham and Women's Hospital, Harvard Medical School, Boston, Massachusetts, United States of America
Division of Genetics, Brigham and Women's Hospital, Harvard Medical School, Boston, Massachusetts, United States of America
Program in Medical and Population Genetics, Broad Institute, Cambridge, Massachusetts, United States of America

Jeffrey D. Greenberg
New York University Hospital for Joint Diseases, New York, New York, United States of America

Faten Mouassess and Walid A. L. Achkar
Molecular Biology and Biotechnology Department, Human Genetics Division, Damascus, Syria

Marieke J. H. Coenen
Department of Human Genetics, Radboud University Medical Centre, Nijmegen, The Netherlands

Robert S. Fulton and Elaine R. Mardis
The Genome Institute, Washington University School of Medicine, St. Louis, Missouri, United States of America

Joshua C. Denny and Robert J. Carroll
Department of Biomedical Informatics, Vanderbilt University School of Medicine, Nashville, Tennessee, United States of America

Namrata Gupta, Daniel Mirel and Stacy Gabriel
Program in Medical and Population Genetics, Broad Institute, Cambridge, Massachusetts, United States of America

Gang Li and Jing Cui
Division of Rheumatology, Immunology, and Allergy, Brigham and Women's Hospital, Harvard Medical School, Boston, Massachusetts, United States of America

Joel M. Kremer
Department of Medicine, Albany Medical Center and The Center for Rheumatology, Albany, New York, United States of America

Dimitrios A. Pappas
Division of Rheumatology, Department of Medicine, New York, Presbyterian Hospital, College of Physicians and Surgeons, Columbia University, New York, New York, United States of America

Anne E. Eyler
Department of Medicine, Vanderbilt University School of Medicine, Nashville, Tennessee, United States of America

Eli A. Stahl
The Department of Psychiatry at Mount Sinai School of Medicine, New York, New York, United States of America

Richa Saxena
Center for Human Genetics Research, Massachusetts General Hospital, Harvard Medical School, Boston, Massachusetts, United States of America

Henk-Jan Guchelaar
Department of Clinical Pharmacy and Toxicology, Leiden University Medical Center, Leiden, The Netherlands

Tom W. J. Huizinga
Department of Rheumatology, Leiden University Medical Centre, Leiden, The Netherlands

Philippe Dieudé
Service de Rhumatologie et INSERM U699 Hôpital Bichat Claude Bernard, Assistance Publique des Hôpitaux de Paris, Paris, France
Université Paris 7-Diderot, Paris, France

Xavier Mariette and Corinne Miceli-Richard
Institut National de la Santé et de la Recherche Médicale (INSERM) U1012, Université Paris-Sud, Rhumatologie, Hôpitaux Universitaires Paris-Sud, Assistance Publique-Hôpitaux de Paris (AP-HP), Le Kremlin Bicêtre, France

Anne Barton
Arthritis Research UK Epidemiology Unit, Centre for Musculoskeletal Research, University of Manchester, Manchester Academic Health Science Centre, Manchester, United Kingdom

Helena Canhão and João E. Fonseca
Rheumatology Research Unit, Instituto de Medicina Molecular, Faculdade de Medicina da Universidade de Lisboa, Lisbon, Portugal
Rheumatology Department, Santa Maria Hospital–CHLN, Lisbon, Portugal

Niek de Vries
Department of Clinical Immunology and Rheumatology & Department of Genome Analysis, Academic Medical Center/University of Amsterdam, Amsterdam, The Netherlands

Paul P. Tak
Department of Clinical Immunology and Rheumatology, Academic Medical Center/ University of Amsterdam, Amsterdam, The Netherlands
GlaxoSmithKline, Stevenage, United Kingdom

Larry W. Moreland
Division of Rheumatology and Clinical Immunology, University of Pittsburgh, Pittsburgh, Pennsylvania, United States of America

S. Louis Bridges, Jr.
Division of Clinical Immunology and Rheumatology, Department of Medicine, University of Alabama at Birmingham, Birmingham, Alabama, United States of America

Mark Lathrop
McGill University and Génome Québec Innovation Centre, Montréal, Canada

Hyon K. Choi
Channing Laboratory,Department of Medicine, Brigham and Women's Hospital, Harvard Medical School, Boston, Massachusetts, United States of America
Section of Rheumatology, Boston University School of Medicine, Boston, Massachusetts, United States of America
Clinical Epidemiology Research and Training Unit, Boston University School of
Medicine, Boston, Massachusetts, United States of America

Yoichiro Kamatani
Laboratory for Statistical Analysis, Center for Integrative Medical Sciences, RIKEN, Yokohama, Japan
Centre d'Etude du Polymorphisme Humain (CEPH), Paris, France

Pilar Galan
Université Paris 13 Sorbonne Paris Cité , UREN (Nutritional Epidemiology Research Unit), Inserm (U557), Inra (U1125), Cnam, Bobigny, France

Towfique Raj and Philip L. De Jager
Division of Genetics, Brigham and Women's Hospital, Harvard Medical School, Boston, Massachusetts, United States of America
Program in Medical and Population Genetics, Broad Institute, Cambridge, Massachusetts, United States of America
Program in Translational NeuroPsychiatric Genomics, Institute for the Neurosciences, Department of Neurology, Brigham and Women's Hospital, Boston, Massachusetts, United States of America

Soumya Raychaudhuri
Division of Rheumatology, Immunology, and Allergy, Brigham and Women's Hospital, Harvard Medical School, Boston, Massachusetts, United States of America
Division of Genetics, Brigham and Women's Hospital, Harvard Medical School, Boston, Massachusetts, United States of America

Program in Medical and Population Genetics, Broad Institute, Cambridge, Massachusetts, United States of America
NIHR Manchester Musculoskeletal Biomedical, Research Unit, Central Manchester NHS Foundation Trust, Manchester Academic Health Sciences Centre, Manchester, United Kingdom

Katherine A. Siminovitch
Lunenfeld-Tanenbaum Research Institute, Mount Sinai Hospital, Toronto, Canada
Toronto General Research Institute, Toronto, Canada
Department of Medicine, University of Toronto, Toronto, Canada

Thurayya Arayssi
Weill Cornell Medical College-Qatar, Education City, Doha, Qatar

Jane Worthington
Arthritis Research UK Epidemiology Unit, Centre for Musculoskeletal Research, University of Manchester, Manchester Academic Health Science Centre, Manchester, United Kingdom
National Institute for Health Research, Manchester Musculoskeletal Biomedical Research Unit, Central Manchester University Hospitals National Health Service Foundation Trust, Manchester Academic Health Sciences Centre, Manchester, United Kingdom

Leonid Padyukov and Lars Klareskog
Rheumatology Unit, Department of Medicine (Solna), Karolinska Institutet, Stockholm, Sweden

Peter K. Gregersen
The Feinstein Institute for Medical Research, North Shore–Long Island Jewish Health System, Manhasset, New York, United States of America

Layla A. Kazkaz
Tishreen Hospital, Damascus, Syria
Syrian Association for Rheumatology, Damascus, Syria

Antonio Mera-Varela and Juan J. Gômez-Reino
Research Laboratory 10 and Rheumatology Unit, Instituto de Investigacion Sanitaria - Hospital Clinico Universitario de Santiago, Santiago de Compostela, Spain
Department of Medicine, University of Santiago de Compostela, Santiago de Compostela, Spain

Aida Ferreiro-Iglesias, Eva Perez-Pampin, Marisol Porto-Silva and Antonio Gonzalez
Research Laboratory 10 and Rheumatology Unit, Instituto de Investigacion Sanitaria - Hospital Clinico Universitario de Santiago, Santiago de Compostela, Spain

Gunter Assmann, Viola Poeschel, Niels Murawski, Jutta Conigliarou and Michael Pfreundschuh
Department of Internal Medicine I, Jose´-Carreras-Centre for Immuno- and Gene Therapy, University Medical School of Saarland, Homburg/Saar, Germany

Klara Shihadeh
Department of Internal Medicine, General Hospital of Herrenberg, Esslingen-Herrenberg, Germany

Mei Fang Ong
Institute of Medical Biometry, Epidemiology and Medical Informatics, Saarland University, Homburg/Saar, Germany

Hao Ye and Jia Wei
R&D Information, AstraZeneca, Shanghai, China

Qi Liu
School of Life Sciences and Technology, Tongji University, Shanghai, China

Shomi Oka, Akiko Komiya, Naoshi Fukui, Shigeto Tohma and Hiroshi Furukawa
Clinical Research Center for Allergy and Rheumatology, Sagamihara Hospital, National Hospital Organization, Sagamihara, Japan

Ikue Ito, Aya Kawasaki and Naoyuki Tsuchiya
Molecular and Genetic Epidemiology Laboratory, Faculty of Medicine, University of Tsukuba, Tsukuba, Japan

Kota Shimada
Department of Rheumatology, Tokyo Metropolitan Tama Medical Center, Fuchu, Japan
Department of Rheumatology, Sagamihara Hospital, National Hospital Organization, Sagamihara, Japan

Shoji Sugii
Department of Rheumatology, Tokyo Metropolitan Tama Medical Center, Fuchu, Japan

Atsushi Hashimoto
Department of Rheumatology, Sagamihara Hospital, National Hospital Organization, Sagamihara, Japan

Yuya Kondo, Takayuki Sumida, Taichi Hayashi and Isao Matsumoto
Department of Internal Medicine, Faculty of Medicine, University of Tsukuba, Tsukuba, Japan

Satoshi Ito
Department of Rheumatology, Niigata Rheumatic Center, Shibata, Japan

Makio Kusaoi, Hirofumi Amano and Yoshinari Takasaki
Department of Internal Medicine and Rheumatology, Juntendo University School of Medicine, Tokyo, Japan

Tatsuo Nagai and Shunsei Hirohata
Department of Rheumatology and Infectious Disease, Kitasato University School of Medicine, Sagamihara, Japan

Keigo Setoguchi
Department of Allergy and Immunological Diseases, Tokyo Metropolitan Cancer and Infectious Diseases Center Komagome Hospital, Tokyo, Japan

Hajime Kono
Department of Internal Medicine, Teikyo University, Tokyo, Japan

Akira Okamoto
Department of Rheumatology, Himeji Medical Center, National Hospital Organization, Himeji, Japan

Noriyuki Chiba
Department of Rheumatology, Morioka Hospital, National Hospital Organization, Morioka, Japan

Eiichi Suematsu
Department of Internal Medicine and Rheumatology, Clinical Research Institute, Kyushu Medical Center, National Hospital Organization, Fukuoka, Japan

Masao Katayama
Department of Internal Medicine, Nagoya Medical Center, National Hospital Organization, Nagoya, Japan

Kiyoshi Migita
Clinical Research Center, Nagasaki Medical Center, National Hospital Organization, Omura, Japan

Akiko Suda
Center for Rheumatic Diseases, Yokohama City University Medical Center, Yokohama, Japan
Department of Rheumatology, Yokohama Minami Kyosai Hospital, Yokohama, Japan

Shigeru Ohno
Center for Rheumatic Diseases, Yokohama City University Medical Center, Yokohama, Japan

Hiroshi Hashimoto
Juntendo University School of Medicine, Tokyo, Japan

Shouhei Nagaoka
Department of Rheumatology, Yokohama Minami Kyosai Hospital, Yokohama, Japan

Alper M. van Sijl, Maarten Boers, Alexandre E. Voskuyl and Michael T. Nurmohamed
Department of Rheumatology, VU University Medical Center, Amsterdam, the Netherlands

Garifallia Sakellariou, Carlo Alberto Sciré, Roberto Caporali and Carlomaurizio Montecucco
Chair and Division of Rheumatology, IRCCS Policlinico San Matteo Foundation, Pavia, Italy

Antonella Zambon
Department of Biostatistics Statistics and Quantitative Methods, University of Milano-Bicocca, Milano, Italy

Masatoshi Sumi
Department of Orthopaedic Surgery, Kobe Rosai Hospital, Chuo-ku, Kobe, Japan

Takashi Yurube, Kotaro Nishida, Yasushi Miura, Hiroaki Hirata and Minoru Doita
Department of Orthopaedic Surgery, Kobe University Graduate School of Medicine, Chuo-ku, Kobe, Japan

Hiroshi Miyamoto
Department of Orthopaedic Surgery, Kobe Medical Center, Suma-ku, Kobe, Japan

Kozo Kohyama
Department of Orthopaedic Surgery, Kohnan Kakogawa Hospital, Kanno-cho, Kakogawa, Japan

Tsukasa Matsubara
Department of Orthopaedic Surgery, Matsubara Mayflower Hospital, Fujita, Kato, Japan

Daisuke Sugiyama
Department of Evidence-Based Laboratory Medicine, Kobe University Graduate School of Medicine, Chuo-ku, Kobe, Japan

Qianwen Lv, Yufeng Yin, Xin Li, Xiangni Wu, Di Liang, Yongzhe Li and Xuan Zhang
Department of Rheumatology & Clinical Immunology, Peking Union Medical College Hospital, Chinese Academy of Medical Sciences and Peking Union Medical College, Beijing, China

Guangliang Shan
Department of Epidemiology and Statistics, Institute of Basic Medical Sciences, Chinese Academy of Medical Sciences and School of Basic Medicine, Peking Union Medical College, Beijing, China

Isabela Goeldner, Angelica B. W. Boldt, Flavia R. Nass and Iara J. Messias-Reason
Department of Medical Pathology, Federal University of Paraná, Curitiba, Brazil

Thelma Skare
Rheumatology Unit, Evangelical University Hospital, Curitiba, Brazil

Shirley R. Utiyama
Department of Clinical Analysis, Federal University of Paraná, Curitiba, Brazil

Dagmar Quandt, Kathrin Rothe, Roger Scholz, Christoph W. Baerwald, Ulf Wagner
Clinics for Gastroenterology and Rheumatology, Division of Rheumatology, University of Leipzig, Leipzig, Saxony, Germany

Kresten Krarup Keller, Kristian Stengaard-Pedersen and Ellen-Margrethe Hauge
Department of Rheumatology, Aarhus University Hospital, Aarhus, Denmark

Jesper Skovhus Thomsen
Department of Biomedicine - Anatomy, Aarhus University, Aarhus, Denmark

Marta Krystyna Kosinska, Heiko Klein, Markus Rickert and Juergen Steinmeyer
Department of Orthopedics, Justus-Liebig-University Giessen, Giessen, Germany

Gerhard Liebisch and Gerd Schmitz
Department of Clinical Chemistry and Laboratory Medicine, University Hospital Regensburg, Regensburg, Germany

Guenter Lochnit
Department of Biochemistry, Justus-Liebig-University Giessen, Giessen, Germany

Jochen Wilhelm
Medical Clinic II/IV, Justus-Liebig-University Giessen, Giessen, Germany

Ulrich Kaesser
Internistisches Praxiszentrum am Krankenhaus Balserische Stiftung, Giessen, Germany

Gabriele Lasczkowski
Institute of Forensic Medicine, Justus-Liebig-University Giessen, Giessen, Germany

Kaini Shen, Daobin Zhou and Jian Li
Department of Hematology, Peking Union Medical College Hospital, Chinese Academy of Medical Sciences and Peking Union Medical College, Beijing, People's Republic of China

Gufeng Xu
Zhejiang University, School of Medicine, Hangzhou, Zhejiang, People's Republic of China

Qing Wu
Division of Health Sciences Research, Mayo Clinic, Scottsdale, Arizona, United States of America

Patrick H. Dessein, Gavin R. Norton and Angela J. Woodiwiss
Cardiovascular Pathophysiology and Genomics Research Unit, School of Physiology, Faculty of Health Sciences, University of the Witwatersrand, Johannesburg, South Africa

Linda Tsang
Milpark Hospital, Johannesburg, South Africa

Ahmed Solomon
Department of Rheumatology, Charlotte Maxeke Johannesburg Academic Hospital, Faculty of Health Sciences, University of the Witwatersrand, Johannesburg, South Africa

Martijn A. H. Oude Voshaar, Peter M. ten Klooster and Erik Taal
Arthritis Center Twente and Psychology, Health & Technology, University of Twente, Enschede, The Netherlands

Cees A. W. Glas
Department of Research Methodology, Measurement and Data Analysis, University of Twente, Enschede, The Netherlands

Harald E. Vonkeman and Mart A. F. J. van de Laar
Arthritis Center Twente and Psychology, Health & Technology, University of Twente, Enschede, The Netherlands
Department of Rheumatology and Clinical Immunology, Medisch Spectrum Twente, Enschede, The Netherlands

Eswar Krishnan
Arthritis, Rheumatism, and Aging Medical Information System Program, Stanford University School of Medicine, Palo Alto, California, United States of
America

Hein J. Bernelot Moens
vDepartment of Rheumatology and Clinical Immunology, Ziekenhuisgroep Twente, Almelo, The Netherlands

Maarten Boers and Caroline B. Terwee
Department of Epidemiology and Biostatistics, Vrije Universiteit Medical Center, Amsterdam, The Netherlands

Piet L. C. M. van Riel
Department of Rheumatic Diseases, Radboud University Medical Centre, Nijmegen, The Netherlands

Yufeng Yin, Di Liang, Lidan Zhao, Yang Li, Yan Ren, Yongzhe Li, Xiaofeng Zeng, Fengchun Zhang, Fulin Tang and Xuan Zhang
Department of Rheumatology, Peking Union Medical College Hospital, Chinese Academy of Medical Sciences and Peking Union Medical College, Beijing, China

Wei Liu
Department of Radiology, Peking Union Medical College Hospital, Chinese Academy of Medical Sciences and Peking Union Medical College, Beijing, China

Guangliang Shan
Department of Epidemiology, Institute of Basic Medical Sciences, Chinese Academy of Medical Sciences and Peking Union Medical College, Beijing, China

Index

CPSIA information can be obtained
at www.ICGtesting.com
Printed in the USA
BVOW07*0749041217
501804BV00017B/9/P

9 781632 424860